Healthy Nutrition as the Key Reference in Special Diets, Quality of Life, and Sustainability

Healthy Nutrition as the Key Reference in Special Diets, Quality of Life, and Sustainability

Editors

António Raposo
Renata Puppin Zandonadi
Raquel Braz Assunção Botelho

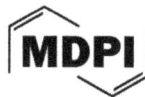

Basel • Beijing • Wuhan • Barcelona • Belgrade • Novi Sad • Cluj • Manchester

Editors
António Raposo
CBIOS
Universidade Lusófona de
Humanidades e Tecnologias
Lisboa
Portugal

Renata Puppin Zandonadi
Department of Nutrition
University of Brasilia
Brasilia
Brazil

Raquel Braz Assunção Botelho
Department of Nutrition
University of Brasilia
Brasilia
Brazil

Editorial Office
MDPI AG
Grosspeteranlage 5
4052 Basel, Switzerland

This is a reprint of articles from the Special Issue published online in the open access journal *Nutrients* (ISSN 2072-6643) (available at: www.mdpi.com/journal/nutrients/special_issues/174ZQ5X30G).

For citation purposes, cite each article independently as indicated on the article page online and as indicated below:

Lastname, A.A.; Lastname, B.B. Article Title. *Journal Name* **Year**, *Volume Number*, Page Range.

ISBN 978-3-7258-2112-9 (Hbk)
ISBN 978-3-7258-2111-2 (PDF)
doi.org/10.3390/books978-3-7258-2111-2

© 2024 by the authors. Articles in this book are Open Access and distributed under the Creative Commons Attribution (CC BY) license. The book as a whole is distributed by MDPI under the terms and conditions of the Creative Commons Attribution-NonCommercial-NoDerivs (CC BY-NC-ND) license.

Contents

About the Editors vii

António Raposo, Renata Puppin Zandonadi and Raquel Braz Assunção Botelho
Healthy Nutrition as the Key Reference in Special Diets, Quality of Life, and Sustainability
Reprinted from: *Nutrients* **2024**, *16*, 2906, doi:10.3390/nu16172906 1

Yu Shen, Mingming Song, Shihao Wu, Hongbo Zhao and Yu Zhang
Plant-Based Dietary Fibers and Polysaccharides as Modulators of Gut Microbiota in Intestinal and Lung Inflammation: Current State and Challenges
Reprinted from: *Nutrients* **2023**, *15*, 3321, doi:10.3390/nu15153321 3

Julyana Nogueira Firme, Priscila Claudino de Almeida, Emanuele Batistela dos Santos, Renata Puppin Zandonadi, António Raposo and Raquel Braz Assunção Botelho
Instruments to Evaluate Food Neophobia in Children: An Integrative Review with a Systematic Approach
Reprinted from: *Nutrients* **2023**, *15*, 4769, doi:10.3390/nu15224769 21

Nathalia Sernizon Guimarães, Marcela Gomes Reis, Luciano de Alvarenga Fontes, Renata Puppin Zandonadi, Raquel Braz Assunção Botelho, Hmidan A. Alturki, et al.
Plate Food Waste in Food Services: A Systematic Review and Meta-Analysis
Reprinted from: *Nutrients* **2024**, *16*, 1429, doi:10.3390/nu16101429 44

Petros C. Dinas, on behalf of the Students of Module 5104 (Introduction to Systematic Reviews), Marianthi Karaventza, Christina Liakou, Kalliopi Georgakouli, Dimitrios Bogdanos and George S. Metsios
Combined Effects of Physical Activity and Diet on Cancer Patients: A Systematic Review and Meta-Analysis
Reprinted from: *Nutrients* **2024**, *16*, 1749, doi:10.3390/nu16111749 63

Camila dos Santos Ribeiro, Rosa Harumi Uenishi, Alessandra dos Santos Domingues, Eduardo Yoshio Nakano, Raquel Braz Assunção Botelho, António Raposo and Renata Puppin Zandonadi
Gluten-Free Diet Adherence Tools for Individuals with Celiac Disease: A Systematic Review and Meta-Analysis of Tools Compared to Laboratory Tests
Reprinted from: *Nutrients* **2024**, *16*, 2428, doi:10.3390/nu16152428 85

Ezequiel Pinto, Carla Viegas, Paula Ventura Martins, Tânia Nascimento, Leon Schurgers and Dina Simes
New Food Frequency Questionnaire to Estimate Vitamin K Intake in a Mediterranean Population
Reprinted from: *Nutrients* **2023**, *15*, 3012, doi:10.3390/nu15133012 101

Xiaoxiao Lin, Shuai Wang and Jinyu Huang
A Bibliometric Analysis of Alternate-Day Fasting from 2000 to 2023
Reprinted from: *Nutrients* **2023**, *15*, 3724, doi:10.3390/nu15173724 111

Xue Li, Can Guo, Yu Zhang, Li Yu, Fei Ma, Xuefang Wang, et al.
Contribution of Different Food Types to Vitamin A Intake in the Chinese Diet
Reprinted from: *Nutrients* **2023**, *15*, 4028, doi:10.3390/nu15184028 124

Zohar Spivak-Lavi, Yael Latzer, Daniel Stein, Ora Peleg and Orna Tzischinsky
Differences in the Factor Structure of the Eating Attitude Test-26 (EAT-26) among Clinical vs. Non-Clinical Adolescent Israeli Females
Reprinted from: *Nutrients* **2023**, *15*, 4168, doi:10.3390/nu15194168 . . . . **134**

Qian Li, Noppawan Piaseu, Srisamorn Phumonsakul and Streerut Thadakant
Effects of a Comprehensive Dietary Intervention Program, Promoting Nutrition Literacy, Eating Behavior, Dietary Quality, and Gestational Weight Gain in Chinese Urban Women with Normal Body Mass Index during Pregnancy
Reprinted from: *Nutrients* **2024**, *16*, 217, doi:10.3390/nu16020217 . . . . **153**

Irene Sánchez Gavilán, Daniela Velázquez Ybarzabal, Vicenta de la Fuente, Rosa M. Cámara, María Cortes Sánchez-Mata and Montaña Cámara
Valorization of *Salicornia patula* Duval-Jouve Young Shoots in Healthy and Sustainable Diets
Reprinted from: *Nutrients* **2024**, *16*, 358, doi:10.3390/nu16030358 . . . . **186**

Cliona Brennan, Julian Baudinet, Mima Simic and Ivan Eisler
The Role of the Dietitian within Family Therapy for Anorexia Nervosa (FT-AN): A Reflexive Thematic Analysis of Child and Adolescent Eating Disorder Clinician Perspectives
Reprinted from: *Nutrients* **2024**, *16*, 670, doi:10.3390/nu16050670 . . . . **196**

Ezequiel Pinto, Carla Viegas, Paula Ventura Martins, Catarina Marreiros, Tânia Nascimento, Leon Schurgers and Dina Simes
Mediterranean Diet Favors Vitamin K Intake: A Descriptive Study in a Mediterranean Population
Reprinted from: *Nutrients* **2024**, *16*, 1098, doi:10.3390/nu16081098 . . . . **207**

Meiling Liu and Sunmin Park
The Role of *PNPLA3*_rs738409 Gene Variant, Lifestyle Factors, and Bioactive Compounds in Nonalcoholic Fatty Liver Disease: A Population-Based and Molecular Approach towards Healthy Nutrition
Reprinted from: *Nutrients* **2024**, *16*, 1239, doi:10.3390/nu16081239 . . . . **219**

Semra Navruz-Varlı, Hande Mortaş and Menşure Nur Çelik
Sociodemographic Trends in Planetary Health Diets among Nutrition Students in Türkiye: Bridging Classroom to Kitchen
Reprinted from: *Nutrients* **2024**, *16*, 1277, doi:10.3390/nu16091277 . . . . **237**

Beatriz Vanessa Díaz-González, Inmaculada Bautista-Castaño, Elisabeth Hernández García, Judith Cornejo Torre, Juan Ramón Hernández Hernández and Lluis Serra-Majem
Bariatric Surgery: An Opportunity to Improve Quality of Life and Healthy Habits
Reprinted from: *Nutrients* **2024**, *16*, 1466, doi:10.3390/nu16101466 . . . . **252**

Semra Navruz-Varlı and Hande Mortaş
Shift Work, Shifted Diets: An Observational Follow-Up Study on Diet Quality and Sustainability among Healthcare Workers on Night Shifts
Reprinted from: *Nutrients* **2024**, *16*, 2404, doi:10.3390/nu16152404 . . . . **265**

About the Editors

António Raposo

António Raposo is an Assistant Professor at Universidade Lusófona de Humanidades e Tecnologias, and he is an Integrated Member of CBIOS (Research Center for Biosciences and Health Technologies). He graduated in Nutritional Sciences from the Instituto Superior de Ciencias da Saúde Egas Moniz, Portugal, in 2009 and obtained his Ph.D. with a European Mention in Animal Health and Food Safety from the University Institute of Animal Health and Food Safety, University of Las Palmas de Gran Canaria, Spain, in 2013. His main research interests are studies on the utilization of Catostylus tagi jellyfish in health sciences, particularly as a food ingredient, food habits, food safety evaluation, food innovation, natural food products, food security, and sustainability. He is a member of the editorial boards and an invited reviewer of relevant international peer-reviewed journals in his research field. He has published more than 155 papers in indexed *JCR* journals, as well as scientific book chapters and a patent model, and co-authored a book in English with a special focus on nutrition, food security, and food safety sciences. He has been a Guest Editor of several Special Issues published in high-impact *JCR* journals such as *Foods*, *Sustainability*, and *International Journal of Environmental Research and Public Health*. He has collaborated as a Visiting Professor at Portuguese, Spanish, Chilean, and Vietnamese universities.

Renata Puppin Zandonadi

Renata Puppin Zandonadi is a researcher and Associate Professor at the University of Brasilia Department of Nutrition and a permanent member of the Postgraduate Program in Human Nutrition (University of Brasilia). She graduated in Nutrition from the University of Brasilia and obtained a Master's degree in Human Nutrition (University of Brasilia) and a Ph.D. in Health Sciences (University of Brasilia). She has co-authored and published one book, fifty book chapters, and 157 articles in peer-reviewed journals. She is a reviewer and member of the editorial board of international journals. Her main research interests are focused on nutrition, food, food-related disorders, eating habits, quality of life, sustainability, food security, and safety.

Raquel Braz Assunção Botelho

Raquel Botelho graduated in Nutrition from the University of Brasilia and obtained a Master's degree in Food Science from the University of Campinas and a Ph.D. in Health Sciences from the University of Brasilia. Currently, she is a researcher and Associate Professor at the Nutrition Department, University of Brasilia, and a member of the Postgraduate Program in Human Nutrition. Professor Raquel Botelho acts as a reviewer and member of the editorial board of international journals and has co-authored and published more than 113 articles in scientific journals, 7 books, and 21 book chapters. Her field of expertise is in nutrition, gastronomy, culinary, food, food-related disorders, eating habits, quality of life, sustainability, food security, and safety.

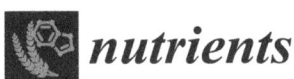

Editorial

Healthy Nutrition as the Key Reference in Special Diets, Quality of Life, and Sustainability

António Raposo [1,*], Renata Puppin Zandonadi [2] and Raquel Braz Assunção Botelho [2]

1. CBIOS (Research Center for Biosciences and Health Technologies), Universidade Lusófona de Humanidades e Tecnologias, Campo Grande 376, 1749-024 Lisboa, Portugal
2. Department of Nutrition, Faculty of Health Sciences, University of Brasilia, Brasilia 70910-900, Brazil; renatapz@unb.br (R.P.Z.); raquelbotelho@unb.br (R.B.A.B.)
* Correspondence: antonio.raposo@ulusofona.pt

Healthy nutrition is considered a key factor in special diets, enhanced quality of life, and sustainability. Nutrition involves eating, which concerns how people relate to food in different contexts, with their food choices influenced by biological, social, cultural, economic, and psychological factors, as well as food availability and access to food [1–3]. Adopting dietary patterns such as the Mediterranean diet and plant-based diets is associated with the optimal intake of some nutrients, the prevention and management of non-communicable chronic diseases and cancer, and health promotion and sustainability [4–9].

Eating decisions can be conscious or subconscious and extend beyond basic physiological and nutritional requirements. Despite being a long-standing international human right, not everyone has access to adequate food; for instance, individuals from low-income families, those who adopt different dietary patterns, and people with dietary restrictions face challenges regarding food availability. Aside from these aspects affecting food choices, people with dietary restrictions are also subject to constraints on food consumption for disease prevention or treatment. Additionally, some individuals refrain from consuming certain types of foods for ethical, moral, religious, health, and environmental reasons. Health-related conditions (such as celiac disease, food allergies, surgeries, and others) may impose lifelong or temporary food restrictions that might be challenging and negatively affect the quality of life, diet quality, and sustainability; thus, health professionals should provide recommendations and guidance to avoid or reduce their impact [8,10,11]. In addition to health-related conditions, eating disorders and food neophobia may impact food choices and nutrient intake, thus affecting health, quality of life, and the environment [12,13]. In this sense, special diets and other dietary patterns should support an individual's nutritional and energy needs with access to pleasing, accessible, and adequate food. A lack of proper instructions on food choices and consumption, as well as a healthy diet, may lead to the inefficacy of special diets or other dietary patterns and therefore can impact sustainability.

Since food consumption involves a complicated amalgam of ingrained habits, social norms, and acquired attitudes and feelings toward food, enhancing nutrition literacy and eating behavior through dietary interventions and strategies concerning food and nutritional education is crucial in all ages to improve nutritional and health status and avoid food waste [14,15]. Food waste is one of the leading causes of environmental decline and has an economic and social impact considering sustainability [16]. Attention to eating consumption and meal selection, variation in food and nutrient intake, avoiding monotony, and the valorization of local food production contribute to sustainability as well as health [16,17].

Acknowledgments: The editors thank and congratulate the authors who published their studies in this Special Issue with *Nutrients*/MDPI for this valuable data collection. We also recognize the valuable work of the reviewers, the Editor-in-Chief, and the MDPI team in constructing this successful Special Issue. Renata Puppin Zandonadi and Raquel Braz Assunção Botelho also thank the Brazilian National Council for Scientific and Technological Development (CNPq) for their scientific support.

Conflicts of Interest: The authors declare no conflicts of interest.

References

1. Navruz-Varlı, S.; Mortaş, H. Shift Work, Shifted Diets: An Observational Follow-Up Study on Diet Quality and Sustainability among Healthcare Workers on Night Shifts. *Nutrients* **2024**, *16*, 2404. [CrossRef] [PubMed]
2. Liu, M.; Park, S. The Role of PNPLA3_rs738409 Gene Variant, Lifestyle Factors, and Bioactive Compounds in Nonalcoholic Fatty Liver Disease: A Population-Based and Molecular Approach towards Healthy Nutrition. *Nutrients* **2024**, *16*, 1239. [CrossRef] [PubMed]
3. Spivak-Lavi, Z.; Latzer, Y.; Stein, D.; Peleg, O.; Tzischinsky, O. Differences in the Factor Structure of the Eating Attitude Test-26 (EAT-26) among Clinical vs. Non-Clinical Adolescent Israeli Females. *Nutrients* **2023**, *15*, 4168. [CrossRef] [PubMed]
4. Pinto, E.; Viegas, C.; Martins, P.V.; Marreiros, C.; Nascimento, T.; Schurgers, L.; Simes, D. Mediterranean Diet Favors Vitamin K Intake: A Descriptive Study in a Mediterranean Population. *Nutrients* **2024**, *16*, 1098. [CrossRef] [PubMed]
5. Pinto, E.; Viegas, C.; Martins, P.V.; Nascimento, T.; Schurgers, L.; Simes, D. New Food Frequency Questionnaire to Estimate Vitamin K Intake in a Mediterranean Population. *Nutrients* **2023**, *15*, 3012. [CrossRef] [PubMed]
6. Shen, Y.; Song, M.; Wu, S.; Zhao, H.; Zhang, Y. Plant-Based Dietary Fibers and Polysaccharides as Modulators of Gut Microbiota in Intestinal and Lung Inflammation: Current State and Challenges. *Nutrients* **2023**, *15*, 3321. [CrossRef] [PubMed]
7. Dinas, P.C.; Karaventza, M.; Liakou, C.; Georgakouli, K.; Bogdanos, D.; Metsios, G.S. Combined Effects of Physical Activity and Diet on Cancer Patients: A Systematic Review and Meta-Analysis. *Nutrients* **2024**, *16*, 1749. [CrossRef] [PubMed]
8. Lin, X.; Wang, S.; Huang, J. A Bibliometric Analysis of Alternate-Day Fasting from 2000 to 2023. *Nutrients* **2023**, *15*, 3724. [CrossRef] [PubMed]
9. Li, X.; Guo, C.; Zhang, Y.; Yu, L.; Ma, F.; Wang, X.; Zhang, L.; Li, P. Contribution of Different Food Types to Vitamin A Intake in the Chinese Diet. *Nutrients* **2023**, *15*, 4028. [CrossRef] [PubMed]
10. Dos, C.; Ribeiro, S.; Uenishi, R.H.; Dos, A.; Domingues, S.; Nakano, E.Y.; Braz, R.; Botelho, A.; Raposo, A.; Zandonadi, R.P. Gluten-Free Diet Adherence Tools for Individuals with Celiac Disease: A Systematic Review and Meta-Analysis of Tools Compared to Laboratory Tests. *Nutrients* **2024**, *16*, 2428. [CrossRef] [PubMed]
11. Díaz-González, B.V.; Bautista-Castaño, I.; Hernández García, E.; Cornejo Torre, J.; Hernández Hernández, J.R.; Serra-Majem, L. Bariatric Surgery: An Opportunity to Improve Quality of Life and Healthy Habits. *Nutrients* **2024**, *16*, 1466. [CrossRef] [PubMed]
12. Brennan, C.; Baudinet, J.; Simic, M.; Eisler, I. The Role of the Dietitian within Family Therapy for Anorexia Nervosa (FT-AN): A Reflexive Thematic Analysis of Child and Adolescent Eating Disorder Clinician Perspectives. *Nutrients* **2024**, *16*, 670. [CrossRef] [PubMed]
13. Firme, J.N.; de Almeida, P.C.; dos Santos, E.B.; Zandonadi, R.P.; Raposo, A.; Botelho, R.B.A. Instruments to Evaluate Food Neophobia in Children: An Integrative Review with a Systematic Approach. *Nutrients* **2023**, *15*, 4769. [CrossRef] [PubMed]
14. Li, Q.; Piaseu, N.; Phumonsakul, S.; Thadakant, S. Effects of a Comprehensive Dietary Intervention Program, Promoting Nutrition Literacy, Eating Behavior, Dietary Quality, and Gestational Weight Gain in Chinese Urban Women with Normal Body Mass Index during Pregnancy. *Nutrients* **2024**, *16*, 217. [CrossRef] [PubMed]
15. Navruz-Varlı, S.; Mortaş, H.; Çelik, M.N. Sociodemographic Trends in Planetary Health Diets among Nutrition Students in Türkiye: Bridging Classroom to Kitchen. *Nutrients* **2024**, *16*, 1277. [CrossRef] [PubMed]
16. Guimarães, N.S.; Reis, M.G.; Fontes, L.d.A.; Zandonadi, R.P.; Botelho, R.B.A.; Alturki, H.A.; Saraiva, A.; Raposo, A. Plate Food Waste in Food Services: A Systematic Review and Meta-Analysis. *Nutrients* **2024**, *16*, 1429. [CrossRef] [PubMed]
17. Sánchez Gavilán, I.; Velázquez Ybarzabal, D.; de la Fuente, V.; Cámara, R.M.; Sánchez-Mata, M.C.; Cámara, M. Valorization of Salicornia Patula Duval-Jouve Young Shoots in Healthy and Sustainable Diets. *Nutrients* **2024**, *16*, 358. [CrossRef] [PubMed]

Disclaimer/Publisher's Note: The statements, opinions and data contained in all publications are solely those of the individual author(s) and contributor(s) and not of MDPI and/or the editor(s). MDPI and/or the editor(s) disclaim responsibility for any injury to people or property resulting from any ideas, methods, instructions or products referred to in the content.

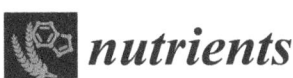

Review

Plant-Based Dietary Fibers and Polysaccharides as Modulators of Gut Microbiota in Intestinal and Lung Inflammation: Current State and Challenges

Yu Shen [1], Mingming Song [1], Shihao Wu [1], Hongbo Zhao [2,*] and Yu Zhang [1,*]

[1] Heilongjiang Provincial Key Laboratory of New Drug Development and Pharmacotoxicological Evaluation, College of Pharmacy, Jiamusi University, Jiamusi 154007, China; shenyu0406@126.com (Y.S.)
[2] College of Rehabilitation Medicine, Jiamusi University, Jiamusi 154007, China
* Correspondence: 368583501@163.com (H.Z.); zhangyu@jmsu.edu.cn (Y.Z.)

Abstract: Recent research has underscored the significant role of gut microbiota in managing various diseases, including intestinal and lung inflammation. It is now well established that diet plays a crucial role in shaping the composition of the microbiota, leading to changes in metabolite production. Consequently, dietary interventions have emerged as promising preventive and therapeutic approaches for managing these diseases. Plant-based dietary fibers, particularly polysaccharides and oligosaccharides, have attracted attention as potential therapeutic agents for modulating gut microbiota and alleviating intestinal and lung inflammation. This comprehensive review aims to provide an in-depth overview of the current state of research in this field, emphasizing the challenges and limitations associated with the use of plant-based dietary fibers and polysaccharides in managing intestinal and lung inflammation. By shedding light on existing issues and limitations, this review seeks to stimulate further research and development in this promising area of therapeutic intervention.

Keywords: dietary fibers; plant polysaccharide; prebiotics; lung inflammation; intestinal inflammation; gut–lung axis; phytotherapy

1. Introduction

Chronic inflammatory diseases affecting mucosal sites, such as the intestine and lungs/airways, are becoming increasingly prevalent worldwide [1,2]. These diseases encompass inflammatory bowel disease (IBD), including ulcerative colitis (UC) and Crohn's disease, as well as lung conditions such as asthma, bronchiectasis, chronic obstructive pulmonary disease (COPD), and cystic fibrosis (CF). COPD, which includes chronic bronchitis and emphysema, has been responsible for 3.23 million deaths in 2019 and emerged as the third leading cause of death globally [3]. Similarly, IBD has witnessed a global increase in prevalence over time and has emerged as a significant health concern [4].

Recent studies focusing on gut and lung inflammatory diseases have revealed a close relationship between the gut and lung microbiota, which is referred to as the gut–lung axis (GLA) [5]. The GLA operates in a bidirectional manner, where lung inflammatory diseases impact the gastrointestinal system, and vice versa [5]. For instance, long-term smoking not only degrades lung tissues and causes inflammation but also leads to the infiltration of circulating immune cells in the gut, resulting in gut dysbiosis and an increased risk of intestinal diseases such as IBD [6]. Likewise, a recent cross-sectional cohort study called Respiratory Health in Northern Europe (RHINE), conducted among participants from North European countries, found an increased risk of asthma in IBD patients, particularly among women [7]. Moreover, it is important to note that genetic susceptibility to inflammatory bowel disease (IBD) can also increase the risk of interstitial lung disease, a condition characterized by inflammation and fibrosis [8,9]. Several factors have been proposed to explain the link between gut and lung diseases, including their shared embryological origin and the influence of gut microbiota and their metabolites on the regulation of lung immunity and inflammatory responses [7]. As a result, the lung and gut exhibit an intricate interconnection, and both should be carefully considered in individuals affected by either disease.

The current management of IBD involves the use of various medications, including corticosteroids, aminosalicylates, immunosuppressive agents, antibiotics, oral small molecules, and biologics such as anti-tumor necrosis factor TNF-α [10]. However, these medications come with a range of side effects, ranging from mild symptoms, like headaches, nausea, and abdominal pains, to more severe complications, such as infertility, photosensitization, opportunistic infections, diabetes mellitus, hemolytic anemia, hypertension, granulocytosis, and osteoporosis [10]. Similar observations have been made in the case of COPD and asthma, where many potential drugs have failed to demonstrate efficacy in clinical trials or have limited application due to side effects such as headaches, nausea, diarrhea, and dose-limiting effects [11].

Due to the intricate connection between the gut and the lungs, and the undesirable side effects of current medications used for gut and lung inflammatory diseases, researchers have shifted their focus towards exploring traditional and alternative medicinal approaches, particularly those based on plant dietary fibers (DFs) and plant polysaccharides. These plant-derived compounds have demonstrated promising potential for preventing and alleviating gut and lung inflammation through their ability to modulate the microbiota. Notably, plant-based polysaccharides exhibit diverse biological functions, including antioxidative, anti-inflammatory, immunomodulatory, antitumor, hypoglycemic, and microbiota modulation capabilities [12]. Such findings hold significant promise for the development of novel therapeutic interventions to address gut–lung-axis diseases.

DFs consist of polymers of monosaccharides that are indigestible and not absorbed in the gastrointestinal tract due to the lack of proper hydrolyzing enzymes. They are primarily found in plants (grains, fruits, and vegetables), fungi, and algae [13–15]. Dietary fibers can be categorized into non-starch polysaccharides (NPSs), such as cellulose, hemicellulose, pectin, beta-glucans, resistant starches, and lignin [15]. Additionally, low-molecular-weight non-digestible oligosaccharides such as fructooligosaccharides (FOSs), galactooligosaccharides (GOSs), xylooligosaccharides (XOSs), and inulin are sometimes included in the definition of dietary fibers [15]. Non-carbohydrate components like lignin, cutin, saponin, and suberin can also function as dietary fibers [14].

This review critically discusses the utilization of plant-based polysaccharides and dietary fibers for ameliorating gut and lung inflammatory diseases, primarily through microbiota modulation. Table 1 provides a summary of alterations in microbial composition associated with intestinal and lung inflammatory diseases within the gut–lung axis. Table 2 presents recent studies on the effects of plant dietary fibers and polysaccharides on intestinal inflammatory diseases through gut microbiota modulation. Furthermore, Table 3 lists examples of plant dietary fibers and polysaccharides that have demonstrated the amelioration of lung inflammation via gut microbiota modulation. Figure 1 provides a summarized mechanism of action for plant-based dietary fibers and polysaccharides against gut and lung inflammatory diseases.

Table 1. Alteration in microbial composition associated with intestinal and lung inflammatory diseases in gut–lung axis.

	Gut Microbiota	Lung Microbiota	
IBD	↓ *Bifidobacterium longum*, ↓ *Eubacterium rectale*, ↓ *Faecalibacterium prausnitzii*, ↓ *Roseburia intestinalis*, ↑ *Bacteroides*, ↑ *Ruminococcus torques*, ↑ *Ruminococcus*, ↓ *Christensenellaceae*, ↓ *Coriobacteriaceae*, ↓ *Clostridium leptum*, ↑ *Actinomyces* spp., ↑ *Veillonella* spp., ↑ *Escherichia coli*, ↓ *Eubacterium rectum*, ↓ *Akkermansia muciniphila*	—	[16]
COPD	*Streptococcus parasanguinis_B* and *Streptococcus salivarius, Streptococcus vestibularis, Streptococcus sp000187445, Lachnospiraceae*	↓ *Veillonella*, ↑ *Actinomyces*, ↑ *Actinobacillus*, ↑ *Megasphaera*, ↑ *Selenomonas*, ↑ *Corynebacterium*, ↑ *Streptococcus pneumoniae*, ↑ *Gemella morbillorum*, ↑ *Prevotella histicola*, ↑ *Streptococcus gordonii*	[17,18]
Asthma	↑ *Haemophilus*, ↑ *Streptococcus*, ↑ *Moraxella*, ↑ *Lactobacillus*	↑ *Haemophilus* spp., ↑ *Moraxella catarrhalis*, ↑ *Streptococcus* spp., *Tropheryma*	[19]
Cystic fibrosis	↑ *Escherichia*, ↑ *Shigella*, ↑ *Enterobacter*, ↑ *Clostridium*, ↑ *Veillonella*, ↑ *Enterococcus*, ↑ *Staphylococcus*, ↓ *Lachnospiraceae*, ↓ *Ruminococcu*, ↓ *Roseburia*, ↓ *Faecalibacterium*, ↓ *Eubacterium*, ↓ *Prevotella*, ↓ *Eggerthella*, ↓ *Alistipes*	*Pseudomonas aeruginosa, Staphylococcus aureus, H. influenzae, Burkholderia cepacia, Actinobacteria, Proteobacteria*	[19,20]

Abbreviations: ↑, increased in abundance; ↓, decreased in abundance; COPD, chronic obstructive pulmonary disease; IBD, inflammatory bowel disease.

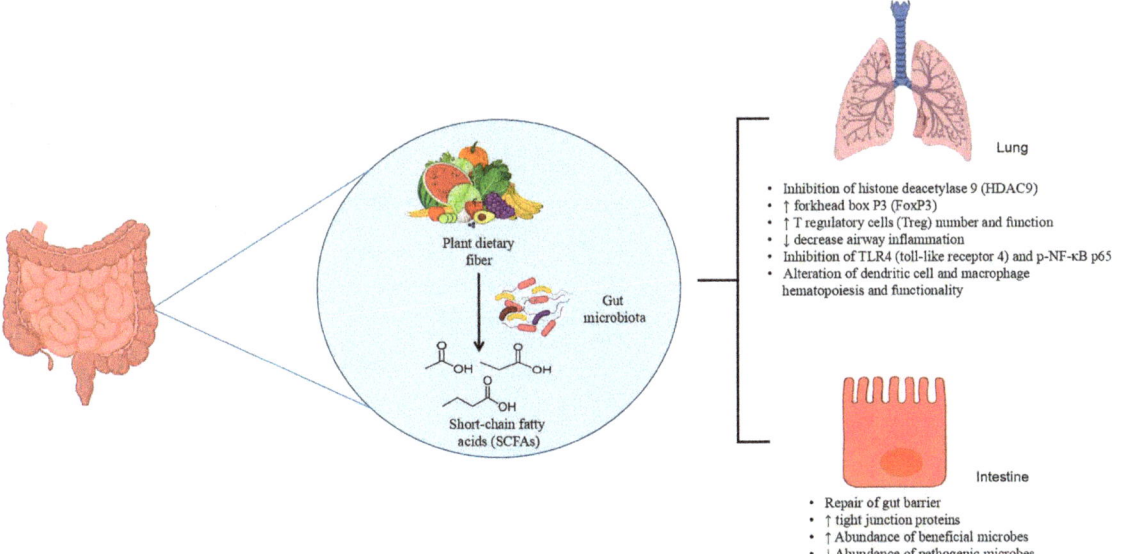

Figure 1. Mechanism of plant dietary fibers and polysaccharides against gut and lung inflammation. Abbreviations: ↑, increased; ↓, decreased.

Table 2. Effect of plant polysaccharides on intestinal inflammatory diseases via gut microbiota modulation.

Natural Source	Model	Effects on Inflammation Related Biomarkers	Intestinal Microbiota Modulation	References
Buckwheat	TNBS-induced colitis	↓ IL-6, IL-1β, and TNF-α	↑ F/B ratio, ↑ Oscillospiraceae, ↑ Oscillibacter, ↑ SCFAs	[21]
Rosa roxburghii Tratt polysaccharide	HFD-induced colitis	↓ TNF-α, IL-6 and IL-1β, ↑ tight junction proteins	↓ Desulfovibrionaceae, ↓ Enterobacteriaceae, ↑ Muribaculaceae, ↑ Bacteroidaceae	[22]
Rubus chingii Hu unripe fruit polysaccharide	HFD-induced colitis	↓ IL-6, ↓ IL-1β, ↓ TNF-α	↑ gut microbial diversity, ↓ Erysipelatoclostridium, ↓ Negativibacillus	[23]
Cyclocarya paliurus polysaccharide	DSS-induced colitis	↑ IL-10, ↓ IL-1β, ↓ TNF-α	↓ Akkermansia, ↓ Sutterella, ↓ AF12, ↓ Clostridiaceae_Clostridium, ↓ Helicobacter, ↓ Prevotella, ↑ Lactobacillus, ↑ Coprococcus	[24]
Smilax china L. polysaccharide	DSS-induced colitis	↓ TNF-α, ↓ IL-6, ↓ IL-1β, ↑ IL-10	↑ Lachnospiraceae, ↑ Muribaculaceae, ↑ Blautia, ↑ Mucispirillum, ↑ Akkermansiaceae, ↓ Deferribacteraceae, ↓ Oscillibacter	[25]
Chinese yam polysaccharide	LPS-stimulated co-culture of Caco-2/Raw264.7 cells	↓ NO, ↓ IL-1β, ↓ TNF-α	↑ Bifidobacterium, ↑ Megasphaera.	[26]
Fuzhuan brick tea polysaccharide	DSS-induced colitis	↓ IL-6, ↓ IL-1β, ↓ IFN-γ, ↓ TNF-α, ↑ tight junction proteins (Occludin, Claudin-1, and ZO-1), ↑ intestinal barrier function	↑ Bacteroides, ↑ Parasutterella, ↑ Collinsella	[27]
Fuc-S (a sulfated α-L-Fucooligosaccharide)	DSS-induced colitis	↓ TNF-α, ↓ IL-1β, ↓ IL-6, ↓ IL-17A	↓ F/B ratio, ↑ Akkermansia, ↑ Prevotellaceae_UCG_001, ↓ Eubacterium xylanophilum, ↓ Intestinimonas, ↓ Ruminococcaceae UCG-014, ↓ Oscillibacter	[28]
Polysaccharide conjugates derived from dried fresh tea leaves, green tea, and black tea	DSS-induced colitis	↓ IL-6, ↓ IFN-γ, ↓ IL-1β, ↓ TNF-α, ↑ IL-10	↑ Bacteroides, ↑ Muribaculaceae, ↓ Helicobacter, ↓ Enterococcus	[29]
Pectin with various esterification degrees	DSS-induced colitis	—	↑ Lactobacillus, ↑ Bifidobacterium	[30]
Rosa roxburghii Tratt	HFD-induced intestinal barrier dysfunction and inflammation	↓ TNF-α, ↓ IL-6, ↓ IL-1β; ↑ tight junction proteins (ZO-1, claudin-1, and occludin); ↓ intestinal permeability; ↓ colonic oxidative stress	↓ F/B ratio, ↓ Ruminococcaceae, ↑ Muribaculaceae, ↑ Akkermansiaceae	[22]
Dendrobium fimbriatum Hook	DSS-induced colitis	↓ IL-1β, ↓ IL-6, ↓ IL-17A, ↓ IL-17F, ↓ IL-21, ↓ IL-23, ↓ IL-5, ↓ IL-10, ↓ IL-22, ↓ IFN-γ, ↑ TNF-α, ↑ TGFβ	↑ Romboutsia, ↓ Lactobacillus, ↑ Odoribacter, ↓ Parasutterella, ↓ Burkholderia-Caballeronia-Paraburkholderia, ↓ Acinetobacter	[31]
Pectin	LPS-induced inflammation in piglets	↓ TNF-α, ↑ IL-10	↓ Helicobacter, ↑ Olsenella, ↑ Bacteroides, ↑ Proteus, ↑ Eubacterium	[32]
Rehmannia glutinosa polysaccharide	DSS-induced colitis	↑tight junction proteins, ↓ IL-10, ↓ IL-6, ↓ TNF-α, ↑ IL-10	↓ Bacteroidaceae, ↑ Lactobacillus, ↑ Alistipes, ↑ Lachnospiraceae_NK4A13	[33]
Polygonatum sibiricum polysaccharide	Aged mouse model	↓ IL-23, ↓ IL-6, ↓ IL-1β, ↓ TNFα, ↓ IL-17, ↓ IL-12, ↓ IL-6, ↑ IL4, ↑ IL-10	↑ Bifidobacterium, ↑ Lactobacillus, ↓ Escherichia coli	[34]
Rhinacanthus nasutus and okra	AA-induced colitis	↓ IL1β, ↓ IL-2, ↓ IL-6, ↑ IL-10	↑ Muribaculaceae, ↓ Bacteroidaceae, ↓ Tannerellaceae	[35]
Houttuynia cordata polysaccharides	DSS-induced colitis	↓ TNF-α, ↓ IL-1β, ↓ IL-6	↑ Firmicutes, ↑ Bacteroides, ↓ Proteobacteria	[36]
Lonicera japonica Thunb	DSS-induced colitis	↑ IL-2, ↑ TNF-α, ↑ IFN-γ	↑ Bifidobacterium, ↑ Lactobacilli, ↓ Escherichia coli, ↓ Enterococcus	[37]
Crataegus pinnatifida	DSS-induced colitis	↓ IL-1β, ↓ IL-6, ↓ TNF-α	↑ Alistipes, ↑ Odoribacter	[38]
Morinda citrifolia L.	DSS-induced colitis	↓ TNF-α, ↓ IL-17	↑ Dubosiella, ↑ Muribaculaceae, ↑ Ruminococcaceae_UGG-014, ↑ Ruminococcus_1, ↓ Bilophila, ↓ Campylobacter, ↓ Escherichia-Shigella, ↓ Ochrobactrum, ↓ Vibrio	[39]
Scutellaria baicalensis Georgi.	DSS-induced colitis	↓IL-6, ↓IL-1β, ↓TNF-α	↑ Bifidobacterium, ↑ Firmicutes, ↑ Lactobacillus, ↑ Roseburia	[40]

Abbreviations: ↑, increased; ↓, decreased; AA, acetic acid; DSS, dextran sulfate sodium; F/B ratio, Firmicutes/Bacteroidetes ratio; HFD, high-fat diet; IL, interleukin; IFN, interferon; LPS, lipopolysaccharide; TGFβ, transforming growth factor β; TNBS, 2,4,6-trinitrobenzene sulfonic acid; TNF, tumor necrosis factor; ZO-1, zonula occludens-1 (also known as Tight junction protein 1).

Table 3. Effect of plant polysaccharides on lung inflammatory diseases mediated via gut microbiota modulation.

Polysaccharide Intervention	Disease	Anti-Inflammatory Outcomes in Lungs	Effects on Intestinal Microflora	Reference
Pear extract	Preclinical asthma mouse model and randomized, double-blind clinical studies	↓ pro-inflammatory cytokines, including IgE, IL-4, IL-5, and IL-13	↑ Bifidobacterium and Eubacterium	[41]
Inulin (10%)	OVA- and Al (OH)3-induced asthma in SD rats	Attenuation of the asthmatic inflammatory response in the offspring	↑ SCFA-producing bacteria (mainly Bifidobacterium) in maternal intestinal microflora; alteration in intestinal microflora composition of offspring	[42]
Astragalus membranaceus polysaccharide (25, 50, and 100 mg/kg)	Bleomycin-induced pulmonary fibrosis	↓ damage and collagen deposition in lung tissue; ↓ inflammatory cytokines TNF-α, IL-6, and IL-1β levels; ↓ apoptosis	Restoration of gut microbiota homeostasis; ↑ Lactobacillus and Akkermansia; ↓ Lachnoclostridium, Clostridium, and Erysipelatoclostridium	[43]
Houttuynia cordata polysaccharides (80 mg/kg) and flavonoids (100 mg/kg) either alone or in combination	Influenza virus H1N1-infected mice	Combined therapy showed more potent effect than monotherapy; inhibition of inflammatory-cell infiltration and production of chemokines or pro-inflammatory cytokines such as MCP-1, IL-8, TNF-α, IL-6, and IL-1 β;	Restoration of microflora composition, ↑ Bacteroidetes-to-Firmicutes (B/F) ratio	[44]
Cellulose-rich diet (30%)	OVA- and Al(OH)3-induced asthma in C57BL/6J mice	↓ inflammatory cell infiltration around the bronchus and blood vessels; normalization of airway epithelial structure; ↓IL-4; ↓ IgE	↑ Peptostreptococcaceae	[45]
Houttuynia cordata polysaccharides (40 mg/kg)	H1N1-induced pneumonia in antibiotic-treated BALB/c mice (termed BALB/c-ABX mice)	Significant amelioration of inflammation in lungs of BALB/c mice	Attenuation of pathological change in intestine; ↓ Bacteroidetes at phylum level; ↓ Bacteroides and ↑ f_Lachnoospiraceae at genus level, ↑ gut microbial diversity; ↑ acetate	[46]
Astragalus polysaccharides	Lipopolysaccharide-induced inflammatory lung injury	Alleviation of histopathological abnormalities in lung tissues; ↓ neutrophils infiltration; inhibition of LPS-induced lung inflammation	Change in colonic microbiota composition; ↑ short-chain fatty acid (SCFA)-producing genera such as Oscillospira, Akkermansia, and Coprococcus	[47]
Platycodon grandiflorus polysaccharide (75, 150, and 300 mg/kg) and platycodin D alone and together	Chronic bronchitis in SD rats induced via smoking	Improvement in histopathological abnormalities; ↓ excess mucus secretion; improved immunological imbalance in lungs of CB model rat	—	[48]
Ephedra sinica polysaccharide	PM- and OVA-induced asthma in mice	↓ eosinophils in BALF; ↓ serum Ig-E, IL-6, TNF-α, and IL-1β; ↓ airway inflammation	↑ Bacteroides, Lactobacillus, Prevotella, Butyricicoccus, and Paraprevotella; ↓ Enterococcus and Ruminococcus; ↓ acetic acid, propionic acid, butyric acid, isobutyric acid, valeric acid, isovaleric acid, and isohexanic acid	[49]
Polysaccharides from Tetrastigma hemsleyanum Diels et Gilg	LPS-induced ARDS in Balb/c mice	↓ IL-6, ↓ TNF-α, inhibition of pulmonary inflammation via TLR2/TLR4 pathway	—	[50]
Polysaccharide-rich ethanol precipitate fraction of black tea	Particulate matter (PM)-induced lung injury in BALB/c mice	↓ oxidative stress and inflammation in the lungs; ↓ IL-6, CXCL1, CXCL15, and MDA	↑ Lachnospiraceae, ↓ Lactobacillaceae	[51]
High-cellulose (20%) or high-pectin diet (20)	Cigarette-smoke (CS)-exposed C57BL/6 mouse emphysema model	↓ Alveolar destruction and inflammation in BALF; ↓ macrophages and neutrophils in BALF; ↓ mRNA expression of IFN-γ, IL-1β, IL-6, IL-18, TNF-α, TGF-β	↑ SCFAs, bile acids, sphingolipids; ↑ Bacteroidetes; ↓ Lactobacillaceae; ↓ Defluviitaleaceae; ↓ Oscillospiraceae	[52]
Cellulose- or pectin-enriched diet	Ozone-induced airway hyperresponsiveness in C57BL/6 mice	↓ ozone-induced AHR, neutrophilic airway inflammation, and airway injury in female but not male mice; cellulose-based diets ameliorated ozone-induced airway hyperresponsiveness in male but not female mice	↓ Firmicutes, ↑ Proteobacteria and Verrucomicrobia in pectin-fed mice; ↑ Proteus and Lactobacillus, and ↓ Parabacteroides, Clostridiales, and Lachnospiraceae in pectin- versus cellulose-fed mice	[53]
Houttuynia cordata polysaccharides	H1N1-induced acute lung injury in C57BL/6 mice	Restoration of Th17/Treg cells balance in the lung, ↓ CCL20 expression	Restoration of Th17/Treg-cell balance of gut mucosa-associated lymphoid tissue (GALT)	[54]
Lycium barbarum polysaccharide	Asthma (OVA-induced mouse model)	↓ lung injury; ↓ TNF, IL-4, IL-6, MCP-1, and IL-17A in plasma and BALF	↑ Lactobacillus and Bifidobacterium; ↓ Firmicutes, Actinobacteria, Alistipes, and Clostridiales	[55]

Table 3. Cont.

Polysaccharide Intervention	Disease	Anti-Inflammatory Outcomes in Lungs	Effects on Intestinal Microflora	Reference
Soluble fiber (inulin 12 g/day), soluble fiber + probiotic (inulin 12 g/day + multi-strain probiotic >25 billion CFU)	Randomized, double-blind, three-way cross-over trial involving asthmatic patients	No differences between groups in asthma control or airway inflammation	No differences between groups in SCFA levels	[56]
Houttuynia cordata polysaccharide (40 mg/kg/day)	H1N1 virus-infected mice	↓ lung inflammation via inhibition of TLR signaling pathway, and IL-1β production and promotion of IL-10 production	↓ intestinal barrier damage; ↑ ZO-1 expression; ↓ relative abundance of pathogenic bacterial genera *Vibrio* and *Bacillus*	[57]
Houttuynia cordata polysaccharide (20 mg/kg; 40 mg/kg)	Influenza A virus (IAV) H1N1-mediated pneumonia in BALB/c mice	Amelioration of pulmonary injury; inhibition of TNF-α, IL-6, IFN-α, RANTES, MCP-1, MIP-1α; and IP-10 production	↓ intestinal goblet cells; ↑ intestinal physical and immune barrier; ↑ tight junction protein (ZO-1) in intestine	[58]
Pectin (30%)	Asthma (ozone-exposed mice)	↓ ozone-induced airway hyperresponsiveness	↑ serum short-chain fatty acids	[59]
GOS (1 or 2.5 w/w%) alone or with budesonide	HDM-induced asthma in BALB/c mice	Budesonide or GOS: ↓ eosinophils in BALF GOS + budesonide: ↓ CCL17, CCL22, and IL-33 protein levels; ↓ allergic inflammatory response	—	[60]
Soluble-fiber meal containing probiotic yoghurt; inulin (3.5 g); and the probiotics Lactobacillus acidophilus, Bifidobacterium lactis, and Lactobacillus rhamnosus	Human subjects with stable asthma	Airway inflammation biomarkers, including sputum total cell count, neutrophils, macrophages, lymphocytes, sputum IL-8, and eNO, significantly decreased; no decrease in airway eosinophils	—	[61]
Soluble pectin/insoluble cellulose (4%)	Asthma (female BALB/c mice; OVA induction)	↓ eosinophil inflammation, ↓ frequency of allergic symptoms, ↓ BALF and NALF total cells and eosinophils, ↓ IL-4 in BALF, ↑ IFN-γ and IL-10 in BALF	↑ Bifidobacteria	[62]
Houttuynia cordata Thunb. polysaccharides (40, 80, and 160 mg/kg)	Lipopolysaccharide-induced acute lung injury in Balb/c mice	↓ pro-inflammatory cytokine (TNF-α, interleukin-6, and interleukin-1β) production	—	[63]
Citrus pectin-derived acidic oligosaccharides (5%)	*Pseudomonas aeruginosa* lung infection in BALB/c mice	↑ M1 macrophage activation, ↑ IL-10 release, ↓ TNF-α release	↑ *Escherichia coli, Allobaculum* species, *Sutturella wadsworthia, Bacteroides vulgatus, Bifidobacterium* species, *Clostridium difficile, Clostridium ramosum, Clostridium sphenoides*; ↑ production of butyrate and propionate	[64]
GOS (1%)	HDM-induced asthma in BALB/c mice	↓ AHR development, ↓ BALF eosinophils, ↓ BALF leukocytes, ↓ CCL5 and IL-13	—	[65]
scGOS/lcFOS (in 9:1 ratio)	OVA-induced asthma in female BALB/c and male C57BL/6	↓ OVA-induced AHR; no significant change in the concentrations of IFN-γ, IL-4, IL-5, IL-10, IL-12(p70), IL-13, IL-17, and TNF-α in BAL fluid and plasma	—	[66]
High-fiber diet	HDM-induced asthma in female C57BL/6 and BALB/C mice	↓ total BALF leukocytes, eosinophils, macrophages, and lymphocytes; ↓ IL-4, -5, -13, −10, and IFN-γ; ↓ airway hyperresponsiveness	↑ Bacteroidetes; ↓ Firmicutes	[67]
Apple pectin (30%)	HDM-induced asthma in BALB/c mice	↓ allergic airway inflammation	Changes in intestinal and lung microbiota; increment in SCFAs; ↑ Bacteroidetes; ↑ Bifidobacteriaceae; ↓ Firmicutes	[68]
Chitosan oligosaccharides	OVA-induced asthma in mice	↓ mRNA and protein levels of IL-4, IL-5, IL-13, TNF-α in lung tissue and BALF	—	[69]
FOS (2.5%)	HDM-induced airway inflammation in male C3H/HeN mice	↓ BALF eosinophils, ↓ IL-5	—	[70]
1% w/w of 9:1 scGOS: lcFOS; 1% w/w of 83% sc-GOS/lcFOS + 17% pAOS	OVA-induced asthma in male BALB/c mice	↓ OVA-induced airway inflammation and hyperresponsiveness, ↓ BALF inflammatory cells	—	[71]

Table 3. *Cont.*

Polysaccharide Intervention	Disease	Anti-Inflammatory Outcomes in Lungs	Effects on Intestinal Microflora	Reference
Raffinose (50 g/kg) and GOS (50 g/kg)	Allergic airway eosinophilia (OVA-sensitized brown Norway rats)	↓ IL-4, ↓ IL-5	↑ total anaerobic bacteria in the colon	[72]
Asian pear pectin (100 µg)	Asthma (OVA-sensitized murine model)	↓ asthmatic reactions in sensitized mice, ↓ IFN-γ, ↓ IL-5	—	[73]
Raffinose (50 g/kg)	Allergic airway eosinophilia (OVA-sensitized brown Norway rats)	↓ IL-4 and IL-5 mRNA expression, ↓ mucus-producing cells, = IFN-γ mRNA expression	↑ bifidobacteria	[74]

Abbreviations: ↑, increased; ↓, decreased; =, no change or no effect; ARDS, acute respiratory distress syndrome; BALF, bronchoalveolar lavage fluid; HDM, house dust mite; TNF-α, tumor necrosis factor alpha; IL-1, interleukin-1; IFN-α, interferon-α; IL-6, interleukin-6; IL-10, interleukin-10; RANTES, regulated on activation, normal-T-cell-expressed and -secreted; IP-10, interferon-inducible protein-10; LPS, lipopolysaccharide; MCP-1, monocyte chemotactic protein-1; MIP-1α, macrophage inflammatory protein-1α; ZO-1, zonula occludens-1, also known as Tight junction protein 1; SD, Sprague–Dawley.

2. Plant Dietary Fibers and Polysaccharides against Gut and Lung Inflammation

2.1. Different Plant Dietary Fibers and Polysaccharides Shape Gut Microbiota and Affect SCFA Production Differently

Despite the availability of various drugs that offer relief for lung inflammation and intestinal inflammatory diseases, tackling gut dysbiosis, a common feature of many gut and lung diseases, as discussed above, remains a significant challenge for these medications. However, dietary fibers (DFs) and polysaccharides have emerged as potential candidates for effectively modulating the gut microbiota and playing a vital role in the prevention and treatment of these conditions. Their ability to target and positively influence the gut microbiota holds promising implications for addressing gut–lung axis diseases more effectively.

A study by Jang et al. [52] demonstrated that different types of DF have differential effects on gut microbial composition and short-chain fatty acid (SCFA) production. In the study, emphysema mice were fed either non-fermentable cellulose or fermentable pectin-rich diets. Both cellulose and pectin lowered pro-inflammatory mediators, including IFN-γ, IL-1β, IL-6, IL-8, IL-18, TNF-α, and TGF-β. However, pectin supplementation (fermentable fiber) exhibited higher anti-inflammatory action than non-fermentable-fiber (cellulose) supplementation in emphysema mice. Regarding gut microbiota composition, at the phylum level, *Bacteroidetes* were the most abundant in the high-pectin diet group. At the family level, *Lactobacillaceae* and *Defluviitaleaceae* were the lowest in the high-pectin diet group compared with the high-cellulose diet group or control.

In addition to the type of dietary fiber (DF), the structural modifications of DF also play a crucial role in its ability to shape the gut microbiota and its preventive effects on lung and gut inflammation. For instance, pectin, a plant-derived water-soluble DF primarily composed of linear chains of galacturonic acid that can be esterified, has been studied in relation to its impact on ulcerative colitis. Research by Fan et al. [75] demonstrated that pectin with a degree of esterification below 50% exhibited a higher preventive potential against ulcerative colitis than pectin with a degree of esterification above 50%. In another study conducted by the same research group, they explored the effects of pectins with different degrees of esterification and dosages on gut microbiota and serum metabolites in a colitis mouse model. These findings highlight the significance of considering structural variations in DF to harness its full potential for modulating gut microbiota and preventing inflammation-related diseases.

The composition changes of major genera, including *Lactobacillus*, *Bifidobacterium*, *Akkermansia*, *Prevotella*, *Ruminococcus*, and *Oscillospira*, vary widely depending on the degree of esterification and pectin dosage. Another comparative study examined three polysaccharide conjugates derived from dried fresh tea leaves (FTPS), green tea (GTPS), and black tea (BTPS) [29]. These conjugates were tested for their capacity to regulate intestinal homeostasis in DSS-induced colitis mice. While all tea polysaccharide conjugates increased the abundance of *Bacteroides* and *Muribaculaceae* and reduced *Helicobacter* and *Enterococcus* abundance, only FTPS and BTPS exhibited inhibitory effects on *Mucispirillum*. Moreover, the production of SCFAs differed among the three conjugates, with FTPS showing the highest SCFA production, followed by BTPS and GTPS. Overall, FTPS demonstrated better efficacy than BTPS and GTPS in preventing colitis.

Cystic fibrosis (CF) is associated with gut dysbiosis and intestinal inflammation. In a pilot study, Wang et al. [76] investigated whether CF patients' depleted microbiota had the potential to utilize a prebiotic substrate, such as high-amylose maize starch (HAMS), for increased SCFA production. Various techniques, including metagenomic sequencing, in vitro fermentation, amplicon sequencing, and metabolomics, were employed to examine the HAMS fermentation capacity of the gut microbiome in adults with CF and controls. CF patients exhibited low abundances of taxa associated with HAMS fermentation (*Faecalibacterium*, *Roseburia*, and *Coprococcus*) and lower levels of acetate production compared to controls. However, there was no difference in the production of butyrate and propionate between CF patients and controls. The study reported that high butyrate production in healthy controls was associated with a high relative abundance of the commensal genus *Faecalibacterium*. Interestingly, in the absence of butyrate-producing *Faecalibacterium* in CF patients, another bacterium, *Clostridium* ss1, competitively fermented HAMS and biosynthesized butyrate. This finding suggests that despite alterations in gut microbiota, the prebiotic effect of DF can be mediated by different taxa, which is in contrast to the notion that the presence of commensal bacteria is necessary to produce the prebiotic effect of DF.

2.2. Plant Dietary Fibers and Polysaccharides Alter the Intestinal Barrier in Both Gut Inflammation and Lung Inflammation

The intestinal barrier serves as an important defense mechanism that maintains a healthy balance of inflammatory factors to prevent the entry of pathogens into the body. It consists of four main barrier systems: mechanical, chemical, immune, and biological barriers [77]. Gut dysbiosis, among other factors, can disrupt the integrity of the intestinal barrier by affecting tight junctions in epithelial cells. This disruption can allow the translocation of gut microbes to other body sites, such as the lungs, and promote lung inflammation [54,78].

Plant polysaccharides have been shown to improve lung inflammation by repairing the intestinal barrier. Zhu et al. [58] extracted *Houttuynia cordata* polysaccharide (HCP), which mainly consists of glucose, galactose, arabinose, and rhamnose in a ratio of 3.40:2.14:1.17:1. The inclusion of HCP in the diet of influenza A virus-infected mice not only repaired the intestinal barrier by increasing secretory immunoglobulin A (sIgA) and the tight junction protein zonula occludens-1 (ZO-1) but also reduced proinflammatory cytokines and chemokines such as TNF-α, IL-6, and IFN-α. Furthermore, the anti-inflammatory properties of HCP in the lung and gut were mediated through the inhibition of toll-like receptor 4 (TLR4) and phosphorylated NF-κB p65 in the lung [58]. However, this study did not explore the effect of HCP on gut microbiota and its role in lung inflammation.

In another study, it was observed that the oral administration of high-amylose cornstarch (HCP) to mice infected with influenza A virus led to improvements in intestinal barrier integrity and alleviated gut inflammation. This effect was attributed to the increased levels of intestinal tight junction proteins and secretory IgA (sIgA) in mice. These findings suggest that HCP may have potential therapeutic benefits in managing gut inflammation and enhancing intestinal barrier function during viral infections. Moreover, HCP corrected the alterations in gut microbiota by reducing the relative abundances of pathogenic bacteria *Vibrio* and *Bacillus* [57].

The protective effects of plant polysaccharides on the intestinal barrier have also been demonstrated for polysaccharides extracted from sources other than *Houttuynia cordata*. These sources include Chinese yam [26], *Rhinacanthus nasutus* and okara [35], *Scutellaria baicalensis* Georgi [40], *Polygonatum sibiricum* [34], *Cyclocarya paliurus* [24], *Rehmannia glutinosa* [33],

Rosa roxburghii Tratt [22,79], *Dendrobium fimbriatum* Hook [31], and tea [29] in animal models of ulcerative colitis and inflammatory bowel disease (IBD).

2.3. Plant-Dietary-Fiber and Polysaccharide Supplementation in Gut and Lung Inflammation in Human Adults (Clinical Studies) and Adult Mice (Preclinical Studies)

Park et al. [80] in a prospective human cohort study (n = 219,123 men and 168,999 women, aged 50–71 years, 9-year follow-up) evaluated the effect of dietary-fiber intake on health outcomes. The study reported that the consumption of dietary fiber was associated with a reduced risk of mortality from respiratory diseases in both men and women. In a three-way, cross-over, double-blind, randomized controlled trial, adults with stable asthma were administered a soluble fiber, inulin (12 g per day), for 7 days, leading to improved asthma control and reduced airway inflammation. Additionally, inulin supplementation was found to modulate the gut microbiome, as evidenced by an increase in the relative abundance and absolute numbers of bifidobacteria [56]. These findings suggest that dietary fiber, particularly inulin, may play a beneficial role in improving respiratory health and gut microbiota composition.

In another randomized, double-blind, placebo-controlled, crossover study, soluble-fiber supplementation in healthy people did not only reduce the levels of pro-inflammatory factors such as TNF-α, IL-6, and IL-8 but also improved gut microbiota composition and increased the production of butyrate [81]. The effect of a soluble-fiber meal (containing 3.5 g of inulin and probiotics) on airway inflammation and free fatty acid receptor activity in adults with stable asthma was examined in a pilot study [61]. Soluble-fiber supplementation alleviated airway inflammation, as shown by reductions in total cell count, neutrophils, macrophages, lymphocytes, and IL-8. Further, the observed anti-inflammatory effect of the soluble-fiber meal was found to improve lung function via the upregulation of free fatty acid receptors, GPR41 and GPR43 gene expression.

In a preclinical study conducted on adult mouse models with allergic airway disease (AAD), a pectin-rich diet was found to alleviate allergic airway inflammation. The pectin-rich diet led to alterations in gut microbiota homeostasis, increasing the abundance of the *Bacteroidaceae* and *Bifidobacteriaceae* families. These bacteria have the capacity to ferment soluble fiber into short-chain fatty acids (SCFAs) such as acetate and propionate. The protective effects of the pectin-rich diet were primarily mediated by SCFAs, which promoted dendritic-cell hematopoiesis and functionality. This, in turn, resulted in reduced Th2-cell response, attenuation of allergic inflammation, and improved lung function [68].

Similarly, SCFAs fermented from an inulin-rich diet have been shown to protect against influenza-induced pathology in adult mice. This protection was achieved by altering macrophage hematopoiesis and functionality and preventing the entry of neutrophils into the airways, thereby ameliorating tissue destruction [82]. These findings indicate that dietary fibers, such as pectin and inulin, can modulate gut microbiota and SCFA production, leading to beneficial effects on respiratory health and inflammation.

Among various plant DFs and polysaccharides, *Houttuynia cordata*-extracted polysaccharide has been frequently used as a gut microbiota modulator to alleviate anti-lung inflammatory agents in lipopolysaccharide-induced acute lung injury [63] and influenza virus infection-induced lung injury [44,46,54,57,58]. Other than *Houttuynia cordata*, polysaccharides derived from *Lycium barbarum* [55] and *Ephedra sinica* [49] can also ameliorate lung inflammation in mice by modulating gut microbiota composition. Polysaccharides extracted from *Platycodon grandiflorus* [48] and *Tetrastigma hemsleyanum* [50] have also been reported to possess lung anti-inflammatory response. *Tetrastigma hemsleyanum* polysaccharides could correct antibiotic-induced intestinal mucosal barrier dysfunction and gut inflammation in mice, thus showing an important role in the management of the gut–lung axis [83].

2.4. Plant-Dietary-Fiber and Polysaccharide Supplementation in Maternal Rodent Models

Dietary fibers (DFs) or polysaccharides have also been investigated for their potential in preventing asthma in offspring by feeding asthmatic mother mice a DF-rich diet during pregnancy and/or lactation. Thorburn et al. [67] fed a high-fiber diet to female mice with house dust mite (HDM)-induced asthma and observed decreased susceptibility to allergic airway disease (AAD) in their offspring. This effect was mediated indirectly through alterations in the gut microbiota, specifically an increase in *Bacteroidetes* and a decrease in *Firmicutes*, as well as directly through the production of short-chain fatty acid (SCFA) metabolites. The intestinal microbiota fermented the high-fiber diet into SCFAs, which inhibited histone deacetylase 9 (HDAC9) and led to epigenetic modifications of the forkhead box P3 (Foxp3) promoter, resulting in increased Foxp3 expression. Foxp3, in turn, led to an increase in the pool and function of T regulatory cells (Tregs), ultimately ameliorating airway inflammation.

In two separate studies conducted by Hogenkamp et al., mice were supplemented with different mixtures of non-digestible oligosaccharides. One study involved a diet supplemented with short-chain galactooligosaccharides (scGOSs) and long-chain fructooligosaccharides (lcFOSs) in a ratio of 9:1, while the other study used a diet supplemented with scGOSs, lcFOSs, and pectin-derived acidic oligosaccharides (pAOSs) in a ratio of 9:1:2 [66,84]. Both studies reported a reduction in allergic asthma in male offspring. However, no significant differences were found in the production of cytokines such as IL-13, IL-4, IL-5, IL-10, IL-17, IFN-γ, and TNF-α between the control group and the non-digestible-oligosaccharide diet group in either study. Additionally, neither study explored whether the therapeutic effect of the oligosaccharide-rich diet on offspring was mediated by the gut microbiota.

However, a recent study by Yuan et al. [42] demonstrated that supplementation with inulin, a soluble dietary fiber, significantly altered the composition of maternal gut microbiota by increasing SCFA-producing *Bifidobacterium*. This supplementation also attenuated the asthmatic inflammatory response in the offspring. The study employed drinking water containing 10% inulin for supplementation.

2.5. Sex Differences in Lung Anti-Inflammatory Effect of Plant DFs and Polysaccharides

Many lung inflammatory diseases, such as asthma, COPD, CF, and acute pneumonia, exhibit sexual dimorphism, with differences in disease susceptibility, severity, and prognosis between males and females [85]. Additionally, sex differences can also impact the microbial populations present in various body parts, including the gut microbiome and lung microbiome, and this is referred to as microgenderome [85]. Therefore, it is possible that dietary interventions involving dietary fiber (DF) against lung inflammation may also show sex-based differences in effectiveness. This hypothesis was recently tested by Tashiro et al. [53] using an ozone-induced airway hyperresponsiveness (AHR) mouse model, where cellulose and pectin were included in the diet. The study found that only the cellulose-rich diet reduced ozone-induced AHR in males, but increased AHR, neutrophilic airway inflammation, and airway injury in females. The sex difference in the efficacy of DF against pulmonary response was attributed to differences in diet-related changes in gut microbiota composition between male and female mice.

Sex-specific effects of DF have also been observed in mouse models of gut inflammation. Isomaltodextrins (IMDs) are starch-based soluble dietary fibers prepared using α-glucosyltransferase and α-amylase enzymes [86]. An interleukin (IL)-10-deficient colitis mouse model was treated with IMDs to examine their effect on colitis and gut microbiota and to assess whether the impact of IMDs was sex-specific [86]. IMD supplementation in female mice reduced alpha diversity and *Coprococcus* abundance, while in male mice, it increased alpha diversity, community richness, and evenness and showed a lesser reduction in *Coprococcus* abundance. These studies highlight the sex-dependent response to DF supplementation of gut microbiota in both gut and pulmonary inflammation, indicating that the therapeutic application of plant DF requires careful adaptation for males and females.

2.6. Combination of Plant Polysaccharides with Other Phytochemicals

There have been only a few studies that have explored the therapeutic effects of plant dietary fibers or plant polysaccharides in combination with other phytochemicals. In an interesting study by Ling et al. [44], the efficacy of polysaccharides and flavonoids isolated from *Houttuynia cordata* was tested either alone or in combination against H1N1-induced pneumonia in mice. The combined administration of polysaccharides (80 mg/kg) and flavonoids (100 mg/kg) demonstrated excellent ability to regulate pulmonary homeostasis compared with either therapy alone.

Budesonide is a corticosteroid drug commonly used for airway and gut inflammation [87]. However, long-term use of this drug can lead to several side effects, such as tuberculosis infection, hypersensitivity reactions, and an increased risk of infections. To enhance the efficacy of budesonide and reduce its side effects by lowering the required dose, Verheijden et al. [60] investigated the use of galactooligosaccharides (GOSs) as a dietary adjunct therapy against pulmonary inflammation in a murine model of house dust mite-induced allergic asthma. The combination of budesonide and GOSs exhibited a more potent anti-allergic inflammation effect than budesonide or GOSs alone. However, one limitation of the study was that the authors did not assess the impact of the various treatments on gut microbiota composition.

2.7. Mechanisms of Polysaccharides and Dietary Fibers in Reducing Intestinal and Lung Inflammation

The underlying mechanisms responsible for the anti-inflammatory effects of plant DFs and polysaccharides on the lungs remain poorly understood. However, among various mechanisms proposed for the lung and intestine anti-inflammatory properties of plant polysaccharides, mostly are mediated via either changes in gut microbiota composition or SCFAs.

T helper type 17 (Th17) and regulatory T (Treg) cells are important subsets of effector cells derived from CD4 T cells, having an important function in maintaining immune homeostasis in the body. Th17 cells are pro-inflammatory in nature, produce pro-inflammatory molecules, such as IL-17, IL-17A, IL-17F, IL-21, and IL-22, and recruit neutrophils; on the other hand, Treg cells help suppress inflammatory and immune responses by producing anti-inflammatory cytokine IL-10 and transforming growth factor (TGF)-β1 [88,89]. Therefore, Th17-/Treg-cell balance is an important factor in determining inflammatory homeostasis in the body, and gut dysbiosis can affect the Th17-/Treg-cell balance in intestinal and lung inflammatory diseases, such as in IBD and asthma [90,91]. Plant-based DFs and polysaccharides can regulate this Th17-/Treg-cell imbalance and improve gut and lung inflammation by modulating gut microbiota and consequently SCFA production [46,54,67]. For example, *Houttuynia cordata* polysaccharide treatment corrected Th17-/Treg-cell imbalance both in gut-associated lymphoid tissue (GALT) and lungs by increasing the total number of Treg cells, reducing the expression of chemokine CCL20 in the lung, and promoting the migration of Treg cells in Peyer's patches–mesenteric lymph nodes–lung axis in H1N1-infected mice [54]. SCFAs, particularly acetate, have been reported to be involved in correcting the balance between Th17 and Treg cells in the gut–lung axis [46]. SCFAs can maintain the Th17-/Treg-cell balance via the following mechanism: SCFAs increase the expression of forkhead box P3 (Foxp3) transcription factor via epigenetic modifications of the Foxp3 promoter by inhibiting the histone deacetylase 9 (HDAC9) enzyme; the increased expression of Foxp3, in turn, leads to an increase in the pool and function of T regulatory cells (Tregs), ultimately ameliorating airway inflammation [67].

However, some studies present an alternative view, suggesting that the alleviation of asthmatic symptoms with high-fiber diets, such as those rich in cellulose, may not be always mediated through increased production of intestinal SCFAs but also via the regulation of intestinal microflora composition, which can affect the body's lipid metabolism [45]. Similarly, Lai et al. [92] showed that oral administration of commensal bacteria *Parabacteroides goldsteinii* MTS01 could significantly inhibit a cigarette-smoke-induced

COPD murine model by correcting disturbed amino acid metabolism, reducing intestinal inflammation, improving ribosomal and mitochondrial functions in the intestines, and ameliorating lung inflammation. Therefore, diets rich in plant polysaccharides that can increase the relative abundance of such beneficial bacteria have the potential to ameliorate lung inflammatory diseases.

Interestingly, other studies highlighted that plant DFs' and polysaccharides' lung and intestinal anti-inflammatory mechanisms were not dependent on either gut microbiota or microbial fermentation of DFs into SCFAs. For example, Sonoyama et al. [72] reported a reduction in eosinophilic infiltration in the lungs and a reduction in the levels of IL-4 and IL-5 mRNA in ovalbumin-sensitized rats supplemented with raffinose (RAF) and α-linked galactooligosaccharide (GOS) diets. These effects were retained even after cecectomy and antibiotic treatment, which led researchers to suggest that the therapeutic effects of RAF and GOS were not due to their fermentation by bacteria. Similarly, for fructan DFs with $\beta 2\rightarrow 1$ linkage, such as inulin and fructooligosaccharides, it was observed that their immunomodulatory effect was mainly dependent on their chemical structure, and this effect was mediated not by the gut microbiota but via increases in the number of type 1 T helper (Th1) cells in Peyer's patches and in the number of dendritic cells and Tregs in mesenteric lymph nodes in mice [93].

As we already discuss above, the gut barrier is an important defense system that prevents the entry of pathogens into the body. The lack of plant DF in diet can increase the permeability of the intestinal barrier to pathogenic microbes and bacterial lipopolysaccharides (LPSs), which, by binding to TLR4, lead to the activation of NF-κB signaling and inflammatory cytokine production [94,95]. Plant DFs and polysaccharides could suppress the expression of TLR4 and p-NF-κB-p65 in the lungs and ultimately inhibit lung inflammation [43,58]. Although bacterial LPSs generally act as activators of TLR4 and play a role in downstream inflammatory activation, in an interesting study, the LPS derived from an intestinal commensal bacterium, *Parabacteroides goldsteinii*, was found to be the main component that ameliorated a cigarette-smoke-induced COPD murine model by acting as an antagonist for TLR4 and consequently reducing the over-expression of proinflammatory cytokines such as IL-1β and TNF-α in the lungs and colon in COPD mice [92].

3. Issues and Challenges

The gut–lung axis represents a bidirectional communication pathway between the respiratory and gastrointestinal tracts. Despite the bidirectional nature of this axis, current research primarily focuses on the impact of gut microbiota on lung diseases, with limited studies investigating the influence of lung microbiota on inflammation and whether dietary interventions using plant-based dietary fibers (DFs) and polysaccharides can affect lung-microbiome diversity. This exploration is necessary, because while the gut and lung microbial populations are similar at the phylum level, they differ significantly at the species level [96].

Another challenge lies in accurately defining plant DFs and polysaccharides. While many studies have demonstrated the therapeutic effects of carbohydrates such as inulin, fructooligosaccharides, and galactooligosaccharides in gut and lung inflammation (refer to Tables 2 and 3), it has been suggested that these low-molecular-weight (LMW) non-digestible carbohydrates should not be considered DFs. Their rapid fermentation in the proximal colon can cause side effects, including flatulence, abdominal distention, and abdominal pain [15]. Therefore, interventions involving polysaccharides should be preferred over oligosaccharide supplementation to maximize the benefits for lung and gut inflammation.

Despite the similarity at the phylum level, the species composition of gut microbiota varies widely among individuals of different races and ethnicities [97]. Generally, studies investigating the therapeutic potential of plant DF and polysaccharide supplementation in gut and lung inflammation have not taken individual variations in microbiota into account, nor have they included an individual's response to such supplementation. It is crucial to understand these variations, because DF supplementation in individuals with gut dysbiosis may inadvertently worsen the dysbiosis. Therefore, prebiotic recommendations cannot be generalized and require proper safety evaluations of plant-based DFs and polysaccharides in populations with gut and lung inflammation.

Compared with research on probiotics and short-chain fatty acids, research exploring the use of plant polysaccharide-based prebiotics against gut and lung inflammation is limited, especially in clinical studies. High-quality, large-scale, well-designed randomized trials are necessary before plant DFs and polysaccharides can be recommended as gut modulator therapies for individuals with gut and lung inflammatory diseases.

4. Conclusions

Plant dietary fibers (DFs) and polysaccharides have shown promising results in preventing gut and lung inflammation by influencing gut microbiota, as supported by both clinical and preclinical studies. This highlights the potential of DFs, including plant polysaccharides, as a prebiotic dietary approach to managing gut and lung inflammation. However, it is essential to address the current research focus, which has been primarily centered on the gut microbiota in the gut–lung axis, with limited attention given to the effects of DFs and plant polysaccharides on the lung microbiome. This knowledge gap is further exacerbated by the predominant emphasis on the bacterial components of the microbiota, while the fungal and viral microbiota of the gastrointestinal tract have been less explored. This limitation hinders a comprehensive understanding of gut and lung inflammation.

Furthermore, there is a scarcity of research on the use of plant polysaccharides, as many studies have predominantly focused on low-molecular-weight (LMW) carbohydrates such as inulin, fructooligosaccharides, and galactooligosaccharides. Therefore, substantial efforts are required to fully explore and harness the prebiotic potential of plant polysaccharides. Addressing these research gaps could not only enhance our understanding of the gut–lung axis but also open new avenues for the development of effective therapeutic interventions using plant-based dietary fibers and polysaccharides to manage gut and lung inflammation.

In conclusion, the modulation of gut microbiota with the administration of plant DFs and polysaccharides shows promise in preventing gut and lung inflammation. However, more research is needed to better understand the effects of DFs and plant polysaccharides on the lung microbiome and to expand our knowledge beyond bacterial microbiota. Additionally, the exploration of plant polysaccharides as prebiotics requires more attention to fully unlock their potential. Advancing our understanding in these areas could facilitate the development of effective dietary strategies for managing gut and lung inflammation.

Author Contributions: Y.S. wrote the first draft of the manuscript; M.S. performed the literature review; S.W. edited the manuscript; H.Z. and Y.Z. gave a scientific contribution and critically revised the manuscript. All authors have read and agreed to the published version of the manuscript.

Funding: This study was supported by North Medicine and Functional Food Characteristic Subject Project in Heilongjiang Province (No. HLJTSXK-2022-03), the excellent youth project of Heilongjiang Natural Science Foundation (No. YQ2023H001), Basic Research Project of Fundamental Research Business Expenses of Education Department in Heilongjiang Province (No. 2021-KYYWF-0586), Basic Research Project of Fundamental Research Business Expenses of Education Department in Heilongjiang Province (No. 2022-KYYWF-0641), the postdoctoral funded project of Heilongjiang Province (No. LBH-Z22292), the Doctoral Special Research Fund launch project of Jiamusi University (No. JMSUBZ2021-10), The Key Laboratory of New Drug Development and Drug Toxicology Evaluation in Heilongjiang Province (No. kfkt2022-14).

Institutional Review Board Statement: Not applicable.

Informed Consent Statement: Not applicable.

Data Availability Statement: This study no new data were created.

Conflicts of Interest: The authors declare that the research was conducted in the absence of any commercial or financial relationships that could be construed as a potential conflict of interest.

References

1. Molodecky, N.A.; Soon, I.S.; Rabi, D.M.; Ghali, W.A.; Ferris, M.; Chernoff, G.; Benchimol, E.I.; Panaccione, R.; Ghosh, S.; Barkema, H.W.; et al. Increasing Incidence and Prevalence of the Inflammatory Bowel Diseases with Time, Based on Systematic Review. *Gastroenterology* **2012**, *142*, 46–54.e42. [CrossRef] [PubMed]
2. Chen, L.; Deng, H.; Cui, H.; Fang, J.; Zuo, Z.; Deng, J.; Li, Y.; Wang, X.; Zhao, L. Inflammatory responses and inflammation-associated diseases in organs. *Oncotarget* **2018**, *9*, 7204. [CrossRef] [PubMed]
3. World Health Organization. Chronic Obstructive Pulmonary Disease (COPD). Available online: https://www.who.int/news-room/fact-sheets/detail/chronic-obstructive-pulmonary-disease-(copd) (accessed on 17 June 2023).
4. Piovani, D.; Danese, S.; Peyrin-Biroulet, L.; Bonovas, S. Inflammatory bowel disease: Estimates from the global burden of disease 2017 study. *Aliment. Pharm. Ther.* **2020**, *51*, 261–270. [CrossRef]
5. Barcik, W.; Boutin, R.C.T.; Sokolowska, M.; Finlay, B.B. The Role of Lung and Gut Microbiota in the Pathology of Asthma. *Immunity* **2020**, *52*, 241–255. [CrossRef] [PubMed]
6. Wang, L.; Cai, Y.; Garssen, J.; Henricks, P.A.J.; Folkerts, G.; Braber, S. The bidirectional gut–lung axis in chronic obstructive pulmonary disease. *Am. J. Respir. Crit. Care Med.* **2023**, *207*, 1145–1160. [CrossRef]
7. Kisiel, M.A.; Sedvall, M.; Malinovschi, A.; Franklin, K.A.; Gislason, T.; Shlunssen, V.; Johansson, A.; Modig, L.; Jogi, R.; Holm, M.; et al. Inflammatory bowel disease and asthma. Results from the RHINE study. *Respir. Med.* **2023**, *216*, 107307. [CrossRef] [PubMed]
8. Antoine, M.H.; Mlika, M. Interstitial lung disease. In *StatPearls*; StatPearls Publishing: Treasure Island, FL, USA, 2023. Available online: http://www.ncbi.nlm.nih.gov/books/NBK541084/ (accessed on 7 June 2023).
9. Luo, Q.; Zhou, P.; Chang, S.; Huang, Z.; Zhu, Y. The gut-lung axis: Mendelian randomization identifies a causal association between inflammatory bowel disease and interstitial lung disease. *Heart Lung* **2023**, *61*, 120–126. [CrossRef]
10. Cai, Z.; Wang, S.; Li, J. Treatment of inflammatory bowel disease: A comprehensive review. *Front. Med.* **2021**, *8*, 765474. [CrossRef]
11. Gross, N.J.; Barnes, P.J. New therapies for asthma and chronic obstructive pulmonary disease. *Am. J. Respir. Crit. Care Med.* **2017**, *195*, 159–166. [CrossRef]
12. Niu, Y.; Liu, W.; Fan, X.; Wen, D.; Wu, D.; Wang, H.; Liu, Z.; Li, B. Beyond cellulose: Pharmaceutical potential for bioactive plant polysaccharides in treating disease and gut dysbiosis. *Front. Microbiol.* **2023**, *14*, 1183130. [CrossRef]
13. Lovegrove, A.; Edwards, C.H.; De Noni, I.; Patel, H.; El, S.N.; Grassby, T.; Zielke, C.; Ulmius, M.; Nilsson, L.; Butterworth, P.J.; et al. Role of polysaccharides in food, digestion, and health. *Crit. Rev. Food Sci. Nutr.* **2017**, *57*, 237–253. [CrossRef] [PubMed]
14. An, Y.; Lu, W.; Li, W.; Pan, L.; Lu, M.; Igor, C.; Li, Z.; Zeng, W. Dietary fiber in plant cell walls—The healthy carbohydrates. *Food Qual. Saf.* **2022**, *6*, fyab037. [CrossRef]
15. Stribling, P.; Ibrahim, F. Dietary fibre definition revisited—The case of low molecular weight carbohydrates. *Clin. Nutr. ESPEN* **2023**, *55*, 340–356. [CrossRef]
16. Qiu, P.; Ishimoto, T.; Fu, L.; Zhang, J.; Zhang, Z.; Liu, Y. The Gut Microbiota in Inflammatory Bowel Disease. *Front. Cell. Infect. Microbiol.* **2022**, *12*, 733992. [CrossRef] [PubMed]
17. Bowerman, K.L.; Rehman, S.F.; Vaughan, A.; Lachner, N.; Budden, K.F.; Kim, R.Y.; Wood, D.L.; Gellatly, S.L.; Shukla, S.D.; Wood, L.G.; et al. Disease-associated gut microbiome and metabolome changes in patients with chronic obstructive pulmonary disease. *Nat. Commun.* **2020**, *11*, 5886. [CrossRef]
18. Russo, C.; Colaianni, V.; Ielo, G.; Valle, M.S.; Spicuzza, L.; Malaguarnera, L. Impact of lung microbiota on COPD. *Biomedicines* **2022**, *10*, 1337. [CrossRef] [PubMed]
19. Magryś, A. Microbiota: A Missing Link in The Pathogenesis of Chronic Lung Inflammatory Diseases. *Pol. J. Microbiol.* **2021**, *70*, 25–32. [CrossRef]
20. Price, C.E.; O'Toole, G.A. The Gut-Lung Axis in Cystic Fibrosis. *J. Bacteriol.* **2021**, *203*, 10–1128. [CrossRef]
21. Yang, J.-Y.; Chen, S.-Y.; Wu, Y.-H.; Liao, Y.-L.; Yen, G.-C. Ameliorative effect of buckwheat polysaccharides on colitis via regulation of the gut microbiota. *Int. J. Biol. Macromol.* **2023**, *227*, 872–883. [CrossRef]
22. Wang, L.; Zhang, P.; Li, C.; Xu, F.; Chen, J. A polysaccharide from *Rosa roxburghii* Tratt fruit attenuates high-fat diet-induced intestinal barrier dysfunction and inflammation in mice by modulating the gut microbiota. *Food Funct.* **2022**, *13*, 530–547. [CrossRef]
23. Luo, H.; Ying, N.; Zhao, Q.; Chen, J.; Xu, H.; Jiang, W.; Wu, Y.; Wu, Y.; Gao, H.; Zheng, H. A novel polysaccharide from Rubus chingii Hu unripe fruits: Extraction optimization, structural characterization and amelioration of colonic inflammation and oxidative stress. *Food Chem.* **2023**, *421*, 136152. [CrossRef]
24. Lu, H.; Shen, M.; Chen, Y.; Yu, Q.; Chen, T.; Xie, J. Alleviative effects of natural plant polysaccharides against DSS-induced ulcerative colitis via inhibiting inflammation and modulating gut microbiota. *Food Res. Int.* **2023**, *167*, 112630. [CrossRef]
25. Li, X.; Qiao, G.; Chu, L.; Lin, L.; Zheng, G. *Smilax china* L. Polysaccharide Alleviates Dextran Sulphate Sodium-Induced Colitis and Modulates the Gut Microbiota in Mice. *Foods* **2023**, *12*, 1632. [CrossRef] [PubMed]
26. Bai, Y.; Zhou, Y.; Zhang, R.; Chen, Y.; Wang, F.; Zhang, M. Gut microbial fermentation promotes the intestinal anti-inflammatory activity of Chinese yam polysaccharides. *Food Chem.* **2023**, *402*, 134003. [CrossRef]

27. Zeng, Z.; Xie, Z.; Chen, G.; Sun, Y.; Zeng, X.; Liu, Z. Anti-inflammatory and gut microbiota modulatory effects of polysaccharides from Fuzhuan brick tea on colitis in mice induced by dextran sulfate sodium. *Food Funct.* **2022**, *13*, 649–663. [CrossRef]
28. Xiao, H.; Feng, J.; Peng, J.; Wu, P.; Chang, Y.; Li, X.; Wu, J.; Huang, H.; Deng, H.; Qiu, M.; et al. Fuc-S-A New Ultrasonic Degraded Sulfated α-l-Fucooligosaccharide-Alleviates DSS-Inflicted Colitis through Reshaping Gut Microbiota and Modulating Host-Microbe Tryptophan Metabolism. *Mar. Drugs* **2022**, *21*, 16. [CrossRef]
29. Xu, A.; Zhao, Y.; Shi, Y.; Zuo, X.; Yang, Y.; Wang, Y.; Xu, P. Effects of oxidation-based tea processing on the characteristics of the derived polysaccharide conjugates and their regulation of intestinal homeostasis in DSS-induced colitis mice. *Int. J. Biol. Macromol.* **2022**, *214*, 402–413. [CrossRef]
30. Wu, Q.; Fan, L.; Tan, H.; Zhang, Y.; Fang, Q.; Yang, J.; Cui, S.W.; Nie, S. Impact of pectin with various esterification degrees on the profiles of gut microbiota and serum metabolites. *Appl. Microbiol. Biotechnol.* **2022**, *106*, 3707–3720. [CrossRef] [PubMed]
31. Wang, Y.-J.; Li, Q.-M.; Zha, X.-Q.; Luo, J.-P. *Dendrobium fimbriatum* Hook polysaccharide ameliorates dextran-sodium-sulfate-induced colitis in mice via improving intestinal barrier function, modulating intestinal microbiota, and reducing oxidative stress and inflammatory responses. *Food Funct.* **2022**, *13*, 143–160. [CrossRef] [PubMed]
32. Wen, X.; Zhong, R.; Dang, G.; Xia, B.; Wu, W.; Tang, S.; Tang, L.; Liu, L.; Liu, Z.; Chen, L.; et al. Pectin supplementation ameliorates intestinal epithelial barrier function damage by modulating intestinal microbiota in lipopolysaccharide-challenged piglets. *J. Nutr. Biochem.* **2022**, *109*, 109107. [CrossRef]
33. Lv, H.; Jia, H.; Cai, W.; Cao, R.; Xue, C.; Dong, N. *Rehmannia glutinosa* polysaccharides attenuates colitis via reshaping gut microbiota and short-chain fatty acid production. *J. Sci. Food Agric.* **2023**, *103*, 3926–3938. [CrossRef] [PubMed]
34. Li, L.-X.; Feng, X.; Tao, M.-T.; Paulsen, B.S.; Huang, C.; Feng, B.; Liu, W.; Yin, Z.-Q.; Song, X.; Zhao, X.; et al. Benefits of neutral polysaccharide from rhizomes of Polygonatum sibiricum to intestinal function of aged mice. *Front. Nutr.* **2022**, *9*, 992102. [CrossRef] [PubMed]
35. Chen, S.; Shen, Y.; Lin, J.; Yen, G. *Rhinacanthus nasutus* and okara polysaccharides attenuate colitis via inhibiting inflammation and modulating the gut microbiota. *Phytother. Res.* **2022**, *36*, 4631–4645. [CrossRef] [PubMed]
36. Cen, L.; Yi, T.; Hao, Y.; Shi, C.; Shi, X.; Lu, Y.; Chen, D.; Zhu, H. *Houttuynia cordata* polysaccharides alleviate ulcerative colitis by restoring intestinal homeostasis. *Chin. J. Nat. Med.* **2022**, *20*, 914–924. [CrossRef]
37. Zhou, X.; Lu, Q.; Kang, X.; Tian, G.; Ming, D.; Yang, J. Protective Role of a New Polysaccharide Extracted from Lonicera japonica Thunb in Mice with Ulcerative Colitis Induced by Dextran Sulphate Sodium. *Biomed Res. Int.* **2021**, *2021*, 8878633. [CrossRef]
38. Guo, C.; Wang, Y.; Zhang, S.; Zhang, X.; Du, Z.; Li, M.; Ding, K. *Crataegus pinnatifida* polysaccharide alleviates colitis via modulation of gut microbiota and SCFAs metabolism. *Int. J. Biol. Macromol.* **2021**, *181*, 357–368. [CrossRef]
39. Jin, M.-Y.; Wu, X.-Y.; Li, M.-Y.; Li, X.-T.; Huang, R.-M.; Sun, Y.-M.; Xu, Z.-L. Noni (*Morinda citrifolia* L.) fruit polysaccharides regulated IBD mice via targeting gut microbiota: Association of JNK/ERK/NF-κB signaling pathways. *J. Agric. Food Chem.* **2021**, *69*, 10151–10162. [CrossRef]
40. Cui, L.; Guan, X.; Ding, W.; Luo, Y.; Wang, W.; Bu, W.; Song, J.; Tan, X.; Sun, E.; Ning, Q.; et al. *Scutellaria baicalensis* Georgi polysaccharide ameliorates DSS-induced ulcerative colitis by improving intestinal barrier function and modulating gut microbiota. *Int. J. Biol. Macromol.* **2021**, *166*, 1035–1045. [CrossRef]
41. Yang, M.; Lee, U.J.; Cho, H.-R.; Lee, K.B.; Shin, Y.J.; Bae, M.-J.; Park, K.-Y. Effects of pear extracts on microbiome and immunocytokines to alleviate air pollution-related respiratory hypersensitivity. *J. Med. Food* **2023**, *26*, 211–214. [CrossRef]
42. Yuan, G.; Wen, S.; Zhong, X.; Yang, X.; Xie, L.; Wu, X.; Li, X. Inulin alleviates offspring asthma by altering maternal intestinal microbiome composition to increase short-chain fatty acids. *PLoS ONE* **2023**, *18*, e0283105. [CrossRef]
43. Wei, Y.; Qi, M.; Liu, C.; Li, L. Astragalus polysaccharide attenuates bleomycin-induced pulmonary fibrosis by inhibiting TLR4/NF-κB signaling pathway and regulating gut microbiota. *Eur. J. Pharmacol.* **2023**, *944*, 175594. [CrossRef]
44. Ling, L.; Ren, A.; Lu, Y.; Zhang, Y.; Zhu, H.; Tu, P.; Li, H.; Chen, D. The synergistic effect and mechanisms of flavonoids and polysaccharides from *Houttuynia cordata* on H1N1-induced pneumonia in mice. *J. Ethnopharmacol.* **2023**, *302*, 115761. [CrossRef] [PubMed]
45. Wen, S.; Yuan, G.; Li, C.; Xiong, Y.; Zhong, X.; Li, X. High cellulose dietary intake relieves asthma inflammation through the intestinal microbiome in a mouse model. *PLoS ONE* **2022**, *17*, e0263762. [CrossRef] [PubMed]
46. Shi, C.; Zhou, L.; Li, H.; Shi, X.; Zhang, Y.; Lu, Y.; Zhu, H.; Chen, D. Intestinal microbiota metabolizing *Houttuynia cordata* polysaccharides in H1N1 induced pneumonia mice contributed to Th17/Treg rebalance in gut-lung axis. *Int. J. Biol. Macromol.* **2022**, *221*, 288–302. [CrossRef] [PubMed]
47. Ming, K.; Zhuang, S.; Ma, N.; Nan, S.; Li, Q.; Ding, M.; Ding, Y. Astragalus polysaccharides alleviates lipopolysaccharides-induced inflammatory lung injury by altering intestinal microbiota in mice. *Front. Microbiol.* **2022**, *13*, 1033875. [CrossRef]
48. Liu, Y.; Chen, Q.; Ren, R.; Zhang, Q.; Yan, G.; Yin, D.; Zhang, M.; Yang, Y. *Platycodon grandiflorus* polysaccharides deeply participate in the anti-chronic bronchitis effects of platycodon grandiflorus decoction, a representative of "the lung and intestine are related". *Front. Pharmacol.* **2022**, *13*, 927384. [CrossRef]
49. Liu, J.-X.; Yuan, H.-Y.; Li, Y.-N.; Wei, Z.; Liu, Y.; Liang, J. *Ephedra sinica* polysaccharide alleviates airway inflammations of mouse asthma-like induced by PM2.5 and ovalbumin via the regulation of gut microbiota and short chain fatty acid. *J. Pharm. Pharmacol.* **2022**, *74*, 1784–1796. [CrossRef]

50. Lu, J.; Zhu, B.; Zhou, F.; Ding, X.; Qian, C.; Ding, Z.; Ye, X. Polysaccharides from the aerial parts of *Tetrastigma hemsleyanum* Diels et Gilg induce bidirectional immunity and ameliorate LPS-induced acute respiratory distress syndrome in mice. *Front. Pharmacol.* **2022**, *13*, 838873. [CrossRef]
51. Zhao, Y.; Chen, X.; Shen, J.; Xu, A.; Wang, Y.; Meng, Q.; Xu, P. Black Tea Alleviates Particulate Matter-Induced Lung Injury via the Gut-Lung Axis in Mice. *J. Agric. Food Chem.* **2021**, *69*, 15362–15373. [CrossRef] [PubMed]
52. Jang, Y.O.; Kim, O.-H.; Kim, S.J.; Lee, S.H.; Yun, S.; Lim, S.E.; Yoo, H.J.; Shin, Y.; Lee, S.W. High-fiber diets attenuate emphysema development via modulation of gut microbiota and metabolism. *Sci. Rep.* **2021**, *11*, 7008. [CrossRef]
53. Tashiro, H.; Kasahara, D.I.; Osgood, R.S.; Brown, T.; Cardoso, A.; Cho, Y.; Shore, S.A. Sex differences in the impact of dietary fiber on pulmonary responses to ozone. *Am. J. Respir. Cell Mol. Biol.* **2020**, *62*, 503–512. [CrossRef] [PubMed]
54. Shi, C.; Zhu, H.; Li, H.; Zeng, D.; Shi, X.; Zhang, Y.; Lu, Y.; Ling, L.; Wang, C.; Chen, D. Regulating the balance of Th17/Treg cells in gut-lung axis contributed to the therapeutic effect of *Houttuynia cordata* polysaccharides on H1N1-induced acute lung injury. *Int. J. Biol. Macromol.* **2020**, *158*, 52–66. [CrossRef] [PubMed]
55. Cui, F.; Shi, C.; Zhou, X.; Wen, W.; Gao, X.; Wang, L.; He, B.; Yin, M.; Zhao, J.-Q. *Lycium barbarum* polysaccharide extracted from *Lycium barbarum* leaves ameliorates asthma in mice by reducing inflammation and modulating gut microbiota. *J. Med. Food* **2020**, *23*, 699–710. [CrossRef] [PubMed]
56. McLoughlin, R.; Berthon, B.S.; Rogers, G.B.; Baines, K.J.; Leong LE, X.; Gibson, P.G.; Williams, E.J.; Wood, L.G. Soluble fibre supplementation with and without a probiotic in adults with asthma: A 7-day randomised, double blind, three way cross-over trial. *EBioMedicine* **2019**, *46*, 473–485. [CrossRef] [PubMed]
57. Chen, M.-Y.; Li, H.; Lu, X.-X.; Ling, L.-J.; Weng, H.-B.; Sun, W.; Chen, D.-F.; Zhang, Y.-Y. *Houttuynia cordata* polysaccharide alleviated intestinal injury and modulated intestinal microbiota in H1N1 virus infected mice. *Chin. J. Nat. Med.* **2019**, *17*, 187–197. [CrossRef]
58. Zhu, H.; Lu, X.; Ling, L.; Li, H.; Ou, Y.; Shi, X.; Lu, Y.; Zhang, Y.; Chen, D. *Houttuynia cordata* polysaccharides ameliorate pneumonia severity and intestinal injury in mice with influenza virus infection. *J. Ethnopharmacol.* **2018**, *218*, 90–99. [CrossRef]
59. Cho, Y.; Abu-Ali, G.; Tashiro, H.; Kasahara, D.I.; Brown, T.A.; Brand, J.D.; Mathews, J.A.; Huttenhower, C.; Shore, S.A. The microbiome regulates pulmonary responses to ozone in mice. *Am. J. Respir. Cell Mol. Biol.* **2018**, *59*, 346–354. [CrossRef]
60. Verheijden KA, T.; Braber, S.; Leusink-Muis, T.; Jeurink, P.V.; Thijssen, S.; Kraneveld, A.D.; Garssen, J.; Folkerts, G.; Willemsen, L.E.M. The combination therapy of dietary galacto-oligosaccharides with budesonide reduces pulmonary Th2 driving mediators and mast cell degranulation in a murine model of house dust mite induced asthma. *Front. Immunol.* **2018**, *9*, 2419. [CrossRef]
61. Halnes, I.; Baines, K.; Berthon, B.; MacDonald-Wicks, L.; Gibson, P.; Wood, L. Soluble fibre meal challenge reduces airway inflammation and expression of GPR43 and GPR41 in asthma. *Nutrients* **2017**, *9*, 57. [CrossRef]
62. Zhang, Z.; Shi, L.; Pang, W.; Liu, W.; Li, J.; Wang, H.; Shi, G. Dietary Fiber Intake Regulates Intestinal Microflora and Inhibits Ovalbumin-Induced Allergic Airway Inflammation in a Mouse Model. *PLoS ONE* **2016**, *11*, e0147778. [CrossRef]
63. Xu, Y.-Y.; Zhang, Y.-Y.; Ou, Y.-Y.; Lu, X.-X.; Pan, L.-Y.; Li, H.; Lu, Y.; Chen, D.-F. *Houttuynia cordata* Thunb. polysaccharides ameliorates lipopolysaccharide-induced acute lung injury in mice. *J. Ethnopharmacol.* **2015**, *173*, 81–90. [CrossRef] [PubMed]
64. Bernard, H.; Desseyn, J.-L.; Bartke, N.; Kleinjans, L.; Stahl, B.; Belzer, C.; Knol, J.; Gottrand, F.; Husson, M.O. Dietary pectin-derived acidic oligosaccharides improve the pulmonary bacterial clearance of *Pseudomonas aeruginosa* lung infection in mice by modulating intestinal microbiota and immunity. *J. Infect. Dis.* **2015**, *211*, 156–165. [CrossRef] [PubMed]
65. Verheijden, K.A.; Willemsen, L.E.; Braber, S.; Leusink-Muis, T.; Delsing, D.J.; Garssen, J.; Kraneveld, A.D.; Folkerts, G. Dietary galacto-oligosaccharides prevent airway eosinophilia and hyperresponsiveness in a murine house dust mite-induced asthma model. *Respir. Res.* **2015**, *16*, 17. [CrossRef] [PubMed]
66. Hogenkamp, A.; Thijssen, S.; Van Vlies, N.; Garssen, J. Supplementing pregnant mice with a specific mixture of nondigestible oligosaccharides reduces symptoms of allergic asthma in male offspring. *J. Nutr.* **2015**, *145*, 640–646. [CrossRef]
67. Thorburn, A.N.; McKenzie, C.I.; Shen, S.; Stanley, D.; Macia, L.; Mason, L.J.; Roberts, L.K.; Wong, C.H.Y.; Shim, R.; Robert, R.; et al. Evidence that asthma is a developmental origin disease influenced by maternal diet and bacterial metabolites. *Nat. Commun.* **2015**, *6*, 7320. [CrossRef]
68. Trompette, A.; Gollwitzer, E.S.; Yadava, K.; Sichelstiel, A.K.; Sprenger, N.; Ngom-Bru, C.; Blanchard, C.; Junt, T.; Nicod, L.P.; Harris, N.L.; et al. Gut microbiota metabolism of dietary fiber influences allergic airway disease and hematopoiesis. *Nat. Med.* **2014**, *20*, 159–166. [CrossRef]
69. Chung, M.J.; Park, J.K.; Park, Y.I. Anti-inflammatory effects of low-molecular weight chitosan oligosaccharides in IgE–antigen complex-stimulated RBL-2H3 cells and asthma model mice. *Int. Immunopharmacol.* **2012**, *12*, 453–459. [CrossRef]
70. Yasuda, A.; Inoue, K.-I.; Sanbongi, C.; Yanagisawa, R.; Ichinose, T.; Yoshikawa, T.; Takano, H. Dietary Supplementation with Fructooligosaccharides Attenuates Airway Inflammation Related to House Dust Mite Allergen in Mice. *Int. J. Immunopath. Pharmacol.* **2010**, *23*, 727–735. [CrossRef]
71. Vos, A.P.; van Esch, B.C.; Stahl, B.; M'Rabet, L.; Folkerts, G.; Nijkamp, F.P.; Garssen, J. Dietary supplementation with specific oligosaccharide mixtures decreases parameters of allergic asthma in mice. *Int. Immunopharmacol.* **2007**, *7*, 1582–1587. [CrossRef]

72. Sonoyama, K.; Watanabe, H.; Watanabe, J.; Yamaguchi, N.; Yamashita, A.; Hashimoto, H.; Kishino, E.; Fujita, K.; Okada, M.; Mori, S.; et al. Allergic airway eosinophilia is suppressed in ovalbumin-sensitized brown norway rats fed raffinose and α-linked galactooligosaccharide1. *J. Nutr.* **2005**, *135*, 538–543. [CrossRef]
73. Lee, J.C.; Pak, S.C.; Lee, S.H.; Na, C.S.; Lim, S.C.; Song, C.H.; Bai, Y.H.; Jang, C.H. Asian pear pectin administration during presensitization inhibits allergic response to ovalbumin in BALB/c mice. *J. Altern. Complement. Med.* **2004**, *10*, 527–534. [CrossRef]
74. Watanabe, H.; Sonoyama, K.; Watanabe, J.; Yamaguchi, N.; Kikuchi, H.; Nagura, T.; Aritsuka, T.; Fukumoto, K.; Kasai, T. Reduction of allergic airway eosinophilia by dietary raffinose in Brown Norway rats. *Br. J. Nutr.* **2004**, *92*, 247–255. [CrossRef]
75. Fan, L.; Zuo, S.; Tan, H.; Hu, J.; Cheng, J.; Wu, Q.; Nie, S. Preventive effects of pectin with various degrees of esterification on ulcerative colitis in mice. *Food Funct.* **2020**, *11*, 2886–2897. [CrossRef]
76. Wang, Y.; Leong, L.E.X.; Keating, R.L.; Kanno, T.; Abell, G.C.J.; Mobegi, F.M.; Choo, J.M.; Wesselingh, S.L.; Mason, A.J.; Burr, L.D.; et al. Opportunistic bacteria confer the ability to ferment prebiotic starch in the adult cystic fibrosis gut. *Gut Microbes* **2019**, *10*, 367–381. [CrossRef]
77. Wang, K.; Wu, L.; Dou, C.; Guan, X.; Wu, H.; Liu, H. Research Advance in Intestinal Mucosal Barrier and Pathogenesis of Crohn's Disease. *Gastroent. Res. Pract.* **2016**, *2016*, 9686238. [CrossRef]
78. Wang, Z.; Li, F.; Liu, J.; Luo, Y.; Guo, H.; Yang, Q.; Xu, C.; Ma, S.; Chen, H. Intestinal microbiota—An unmissable bridge to severe acute pancreatitis-associated acute lung injury. *Front. Immunol.* **2022**, *13*, 913178. [CrossRef]
79. Wang, L.; Zhang, P.; Chen, J.; Li, C.; Tian, Y.; Xu, F. Prebiotic properties of the polysaccharide from *Rosa roxburghii* Tratt fruit and its protective effects in high-fat diet-induced intestinal barrier dysfunction: A fecal microbiota transplantation study. *Food Res. Int.* **2023**, *164*, 112400. [CrossRef]
80. Park, Y.; Subar, A.F.; Hollenbeck, A.; Schatzkin, A. Dietary Fiber Intake and Mortality in the NIH-AARP Diet and Health Study. *Arch. Intern. Med.* **2011**, *171*, 1061–1068. [CrossRef]
81. Macfarlane, S.; Cleary, S.; Bahrami, B.; Reynolds, N.; Macfarlane, G.T. Synbiotic consumption changes the metabolism and composition of the gut microbiota in older people and modifies inflammatory processes: A randomised, double-blind, placebo-controlled crossover study. *Aliment. Pharm. Ther.* **2013**, *38*, 804–816. [CrossRef]
82. Trompette, A.; Gollwitzer, E.S.; Pattaroni, C.; Lopez-Mejia, I.C.; Riva, E.; Pernot, J.; Ubags, N.; Fajas, L.; Nicod, L.P.; Marsland, B.J. Dietary Fiber Confers Protection against Flu by Shaping Ly6c− Patrolling Monocyte Hematopoiesis and CD8+ T Cell Metabolism. *Immunity* **2018**, *48*, 992–1005.e8. [CrossRef]
83. Zhou, F.; Lin, Y.; Chen, S.; Bao, X.; Fu, S.; Lv, Y.; Zhou, M.; Chen, Y.; Zhu, B.; Qian, C.; et al. Ameliorating role of *Tetrastigma hemsleyanum* polysaccharides in antibiotic-induced intestinal mucosal barrier dysfunction in mice based on microbiome and metabolome analyses. *Int. J. Biol. Macromol.* **2023**, *241*, 124419. [CrossRef]
84. Hogenkamp, A.; Knippels LM, J.; Garssen, J.; van Esch, B.C.A.M. Supplementation of mice with specific nondigestible oligosaccharides during pregnancy or lactation leads to diminished sensitization and allergy in the female offspring. *J. Nutr.* **2015**, *145*, 996–1002. [CrossRef]
85. Beauruelle, C.; Guilloux, C.-A.; Lamoureux, C.; Héry-Arnaud, G. The human microbiome, an emerging key-player in the sex gap in respiratory diseases. *Front. Med.* **2021**, *8*, 600879. [CrossRef] [PubMed]
86. Zhang, Z.; Hyun, J.E.; Thiesen, A.; Park, H.; Hotte, N.; Watanabe, H.; Higashiyama, T.; Madsen, K.L. Sex-Specific Differences in the Gut Microbiome in Response to Dietary Fiber Supplementation in IL-10-Deficient Mice. *Nutrients* **2020**, *12*, 2088. [CrossRef]
87. Kalola, U.K.; Ambati, S. Budesonide. In *StatPearls*; StatPearls Publishing: Treasure Island, FL, USA, 2023. Available online: http://www.ncbi.nlm.nih.gov/books/NBK563201/ (accessed on 8 June 2023).
88. Lee, G.R. The Balance of Th17 versus Treg Cells in Autoimmunity. *Int. J. Mol. Sci.* **2018**, *19*, 730. [CrossRef] [PubMed]
89. Zhang, S.; Gang, X.; Yang, S.; Cui, M.; Sun, L.; Li, Z.; Wang, G. The Alterations in and the Role of the Th17/Treg Balance in Metabolic Diseases. *Front. Immunol.* **2021**, *12*, 678355. [CrossRef] [PubMed]
90. Barnig, C.; Bezema, T.; Calder, P.C.; Charloux, A.; Frossard, N.; Garssen, J.; Haworth, O.; Dilevskaya, K.; Levi-Schaffer, F.; Lonsdorfer, E.; et al. Activation of Resolution Pathways to Prevent and Fight Chronic Inflammation: Lessons from Asthma and Inflammatory Bowel Disease. *Front. Immunol.* **2019**, *10*, 1699. [CrossRef]
91. Cheng, H.; Guan, X.; Chen, D.; Ma, W. The Th17/Treg Cell Balance: A Gut Microbiota-Modulated Story. *Microorganisms* **2019**, *7*, 583. [CrossRef]
92. Lai, H.-C.; Lin, T.-L.; Chen, T.-W.; Kuo, Y.-L.; Chang, C.-J.; Wu, T.-R.; Shu, C.C.; Tsai, Y.H.; Swift, S.; Lu, C.C. Gut microbiota modulates COPD pathogenesis: Role of anti-inflammatory Parabacteroides goldsteinii lipopolysaccharide. *Gut* **2022**, *71*, 309–321. [CrossRef]
93. Fransen, F.; Sahasrabudhe, N.M.; Elderman, M.; Bosveld, M.; El Aidy, S.; Hugenholtz, F.; Theo, B.; Ben, K.; Simon, W.; van der Gaast-de Jongh, C.; et al. β2→1-Fructans Modulate the Immune System In Vivo in a Microbiota-Dependent and -Independent Fashion. *Front. Immunol.* **2017**, *8*, 154. [CrossRef]
94. Liu, T.; Zhang, L.; Joo, D.; Sun, S.-C. NF-κB signaling in inflammation. *Signal Transduct. Target. Ther.* **2017**, *2*, 17023. [CrossRef] [PubMed]

95. Schroeder, B.O.; Birchenough, G.M.H.; Ståhlman, M.; Arike, L.; Johansson, M.E.V.; Hansson, G.C.; Bäckhed, F. Bifidobacteria or Fiber Protects against Diet-Induced Microbiota-Mediated Colonic Mucus Deterioration. *Cell Host Microbe* **2018**, *23*, 27–40.e7. [CrossRef] [PubMed]
96. Dumas, A.; Bernard, L.; Poquet, Y.; Lugo-Villarino, G.; Neyrolles, O. The role of the lung microbiota and the gut-lung axis in respiratory infectious diseases. *Cell. Microbiol.* **2018**, *20*, e12966. [CrossRef] [PubMed]
97. Gupta, V.K.; Paul, S.; Dutta, C. Geography, ethnicity or subsistence-specific variations in human microbiome composition and diversity. *Front. Microbiol.* **2017**, *8*, 1162. [CrossRef]

Disclaimer/Publisher's Note: The statements, opinions and data contained in all publications are solely those of the individual author(s) and contributor(s) and not of MDPI and/or the editor(s). MDPI and/or the editor(s) disclaim responsibility for any injury to people or property resulting from any ideas, methods, instructions or products referred to in the content.

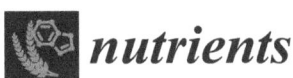

Review

Instruments to Evaluate Food Neophobia in Children: An Integrative Review with a Systematic Approach

Julyana Nogueira Firme [1], Priscila Claudino de Almeida [1], Emanuele Batistela dos Santos [1,2], Renata Puppin Zandonadi [3], António Raposo [4,*] and Raquel Braz Assunção Botelho [3,*]

1. Human Nutrition Graduate Program, Nutrition Department, University of Brasília, Brasília 70910-900, Brazil; julyanafirme@gmail.com (J.N.F.); nprialmeida@gmail.com (P.C.d.A.); emanuelebatistela.ufmt@gmail.com (E.B.d.S.)
2. Department of Food and Nutrition, Federal University of Mato Grosso, Cuiabá 78060-900, Brazil
3. Nutrition Department, University of Brasília, Brasília 70910-900, Brazil; renatapz@unb.br
4. CBIOS (Research Center for Biosciences and Health Technologies), Universidade Lusófona de Humanidades e Tecnologias, Campo Grande, 376, 1749-024 Lisboa, Portugal
* Correspondence: antonio.raposo@ulusofona.pt (A.R.); raquelbotelho@unb.br (R.B.A.B.)

Abstract: Food neophobia (FN), a frequent disorder in childhood, profoundly impacts the quality of a diet, restricting the intake of nutrients to maintain proper nutrition. Therefore, using the appropriate tools to assess FN in children to promote healthy eating habits is essential. The study aimed to develop an integrative review with a systematic approach to identify the instruments to measure FN in children and analyze their differences. The included studies (n = 17) were more concentrated in Europe, demonstrating the possible lack of dissemination of the topic at a global level. Among the 18 tools, 6 were represented by adaptations of the Food Neophobia Scale (FNS) and the Children's Food Neophobia Scale (CFNS), and one was the CFNS itself, demonstrating the relevance of these pioneering tools. The need to meet mainly cultural and cognitive criteria led to the creation of other instruments (n = 11). A diversity of approaches concerning the respondents, age range, items, scales, and validation methods was revealed. Modifications to the tools in some nations highlighted their adaptability and effectiveness in addressing regional variations. The instruments can contribute to additional research to help us better understand the prevalence of FN in children, resulting in their health and well-being.

Keywords: food neophobia; children; instruments; evaluation

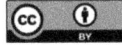

1. Introduction

Food neophobia (FN) is a frequent disorder in childhood, defined as a behavior related to the reluctance to eat new foods and accept newly introduced flavors or those with a different consistency [1]. FN is a considerable factor in determining food choices that profoundly impact the quality of a diet and plays a significant role in determining food preference [2]. All ages have an impact of FN on food preferences; although it is primarily researched in children, there is growing evidence linking fear of food to unhealthy eating habits in adults [3]. In the case of children, if they do not receive adequate treatment, the FN can follow them into adulthood. FN can be reduced in adulthood with successful management in childhood, such as using cooking-related activities or promoting flexibility and adaptation in food-related situations [4,5].

The adverse impacts of FN on children's daily food intake [6] involve an increase in foods rich in calories but poor in nutrients [7]. Children who show neophobic behavior are more likely to be overweight because they generally eat less variety and quantity of fruit and vegetables [7]. The lack of variety in the diet, caused by FN, restricts the intake of nutrients to maintain proper nutrition in the body. When the imbalance is severe and/or long-lasting, it tends to affect various body systems, such as the nervous system, impairing the child's cognitive and physical abilities [8]. Therefore, it is essential to choose and use the appropriate tools to assess FN [9].

The Food Neophobia Scale (FNS), created by Plinner and Hobden in 1992, was the first successful attempt to create an instrument specifically dedicated to evaluating the levels of FN in humans [10]. With ten items and evaluated by a 7-point Likert scale, the scale was validated in Canada with a sample of psychology undergraduate students [1]. The FNS has been widely used and has produced reliable results [11–13]; however, it consists of ten items that were created over 30 years ago [9].

Later, Pliner [14] evaluated neophobic behavior in 5-, 8-, and 11-year-old children and adjusted the FNS, developing the Food Neophobia Scale for Children (CFNS). Since 1994, the CFNS has been adjusted for many scenarios and used to assess FN levels in children [7,11,15,16]. However, other tools to measure FN in children have been created over the past decade. Some examples are the Instrument to Identify Food Neophobia in Brazilian Children by Their Caregivers [7], the Child Food Rejection Scale [17], the Trying New Foods Scale [18], and the Food Neophobia Test Tool [9]. These differ according to the respondents (child or caregiver), age group, number of items and response scale, and cultural issues.

Research into FN in children is necessary in order to understand and manage the complexity of this issue in the child development process. A previous review by Damsbo-Svendsen, Frøst, and Olsen [9] evaluated thirteen reviews of designs to assess food neophobia and willingness to try unfamiliar foods. However, the limitation was that the search was carried out in only two databases, and may have missed important information about the FN assessment tools available in other databases. Therefore, there is a need for a recent review of tools to access FN in children to provide a more complete and updated understanding of this topic.

Understanding the prevalence of FN in children is critical for promoting healthy eating habits. However, no studies have combined the available tools for assessing childhood FN. Thus, it is essential to analyze the different existing instruments, considering their particularities, because examining these differences increases the precision and comparability of research results. Moreover, understanding the characteristics of the different available instruments can help to choose the appropriate instrument according to different realities, leading to a better understanding of the impact of FN on nutrition and child development.

2. Materials and Methods

This is an integrative review with a systematic search. It is a thorough review of the body of literature that combines the integrative methodology of multiple sources of evidence with the systematic method of an organized and rigorous search process. To ensure openness and repeatability, this hybrid strategy involves carefully designing study questions, using well-defined inclusion and exclusion criteria, conducting exhaustive literature searches across different databases, and implementing systematic review protocols. The phases followed for the elaboration process of the integrative review were elaboration of the guiding question, search or sampling in the literature, data collection, critical analysis of the included studies, and discussion of the results.

2.1. Inclusion and Exclusion

Inclusion criteria were studies that included data on instruments used to identify food neophobia and its prevalence in children. It is worth mentioning that the age group varies among the studies, and all studies on food neophobia instruments for children were included independently of the age group. Exclusion criteria were: (1) letters, conferences, books, review studies, editorials, undergraduate works, and case reports; (2) studies whose target population did not involve children; and (3) studies that did not contemplate original instruments for the assessment of food neophobia in children. In the selection of studies, instruments developed for a specific population (originals) and their adaptations for children from other countries were considered as long as they met instrument validation criteria.

2.2. Database

Individual search strategies were developed for each database: Embase, Lilacs, Scopus, Pubmed, and Web of Science. The search for gray literature was performed on Google Scholar and ProQuest, with dissertations and theses. In addition, reference lists of studies were consulted to read the full texts of any potentially pertinent studies. The last search across all databases was performed on 24 January 2023.

2.3. Search Strategy

The search in each database was customized using the food neophobia and children keyword combinations and the Boolean operators OR and AND. All references were managed by Mendeley Reference Manager v2.103.0 software, and duplicate publications were excluded using Rayyan software (Qatar Computing Research Institute-QCRI; https://rayyan.ai/cite, accessed on 11 November 2023).

2.4. Study Selection

The process of screening the studies was performed in two phases: In Phase 1, two researchers (JNF, PCA) separately reviewed the titles and abstracts of all references detected in the databases. Only those who met the inclusion criteria were included in the next phase. In Phase 2, the same reviewers (JNF and PCA) evaluated the full texts of the articles included in Phase 1. The third reviewer (EBS) gave the final opinion in disagreement cases. The EBS researcher carefully analyzed the reference list of the selected articles. Disagreements between JNF, PCA, and EBS were resolved by expert investigators RBAB and RPZ.

2.5. Data Extraction

Of the selected studies, two reviewers (JNF and PCA) collected the following characteristics of the publications: research country, authors, year of publication, title, objective, type of study, sample, method used, variables, results, and conclusions. To ensure consistency between reviewers, calibration activities were performed before the review. Disagreements were resolved through discussion, and the third reviewer (EBS) decided on issues that could not be resolved by the two reviewers (JNF and PCA). Data were systematized in tables by the reviewers.

3. Results and Discussion

The search strategies are presented in Appendix A. A total of 6510 articles were found in the databases. After excluding 3558 duplicates, 2952 articles were reviewed through their titles and abstracts. Of these, 2665 were excluded because they did not meet the eligibility criteria. Therefore, 287 studies were selected for complete reading. Of these, 17 studies were included. The selection process is described in the flowchart of the integrative review with a systematic search (Figure 1).

3.1. Instruments

The selected studies (n = 17) included children from 1 to 16 years old and were developed between 1994 and 2021 in the following countries: Brazil (n = 1), Canada (n = 2), China (n = 1), Denmark (n = 1), France (n = 3), Italy (n = 1), Portugal (n = 2), South Korea (n = 1), Spain (n = 1), Turkey (n = 1), United Kingdom and France (n = 1), and United States (n = 2), as shown in Figure 2.

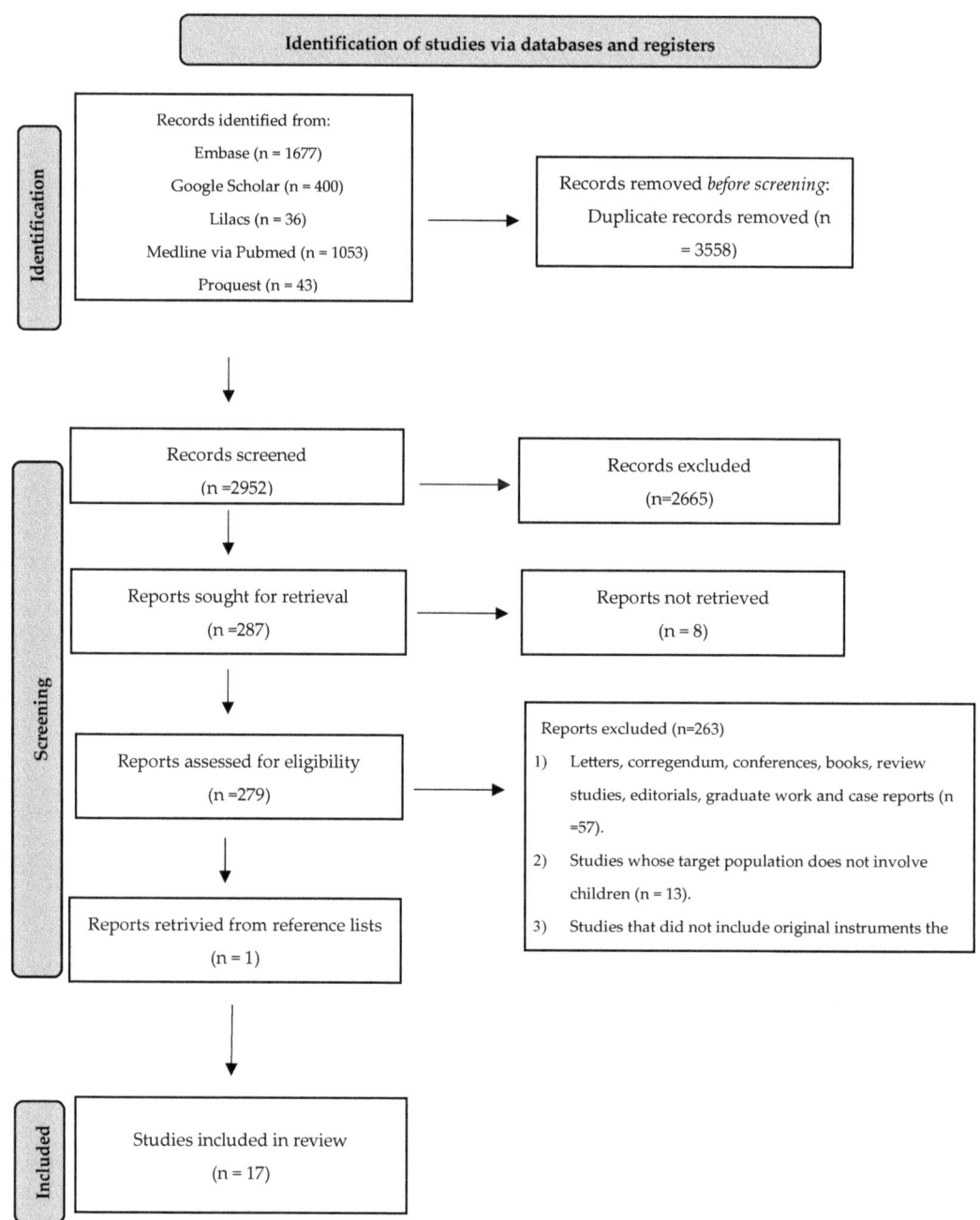

Figure 1. Flowchart of the integrative review with a systematic search. Adapted from PRISMA protocol [19].

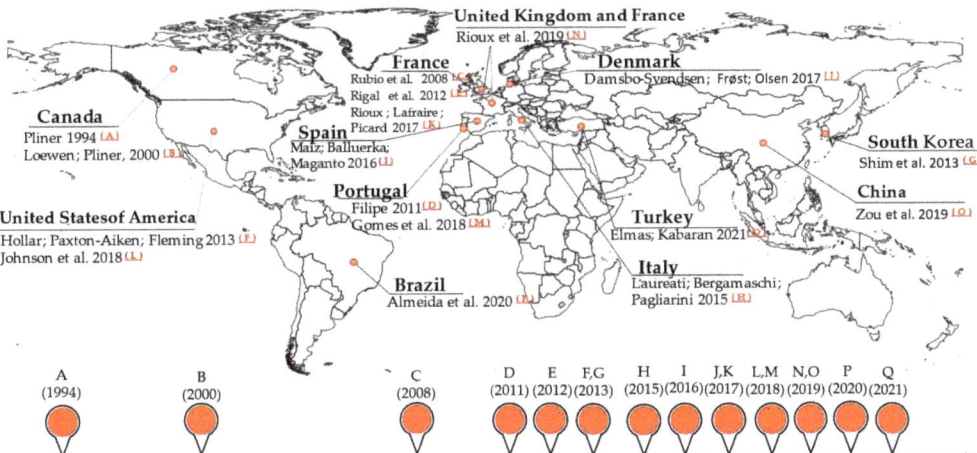

Figure 2. Instruments to assess food neophobia in children worldwide, 1994–2021, in chronological order.

Childhood FN has seen a remarkable transformation in understanding and treatment over the years, reflecting the global attention and concern on this issue. However, the importance of this phenomenon expanded over time, and it has caused a gradual spread of these instruments to other nations.

Figure 2 represents the availability of instruments to assess FN in several countries from 1994 to 2021. The image highlights the geographic diversity of research on FN and confirms how this phenomenon crosses cultural and geographic borders and how assessment methods have been developed throughout time precisely because of the complexity of this behavior in children. Few nations initially developed specialized tools to assess childhood FN; for example, no studies have been conducted on Oceania and Africa. Furthermore, the developed tools are concentrated in the United States, Canada, and some European countries. The illustration demonstrates the evolution of the research on FN, its global dissemination, and the continued need for updated assessment tools to understand and address this challenge.

3.2. Instruments and Features

The original instruments and their corresponding adaptations for children from different countries and the original instruments that were not adjusted were divided into groups to highlight the results better. The characteristics of the analyzed studies are shown in Table 1.

Table 1. Main descriptive characteristics and results from the included instrument (n = 18).

Author; (Year); Country	Tool	Items	Validation	Likert Scale	Respondent	Age Group
Pliner [14] (1994) Canada	CFNS (Child Food Neophobia Scale)	10 items	Convergent validity (behavioral measure of neophobia)	7 points	Caregiver	5, 8, 11 years
Filipe [20] (2011) Portugal	CFNS (Portuguese version of Child's Food Neophobia Scale)	10 items	Analysis of psychometric properties: Correlation analysis between items Determination of the percentage of response to the alternatives for each item Factor analysis Internal consistency Item-total correlation	5 points	Caregiver	5–6 years
Gomes et al.; [6] (2018) Portugal	CFNS (Portuguese version Child's Food Neophobia Scale)	8 items	Construct validity: factor analysis Convergent and discriminant validity Forward-backward translation process Internal consistency Invariance analysis Test-retest reliability	5 points	Caregiver	2–6 years
Zou et al.; [21] (2019) China	CFNS (Chinese version of the Child Food Neophobia Scale)	6 items	Forward-backward translation Factor analysis Internal consistency Test-retest reliability	7 points	Caregiver	1–3 years
Laureati; Bergamaschi; Pagliarini; [15] (2015) Italy	ICFNS (Italian Child Food Neophobia Scale)	3 versions: 10 items, 9 items, 6 items	Predictive validity Internal consistency Test-retest reliability	5 points + figures with facial expressions	Child	6–9 years
Damsbo-Svendsen; Frost; Olsen; [9] (2017) Denmark	FNTT (Food Neophobia Test Tool)	8 items	Behavioral validation test Correlations between FNS and FNTT Forward-backward translation process Internal consistency Item-item and item–rest correlations Behavioral validation	5 points	Child	9–13 years
	Shortened 6-item version of the FNS	6 items	Internal consistency Test-retest reliability	5 points	Child	9–13 years

Table 1. *Cont.*

Author; (Year); Country	Tool	Items	Validation	Likert Scale	Respondent	Age Group
Elmas; Kabaran; [22] (2021) Turkey	FNS (Turkish version of the Food Neophobia Scale FNS)	9 items	Construct validity (factor analysis) Content validity Forward–backward translation process Internal consistency Test-retest reliability	5 points + figures with facial expressions	Child	9–11 years
Loewen; Pliner; [23] (2000) Canada	FSQ (The Food Situations Questionnaire)	10 items	Convergent validity (correlation between behavior and FSQ scores) Factor analysis Internal consistency Test-retest reliability	5 points + figures with facial expressions	Child	7–12 years
Maiz; Balluerka; Maganto; [24] (2016) Spain	SFSQ (Spanish Food Situations Questionnaire)	10 items	Convergent validity Dimensionality External validity Factor analysis Forward–backward translation process Internal consistency Temporal stability	5 points + figures with facial expressions	Child	8–16 years
Rubio et al.; [25] (2008) France	QENA (Questionnaire on Food Neophobia among French-speaking Children)	13 items	Factor analysis Internal consistency Predictive validity (food task) Test-retest reliability	4 points	Child	5–8 years
Rigal et al.; [26] (2012) France	Children's Eating Difficulties Questionnaire	12 items (3 for neophobia)	Factor analysis (structural equation modeling) Internal consistency	5 points	Caregiver	1.6–3 years
Hollar; Paxton-Aiken; Fleming; [27] (2013) United States	FVNI (Fruit and Vegetable Neophobia Instrument)	18 items	Construct (convergent) Validation—factor analysis	4 points	Child	8–10 years

Table 1. Cont.

Author; (Year); Country	Tool	Items	Validation	Likert Scale	Respondent	Age Group
Shim et al.; [28] (2013) South Korea	An assessment tool to evaluate the multifaceted characteristics of picky eating habits in children aged 1 to 5 years	21 items (2 for food neophobia)	Facial validity Internal consistency	7 points	Caregiver	1–5 years
Rioux; Lafraire; Picard; [17] (2017) France	CFRS (Child Food Rejection Scale)	11 items (6 for neophobia)	Convergent and discriminant validity Internal consistency Test–retest	5 points	Caregiver	2–7 years
Rioux et al.; [29] (2019) United Kingdom and France	CFRS (English version of The Child Food Rejection Scale)	8 items (Neophobia subscale: N1 N2 N6 N7 N10)	Construct validity Convergent validity Internal consistency	5 points	Caregiver	2–7 years
Jonhson et al.; [18] (2018) United States	The Trying New Foods Scale	9 items	Component analysis Criterion validity Internal consistency Test–retest reliability	4 points + figures with facial expressions	Child	3–5 years
Almeida et al.; [7] (2020) Brazil	Instrument to Identify Food Neophobia in Brazilian Children by Their Caregivers by their caregivers	25 items	Content validity (panel of experts) Internal consistency Semantic evaluation (panel of experts) Test–retest and interobserver reliability	5 points	Caregiver	4–11 years

3.2.1. Child Food Neophobia Scale (CFNS) and Its Adaptations

The Children's Food Neophobia Scale (CFNS) comprises 10 items and were developed in 1994 by Pliner [14], and emerged from the adaptation of the Food Neophobia Scale for Adults (FNS) by Pliner and Hobden [1]. Believing that FN corresponds to a human personality trait, Pliner and Hobden [1] developed this paper-and-pencil measure of FN, which showed a high correlation with the measure of behavioral neophobia in laboratory situations. The measure presented satisfactory internal consistency ($\alpha = 0.88$) and test–retest data results when applied to adults.

Previous research has shown evidence of different motivations for children (compared to adults) to reject familiar foods, motivations that also differ according to the child's age group. Given this, Pliner proposed adapting the behavioral and paper-and-pencil measures initially intended for adults [1]. Using these new measures, the author sought to identify whether there were differences in the degree of FN concerning the age group and sex of the children, and to investigate whether child FN levels differed between foods of animal and non-animal origin and whether there were similarities between the FN of parents and children [14]. Like the FNS, the CFNS is composed of 10 items using a 7-point Likert scale, but the terms and pronouns of the FNS were modified to refer to children's behavior reported by their caregivers. The CFNS was intended to assess the FN of Canadian children aged 5, 8, and 11 years old. The FN level is identified from the sum of the responses to each item by inverting the classifications of the neophilic items. The score can range from 10 to 70. The CFNS obtained evidence of convergent validity since the willingness to try new foods ratio and FN were correlated ($r101 = 0.38$, $p < 0.001$). The willingness to try new foods ratio was developed to assess behavioral neophobia.

Since its development, CFNS has been widely used worldwide [30–33]. However, in some countries, the instrument was validated for its respective population, undergoing modifications in the number of items or the response scale due to local cognitive and cultural aspects [6,9,15,20–22]. In the present study, adaptations aimed at children of both FNS and CFNS were identified in the continents of Europe [6,9,15,20] and Asia. Table 1 presents details of these adaptations in different countries.

Filipe [20] used the CFNS to assess FN among Portuguese children aged 5 to 6. Although the author did not make any changes to the wording or number of items of the original instrument, the author modified the response scale from 7 to 5 points on the Likert scale ("I completely agree", "I agree", "I neither agree nor disagree", "Disagree", and "Completely disagree") and the total score varied between 10 and 50 points. In the factor analysis, the organization was maintained in one factor because the second factor included only one item, whose content was not differentiated from the first factor. The author determined the percentage of responses to the alternatives for each item (there was no need to eliminate items, as no alternative had a proportion of responses > 95%, and all alternatives were completed). They analyzed the item–total correlation (no value presented <0.20), with internal consistency ($\alpha = 0.872$). Removing any item did not increase this value, and the correlation between items (items moderately correlated with each other and no value above 0.8/0.85, indicating that all items evaluated different questions).

Still in Portugal, [6] validated a Portuguese version of the CFNS for children aged 2 to 6. The authors, in addition to changing the Likert scale to 5 points (to better adapt to the characteristics of the population), excluded 2 of the 10 items of the original Canadian version due to issues related to the exploratory factor analysis, which also revealed a two-factor structure (food neophobia and food neophilia). The removed items were 5, "Ethnic food looks too weird to eat," and 9, "I will eat almost anything". According to the authors, the two subscales presented satisfactory internal consistency—Food Neophobia ($\alpha = 0.81$; inter-item correlation mean = 0514) and Food Neophilia ($\alpha = 0.68$; inter-item correlation mean = 0354)—and the subscales were significantly, moderately, and negatively correlated ($rs = -0.451$; $p < 0.01$). The authors described excellent test–retest reliability coefficients ($rs = 0.92$, $p < 0.01$ for Food Neophobia; and $rs = 0.91$, $p < 0.01$ for Food Neophilia). Regarding the invariance analysis, the food neophobia construct had the same structure for the two analyzed age groups. However, only partial metric invariance was found between the sexes, and concerning the convergent and discriminant validity, weak to moderate associations were found between the two subscales and other analyzed variables.

Zou [21] cross-culturally adapted the CFNS for Chinese children aged 12–36 months. The authors informed that the CFNS was translated and adapted into a Chinese version (CFNS-CN) through a forward translation, reconciliation, back-translation, expert review, and pretesting. The adaptation of this instrument, completed by caregivers, involved removing 4 of the 10 items from the original Canadian version, which were considered inappropriate by the authors for the sample's age group. The instrument presented good internal consistency ($\alpha = 0.91$) and substantial-to-good agreement between the test and retest (kappa coefficients ranged from 0.616 to 0.834).

In Italy, Laureati, Bergamaschi, and Pagliarini [15] developed and validated a self-report measure of FN for children aged 6 to 9 years old based on the adaptation of the FNS. The authors made several modifications, including the number of items, the format of the response scale, and the respondents (by the children themselves). The Italian version of the instrument (ICFNS) contains eight items (four related to neophilic attitudes and four related to neophobic attitudes). Concerns about children not understanding terms such as "ethnic" resulted in the removal of three items, replaced by one new item "I like trying new food and tastes from other countries". The authors also changed the answer options from 7 to 5 points on the Likert scale, justifying that younger children might have difficulty discriminating between the seven options. Furthermore, they added facial figures in each answer option to help children express their opinions.

The internal consistency of the ICFNS was satisfactory ($\alpha = 0.71$), and the instrument had good repeatability over the two sessions, except for younger children (6 years old). The ICFNS predicted the children's willingness to taste and like novel food, but the ICFNS scores for the 6- and 7-year-old children were not significantly correlated with either willingness to taste or liking one of the two tested novel foods. Therefore, the authors informed that the ICFNS can be reliably used with Italian primary school children starting from eight years and most likely as early as seven years.

Aiming to develop new tools to measure FN in children aged 6 to 13 in Denmark, Damsbo-Svendsen, Frøst, and Olsen [9] presented a shortened 6-item version of the FNS [1]. In this tool, answered by the children, the exclusion of 4 items also resulted from problems with the target audience understanding terms such as "ethnic", as well as "trust" and "particular". The authors also changed the answer options from 7 to 5 points on the Likert scale. The results of the behavioral validation suggested that scores in 6- and 10-item versions of FNS were predictive of neophobic behavior. The authors informed that, when administered to children, the original 10-item version of FNS appeared reliable ($\alpha = 0.80$) and valid (item–rest correlations, r = 0.41–0.57), but comprehension issues were evident. The shortened 6-item version of the FNS was sufficiently reliable ($\alpha = 0.72$) and valid (item–rest correlations, r = 0.35–0.55). The authors found evidence for the usefulness of this shortened version to measure food neophobia without leading to comprehension issues related to items.

The most recent identified adaptation was conducted in Turkey, adapting the FNS for Turkish children aged 9 to 11 [22]. This instrument remained with 9 of the 10 items in the original version since item 10, "I like to try ethnic restaurants," was excluded because the analysis demonstrated that it was repetitive. The response scale was modified from 7 to 5 points, using emojis to keep children's attention. Furthermore, unlike the original version for adults, this version had children themselves as respondents. Regarding the test–retest reliability and internal consistency, the authors informed that there was no difference between the first and second test scores of all items ($p > 0.05$), and the Cronbach alpha was found to be very good for the first ($\alpha = 0.890$) and for the second stage ($\alpha = 0.885$).

3.2.2. Food Neophobia Test Tool—FNTT

The Food Neophobia Test Tool (FNTT) was developed by Damsbo-Svendsen, Frøst, and Olsen [9] in Denmark in a study that proposed creating valid, reliable, and currently relevant tools to measure the food neophobia trait among children aged 9 to 13 years. The initial items were selected from a literature review of 13 designs created to measure food neophobia and willingness to try unfamiliar foods (134 items). The next step involved deleting items because they were not relevant to children, they were too long, or they assessed multiple topics in a single item. New items were also added by the authors, and the version at this developmental stage consisted of 19 items.

The questionnaire applied to children contained the FNTT tool and the FNS, items about willingness to try novel foods in different surroundings and a behavioral test. The questionnaire was initially developed in English, translated into Danish, and back-translated into English, so inconsistencies between words were evaluated to generate the final version in Danish. After conducting a pilot, 3 of the 19 questions of FNTT were deleted, and 3 new ones were included because the authors observed that certain aspects of food neophobia were not covered by the remaining items. Total FNTT19 scores could range from 19 to 95.

To reduce the number of items in the FNTT in order to not make it more complicated and time-consuming compared to the FNS, the authors developed three versions of the tool, containing 10, 9, and 6 items. The criteria for excluding items involved the evidence of prominent comprehension issues (in >58% of 12 classes), item–rest correlations $r \leq 0.5$, a decrease in Cronbach's α, and/or few significant item–item correlations (≥ 2 non-significant). The reliability of the FNTT (Cronbach's alpha) and its validity (item–item and item–rest correlations, behavioral validation, and correlations between FNS and FNTT) were evaluated.

The authors reported that the FNTT10 and the FNTT9 were the most reliable ($\alpha = 0.91$) tools, and the FNTT6 was the most valid (item–rest correlations, $r = 0.67$–0.80). Furthermore, they found evidence of the construct and criterion validity of the FNTT. It is important to highlight that, in the FNTT9 and FNTT10, items included led to comprehension issues in 8–75% of 12 classes, while the FNTT6 led to comprehension issues in only 8–17% of 12 classes. Therefore, the authors pondered that the latter may be a more appropriate tool, as it potentially leads to less bias than the FNTT9 and FNTT10, recommending its use in measuring food neophobia in children. In circumstances where more information is requested, they suggested the use of the FNTT9 [9].

3.2.3. Food Situation Questionnaire (FSQ) and Its Adaptation

The Food Situation Questionnaire (FSQ) was developed and validated in Canada by Loewen and Pliner [23]. Before its creation, no tools measured the level of FN through children's self-reports. Previous experiences by the authors and other groups of researchers had already demonstrated that the CFNS had some limitations due to the presence of items that addressed unusual situations and expressions not understood by children. Reports of difficulties using the 7-point Likert scale were also common. The FSQ arose from the need to address this gap, providing an easy-to-complete, self-reported measure of FN, in which the items described familiar situations and a vocabulary suitable for children.

The FSQ is an instrument comprising 10 items, which begin by describing a hypothetical situation in which new foods could be presented to children and end with a general question about the affective response, addressing different situations that may vary in terms of how to describe the food, the occasion, and who presents it. Factor analysis generated two factors that were moderately correlated (all children: $r = 0.42$; younger children: $r = 0.39$; and older children: $r = 0.52$) and which were retained as the following subscales: 1—Willingness to Try Novel Foods in Stimulating Circumstances (HI-STIM) represents the willingness to try new foods in highly stimulating circumstances, such as festive occasions, eating out, and accompanied by adults other than parents; and 2—Willingness to Try Novel Foods in Non-Stimulating Circumstances (LO-STIM) refers to the willingness to try new foods in non-stimulating circumstances, such as in the presence of family members, on non-festive occasions and involving "mundane" foods in meals, instead of treats.

Five facial expressions can respond to the instrument, ranging from "very sad" to "very happy". Scores are obtained by adding the score for each subscale and the overall score of the instrument, ranging from 5 to 25 in the case of subscales and from 10 to 50 for the total scale. Higher scores indicate less neophobia as the items were described considering the willingness to try the foods. The FSQ could predict children's real willingness to try new foods in a laboratory situation better than parents' reports. Furthermore, it presented satisfactory reliability properties. The mean internal consistency coefficient was 0.80, and the correlation between the first and second administrations of the whole scale was 0.64.

To develop and validate a self-reported FN measurement tool for Spanish children and adolescents, Maiz, Balluerka, and Maganto [24] translated the FSQ into Spanish using the back-translation procedure. The Spanish Food Situations Questionnaire (SFSQ) was administered to a sample of 831 participants between 8 and 16 years old. The SFSQ maintained the same number of items, and factor analysis revealed a two-factor structure (as in the original instrument), but, for cross-cultural adequacy, some foods and situations described in the Spanish instrument differ from the original version (examples: cassava chips versus umami flavored chips; Halloween versus carnival; and lunch box versus afternoon snack). Furthermore, the order of the response scale was changed, starting from "very good" to "very bad". Therefore, the higher the score, the higher the FN level, unlike the original instrument, in which the higher the score, the lower the FN level. The instrument presented satisfactory results concerning internal consistency (α = 0.77 for both the low- and high-stimulation subscales) and moderate temporal stability (Pearson correlation indices: 0.52 for the low-stimulation and 0.45 for the high-stimulation subscales). Furthermore, the Pearson correlation coefficients were used to investigate the instrument's convergent and external validity. Total food neophobia, as measured by the Spanish version of the CFNS, had a moderate and positive correlation with the total SFSQ score (r = 0.49; $p < 0.001$) and with high-stimulation situations (r = 0.31; $p < 0.001$), and a high and positive correlation with low-stimulation situations (r = 0.57; $p < 0.001$). Concerning the external validity, the dimensions of the SFSQ were negatively correlated (in a low way) with the two subscales of the Sensation Seeking Scale.

3.2.4. Questionnaire on Food Neophobia among French-Speaking Children—"QENA"

Rubio et al. [25] developed a questionnaire on food neophobia among French-speaking children (QENA). This self-reported image-based instrument has 13 items aimed at children aged 5 to 8 years old. The authors justified the need to create the instrument due to the differences in the eating habits of French children compared to those in other Western countries, for which tools such as the FSQ were created. Furthermore, they cited children's difficulties understanding specific terms in the FSQ.

According to the authors, QENA brings together a series of unique characteristics that favor its use among French children. It uses pictures to represent foods, facilitating understanding for young children and activating brain regions that produce conceptual inferences to prove. Furthermore, the administration method (self-reported questionnaire), different consumption contexts, and the response scale (based on different types of FN) are also highlighted as strengths of the tool.

In developing the questionnaire items, the authors considered methods known to alter neophobic behavior (imitation, information, taste principle, and external stimulation). To validate the QENA, two steps were necessary. Children also completed a food task to assess the predictive validity of the questionnaire based on Pliner's [14] methodology. In the final version of the instrument, two items use general statements about reluctance to try new foods, answered on a 4-point scale ranging from "strongly disagree" to "strongly agree". Six items assess children's willingness to try new foods, and five assess the FN typology.

This typology varies between without FN (referring to the child who shows a desire to try new foods), flexible FN (a child who agrees to consume the new food after trying a small piece), rigid FN (a child who consumes the new food under a pressure situation), and strong FN (a child who refuses to consume the new food). Factor analysis demonstrated a single-factor structure. The score to assess each child's FN is obtained by averaging the item scores so that a high score indicates a strong FN. The QENA achieved satisfactory internal consistency (α = 0.84), test–retest results (r = 0.74, p < 0.001), and predictive validity, with scores moderately correlated with the choice of new foods (r = -0.34, p < 0.001) and willingness to try them (r = -0.47, p < 0.001). These results suggest that it is an efficient instrument for measuring NA among French children aged 5 to 8 years old.

3.2.5. Children's Eating Difficulties Questionnaire

This instrument was created by Rigal et al. [26], in a study that had the objective to validate measures of young children's eating difficulties and maternal feeding practices in a French sample (children aged 20 to 36 months). The same study validated three other questionnaires: The Feeding Style Questionnaire, The Feeding Strategy Questionnaire, and the questionnaire relating to parental motivations when buying food for children. The study still assessed the links between maternal practices and children's eating difficulties.

To prepare the items that made up the Children's Eating Difficulties Questionnaire, answered by parents, and the other study questionnaires, a sample of mothers of French children aged 20 to 26 months were interviewed to investigate their children's possible difficulties during meals and the strategies used to overcome these difficulties.

The final version of the Children's Eating Difficulties Questionnaire, with 12 items, covers four dimensions: neophobia, pickiness, low appetite, and low enjoyment in food, but the high correlation between neophobia and pickiness and enjoyment and appetite suggested the existence of two underlying dimensions, namely, "Narrow food repertoire" and "Low drive-to-eat". The answer options range from 5 points, "very wrong" (1) to "very true" (5) for the child. The scores of six items were reversed to enable comparison.

The questionnaire was validated using a structural equation modelling (SEM) approach (with four constructs) and underwent internal consistency analysis, with a Cronbach alpha greater than 0.70 for all dimensions. The neophobia dimension, especially, presented α = 0.85.

3.2.6. Fruit and Vegetable Neophobia Instrument—FVNI

The Fruit and Vegetable Neophobia Instrument (FVNI) was developed by Hollar, Paxton-Aiken, and Fleming [27] to measure students' attitudes toward new fruits and vegetables. The study sample was students aged 8 to 10 years old, from the third to the fifth grade, collected from two evaluations of the Farm-to-School program in the United States. The FVNI, an 18-item self-report questionnaire, was adapted from the FNS. The FVNI has two subscales: a fruit subscale that asks about the child's willingness to try new fruits in different circumstances and an analogous vegetable subscale.

Questions from Pliner and Hobden [1] were used to design the FVNI and to meet the needs of the Farm-to-School assessment [1]. Based on the FNS, two subscales, each consisting of nine items, were created in which "fruit" and "vegetable" replaced "food" in the original scale. The FVNI was scored on a scale of 1 to 4 for each item, with a higher score indicating greater FN.

The items dealing with foods from other countries and "constantly trying new foods" were not used because the children in the study sample had limited control over their exposure to culturally varied foods. Pliner's [14] FN guided the development of additional items that asked about tasting or experiencing fruits and vegetables in various settings [14]. The study suggests that separate fruit and vegetable subscales should be employed according to the fit indices of the modified two-factor FVNI model to assess childhood neophobia.

3.2.7. Assessment Tool to Evaluate the Multifaceted Characteristics of Picky Eating Habits in Children Aged 1 to 5 Years

The instrument developed by Shim et al. [28] in South Korea does not exclusively assess FN, expanding the analysis to the components of picky eating habits. However, one of these components refers to the refusal of new foods. The authors' objective in the study that originated the tool was to evaluate the relationship between picky eating habits and the growth status of South Korean children aged 1 to 5 years old.

The authors argued that most instruments for measuring FN extracted the components through factor analysis, resulting in the union of highly related items through the subjects' similar responses, which often had no conceptual relationship. Furthermore, they cited the existence of a study that evaluated the presence of picky eating habits in babies and young children, in which the "lack of intake" component was not evaluated and where the other components were evaluated through a question, highlighting, therefore, the need for an instrument that could solve these gaps.

The tool presents 21 items answered by parents, referring to specific eating habits reported in previous studies. Four constructs are covered: "eating a small amount" (3 items), "neophobic behavior" (2 items), "refusal of specific food groups" (9 items), and "preference for foods with specific preparation methods" (7 items). As the questions related to neophobic behavior were worded with negative words, they were scored inverted. The items referring to FN are described as "How willing is your child to enjoy new and unfamiliar food when offered?" and "How often does your child try new and unfamiliar foods at home?". The authors use a 7-point response scale for all items. The higher the instrument score, the greater the degree of picky eating habits.

The instrument underwent a facial validity analysis, being submitted to a panel of experts in children's eating habits, and an internal consistency assessment ($\alpha = 0.79$ for questions related to the reluctance to try new foods). The authors highlighted that the tool could reflect well the multifaceted aspects of picky eating habits in children.

3.2.8. Child Food Rejection Scale—CFRS

The Child Food Rejection Scale (CFRS) was developed by Rioux et al. [17] to assess FN in French children aged 2 to 7 years old. A combination of instruments was used: FNS [1], Questionnaire of Eating and Weight in Spanish Children—QENA [25], Child Eating Behavior Questionnaire—CEBQ [34], and Children's Eating Difficulties Questionnaire—CEDQ [26]. The FN assessment instruments that existed before the creation of the CFRS were primarily developed for adults and did not sufficiently address the age range of children. As a result, the scientific literature lacked the correct assessment of FN in children.

The CFRS comprises 11 items, 6 for FN and 5 for food selectivity. The items are evaluated using a 5-point Likert scale, with coded responses ranging from 11 to 55 points. Children were presented with eight food images, four measuring selectivity and four measuring NA. The images were fixed on a plate for better understanding by the target audience.

The instrument's two-dimensional structure, internal consistency, test–retest reliability, and convergent and discriminant validity were investigated to determine the instrument's validity. Convergent and discriminant validity were assessed using the methodology of Pliner and Hobden [1] The results demonstrated that the CFRS scale presented good psychometric properties, is brief and straightforward, and is useful for examining FN tendencies in French children. It is essential to highlight that, in the final scale, half of the items retained for the neophobia subscale were adapted from the FNS [1], while all items retained for the selectivity subscale were explicitly created for this study.

Similar to the methodology used by Rioux et al. [17], Rioux et al. [29] validated the CFRS for the English version with caregivers of children aged 2 to 7 years old and compared the levels of selectivity and FN in children between France and the United Kingdom. English caregivers rated each item based on their child's behavior using a 5-point Likert scale (ranging from "Strongly Disagree" to "Strongly Agree"). These responses were then quantitatively coded. For each child, three distinct scores were calculated: a FN subscore (ranging from 6 to 30), a food selectivity subscore (ranging from 5 to 25), and a total food rejection score (ranging from 11 to 55).

The authors translated and back-translated the CFRS into English before moving on to the validation and reliability assessment phases. They evaluated their construct validity, convergent validity, and reliability and conducted a confirmatory factor analysis to verify that the two-factor model found for the original CFRS by Rioux et al. [17] combined English data to assess their construct validity. The authors calculated the correlation between the CFRS and FNS points (Spearman correlation coefficient) to determine their convergent validity. Cronbach's alpha coefficient was used to measure its consistency and reliability. The English version of the CFRS consists of 8 items, unlike the French version of the CFRS, with 11 items.

The results demonstrated that the CFRS is valid outside of France, considering that the 8-item English CFRS showed good convergent validity (CFRS scores and FNS scores highly correlated, $r = 0.79$, $p < 0.001$) and also good reliability (Cronbach's alpha of 0.85). Interestingly, a reduction in the number of pertinent items is not uncommon after cross-cultural adaptation and validation [15]. These cultural variations can help guide specific actions to improve the eating habits of populations.

3.2.9. Trying New Foods Scale

The Trying New Foods Scale was created by Johnson et al. [18] in the United States. This instrument assesses FN in children from the perspective of their self-competence in trying new foods. Their proposition was justified by the fact that hitherto existing measures were based, according to the authors, on the caregivers' point of view, and the items related to feelings of fear and disgust had their origin in observations of children's behavior or adults' assumptions about the cause of reluctance to consume food. The authors argued that the tool could perform this measure, eliminating the need to rely on reports provided by caregivers (since it is a self-reported measure) and direct observations. The Trying New Foods Scale was developed so children can report the challenges and experiences of trying new foods.

Based on interviews with children aged 3 to 5 years old, the authors used playful resources to investigate their experience when asked to try new foods using an instrument containing a 9-item scale. The scale assesses various aspects of children's experience, including the reasons for rejection, feelings, and consequences of trying new foods.

The description of each item is through positive and negative propositions, represented by figures that explain the content of that item (for example, "This girl likes the taste of new foods. This girl does not like the taste of new foods. Which girl is more like you?"). Each image is accompanied by a pair of circles (one large and one small) that represent the child's frequency of identification with the given situation, such as "Always" (the large circle), "Normally" (the smaller circle) for the positive statements, and "Sometimes" (smaller circle) or "Never" (large circle) for negative statements. Thus, the answer options vary between 4 points: less neophobic/more willing to try = 4; and more neophobic/less willing to try = 1).

The principal components analysis (PCA) results demonstrated a single component with strong item–total correlations (mean $\pm$ s.d. $= 3.08 \pm 0.70$). The instrument showed strong internal consistency ($\alpha = 0.88$) and initial evidence of criterion validity, but it did not show significance in test–retest reliability ($r = 0.52$, $p = 0.086$). The authors attributed this fact to the small sample size involved in the test.

3.2.10. Instrument to Identify Food Neophobia in Brazilian Children by Their Caregivers

The scarcity of information about FN in Brazilian children due to the lack of culturally appropriate instruments for this population led Almeida et al. [7] to develop and validate a tool capable of evaluating which types of food children are most reluctant to try. The instrument to identify FN in Brazilian children was developed from an extensive literature review, which allowed the identification and use of three tools as a basis for its preliminary version: the FN scale for adults 1992 [1], the FNTT [9]. and the FVNI [27].

After translation, these tools had their items carefully analyzed to adapt to the cultural aspects of Brazilian children. Similar items were merged, and those that did not meet the cultural issues or those not related to the age group of the sample were excluded. The researchers developed additional items. Authors describe that these additional items consider that the environment may influence eating behavior. The created items considered if the child would taste foods in different ambiances such as a friend's house, school, or parties.

Intended to assess FN in children aged 4 to 11 years old, the instrument contains 25 items to be answered by caregivers. This has variables related to food neophobia in different environments (home, friends' houses, school, or social events) and situations (birthday parties or friends' meetings). Furthermore, it has three domains: general FN, FN with an emphasis on fruits, and FN focusing on vegetables. Responses vary on a 5-point scale, ranging from "Strongly Disagree" to "Strongly Agree". The instrument's overall score can vary between 25 and 125, so the lower the score, the greater the neophobic behavior.

The instrument presented excellent internal consistency ($\alpha = 0.958$, $p < 0.001$) and reproducibility when answered by the caregiver who knows the child's eating habits (intraclass correlation coefficient = 0.987, $p < 0.001$). Furthermore, the reproducibility analysis showed that both caregivers can also answer the instrument (intraclass correlation coefficient = 0.712, $p = 0.003$). The three domains have a similar number of items, which allows for an adequate analysis of the general score and those domains. The instrument is valid and reliable for assessing FN among Brazilian children.

3.3. Instrument Approach: Respondents, Age Range, Items, Scales, and Validation Methods

The discussion of the instruments used to assess FN in children revealed a diversity of approaches concerning the respondents, the studied age range, and the validation methods. The descriptors were previously studied, so the search reflected the largest number of studies with children as the target audience.

Most of the instruments (n = 14, 78%) were built to assess FN exclusively [6,7,9,14,15,18,20–25,27]. However, it is important to highlight that there is variability in how FN is measured through these different instruments. An example of these differences is that some tools have subscales specific for fruits and vegetables [7,27], differing from others like CFNS, and adaptations [14], which evaluate the general FN.

Besides that, four tools did not evaluate FN exclusively. The Children's Eating Difficulties Questionnaire [26] involves, in addition to FN, the assessment of other possible difficulties during meals (pickiness, low appetite, and low enjoyment of food). The instrument from Shim et al. [28] evaluates, besides FN, three other dimensions: eating a small amount, refusal of specific food groups, and preference for foods with specific preparation methods. The instruments of Rioux et al. [17,29] evaluate FN and pickiness. These instruments were included because they evaluated, although not exclusively, the FN.

It is crucial to distinguish "picky eating habits", "avoidant restrictive food intake disorder (ARFID)", and "food neophobia" when discussing children's eating habits [26]. A child's selective preferences for particular foods, frequently motivated by flavor, texture, or familiarity, are considered picky eating. It is a typical stage of childhood development that most kids outgrow later. Contrarily, FN extends beyond basic fussiness [13]. It is defined by a dislike of tasting new or strange foods, frequently accompanied by apprehension or dread of unusual tastes or components. According to the Diagnostic and Statistical Manual, 5th Edition (DSM-5), ARFID is a more serious eating disorder characterized by significant dietary restrictions that can negatively impact health and development [35]. It is a disturbed pattern of feeding or eating that needs one of these characteristics to be diagnosed: failure to achieve growth in children, significant nutrition deficiency, dependence on tube feeding, or interference with an individual's psychosocial functioning. The FN can be more enduring and hinder a child's openness to new foods, which may impact their dietary diversity and nutritional intake [7]. Some instruments assess FN and picky eating, probably because FN is one constituent part of picky eating [36]. Recognizing and effectively resolving feeding issues in children requires understanding these variances.

Respondent-related questions are important because parents play a crucial role in feeding their children, but evaluating FN from the perspective of children has been the justification for the development of some instruments in recent years [9,15,18,25]. Relying solely on parents' reports of their child's FN underestimates the child's role in the process [15,36]. Even so, half of the analyzed instruments chose to evaluate the perspective of parents or caregivers, which reflects the perception of only one side. This can be explained, in part, by the fact that some of these tools are old, such as CFNS (which, despite being widely used, is approximately 30 years old), and others are products of its adaptations [6,14,20]. Furthermore, some instruments were applied to babies, and very young children [21,26] and, in some cases, the online method was used to obtain answers, situations that would make it difficult for the children themselves to fill out the instruments [7]. It should be noted that, when creating questions for children, some attention should be taken, such as changing items to describe situations that children are likely to be familiar with, using age-appropriate language, and providing a clear response format [15,23]. In addition, there are concerns about how different groups and cultures might perceive and understand specific FN statements [15,37].

As a result of the search and data analysis, the children's age ranged between 1 and 16 years old since one of the instruments was built to evaluate FN in children and adolescents. In this sense, the study that included adolescents was selected since the authors also evaluated children's FN. Concerning the age group, we observed an emphasis on instruments that investigated children of preschool and school ages (3 to 10 years old), predominantly among children aged 5 [6,7,14,17,18,20,25,28,29] and 9 [7,9,15,22–24,27]. This concentration can be attributed to the perception that these age groups are more susceptible to the understanding and cognitive manifestation of FN, given their stage of development and food exploration [2].

In the review, 70% of the studies evaluated the effect of age on FN. Among the included studies, 67% observed no difference concerning the age groups assessed [6,9,14,17,18,20,28,29]. Zou [21] and Rigal [26] evaluated children aged 1 to 3 years and observed that children from 2 years were more neophobic. For older age groups, Loewen and Pliner [23] described greater neophobia among children aged 7 to 9 than those aged 10 to 12, and Elmas and Kabaran [22] identified that children aged 10 were less neophobic than those aged 9 and 11. Even though some studies have presented differences in age groups, as the present review did not aim to evaluate the prevalence of FN among children, it is impossible to affirm that the prevalence of FN varies according to age because most studies showed equal behavior regardless of age group.

Some studies (n = 4; 23%) presented the prevalence of FN varying from 21% to 56% [15,20,21,28]. However, it is impossible to compare the prevalence since the authors used different instruments and forms of classification.

Sex differences were also explored in 70% of the studies. Among these, 83% did not find different levels of FN between sexes [6,9,14,17,20–23,29]. Among the studies that found some difference, FN was higher among boys aged 1 to 3 years [26] and higher among girls aged 3 to 5 years [18]. Not all studies explicitly included data that would allow an exploration of FN prevalence based on sex or age.

This lack of pattern regarding sex or age with higher degrees of FN represents an important consideration for the conclusions of our study [23]. There was no standard classification among the studies, whether in percentage or degree of FN. We suggest it is an important gap in research and providing valuable information about possible variations in FN between different demographic groups would offer a favorable avenue for future investigations on the topic.

The acceptance or rejection of food can be strongly influenced by the culture and context in which the child grows up [8]. Some foods may be considered taboo in certain cultures, while others may be celebrated. It is essential to consider the cultural context when creating an assessment tool and adapt it, if necessary, to reflect cultural specificities.

Authors like Maiz et al. [24] modified items of the instrument to make them more appropriate to Spanish culture. The foods listed in items 7 and 10 of the original FSQ are cassava and chayote, respectively; they are translated as "cassava" and "chayote" in Spanish. Because the purpose of these items is to introduce new and unfamiliar foods, and because some Spanish-speaking children may be familiar with these two foods, the "umami flavor" is replaced with "cassava" (cassava) and "chucander" (an Indian flavor vegetable) to "chayote". The review revealed a variety of options for the most popular rating scales, including 4-, 5-, and 7-point rating scales.

In the Brazilian instrument, categories that were not representative of the Brazilian scenario or had no influence on assessing children's FN were eliminated. There were no synonyms because Brazil is a country with a wide variety of cuisines and strong cultural influences, so items that mentioned ethnic foods or restaurants, for example, were excluded [7].

The study by Rubio et al. [25] emphasized the influence of cultural factors on food selection and highlighted differences in rules, consumption conditions, beliefs, meal preparation, and meal preferences between cultures. The instrument included items that described various contexts of food consumption, aiming to integrate the context in which children can find new foods and increase the instrument's validity.

The most common scale was the 5-point scale (67%) [6,7,9,17,20,22–24,26,29], followed equally by the 4-point [18,25,27] and 7-point scales [14,18,21] with 16.5% each. Some scales also had facial expressions to facilitate comprehension by the children (28%) [15,18,22–24]. Regarding the number of items to measure FN, there was a notable variation, with a predominance of scales with ten items, totaling 25% [9,14,20,23,24]. Other instruments present few items, with the predominance of six items of FN assessment (20%) [9,17,21], and others, such as Brazil, use more extensive instruments, with 25 items [7]. This highlights the need to balance the breadth of assessment with the practicality of use while considering each research situation's unique characteristics.

All instruments included in the present study showed evidence of validity and reliability. The most common validation steps in the instruments included construct and convergent validation, but other approaches were described as criterion, external, content, discriminant, predictive, and facial validation. Regarding reliability, the most evaluated properties were internal consistency and reproducibility, usually temporal stability.

Both validity and reliability are considered important factors to guarantee the quality of measurement instruments. Therefore, their rigorous evaluation is necessary [38,39]. Validity concerns the instrument measuring precisely what it purports to measure [40]. Construct validity assesses the degree to which an instrument can measure a concept that cannot be measured directly, the construct. Predictive validity (the ability of the instrument to predict an evaluated criterion) and concurrent validity (where scores of the measure under evaluation are correlated with the scores of another measure that evaluates the same construct) are categories of criterion validity. All evidence of validity leads to evidence of construct validity [38].

Classical test theory emphasizes the importance of reliability in measurement, asserting that any measurement result comprises both the "true" score and measurement error. Achieving a perfect score requires eliminating measurement errors, making instrument development crucial [38]. Test–retest reliability and internal consistency are key aspects of reliability assessment, evaluating item equivalence and interrater reliability [41,42].

Higher reliability coefficients (ranging from 0.00 to 1.00) signify more excellent reliability. Internal consistency, often assessed with Cronbach's alpha, gauges item comparability and accuracy, with increased items improving measurement precision. Employing multiple items enhances measurement reliability and accuracy [38].

It is important to highlight that, despite all tools evaluating FN and most of them being developed based on the same previous tool, they differ among the number of items and scales, and some use different domains and types of items. In this sense, studies that used different tools cannot be compared since they evaluate FN in different ways.

Finally, it is essential to emphasize that this review has some limitations, including language barriers, as studies written in languages other than English were translated on virtual platforms, which may have led to the loss of some information. Furthermore, the focus of the study was to present the tools available for assessing FN in children, not including a set of studies that used these tools and their respective results. Future research could focus on gathering evidence on the results of applying these tools to different populations. As strengths, the study provides the first comprehensive and critical view of the tools used to measure children's dietary FN, highlighting their strengths and contributions to understanding this issue. Future research can benefit from reviews such as this one by exploring the causes of childhood FN, improving the assessment tools already available to deal with it more effectively, and expanding the foundation for building future instruments, especially in countries that do not have this type of study.

4. Conclusions

This study presented a complete overview of the tools used to measure children's FN by an integrative review with a systematic approach. The geographic distribution of these studies, more concentrated in Europe, demonstrated the possible lack of dissemination of the topic globally, making it challenging to identify the prevalence of FN in children in countries where validated tools are unavailable.

Among the 18 tools found in this study, six were represented by adaptations of FNS and CFNS [1,15], demonstrating the relevance of this pioneering tool in detecting FN. However, there is a need to make more current instruments available, capable of being answered by children, involving appropriate language and experiences common to this audience. Instruments that consider this group's specificities include different age groups (from babies to older children), considering the cultural characteristics specific to each country. It is essential to highlight that cultural issues must be considered when producing an instrument to assess FN. Modifications made in the tools in many nations highlight their adaptability and effectiveness in addressing regional variations in cognition and culture.

The preponderance of measures reported by caregivers highlights the importance of parents and other caregivers in this situation. Nevertheless, it is also important to emphasize the value of considering children's views. We can understand more about FN if we consider age-related differences, as well as the wide range of rating scales and items of the instruments.

The review also highlighted the value of using standardized tests to identify children's FN. Even with the effort made to detect only validated instruments in the literature, it is noteworthy that it is impossible to list the best or most appropriate instrument to measure FN, because this choice will depend on specific conditions, such as information relating mainly to the age group to be studied, the country, and the individual who will respond to the instrument (child/caregiver).

Considering the study's objective of identifying instruments to measure FN in children and analyzing their differences, the importance of considering cultural influences in the development and adaptation of such assessment tools should be considered. The impact of culture on the acceptance and rejection of foods is evident, as different societies may have different attitudes towards different foods. This requires careful consideration of the cultural context when developing instruments to assess food consumption, especially FN. In summary, this study highlights the importance of incorporating cultural adaptations in developing assessment instruments to ensure their relevance and effectiveness in diverse cultural contexts.

Childhood FN is significantly complex, needing special attention and care for a thorough and accurate assessment. Thus, using validation approaches ensures the quality of instruments to obtain diagnostic measures that support the treatment. Healthcare professionals, especially nutritionists, must keep up with the most recent assessment techniques as understanding the subject improves the design of effective feeding patterns and support systems for kids with FN. The studied instruments can contribute to additional research to help better understand and address the prevalence of FN in children, resulting in their health and well-being.

Author Contributions: J.N.F.: conceptualization, investigation, methodology, writing—original draft, and writing—review and editing; P.C.d.A. and E.B.d.S.: investigation and methodology; R.P.Z. and A.R.: data curation, formal analysis, supervision, validation, and writing—review and editing; and R.B.A.B.: data curation, formal analysis, supervision, validation, and writing—review and editing. All authors have read and agreed to the published version of the manuscript.

Funding: This research received no external funding.

Data Availability Statement: No data availability.

Acknowledgments: The authors would like to acknowledge the "Higher Improvement Commission—CAPES".

Conflicts of Interest: The authors declare no conflict of interest.

Appendix A

Table A1. Databases and terms used to search reference instruments used in the world to identify the prevalence of FN in children.

Database	Search (24 January 2023)
MEDLINE via Pubmed	("Avoidant Restrictive Food Intake Disorder"[MeSH Terms] OR "Avoidant Restrictive Food Intake Disorder"[Title/Abstract] OR "food neophobia"[Title/Abstract] OR "choosy eating"[Title/Abstract] OR "food refusal"[Title/Abstract] OR "food rejection"[Title/Abstract] OR "food aversion"[Title/Abstract] OR "feeding neophobia"[Title/Abstract] OR "picky eating"[Title/Abstract] OR "picky eaters"[Title/Abstract]) AND ("child"[MeSH Terms] OR "child"[Title/Abstract] OR "children"[Title/Abstract] OR "infant"[Title/Abstract] OR "child preschool"[Title/Abstract] OR "schoolchildren"[Title/Abstract] OR "child nutrition"[Title/Abstract] OR "child feeding"[Title/Abstract] OR "parent"[Title/Abstract] OR "parents"[Title/Abstract] OR "guardian"[Title/Abstract] OR "guardians"[Title/Abstract] OR "caregiver"[Title/Abstract] OR "caregivers"[Title/Abstract] OR "mother"[Title/Abstract] OR "mothers"[Title/Abstract] OR "father"[Title/Abstract] OR "fathers"[Title/Abstract] OR "son"[Title/Abstract] OR "sons"[Title/Abstract] OR "daughter"[Title/Abstract] OR "daughters"[Title/Abstract] OR "sibling"[Title/Abstract] OR "siblings"[Title/Abstract] OR "family"[Title/Abstract] OR "families"[Title/Abstract])
Embase	'('avoidant restrictive food intake disorder'/exp OR 'avoidant restrictive food intake disorder' OR 'food neophobia':ti,ab,kw OR 'choosy eating':ti,ab,kw OR 'food refusal':ti,ab,kw OR 'food rejection':ti,ab,kw OR 'food aversion':ti,ab,kw OR 'feeding neophobia':ti,ab,kw OR 'picky eating':ti,ab,kw OR 'picky eaters':ti,ab,kw) AND ('child' OR 'child'/exp OR child OR children:ti,ab,kw OR infant:ti,ab,kw OR 'child preschool':ti,ab,kw OR schoolchildren:ti,ab,kw OR 'child nutrition':ti,ab,kw OR 'child feeding':ti,ab,kw OR parent:ti,ab,kw OR parents:ti,ab,kw OR guardian:ti,ab,kw OR guardians:ti,ab,kw OR caregiver:ti,ab,kw OR caregivers:ti,ab,kw OR mother:ti,ab,kw OR mothers:ti,ab,kw OR father:ti,ab,kw OR fathers:ti,ab,kw OR son:ti,ab,kw OR sons:ti,ab,kw OR daughter:ti,ab,kw OR daughters:ti,ab,kw OR sibling:ti,ab,kw OR siblings:ti,ab,kw OR family:ti,ab,kw OR families:ti,ab,kw)

Table A1. Cont.

Database	Search (24 January 2023)
Web of Science	TS = ("School Feeding" OR "Nutrition Programs and Policies" OR "School Meal" OR "School Meals" OR "School Meal Quality" OR "School Lunch" OR "School Lunches" OR "School Food Service" OR "School Food Services" OR "Brazilian National School Feeding Program" OR "National School Food Program" OR "School Feeding Program" OR "School Feeding Programs" OR "School Feeding Programmes" OR "School Nutrition" OR "School canteens" OR "School canteen") AND TS = ("Sustainable development" OR "Waste management" OR "Sustainable" OR "Sustainability" OR "Environmental Sustainability" OR "Economic Sustainability" OR "Social Sustainability")
Scopus	(TS = ("Avoidant Restrictive Food Intake Disorder") OR TS = ("food neophobia") OR TS = ("choosy eating") OR TS = ("food refusal") OR TS = ("food rejection") OR TS = ("food aversion") OR TS = ("feeding neophobia") OR TS = ("picky eating") OR TS = ("picky eaters")) AND (TS = (child) OR TS = (children) OR TS = (infant) OR TS = ("child preschool") OR TS = (schoolchildren) OR TS = ("child nutrition") OR TS = ("child feeding") OR TS = (parent) OR TS = (parents) OR TS = (guardian) OR TS = (guardians) OR TS = (caregiver) OR TS = (caregivers) OR TS = (mother) OR TS = (mothers) OR TS = (father) OR TS = (fathers) OR TS = (son) OR TS = (sons) OR TS = (daughter) OR TS = (daughters) OR TS = (sibling) OR TS = (siblings) OR TS = (family) OR TS = (families))
Lilacs	'((("Avoidant Restrictive Food Intake Disorder") OR ("food neophobia") OR ("choosy eating") OR ("food refusal") OR ("food rejection") OR ("food aversion") OR ("feeding neophobia") OR ("picky eating") OR ("picky eaters") OR ("transtorno da evitação ou restrição da ingestão de alimentos") OR ("neofobia alimentar") OR ("Trastorno de la Ingesta Alimentaria Evitativa/Restrictiva") OR ("F03.400.157")) AND ((child) OR (Niño) OR (children) OR (infant) OR ("child preschool") OR (schoolchildren) OR ("child nutrition") OR ("child feeding") OR (parent) OR (parents) OR (guardian) OR (guardians) OR (caregiver) OR (caregivers) OR (mother) OR (mothers) OR (father) OR (fathers) OR (son) OR (sons) OR (daughter) OR (daughters) OR (sibling) OR (siblings) OR (family) OR (families) OR (criança) OR (crianças) OR ("M01.060.406") OR ("pré-escolar") OR ("pré-escolares") OR (escolar) OR (escolares))

References

1. Pliner, P.; Hobden, K. Development of a Scale to Measure the Trait of Food Neophobia in Humans. *Appetite* **1992**, *19*, 105–120. [CrossRef] [PubMed]
2. Lafraire, J.; Rioux, C.; Giboreau, A.; Picard, D. Food Rejections in Children: Cognitive and Social/Environmental Factors Involved in Food Neophobia and Picky/Fussy Eating Behavior. *Appetite* **2016**, *96*, 347–357. [CrossRef] [PubMed]
3. Hazley, D.; McCarthy, S.N.; Stack, M.; Walton, J.; McNulty, B.A.; Flynn, A.; Kearney, J.M. Food Neophobia and Its Relationship with Dietary Variety and Quality in Irish Adults: Findings from a National Cross-Sectional Study. *Appetite* **2022**, *169*, 105859. [CrossRef] [PubMed]
4. Shimshoni, Y.; Lebowitz, E.R. Childhood Avoidant/Restrictive Food Intake Disorder: Review of Treatments and a Novel Parent-Based Approach. *J. Cogn. Psychother.* **2020**, *34*, 200–224. [CrossRef] [PubMed]
5. Maiz, E.; Urkia-Susin, I.; Urdaneta, E.; Allirot, X. Child Involvement in Choosing a Recipe, Purchasing Ingredients, and Cooking at School Increases Willingness to Try New Foods and Reduces Food Neophobia. *J. Nutr. Educ. Behav.* **2021**, *53*, 279–289. [CrossRef]
6. Gomes, A.I.; Barros, L.; Pereira, A.I.; Roberto, M.S.; Mendonça, M. Assessing Children's Willingness to Try New Foods: Validation of a Portuguese Version of the Child's Food Neophobia Scale for Parents of Young Children. *Food Qual. Prefer.* **2018**, *63*, 151–158. [CrossRef]
7. de Almeida, P.C.; Rosane, B.P.; Nakano, E.Y.; Vasconcelos, I.A.L.; Zandonadi, R.P.; Botelho, R.B.A. Instrument to Identify Food Neophobia in Brazilian Children by Their Caregivers. *Nutrients* **2020**, *12*, 1943. [CrossRef]

8. de Oliveira Torres, T.; Gomes, D.R.; Mattos, M.P. Factors Associated with Food Neophobia in Children: Systematic Review. *Rev. Paul. De Pediatr.* **2020**, *39*, e2020089. [CrossRef]
9. Damsbo-Svendsen, M.; Frøst, M.B.; Olsen, A. Development of Novel Tools to Measure Food Neophobia in Children. *Appetite* **2017**, *113*, 255–263. [CrossRef]
10. Rabadán, A.; Bernabéu, R. A Systematic Review of Studies Using the Food Neophobia Scale: Conclusions from Thirty Years of Studies. *Food Qual. Prefer.* **2021**, *93*, 104241. [CrossRef]
11. Mustonen, S.; Oerlemans, P.; Tuorila, H. Familiarity with and Affective Responses to Foods in 8-11-Year-Old Children. The Role of Food Neophobia and Parental Education. *Appetite* **2012**, *58*, 777–780. [CrossRef] [PubMed]
12. Knaapila, A.; Tuorila, H.; Silventoinen, K.; Keskitalo, K.; Kallela, M.; Wessman, M.; Peltonen, L.; Cherkas, L.F.; Spector, T.D.; Perola, M. Food Neophobia Shows Heritable Variation in Humans. *Physiol. Behav.* **2007**, *91*, 573–578. [CrossRef] [PubMed]
13. Galloway, A.T.; Lee, Y.; Birch, L.L. Predictors and Consequences of Food Neophobia and Pickiness in Young Girls. *J. Am. Diet. Assoc.* **2003**, *103*, 692–698. [CrossRef] [PubMed]
14. Pliner, P. Development of Measures of Food Neophobia in Children. *Appetite* **1994**, *23*, 147–163. [CrossRef] [PubMed]
15. Laureati, M.; Bergamaschi, V.; Pagliarini, E. Assessing Childhood Food Neophobia: Validation of a Scale in Italian Primary School Children. *Food Qual. Prefer.* **2015**, *40*, 8–15. [CrossRef]
16. Howard, A.J.; Mallan, K.M.; Byrne, R.; Magarey, A.; Daniels, L.A. Toddlers' Food Preferences. The Impact of Novel Food Exposure, Maternal Preferences and Food Neophobia. *Appetite* **2012**, *59*, 818–825. [CrossRef]
17. Rioux, C.; Lafraire, J.; Picard, D. L'échelle de Rejets Alimentaires Pour Enfant: Développement et Validation d'une Nouvelle Échelle Pour Mesurer La Néophobie et La Sélectivité Alimentaire Chez Les Jeunes Enfants Français de 2 à 7 Ans. *Rev. Eur. Psychol. Appl.* **2017**, *67*, 67–77. [CrossRef]
18. Johnson, S.L.; Moding, K.J.; Maloney, K.; Bellows, L.L. Development of the Trying New Foods Scale: A Preschooler Self-Assessment of Willingness to Try New Foods. *Appetite* **2018**, *128*, 21–31. [CrossRef]
19. Page, M.J.; McKenzie, J.E.; Bossuyt, P.M.; Boutron, I.; Hoffmann, T.C.; Mulrow, C.D.; Shamseer, L.; Tetzlaff, J.M.; Akl, E.A.; Brennan, S.E.; et al. The PRISMA 2020 Statement: An Updated Guideline for Reporting Systematic Reviews. *Int. J. Surg.* **2021**, *18*, 105906. [CrossRef]
20. Patrícia, A.; Da, P.; Filipe, S.P. Neofobia Alimentar e Hábitos Alimentares Em Crianças Pré-Escolares e Conhecimentos Nutricionais Parentais. Master's Thesis, Universidade de Lisboa, Lisboa, Portugal, 2011.
21. Zou, J.; Liu, Y.; Yang, Q.; Liu, H.; Luo, Y.; Ouyang, Y.; Wang, J.; Lin, Q. Cross-Cultural Adaption and Validation of the Chinese Version of the Child Food Neophobia Scale. *BMJ Open* **2019**, *9*, e026729. [CrossRef]
22. Elmas, C.; Kabaran, S. Food Neophobia Scale (Fns): Testing the Validity and Reliability of the Turkish Version in School-Age Children. *Progress. Nutr.* **2021**, *23*. [CrossRef]
23. Loewen, R.; Pliner, P. The Food Situations Questionnaire: A Measure of Children's Willingness to Try Novel Foods in Stimulating and Non-Stimulating Situations. *Appetite* **2000**, *35*, 239–250. [CrossRef] [PubMed]
24. Maiz, E.; Balluerka, N.; Maganto, C. Validation of a Questionnaire to Measure the Willingness to Try New Foods in Spanish-Speaking Children and Adolescents. *Food Qual. Prefer.* **2016**, *48*, 138–145. [CrossRef]
25. Rubio, B.; Rigal, N.; Boireau-Ducept, N.; Mallet, P.; Meyer, T. Measuring Willingness to Try New Foods: A Self-Report Questionnaire for French-Speaking Children. *Appetite* **2008**, *50*, 408–414. [CrossRef]
26. Rigal, N.; Chabanet, C.; Issanchou, S.; Monnery-Patris, S. Links between Maternal Feeding Practices and Children's Eating Difficulties. Validation of French Tools. *Appetite* **2012**, *58*, 629–637. [CrossRef]
27. Hollar, D.; Paxton-Aiken, A.; Fleming, P. Exploratory Validation of the Fruit and Vegetable Neophobia Instrument among Third- to Fifth-Grade Students. *Appetite* **2013**, *60*, 226–230. [CrossRef]
28. Shim, J.E.; Yoon, J.H.; Kim, K.; Paik, H.Y. Association between Picky Eating Behaviors and Growth in Preschool Children. *J. Nutr. Health* **2013**, *46*, 418–426. [CrossRef]
29. Rioux, C.; Lafraire, J.; Picard, D.; Blissett, J. Food Rejection in Young Children: Validation of the Child Food Rejection Scale in English and Cross-Cultural Examination in the UK and France. *Food Qual. Prefer.* **2019**, *73*, 19–24. [CrossRef]
30. Moroshko, I.; brennan, L. Maternal Controlling Feeding Behaviours and Child Eating in Preschool-Aged Children. *Nutr. Diet.* **2013**, *70*, 49–53. [CrossRef]
31. Kaar, J.L.; Shapiro, A.L.; Fell, D.M.; Johnson, S.L. Parental Feeding Practices, Food Neophobia, and Child Food Preferences: What Combination of Factors Results in Children Eating a Variety of Foods? *Food Qual. Prefer.* **2016**, *50*, 57–64. [CrossRef]
32. Maslin, K.; Grimshaw, K.; Oliver, E.; Roberts, G.; Arshad, S.H.; Dean, T.; Grundy, J.; Glasbey, G.; Venter, C. Taste Preference, Food Neophobia and Nutritional Intake in Children Consuming a Cows' Milk Exclusion Diet: A Prospective Study. *J. Human. Nutr. Diet.* **2016**, *29*, 786–796. [CrossRef] [PubMed]
33. Rahmaty, A. *Individual, Caregiver, and Family Characteristics Associated with Obesity in Preschool-Age Children Item Type Dissertation*; University of Maryland: Baltimore, MD, USA, 2021.
34. Wardle, J.; Guthrie, C.A.; Sanderson, S.; Rapoport, L. Development of the Children's Eating Behaviour Questionnaire. *J. Child Psychol. Psychiatry* **2001**, *42*, 963–970. [CrossRef] [PubMed]
35. Kocsis, R.N. Book Review: Diagnostic and Statistical Manual of Mental Disorders: Fifth Edition (DSM-5). *Int. J. Offender Ther. Comp. Criminol.* **2013**, *57*, 1546–1548. [CrossRef]
36. Aldridge, V.; Dovey, T.M.; Halford, J.C.G. The Role of Familiarity in Dietary Development. *Dev. Rev.* **2009**, *29*, 32–44. [CrossRef]

37. Fernández-Ruiz, V.; Claret, A.; Chaya, C. Testing a Spanish-Version of the Food Neophobia Scale. *Food Qual. Prefer.* **2013**, *28*, 222–225. [CrossRef]
38. Kimberlin, C.L.; Winterstein, A.G. Validity and Reliability of Measurement Instruments Used in Research. *Am. J. Health-Syst. Pharm.* **2008**, *65*, 2276–2284. [CrossRef]
39. Souza, A.C.d.; Alexandre, N.M.C.; Guirardello, E.d.B. Propriedades Psicométricas Na Avaliação de Instrumentos: Avaliação Da Confiabilidade e Da Validade. *Epidemiol. Serviços Saúde* **2017**, *26*, 649–659. [CrossRef]
40. Mokkink, L.B.; Terwee, C.B.; Patrick, D.L.; Alonso, J.; Stratford, P.W.; Knol, D.L.; Bouter, L.M.; de Vet, H.C.W. The COSMIN Study Reached International Consensus on Taxonomy, Terminology, and Definitions of Measurement Properties for Health-Related Patient-Reported Outcomes. *J. Clin. Epidemiol.* **2010**, *63*, 737–745. [CrossRef]
41. Cohen; Swerdlik; Sturman. *Testagem e Avaliação Psicológica—Introdução a Testes e Medidas*, 8th ed.; 2014. Available online: https://seer.uscs.edu.br/index.php/revista_ciencias_saude/article/view/3391 (accessed on 11 November 2023).
42. Cunha, C.M.; De Almeida Neto, O.P.; Stackfleth, R. Principais Métodos de Avaliação Psicométrica Da Validade de Instrumentos de Medida. *Rev. Bras. Ciências Saúde USCS* **2016**, *14*, 75–83. [CrossRef]

Disclaimer/Publisher's Note: The statements, opinions and data contained in all publications are solely those of the individual author(s) and contributor(s) and not of MDPI and/or the editor(s). MDPI and/or the editor(s) disclaim responsibility for any injury to people or property resulting from any ideas, methods, instructions or products referred to in the content.

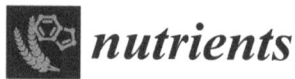

Review

Plate Food Waste in Food Services: A Systematic Review and Meta-Analysis

Nathalia Sernizon Guimarães [1,*], Marcela Gomes Reis [1], Luciano de Alvarenga Fontes [2], Renata Puppin Zandonadi [3], Raquel Braz Assunção Botelho [3], Hmidan A. Alturki [4], Ariana Saraiva [5] and António Raposo [6,*]

[1] Department of Nutrition, Nursing School, Universidade Federal de Minas Gerais, Alfredo Balena Avenue, 190, Room 314, Santa Efigênia, Belo Horizonte 30130-100, Minas Gerais, Brazil; reis.marcelanutri@gmail.com
[2] Department of Agricultural Engineering, Vaz de Mello Consultoria e Perícia, Gonçalves Dias Street, 1181, Funcionários, Belo Horizonte 30140-091, Minas Gerais, Brazil; consultorfundiario@gmail.com
[3] Department of Nutrition, School of Health Sciences, University of Brasilia (UnB), Campus Darcy Ribeiro, Asa Norte 70910-900, Brasilia, Brazil; renatapz@unb.br (R.P.Z.); raquelbotelho@unb.br (R.B.A.B.)
[4] King Abdulaziz City for Science & Technology, Wellness and Preventive Medicine Institute—Health Sector, Riyadh 11442, Saudi Arabia; halturki@kacst.edu.sa
[5] Department of Animal Pathology and Production, Bromatology and Food Technology, Faculty of Veterinary, Universidad de Las Palmas de Gran Canaria, Trasmontaña s/n, 35413 Arucas, Spain; ariana_23@outlook.pt
[6] CBIOS (Research Center for Biosciences and Health Technologies), Universidade Lusófona de Humanidades e Tecnologias, Campo Grande 376, 1749-024 Lisboa, Portugal
* Correspondence: nasernizon@gmail.com (N.S.G.); antonio.raposo@ulusofona.pt (A.R.); Tel.: +55-031-997772844 (N.S.G.)

Abstract: Food waste is considered to be a social, environmental, administrative, and economic problem. Given the large-scale production and distribution of food, food waste in food services has been widely discussed by experts, professors, and scientists in the field. This systematic review aimed to understand which food service has the highest percentage of plate food waste. A systematic review and meta-analysis were conducted until January 2024 in ten electronic databases: MEDLINE, Embase, IBECS, BINACIS, BDENF, CUMED, BDNPAR, ARGMSAL, Cochrane Library, Sustainable Development Goals, and the gray literature. The protocol was previously registered with PROSPERO under the code CRD42024501971. Studies that have assessed plate food waste in food services were included. There were no restrictions on language, publication location, or date. The risk of bias analysis was carried out using the JBI instrument. A proportion meta-analysis was carried out using R software (version 4.2.1). This systematic review with meta-analysis showed that the type of distribution and the food service are the factors that have the greatest impact on the percentage and per capita of plate food waste. In the face of increased waste, interventions should be targeted by type and distribution system, diners, and meals in order to lessen the impact of these factors.

Keywords: food waste; food services; sustainability; collective feeding

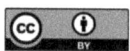

1. Introduction

Food services include commercial and institutional establishments, and they aim to manage the production of nutritionally balanced meals with good hygienic and sanitary standards for consumption outside the home. They may contribute to maintaining or recovering the health of groups and help to develop eating habits [1,2].

The success of a food service operation lies in the precise definition of its objectives, its administrative structure, its physical facilities and human resources, and, above all, the standardization of all the operations carried out, which must be supported by the five elements of the administrative process: forecasting, organization, command, coordination and control. Processes are a set of inter-related activities designed to optimize quality customer service. For a process to take place, the transformation of food and drink (input) into products/meals (outputs) must occur [3]. Given the production process carried out on a large scale in food services, the waste of food, water, materials, and energy, among other things, has been one of the biggest problems due to leftovers and food scraps [4].

In the area of food, the impact of waste is a social, environmental, administrative, and economic problem, leading to an annual global cost of USD 2.65 billion, so that almost a third of all food produced is wasted annually [5]. This not only represents a huge waste of natural resources such as water, energy, and land, but also contributes significantly to greenhouse gas emissions associated with food production. Studies show the relationship between waste and the reallocation of wasted food to cover hunger in various nations [6–8]. According to the data described by some studies, 10 tons of food that have been wasted could feed 12,470 people [9–11].

In this way, reducing food waste worldwide is directly associated with the amount of wasted food that could feed countless families in situations of hunger and food and nutritional insecurity. At a global level, food and nutritional insecurity affect not only low- and middle-income countries but also high-income countries such as the United States of America [12,13].

To quantify food waste, the percentage of leftovers, i.e., the ratio between the leftovers returned on the trays by the diner and the amount of food and food preparations offered, is used and expressed as a percentage. The control of leftovers aims to assess the adequacy of the quantities prepared concerning consumption needs, portioning in distribution, and acceptance of the menu. In healthy groups, less than 10% rates are acceptable as a percentage of leftover intake [14]. Food waste in food services can serve as a measure of the quality of the service. The variables of food seasonality and handler training should be considered in any food service that aims to optimize its actions in the use of food [15].

Considering that leftover food interferes in many social, environmental, and economic areas, resulting in significant impacts on sustainability, this systematic review aimed to understand which food service has the highest percentage of plate food waste. The data from this study will be important for adopting specific campaigns and actions according to the frequency of waste.

2. Materials and Methods

A systematic review and meta-analysis were carried out according to the recommendations of the Cochrane Collaboration [16] and written according to the PRISMA checklist [17]. The study protocol was previously registered on the PROSPERO platform under the code CRD42024501971.

2.1. Search Strategy

To answer the question "Does the frequency of food waste differ by type of food service?", we searched ten different independent databases: MEDLINE (PubMed), Embase; Cochrane Library Collaboration; Índice Bibliográfico Espanhol em Ciências de la Salud (IBECS), Bibliografía Nacional en Ciencias de la Salud Argentina (BINACIS), Base de dados de Enfermagem (BDENF), Committee on Undergraduate Medical Education (CUMED), Base de Datos Nacional del Paraguay (BDNPAR), Revista Argentina de Salud Pública (ARGMSAL), and Sustainable Development Goals (SDGs). In addition, a manual search was carried out in the included reference lists to understand local studies published in journals not indexed in the databases evaluated.

There were no language, date, document type, or publication status restrictions to including records. The search for studies was carried out in January 2024 and included studies up to this date. The descriptors were identified in Medical Subject Headings (MeSHs), Health Sciences Descriptors (DeCSs), and Embase Subject Headings (Emtree). Subsequently, the descriptors were combined with the Boolean operator AND, while their synonyms were combined with the Boolean operator OR. The search strategy adopted for each database is presented in Table S1.

2.2. Outcomes

The primary outcomes were plate food waste (or leftover food intake) (%) and per capita plate food waste (or per capita leftover food intake) (kg), following Equations (1) and (2) [10]:

$$\% \text{ plate food waste} = \frac{\text{weight of plate food waste} \times 100}{\text{weight of meal distributed}} \quad (1)$$

$$\text{Per plate food waste(kg)} = \frac{\text{weight of plate food waste(kg)}}{\text{number of served meals}} \quad (2)$$

2.3. Eligibility Criteria

Observational studies (cross-sectional, case-control, or cohort) and intervention studies were included. Studies at food services such as hospital food service, school canteens, restaurants, university restaurants, and popular restaurants that evaluated plate food waste were included. Experimental studies, case series or case reports, trials, reviews, in vitro or experimental animal studies, cost-effectiveness analyses, letters, comments, or editorials were excluded.

2.4. Study Selection and Data Extraction

The studies found in the electronic search of the databases were exported in "ris" format to the Rayyan Qatar Computing Research Institute application for systematic reviews [18]. Two reviewers (NSG, MGR) screened the studies independently to determine whether they met the inclusion criteria.

Two reviewers (NSG, MGR) independently examined the titles and abstracts to determine whether they met the inclusion criteria. After this stage, a textual analysis of the studies was carried out independently. An independent reviewer analyzed any discrepancies. To create the extraction table, the following data were collected: reference (author, year, title), study location, research design, follow-up period (weeks), population characteristics (type of food service, diners, distribution method, and system), type of menu served, number of served meals, definition plate food waste, and main results for the outcomes assessed.

2.5. Quality Assessment

The Joanna Briggs Institute (JBI) tool was used to assess the methodological quality of the systematic prevalence review [19]. Two researchers independently assessed the risk of bias in the chosen studies. Disagreements between reviewers regarding potential bias in specific studies were resolved through discussion, occasionally involving a third review author. Studies were classified as having a low risk of bias if the total score was up to 49.0%, moderate risk of bias if the score fell between 50.0% and 70.0%, and high risk of bias if it was above 70.0%. The risk of bias in each study is described in Table S2 [20].

2.6. Meta-Analysis

This meta-analysis estimated the proportion of food waste using the crude proportions (PRAW) method with random effect. We chose this method because it corrected for overestimations of the weight of studies with estimates very close to 0% or 100% [21]. Subgroup analyses were carried out by type of food service, diners, distribution method, food service management, type of meal, and distribution system. The random effects model assessed heterogeneity, the chi-squared test was applied with a significance of $p < 0.10$, and its magnitude was determined by the I-squared (I^2). In the all analyses, a p-value < 0.05 was considered statistically significant. The analyses were carried out using the 'Meta' packages in the Rstudio software, version 4.2.1 (R: A Language and Environment for Statistical Computing, Vienna, Austria).

3. Results

A total of 4459 studies were found. After excluding 4379 duplicates, 80 titles and abstracts were examined. Of these 80 records evaluated by full text, 49 were excluded according to the eligibility criteria, as described in Table S3. Further, 31 were included in the review studies via electronic database and 12 studies were added after a manual search of the gray literature. For the meta-analysis, in total of 21 studies via the electronic database and 9 of the gray literature were included. Therefore, 43 studies were included in the systematic review, and 30 studies were eligible for meta-analysis (Figure 1).

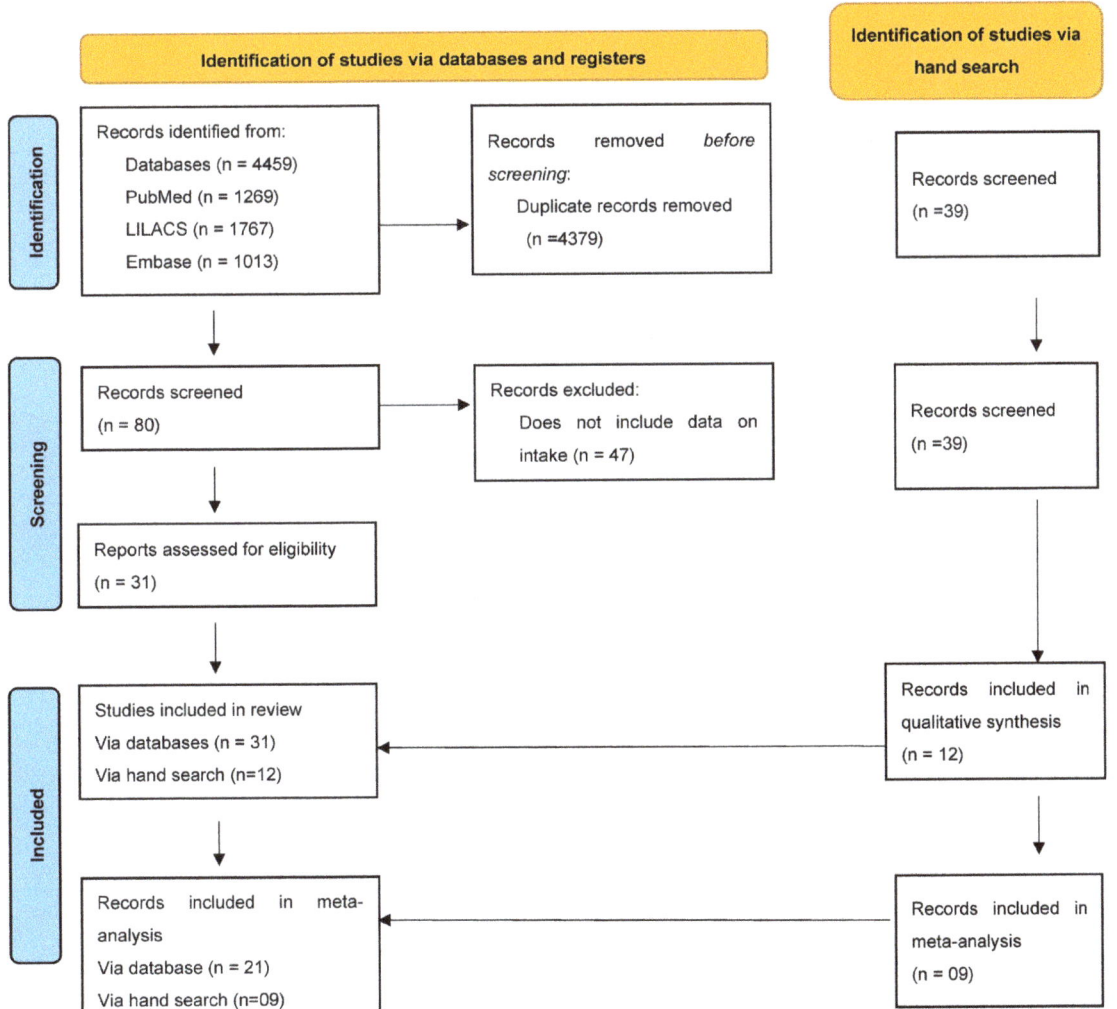

Figure 1. Flowchart for the selection of studies, 2024.

3.1. Characteristics of the Studies

Table 1 summarizes the main characteristics of the included studies. According to the location of the study, 32 (74.4%) were carried out in America (Brazil and USA), five (11.6%) in Asia (Indonesia, Taiwan, Libano, and China), five (11.6%) in Europe (Croatia, Denmark, Latvia, Lithuania, and Finland), and one in South Africa (2.32%).

Table 1. Characteristics of the included studies.

Author and Year	Local	Design	Foodservice Type	Diners	Self-Managed or Outsourcing	Utensils	Distribution System	Meal	Period of Data Collection (Weeks)
Aranha et al., 2018 [9]	Brazil	Cross-sectional	n.i.	n.i.	n.i.	Trays	Mixed	Lunch	1
Augustini et al., 2008 [10]	Brazil	Cross-sectional	Restaurant	Food Service Workers	n.i.	Plate + Trays	Self-Service	Lunch + dinner	14
Barbosa et al., 2021 [22] *	Brazil	Cross-sectional	Restaurant	Food Service Workers	n.i.	Plate	Self-Service	n.i.	n.i.
Bardini et al., 2014 [23]	Brazil	Cross-sectional	n.i.	Food Service Workers	n.i.	Plate	Self-Service	Lunch	$\frac{1}{2}$
Bicalho et al., 2013 [24]	Brazil	Cohort	University Restaurant	n.i.	n.i.	Plate	Self-Service	Lunch	17
Borges et al., 2019 [25]	Brazil	Case report	University Restaurant	Diners + Food Service Workers	Outsourcing	Plate	Mixed	Lunch + dinner	17
Byker et al., 2014 [26]	USA	Cross-sectional	Primary School	Diners	n.i.	Plate	Self-Service	Lunch	1
Carvalho et al., 2013 [11]	Brazil	Cross-sectional	Restaurant	Food Service Workers	Outsourcing	n.i.	Self-Service	Lunch	1
Chang, 2021 [27]	Taiwan	Case-control	Restaurant	Diners	n.i.	Plate	Mixed	n.i.	
Chaves et al., 2019 [28]	Brazil	Cohort	Hospital Food Service	Food Service Workers	n.i.	Plate	v	Lunch	3
Coimbra et al., 2019 [29]	Brazil	Cross-sectional	University Restaurant	n.i.	n.i.	Plate	Mixed	Lunch	1
Dagiliūtė and Musteikytė, 2019 [30]	Lithuania	Cohort	Restaurant	Diners	Self-managed and outsourcing	Plate	Mixed	n.i.	24
Delazeri et al., 2015 [31] *	Brazil	Cohort	Restaurant	n.i.	n.i.	Trays	Self-Service	Lunch	1
Galego et al., 2014 [32] *	Brazil	Cross-sectional	n.i.	Food Service Workers	Self-managed	n.i.	n.i.	Lunch	2

Table 1. Cont.

Author and Year	Local	Design	Foodservice Type	Diners	Self-Managed or Outsourcing	Utensils	Distribution System	Meal	Period of Data Collection (Weeks)
Ilic et al., 2022 [33]	Croatia	Cross-sectional	Primary School	Diners	n.i.	Plate + Trays	A la carte	Lunch	1
Liu et al., 2016 [34]	China	Pilot study	Primary School	Diners	n.i.	Plate + Trays	A la carte	Lunch	n.i.
Lonska et al., 2022 [35]	Latvia	Cross-sectional	Primary School	Diners	n.i.	Plate + Trays	A la carte	Lunch	1
Machado et al., 2014 [36] *	Brazil	Case report	Restaurant	Food Service Workers	n.i.	Plate	n.i.	Lunch	2
Marais et al., 2017 [37]	South Africa	Cross-sectional	Restaurant	Diners + Food Service Workers	Outsourcing	n.i.	n.i.	Lunch + dinner	$\frac{1}{5}$
Matzembacher et al., 2020 [38] *	Brazil	Cohort	Restaurant	n.i.	Self-managed	Plate	Mixed	Lunch	4
Medeiros et al., 2014 [39]	Brazil	Cross-sectional	n.i.	n.i.	n.i.	Plate	n.i.	Lunch	$\frac{1}{2}$
Mello et al., 2011 [40]	Brazil	Cross-sectional	Restaurant	n.i.	Outsourcing	Plate	Mixed	Lunch + dinner	3
Nonino Borges et al., 2006 [41]	Brazil	Cross-sectional	Hospital Food Service	Diners + Food Service Workers	n.i.	n.i.	Self-Service	Lunch + dinner	2
Ofei et al., 2015 [42]	Denmark	Cross-sectional	Hospital Food Service	Diners	Self-managed	Plate	A la carte	Lunch + Supper	5 days
Pistorello et al., 2015 [43]	Brazil	Cross-sectional	Restaurant	Diners	n.i.	Plate	n.i.	Snacks	9
Pontes et al., 2022 [44]	Brazil	Cross-sectional	Restaurant	Diners	n.i.	Plate	Mixed	Lunch + dinner + Snacks	40
Quemelli et al., 2020 [45]	Brazil	Cross-sectional	Hospital Food Service	Food Service Workers	Outsourcing	Plate	Mixed	Lunch	2
Rabelo et al., 2016 [46]	Brazil	Cohort	Restaurant	Food Service Workers	Self-managed	Plate + Trays + lunchbox	Mixed	Lunch	4

Table 1. Cont.

Author and Year	Local	Design	Foodservice Type	Diners	Self-Managed or Outsourcing	Utensils	Distribution System	Meal	Period of Data Collection (Weeks)
Rodrigues et al., 2015 [47]	Brazil	Cross-sectional	Popular Food Service	n.i.	n.i.	Trays	n.i.	Lunch	13
Sabino et al., 2016 [48]	Brazil	Cross-sectional	Hospital Food Service	Diners + Food Service Workers	n.i.	Lunchbox	n.i.	n.i.	2
Santana et al., 2019 [49]	Brazil	Cross-sectional	Hospital Food Service	Food Service Workers	Outsourcing	Trays	Mixed	Lunch	1
Saputri et al., 2019 [50] *	Indonésia	Cross-sectional	University Restaurant	Diners + Food Service Workers	n.i.	n.i.	n.i.	n.i.	1
Scholz et al., 2019 [51] *	Brazil	Cross-sectional	Restaurant	Food Service Workers	Outsourcing	Trays	n.i.	Lunch	8
Silva et al., 2010 [52] *	Brazil	Cohort	Hospital Food Service	Food Service Workers	Self-managed	Trays	Self-Service	Lunch	8
Silvennoinen et al., 2015 [53] *	Finland	Case studies	Schools, day-care centers, University Restaurants, Restaurants, Cafes and petrol stations	n.i	n.i	Plate + Trays + lunch box	Mixed		
Strapazzon et al., 2016 [54] *	Brazil	Cross-sectional	n.i.	n.i.	n.i.	Trays	n.i.	n.i.	n.i.
Souza et al., 2022 [55]	Brazil	Cross-sectional	Hospital Food Service	Diners + Patient companion	Self-managed	Trays	Self-Service	Breakfast, morning snack, lunch, afternoon snack, dinner, and night snack	5 days
Thiagarajah et al., 2013 [56] *	USA	Cohort	University Restaurant	Diners + Food Service Workers	Self-managed	Plate	Self-Service	Lunch + dinner	17
Viana et al., 2016 [57]	Brazil	Cross-sectional	Hospital Food Service	Diners + Food Service Workers	n.i.	Plate	Self-Service	Lunch	1

Table 1. *Cont.*

Author and Year	Local	Design	Foodservice Type	Diners	Self-Managed or Outsourcing	Utensils	Distribution System	Meal	Period of Data Collection (Weeks)
Viana et al., 2017 [58]	Brazil	Cross-sectional	School Canteens	Food Service Workers	n.i.	Trays	Mixed	Lunch	$\frac{1}{2}$
Zandonadi et al., 2012 [59]	Brazil	Cross-sectional	Restaurant	Food Service Workers	n.i.	Plate	Mixed	Lunch	2
Zeineddine et al., 2021 [60] *	Lebanon	Ecologic study	Restaurant	Diners	Self-managed and outsourcing	Plate	Mixed	Dinner	76
Wang et al., 2017 [61] *	China	Survey study	Restaurant	Diners	Self-managed and outsourcing	Plate	Mixed	Dinner	52

Note: n.i. = not informed. Mixed is self-service and thermal counter. * Articles excluded from the meta-analysis.

3.2. Meta-Analysis

In the analysis of plate food waste (%), 30 studies were included, evaluating 117,819 meals and per capita plate food waste (kg). In the final column of Table 2, we have included the percentage of interpretation of the most frequent case within the subgroup evaluated in the meta-analysis to make it clearer. Studies not included in the meta-analysis due to lack of data are described in Table S3.

Table 2. Food waste and total waste by type of food service, type of diners, type of distribution of meals, and distribution system.

	Number of Meals Offered (Absolute Number)	Plate Food Waste (kg) *	Weight of Studies	Plate Food Waste (%) by Subgroup Categories
Food Service Type: Hospital Food Service				
Chaves et al., 2019 [28]	152	7.76	2.9%	
Nonino Borges et al., 2006 [41]	650	24.0	3.8%	
Ofei et al., 2015 [42] (1)	142	8.62	2.7%	
Ofei et al., 2015 [42] (2)	114	6.1	2.6%	
Quemelli et al., 2020 [45]	184	7.15	3.2%	77.7%
Sabino et al., 2016 [48]	505	39.62	3.4%	
Santana et al., 2019 [49]	221	7.25	3.4%	
Souza et al., 2022 [55]	1472	7.7	4.0%	
Viana et al., 2016 [57]	67	3.0	2.2%	
Total	3507	111.2	28.1%	
Food Service Type: School Canteens				
Byker et al., 2014 [26]	304	45.3	2.6%	
Ilic et al., 2022 [33]	17,163	21	4.0%	
Liu et al., 2016 [34]	923	11.99	3.9%	10.5%
Lonska et al., 2022 [35]	7064	28.75	4.0%	
Viana et al., 2017 [58]	2329	13.74	4.0%	
Total	27,783	120.78	18.6%	
Food Service Type: Restaurant (Commercial Food Service)				
Augustini et al., 2008 [10]	4803	6.45	4.0%	
Carvalho et al., 2013 [11]	5849	6.87	4.0%	
Chang, 2021 [27]	360	0.93	4.0%	
Dagiliūtė and Musteikytė, 2019 [30]	174	14.74	2.6%	
Marais et al., 2017 [37]	586	16.90	3.8%	
Mello et al., 2011 [40]	3500	10.71	4.0%	7.3%
Pistorello et al., 2015 [43]	8389	30.71	4.0%	
Pontes et al., 2022 [44]	7997	6.67	4.0%	
Rabelo et al., 2016 [46]	440	9.45	3.8%	
Zandonadi et al., 2012 [59]	1646	4.39	4.0%	
Total	33,744	101.15	38.2%	
Food Service Type: University Restaurant				
Bicalho et al., 2013 [24]	193	10.67	3.0%	
Borges et al., 2019 [25]	1150	8.68	4.0%	2.7%
Coimbra et al., 2019 [29]	23,195	7.51	4.0%	
Total	24,538	26.86	11.0%	

Table 2. Cont.

	Number of Meals Offered (Absolute Number)	Plate Food Waste (kg) *	Weight of Studies	Plate Food Waste (%) by Subgroup Categories
		Food Service Type: Popular Food Service		
Rodrigues et al., 2015 [47]	26,110	18.97	4.0%	1.7%
Total overall	1,115,682	378.96	100.0%	100.0%
	Diners type: Diners and food service workers			
Borges et al., 2019 [25]	1150	8.68	4.5%	
Marais et al., 2017 [37]	586	16.9	4.3%	
Nonino Borges et al., 2006 [41]	650	24	4.2%	69.95%
Sabino et al., 2016 [48]	505	39.62	3.8%	
Viana et al., 2016 [57]	67	3.0	2.6%	
Total	2958	92,2	19.3%	
	Diners type: Food Service Workers			
Augustini et al., 2008 [10]	4803	6.45	4.5%	
Bardini et al., 2014 [23]	1125	8.67	4.5%	
Carvalho et al., 2013 [11]	5849	6.87	4.5%	
Chaves et al., 2019 [28]	152	7.76	3.3%	9.41%
Quemelli et al., 2020 [45]	184	7.15	3.6%	
Rabelo et al., 2016 [46]	440	9.45	4.3%	
Santana et al., 2019 [49]	221	7.25	3.8%	
Total	12,774	53.6	28.4%	
	Diners type: Diners			
Byker et al., 2014 [26]	304	45.3	3.0%	
Chang, 2021 [27]	360	0.93	4.5%	
Dagiliūtė and Musteikytė, 2019 [30]	174	14.74	2.9%	
Ilic et al., 2022 [33]	17,163	21	4.5%	
Liu et al., 2016 [34]	923	11.99	4.4%	
Lonska et al., 2022 [35]	7064	28.75	4.5%	
Ofei et al., 2015 [42] (1)	142	8.62	3.0%	8.96%
Ofei et al., 2015 [42] (2)	114	6.1	2.9%	
Pistorello et al., 2015 [43]	8389	30.71	4.5%	
Pontes et al., 2022 [44]	7997	6.67	4.5%	
Viana et al., 2017 [58]	2329	13.74	4.5%	
Zandonadi et al., 2012 [59]	1646	4.395	4.5%	
Total	46,605	186	47.8%	
	Diners type: Diners and patients' companions			
Souza et al., 2022 [55]	1472	7.7	4.5%	11.65%
Total overall	63,809	339.77	100.0%	100.0%
	Type of distribution: Lunch Box			
Sabino et al., 2016 [48]	505	39.62	3.6%	72.82%
	Type of distribution: Lunch Box + Plate + Tray			
Rabelo et al., 2016 [46]	440	9.45	4.0%	19.94%
	Type of distribution: Plate			
Bardini et al., 2014 [23]	1125	8.67	4.2%	
Bicalho et al., 2013 [24]	193	10.67	3.2%	3.33%
Borges et al., 2019 [25]	1150	8.68	4.2%	

Table 2. Cont.

	Number of Meals Offered (Absolute Number)	Plate Food Waste (kg) *	Weight of Studies	Plate Food Waste (%) by Subgroup Categories
Byker et al., 2014 [26]	304	45.3	2.8%	
Chaves et al., 2019 [28]	152	7.76	3.1%	
Coimbra et al., 2019 [29]	23,195	7.51	4.2%	
Dagiliūtė and Musteikytė, 2019 [30]	174	14.74	2.8%	
Mello et al., 2011 [40]	3500	10.71	4.2%	
Ofei et al., 2015 [42] (1)	142	8.62	2.9%	
Ofei et al., 2015 [42] (2)	114	6.1	2.8%	3.33%
Pistorello et al., 2015 [43]	8389	30.71	4.2%	
Pontes et al., 2022 [44]	7997	6.67	4.2%	
Quemelli et al., 2020 [45]	184	7.15	3.4%	
Souza et al., 2022 [55]	1472	7.7	4.2%	
Viana et al., 2016 [57]	67	3.0	2.4%	
Zandonadi et al., 2012 [59]	1646	4395	4.2%	
Total	49,804	181.71	56.7%	
Type of distribution: Tray				
Aranha et al., 2018 [9]	152	8.73	3.0%	
Medeiros et al., 2014 [39]	896	9.96	4.1%	
Rodrigues et al., 2015 [47]	26,110	18.97	3.6%	1.85%
Santana et al., 2019 [49]	221	7.25	4.2%	
Viana et al., 2017 [58]	2329	13.74	4.2%	
Total	29,708	58.65	19.1%	
Type of distribution: Plate + Tray				
Augustini et al., 2008 [10]	4803	6.45	4.2%	
Ilic et al., 2022 [33]	17,163	21	4.2%	
Liu et al., 2016 [34]	923	11.99	4.1%	2.13%
Lonska et al., 2022 [35]	7064	28.75	4.2%	
Total	29,953	68.19	16.7%	
Total overall	110,410	357.62	100.0%	100.0%
Management Mode: Self-Management				
Borges et al., 2019 [25]	1150	8.68	14.8%	
Carvalho et al., 2013 [11]	5849	6.87	15.1%	
Marais et al., 2017 [37]	586	16.9	12.8%	
Mello et al., 2011 [40]	3500	10.71	15.1%	87.40%
Quemelli et al., 2020 [45]	184	7.15	8.4%	
Santana et al., 2019 [49]	221	7.25	9.7%	
Total	696	24.17	75.9%	
Management Mode: Outsourcing				
Ofei et al., 2015 [42] (1)	142	8.62	5.9%	
Ofei et al., 2015 [42] (2)	114	6.1	5.5%	12.60%
Rabelo et al., 2016 [46]	440	9.45	12.8%	
Total	11,490	57.56	24.1%	
Total overall	12,186	81.73	100.0%	100.0%
Meal type: Lunch and Dinner				
Augustini et al., 2008 [10]	4803	6.45	4.1%	5.24%
Borges et al., 2019 [25]	1150	8.68	4.1%	

Table 2. Cont.

	Number of Meals Offered (Absolute Number)	Plate Food Waste (kg) *	Weight of Studies	Plate Food Waste (%) by Subgroup Categories
Marais et al., 2017 [37]	586	16.9	3.8%	
Mello et al., 2011 [40]	3500	10.71	4.1%	
Nonino Borges et al., 2006 [41]	650	24	3.8%	5.24%
Pontes et al., 2022 [44]	7997	6.67	4.1%	
Total	18,686	66.74	24.0%	
Meal type: Snacks				
Pistorello et al., 2015 [43]	8389	30.71	4.1%	5.38%
Meal type: Lunch				
Aranha et al., 2018 [9]	152	8.73	2.5%	
Bardini et al., 2014 [23]	1125	8.67	4.1%	
Bicalho et al., 2013 [24]	193	10.67	2.7%	
Byker et al., 2014 [26]	304	45.3	2.3%	
Carvalho et al., 2013 [11]	5849	6.87	4.1%	
Chaves et al., 2019 [28]	152	7.76	2.6%	
Coimbra et al., 2019 [29]	23,195	7.51	4.1%	
Ilic et al., 2022 [33]	17,163	21	4.1%	
Liu et al., 2016 [34]	923	11.99	4.0%	
Lonska et al., 2022 [35]	7064	28.75	4.1%	2.91%
Medeiros et al., 2014 [39]	896	9.96	4.0%	
Ofei et al., 2015 [42] (1)	142	8.62	2.4%	
Quemelli et al., 2020 [45]	184	7.15	3.0%	
Rabelo et al., 2016 [46]	440	9.45	3.8%	
Rodrigues et al., 2015 [47]	26,110	18.97	4.1%	
Santana et al., 2019 [49]	221	7.25	3.3%	
Viana et al., 2016 [57]	67	3.0	1.9%	
Viana et al., 2017 [58]	2329	13.74	4.1%	
Zandonadi et al., 2012 [59]	1646	4395	4.1%	
Total	62,559	124.12	65.5%	
Meal type: Supper				
Ofei et al., 2015 [42] (2)	114	6.1	2.2%	77.87%
**Meal type: Small and large meals ** **				
Souza et al., 2022	1472	7.7	4.1%	7.56%
Total overall	**116,816**	**351.03**	**100.0%**	**100.0%**
Distribution system: Self-Service				
Bardini et al., 2014 [23]	1125	8.67	4.4%	
Bicalho et al., 2013 [24]	193	10.67	3.2%	
Byker et al., 2014 [26]	30.10	45.3	2.8%	
Carvalho et al., 2013 [11]	5849	6.87	4.4%	61.42%
Chaves et al., 2019 [28]	152	7.76	3.1%	
Nonino Borges et al., 2006 [41]	650	24	4.1%	
Viana et al., 2016 [57]	67	3.0	2.4%	
Total	13,143	112.72	24.5%	
Distribution system: *A la carte*				
Ilic et al., 2022 [33]	27.12	21	4.4%	22.14%
Liu et al., 2016 [34]	11.7	11.99	4.3%	

Table 2. Cont.

	Number of Meals Offered (Absolute Number)	Plate Food Waste (kg) *	Weight of Studies	Plate Food Waste (%) by Subgroup Categories
Lonska et al., 2022 [35]	4.5	28.75	4.4%	
Ofei et al., 2015 [42] (1)	21.5	8.62	2.9%	
Ofei et al., 2015 [42] (2)	23.4	6.1	2.8%	22.14%
Souza et al., 2022 [55]	11.1	7.7	4.4%	
Total	26,878	84.16	23.2%	
Distribution system: Mixed * **				
Aranha et al., 2018 [9]	152	8.73	3.0%	
Augustini et al., 2008 [10]	23.2	6.45	4.4%	
Borges et al., 2019 [25]	1150	8.68	4.4%	
Chang, 2021 [27]	25.12	0.93	4.4%	
Coimbra et al., 2019 [29]	23,195	7.51	4.4%	
Dagiliūtė and Musteikytė, 2019 [30]	22.6	14.74	2.8%	
Mello et al., 2011 [40]	31.7	10.71	4.4%	16.42%
Pontes et al., 2022 [44]	22.11	6.67	4.4%	
Quemelli et al., 2020 [45]	184	7.15	3.5%	
Rabelo et al., 2016 [46]	440	9.45	4.2%	
Santana et al., 2019 [49]	221	7.25	3.7%	
Viana et al., 2017 [58]	2329	13.74	4.4%	
Zandonadi et al., 2012 [59]	1646	4.39	4.4%	
Total	41,348	93.28	52.3%	
Total overall	**81,369**	**290.16**	**100.0%**	**100.0%**

Note: * Weight of plate food waste is total weight for the amount of people; ** Breakfast, snacks, lunch, dinner, and supper. Small meal is snacks + supper. Large dinner is breakfast + lunch + dinner. *** Mixed is a self-service and thermal counter.

3.3. Plate Food Waste (in Percentual)

Table 2 summarizes the analysis of the included studies. Analyzing the percentage of plate food waste according to the type of food service, hospital food service (n = eight studies) is the type of service with the highest rate of plate waste (77.7%) and popular restaurants has the lowest rate (1.7%). The second highest percentage of plate food waste was observed in school canteens (n = five; 10.5%), commercial food service (n = ten studies; 7.3%), and university canteens (n = three studies; 2.7%), respectively.

Concerning the diners' groups, diners and food service workers (n = five studies) had the highest percentage of plate waste, 69.95%, followed by diners and patient companions, 11.65%.

According to the forms of distribution, the study that only analyzed the distribution of meals in lunchboxes (n = 1 study) obtained a percentage approximately 3× higher, with 72.82% of plate waste, compared to the second highest type of waste, which would be distribution by plates, trays, and lunchboxes (n = 1 study) with 19.94%. With even lower percentages are distribution on plates (n = 15 studies; 3.33%), followed by trays (n = 4 studies; 1.85%), and the lowest percentage represented by the trays and plates subgroup (n = 4 study; 2.13%).

According to the type of management, they were classified as self-management (n = two studies) and outsourced (n = six studies). Self-management had the highest percentage of leftover food, with 87.40%, followed by outsourced management (12.60%).

According to the meal type, we used data from lunch (n = 19 studies), large meals (n = 6 studies), small and large meals and supper (n = 1 study), and snacks in general (n = 1 study). Supper accounted for the highest percentage of leftovers (77.87%), followed by small and large meals (7.56%), and lunch had the lowest percentage of plate waste food (2.91%).

According to the distribution system, they were classified as self-service (n = 8 studies), a la carte (n = 5 studies), and mixed (n = 12 studies), with the former having a higher percentage of plate waste (61.42%) and the latter a lower percentage of plate waste (16.42%).

3.4. Per Capita Waste (kg)

When analyzing the per capita number of leftovers according to the type of food service, it was possible to see that hospital food service and university canteens are the types of service with the highest per capita waste of leftovers (0.03 kg/per capita/meal). However, the other services, such as popular restaurants, school canteen food service, and commercial food service, obtained a per capita equal to zero, given the lower waste in their analysis (Table 3). The study by Chang and collaborators (2021) evaluating buffet restaurants [27] did not present per capita value.

Table 3. Number of meals offered, plate food waste per capita (kg and %) by type of food service, type of diners, type of distribution, type of meal, and distribution system.

	Number of Meals Offered (Absolute Number)	Per Capita (kg) Plate Food Waste in the Period of the Study	Plate Food Waste per Capita (%)
	Food Service Type		
University Restaurant	37,788	9.92	0.03
Hospital Food Service	4222	0.95	0.02
Restaurant	54,685	4.00	0.01
School Canteens	20,415	0.08	0.00
Popular Food Service	26,110	0.09	0.00
	Type of diners		
Food Service Workers	25,175	2.37	0.01
Diners and Food Service Workers	16,208	0.57	0.00
Diners	38,621	0.23	0.00
Diners and Companies	1472	0.03	0.00
	Type of distribution		
Lunchbox	505	0.17	0.03
Plate + Tray	22,889	0.74	0.00
Plate	69,546	3.92	0.01
Lunch Box + Plate + Tray	440	0.06	0.01
Tray	40,498	1.01	0.00
	Distribution Modality		
Self-Management	15,005	3.77	0.03
Outsourcing	16,078	0.54	0.00
	Type of Meal		
Lunch	102,599	5.52	0.01
Lunch and Dinner	27,866	1.11	0.00
Snacks	8389	0.07	0.00
Small and Large meals *	1472	0.03	0.00
	Distribution System		
Mixed **	45,335	4.05	0.01
Self-Service	28,246	1.55	0.01
Assisted service	19,558	0.03	0.00

Note: * Breakfast, snacks, lunch, dinner, and supper. Small meal is snacks + supper. Large dinner is breakfast + lunch + dinner. ** Mixed is self-service and thermal counter.

Concerning the diners' groups, the food service workers group obtained a per capita leftovers (per capita waste) of 0.01 kg, and the other subgroups, such as customers and employees as well as only customers, obtained a per capita equal to zero, given the lower waste in their analysis (Table 3).

According to the forms of distribution, the distribution in lunch boxes had a per capita leftover intake of 0.03 kg, followed by the trays and plates subgroup (0.02 kg), and 0.01 kg of the plates subgroup, and the distribution on plates, trays, and lunch boxes. It is worth noting that distribution on trays, due to their lower waste, accounted for zero kg in the analysis (Table 3). According to the management method, only the self-management had a per capita leftover different from zero (0.03 kg). For the type of meal, only lunch and large meals had a per capita different from zero (0.01 kg), while the snacks had zero kg/per capita. Even so, regarding the distribution system, both self-service and mixed service had 0.01 kg/per capita.

4. Discussion

Food waste is not only ethically unacceptable but has essential impacts on human health, food safety, and the environment. Plate food waste can be avoided, and its prevention is fundamental, but it depends on an individual's awareness [61]. Studying data about plate food waste is essential to raise public awareness about the need for change.

This systematic review aimed to understand which food service has the highest plate food waste. It is estimated that in developing countries, food loss occurs mainly during the first stages of the food supply chain (post-harvest production and distribution due to lack of financial, technical, and management resources), while food waste in consumption tends to be lower than that of developed countries [61]. Despite not being studied, it probably occurs due to the food insecurity experienced in some developing countries and the concern about food waste in this context. Therefore, it is expected that there will be more studies on food waste in countries that suffer from food insecurity, as seen in this systematic review, in which around 70% of the studies were carried out in Brazil (Table 1).

This systematic review showed that hospital food service (n = nine studies) is the type of service with the highest rate of plate food waste (4.9%), and popular restaurants presented the lowest rate (0.07%). Hospital food service also has the highest per capita plate food waste (0.03 kg), which is justified by patients' health conditions, the menus served, service, and hospital environmental issues [42]. These results can also be expected since hospital consumers are generally affected by illness or taking medications that can impair their appetite [28,41,45,48,49,52,57]. It is important to mention that five studies only evaluated the lunch meal, and others evaluated lunch and dinner or supper or all the meals. On the other hand, popular restaurants (or community restaurants) are part of a Brazilian assistance program that offers cheap and healthy meals to low-income populations. They mainly attend to people at risk of food insecurity, who are expected to eat all the food on their plates [62]. One study in this review was conducted in popular restaurants and evaluated just lunch. Therefore, it is difficult to compare studies because they served different types of meals, and the attending population is not the only criterion to be analyzed. The second highest percentage of plate food waste was observed in the school canteen food service (0.43%), which was also expected to be high since, in childhood, there is frequent food neophobia and a lack of sustainable and health knowledge, which can determine food choices, impact the quality of a diet, and influence unfinished plates [63]. Also, children are exposed to a greater variety of food in school canteens as part of the nutrition education process. Exposure to new ingredients and preparations is expected to cause more plate food waste.

Meal distribution in lunchboxes presented the highest percentage of plate food waste compared to distribution by plates and/or trays. Considering that lunchboxes are pre-prepared and do not allow the client to choose the dishes (and quantity) composing their meal, lunchbox food waste is expected to be higher than the distribution system in which clients may select dishes among served options and the amount that will compose their plate. Three studies evaluated lunchboxes in commercial restaurants, university restaurants, and school canteens.

Self-management food services presented a higher percentage of plate food waste (3.47%) than outsourced management (0.50%). Outsourced restaurants, that do not have their own management, need to comply with the criteria established by the contract manager, which are often associated with the menu's quality aspects (nutritional, sensorial, microbiological, and economic). Furthermore, for a restaurant to make a profit, it needs to reduce waste in general, which involves good acceptance of the dishes by consumers. These aspects may explain the data from studies comparing outsourced and self-management restaurants.

According to the type of meal, supper accounted for the highest percentage of leftovers (5.35%). However, it is important to consider that the only study evaluating supper [42] and the study evaluating small and large meals [55] were performed in hospital restaurants, in which consumers are generally affected by illness or taking medications impairing their appetite in addition to being in the hospital environment [42]. Lunch presented the lowest percentage of plate waste food (0.27%). It is essential to highlight that only 26% (n = 5) of the studies only evaluated lunch and were performed in hospitals [28,45,49,52,57]. Almost half of the studies evaluating lunch were performed in restaurants in Brazil [11,23,31,38,42,46,47,51,59]. In Brazil, lunch is considered the main and largest meal during the day. It mainly comprises traditional and well-accepted dishes such as rice, beans, meat, and some vegetables. Considering the importance of lunch in Brazil and the food insecurity experienced in this country, these factors probably impacted the small percentage of lunch plate waste in this review.

Self-service restaurants had a higher percentage of plate food waste (0.86%), and mixed-service restaurants had a lower percentage (0.23%). A study showed that buffet (self-service) restaurants cause more plate food waste than other food services [64], which is similar to the findings in our review. Self-service restaurants can charge by plate weight or charge per person (regardless of the amount they will eat). When a meal is charged per person there tends to be greater waste, as the value is the same no matter how much food is put on the plate. When charged according to plate weight, consumers tend to be more attentive when choosing food and put less food on the plate, tending to create less food waste. However, many studies do not specify the type of self-service analyzed, which impairs discussion of this topic. However, the type of distribution service is a critical topic in plate food waste prevention, since this review showed it has the second greatest impact on the percentage of plate food waste.

It is important to highlight that most of the studies included in this review are from Brazil, which might skew the general applicability of the results to other global contexts, especially in countries with different eating habits and food service operations. It is also essential to note that the studies used different methodologies, which may affect the overall analysis, so the data must be analyzed cautiously. However, the knowledge about the type of food service, meal distribution system, and dinners that produce the most plate food waste may help managers plan educational actions to prevent and correct waste, as well as to identify the dishes that are most wasted (whether due to low acceptance, excessive portion size, or for another reason), allowing them to make changes to the menu to reduce plate food waste.

5. Conclusions

Plate food waste causes high financial waste, lower valuable nutrient intake by consumers, and a negative environmental impact. Several individuals' factors may influence plate food waste, such as age, serving size, sex, food preferences, eating behaviors, competitive foods during meals, how long meals last, and educational and economic levels, among others. However, this review showed that aspects of food service also impact plate food waste. The type of distribution and the food service are factors that have the greatest impact on percentage and per capita of plate food waste. In contrast, the type and system of distribution, the types of diners, and the types of meals have less impact, but they are still relevant factors that need to be analyzed. Therefore, this review highlights the need for targeted interventions that reduce plate food waste and for understanding of the specific conditions of each food service type to help design effective waste reduction strategies.

Supplementary Materials: The following supporting information can be downloaded at: https://www.mdpi.com/article/10.3390/nu16101429/s1, Table S1: Indexers used to select publications; Table S2: JBI Critical Appraisal Checklist (Risk of Bias); Table S3: Full-text excluded articles and reasons.

Author Contributions: Conceptualization, N.S.G., M.G.R. and L.d.A.F.; methodology, N.S.G., M.G.R. and L.d.A.F.; validation, N.S.G., R.P.Z., R.B.A.B. and A.R.; formal analysis, N.S.G., M.G.R. and L.d.A.F.; investigation, N.S.G., M.G.R. and L.d.A.F.; writing—original draft preparation, N.S.G., M.G.R. and L.d.A.F.; writing—review and editing, N.S.G., M.G.R., L.d.A.F., R.P.Z., R.B.A.B., H.A.A., A.S. and A.R.; supervision, A.R.; project administration, A.R.; funding acquisition, H.A.A. and A.R. All authors have read and agreed to the published version of the manuscript.

Funding: This research received no external funding.

Acknowledgments: We thank all the authors contacted who clarified questions or sent us additional information about their studies.

Conflicts of Interest: The authors declare no conflicts of interest.

References

1. Colares, L.G.T.; de Freitas, C.M. Work Process and Workers' Health in a Food and Nutrition Unit: Prescribed versus Actual Work. *Cad. Saude Publica* **2007**, *23*, 3011–3020. [CrossRef] [PubMed]
2. Ribeiro, J.S. Food Waste Indicators in Commercial Restaurants [Brazil]. *Rev. Rosa Ventos—Turismo Hosp.* **2020**, *12*, 350–365. [CrossRef]
3. De Abreu, E.S.; Spinelli, M.G.N.; Pinto, M.A.S. *Gestão de Unidades de Alimentação e Nutrição: Um Modo de Fazer*; Metha, Ed.: São Paulo, Brasil, 2016.
4. Mouat, A.R. Sustainability in Food-Waste Reduction Biotechnology: A Critical Review. *Curr. Opin. Biotechnol.* **2022**, *77*, 102781. [CrossRef] [PubMed]
5. Teixeira, F.; Nunes, G.; Antonovicz, S. Principais Fatores Associados Aos Índices de Desperdício em Unidades de Alimentação e Nutrição: Uma Revisão Integrativa. *Saúde Rev.* **2017**, *17*, 42–50. [CrossRef]
6. Ishangulyyev, R.; Kim, S.; Lee, S.H. Understanding Food Loss and Waste—Why Are We Losing and Wasting Food? *Foods* **2019**, *8*, 297. [CrossRef] [PubMed]
7. Parsa, A.; Van De Wiel, M.; Schmutz, U.; Fried, J.; Black, D.; Roderick, I. Challenging the food waste hierarchy. *J. Environ. Manag.* **2023**, *344*, 118554. [CrossRef] [PubMed]
8. Wani, N.R.; Rather, R.A.; Farooq, A.; Padder, S.A.; Baba, T.R.; Sharma, S.; Mubarak, N.M.; Khan, A.H.; Singh, P.; Ara, S. New insights in food security and environmental sustainability through waste food management. *Environ. Sci. Pollut. Res.* **2023**, *31*, 17835–17857. [CrossRef] [PubMed]
9. Aranha, F.Q.; Flora Silva Gustavo, A. Avaliação Do Desperdício De Alimentos Em Uma Unidade De Alimentação E Nutrição Na Cidade De Botucatu. *Hig. Aliment.* **2018**, *32*, 28–32.
10. De Menezes Augustini, V.C.; Kishimoto, P.; Tescaro, T.C.; de Almeida, F.Q.A. Avaliação Do Índice De Resto-Ingesta E Sobras Em Unidade De Alimentação E Nutrição (UAN) De Uma Empresa Metalúrgica Na Cidade De Piracicaba/SP. *Rev. Simbio-Logias* **2008**. Available online: https://simbiologias.ibb.unesp.br/index.php/files/article/view/7/33 (accessed on 22 April 2024).
11. De Carvalho, E.M.; Fonseca, C.S.; Castro, L.C.V.; Costa, A.C. Avaliação Do Índice de Resto-Ingestão e Sobras Em Uma Unidade Produtora de Refeição (UPR). *Hig. Aliment.* **2013**, *27*, 19–22.
12. Hazzard, V.M.; Loth, K.A.; Hooper, L.; Becker, C.B. Food Insecurity and Eating Disorders: A Review of Emerging Evidence. *Curr. Psychiatry Rep.* **2020**, *22*, 74. [CrossRef]
13. Brasil—Ministério do Desenvolvimento Social Fome No Brasil Piorou Nos Últimos Três Anos, Mostra Relatório Da FAO—Ministério Do Desenvolvimento e Assistência Social, Família e Combate à Fome. Available online: https://www.gov.br/mds/pt-br/noticias-e-conteudos/desenvolvimento-social/noticias-desenvolvimento-social/fome-no-brasil-piorou-nos-ultimos-tres-anos-mostra-relatorio-da-fao (accessed on 25 March 2024).
14. Maistro, L.C. Estudo Do Índice De Resto Ingestão Em Serviços De Alimentação. Nutrição Em Pauta. *Nutr. Pauta* **2000**, *8*, 40–43.
15. Martins, M.T.S.; Epstein, M.; de Oliveira, D.R.M. Parâmetros de Controle e/Ou Monitoramento Da Qualidade Do Serviço Empregado Em Uma Unidade de Alimentação e Nutrição. *Hig. Aliment.* **2006**, *20*, 52–57.
16. Higgins, J.; Thomas, J.; Chandler, J.; Cumpston, J.; Li, T.; Page, M. (Eds.) *Cochrane Handbook for Systematic Reviews of Interventions*; John Wiley & Sons: Chichester, UK, 2021; Volume 1.
17. Page, M.J.; McKenzie, J.E.; Bossuyt, P.M.; Boutron, I.; Hoffmann, T.C.; Mulrow, C.D.; Shamseer, L.; Tetzlaff, J.M.; Akl, E.A.; Brennan, S.E.; et al. The PRISMA 2020 Statement: An Updated Guideline For Reporting Systematic Reviews Systematic Reviews And Meta-Analyses. *BMJ* **2021**, *372*, 71. [CrossRef] [PubMed]
18. Ouzzani, M.; Hammady, H.; Fedorowicz, Z.; Elmagarmid, A. Rayyan—A Web and Mobile App for Systematic Reviews. *Syst. Rev.* **2016**, *5*, 210. [CrossRef]

19. Munn, Z.; Moola, S.; Lisy, K.; Riitano, D.; Tufanaru, C. Methodological Guidance for Systematic Reviews of Observational Epidemiological Studies Reporting Prevalence and Cumulative Incidence Data. *Int. J. Evid.-Based Healthc.* **2015**, *13*, 147–153. [CrossRef]
20. de Azevedo, Y.J.; Ledesma, A.L.L.; Pereira, L.V.; Oliveira, C.A.; Junior, F.B. Vestibular Implant: Does It Really Work? A Systematic Review. *Braz. J. Otorhinolaryngol.* **2019**, *85*, 788–798. [CrossRef]
21. Hunter, J.P.; Saratzis, A.; Sutton, A.J.; Boucher, R.H.; Sayers, R.D.; Bown, M.J. In meta-analyses of proportion studies, funnel plots were found to be an inaccurate method of assessing publication bias. *J. Clin. Epidemiol.* **2014**, *67*, 897–903. [CrossRef] [PubMed]
22. Barbosa, A.K.d.S.; Lima, M.F.; Lima, W.L. Avaliação Do Resto E Ingesta de Refeições Em Um Restaurante de Empresa Privada. *Hig. Aliment.* **2021**, *35*, e1027. [CrossRef]
23. Bardini, M.M.V.; Cruz, A. Determinação Do Índice de Resto-Ingestão Em Unidade de Alimentação e Nutriçao Do Município de Tubarão, SC. *Hig. Aliment.* **2014**, *28*, 53–57.
24. Bicalho, A.H.; Lima, V.O.B. Impacto De Uma Intervenção Para Redução Do Desperdício Em Uma Unidade De Alimentação E Nutrição. *Nutrire* **2013**, *38*, 269–277. [CrossRef]
25. Borges, M.P.; Souza, L.H.R.; De Pinho, S.; De Pinho, L. Impacto De Uma Campanha Para Redução De Desperdício De Alimentos Em Um Restaurante Universitário. *Eng. Sanit. Ambient.* **2019**, *24*, 843–848. [CrossRef]
26. Byker, C.J.; Farris, A.R.; Marcenelle, M.; Davis, G.C.; Serrano, E.L. Food Waste in a School Nutrition Program After Implementation of New Lunch Program Guidelines. *J. Nutr. Educ. Behav.* **2014**, *46*, 406–411. [CrossRef]
27. Chang, Y.Y.-C. All You Can Eat Or All You Can Waste? Effects Of Alternate Serving Styles And Inducements On Food Waste In Buffet Restaurants. *Curr. Issues Tour.* **2022**, *25*, 727–744. [CrossRef]
28. Chaves, V.S.; Carolina, C.; Machado, B.; de Abreu, S.V. Índice De Resto Ingestão Antes E Após Campanha De Conscientização De Comensais. *Rev. EVS-Rev. Ciências Ambient. Saúde* **2019**, *46*, 1–7. [CrossRef]
29. Coimbra, A.L.Q.; Silva, L.K.R.; Lacerda, R.S.; Chagas, G.V.; Trindade, S.N.C. Índice de Resto-Ingestão e Avaliação Qualitativa Das Preparações Do Cardápio de Um Restaurante Universitário Do Município de Barreiras-BA/Rest Index-Ingestion and Qualitative Evaluation of the Preparations of the Menu of a University Restaurant in Barreiras-BA. *Hig. Aliment.* **2019**, *33*, 398–402.
30. Dagiliūtė, R.; Musteikytė, A. Food waste generation: Restaurant data and consumer attitudes. *Environ. Res. Eng. Manag.* **2019**, *75*, 7–14. [CrossRef]
31. Delazeri, P.C.; Batisti, S.L.; Silva, A.B.G. Avaliação E Campanha Para Diminuição Do Resto Em Uma Unidade De Alimentação E Nutrição De Uma Empresa Do Vale Do Taquari. RS. *Hig. Aliment.* **2015**, *29*, 37–43.
32. Galego, B.V.; Russo, C.B.; Moura, P.N. Síntese Avaliação Do Índice De Desperdício Do Refeitório De Uma UAN Do Município De Guarapuava-PR. *Hig. Aliment.* **2014**, *28*, 202–204.
33. Ilić, A.; Bituh, M.; Brečić, R.; Barić, I.C. Relationship Between Plate Waste and Food Preferences Among Primary School Students Aged 7–10 Years. *J. Nutr. Educ. Behav.* **2022**, *54*, 844–852. [CrossRef]
34. Liu, Y.; Cheng, S.; Liu, X.; Cao, X.; Xue, L.; Liu, G. Plate Waste in School Lunch Programs in Beijing, China. *Sustainability* **2016**, *8*, 1288. [CrossRef]
35. Lonska, J.; Zvaigzne, A.; Kotane, I.; Silicka, I.; Litavniece, L.; Kodors, S.; Deksne, J.; Vonoga, A. Plate Waste in School Catering in Rezekne, Latvia. *Sustainability* **2022**, *14*, 4046. [CrossRef]
36. Machado, C.C.B.; Mendes, C.K.; Souza, P.G.; Martins, K.S.R.; Silva, K.C.C. Avaliação Do Índice De Resto Ingesta de Uma Unidade de Alimentação e Nutrição Institucional de Anápolis-GO. *Ens. Ciência C Biológicas Agrárias Saúde* **2012**, *16*, 151–162.
37. Marais, M.; Smit, Y.; Koen, N.; Lötze, E. Are The Attitudes And Practices Of Foodservice Managers, Catering Personnel And Students Contributing To Excessive Food Wastage At Stellenbosch University? *S. Afr. J. Clin. Nutr.* **2017**, *30*, 60–67. [CrossRef]
38. Matzembacher, D.E.; Brancoli, P.; Maia, L.M.; Eriksson, M. Consumer's Food Waste in Different Restaurants Configuration: A Comparison between Different Levels of Incentive and Interaction. *Waste Manag.* **2020**, *114*, 263–273. [CrossRef] [PubMed]
39. Medeiros, L.B.; Saccol, A.L.F. Avaliação Do Índice De Resto E Sobras Em Serviços De Alimentação. *Hig. Aliment.* **2014**, *28*, 64–68.
40. De Mello, A.G.; Back, F.d.S.; Baratta, R.; Pires, L.A.; Colares, L.G.T. Avaliação Do Desperdício de Alimentos Em Unidade de Alimentação e Nutrição Localizada Em Um Clube Da Cidade Do Rio de Janeiro. *Hig. Aliment.* **2011**, *25*, 33–39.
41. Nonino-Borges, C.B.; Rabito, E.I.; da Silva, K.; Ferraz, C.A.; Chiarello, P.G.; dos Santos, J.S.; Marchini, J.S. Desperdício De Alimentos Intra-Hospitalar. *Rev. Nutr.* **2006**, *19*, 349–356. [CrossRef]
42. Ofei, K.T.; Holst, M.; Rasmussen, H.H.; Mikkelsen, B.E. Effect Of Meal Portion Size Choice On Plate Waste Generation Among Patients With Different Nutritional Status. An Investigation Using Dietary Intake Monitoring System (DIMS). *Appetite* **2015**, *91*, 157–164. [CrossRef]
43. Pistorello, J.; De Conto, S.M.; Zaro, M. Geração De Resíduos Sólidos Em Um Restaurante De Um Hotel Da Serra Gaúcha, Rio Grande Do Sul, Brasil. *Eng. Sanit. Ambient.* **2015**, *20*, 337–346. [CrossRef]
44. Pontes, T.d.O.; César, A.d.S.; Conejero, M.A.; Deliberador, L.R.; Batalha, M.O. Food waste measurement in a chain of industrial restaurants in Brazil. *J. Clean. Prod.* **2022**, *369*, 133351. [CrossRef]
45. Quemelli, C.A.; Nogueira, G.B. Avaliação Da Sobra E Do Resto Ingesta Como Estratégia Na Redução Do Desperdício De Alimentos. *Saber Científico* **2020**, *9*, 30–42. [CrossRef]
46. Rebelo, N.M.L.; Alves, T.C.U. Avaliação Do Percentual de Resto-Ingestão e Sobra Alimentar Em Uma Unidade de Alimentação e Nutrição Institucional. *Rev. Bras. Tecnol. Agroind.* **2016**, *10*, 2025–2039. [CrossRef]

47. Rodrigues, A.N.; Mendonça, X.M.F.D.; Nascimento, F.C.A. Estudo Do Desperdício de Alimentos Em Um Restaurante Popular de Belém—PA: Foco Na Sustentabilidade e Qualidade de Vida. *Hig. Aliment.* **2015**, *29*, 133–137.
48. Sabino, J.B.; Brasileiro, N.P.M.; Souza, L.T. Pesquisa de Resto-Ingesta Em Uma Unidade de Alimentação e Nutrição Hospitalar de Teófilo Otoni—MG. *Hig. Aliment.* **2016**, *30*, 24–27.
49. Santana, K.L.; Fernandes, C.E.; Oliveira, L.G.B.; Santos, V.V.; Guerra, J.M.C. Análise Do Índice De Resto-Ingesta E De Sobra Suja Em Uma UAN Hospitalar De Recife—PE. *Hig. Aliment.* **2019**, *33*, 133–137.
50. Saputri, E.M.; Tangsuphoom, N.; Rojroongwasinkul, N. Nutritional Impact of Plate Waste in University Canteens: An Assessment at Mulawarman University. *Abstr. Ann. Nutr. Metab.* **2019**, *75*, 424.
51. Scholz, F.; Adami, F.S.; Rosolen, M.D.; Fassina, P. Avaliação Do Resto-Ingesta Antes E Durante Uma Campanha De Conscientização Contra O Desperdício De Alimentos. *Nutr.-Rev. Nutr. Vigilância Saúde* **2019**, *6*, 1–9. [CrossRef]
52. Silva, A.M.D.; Silva, C.P.; Pessina, E.L. Avaliação Do Índice De Resto Ingesta Após Campanha De Conscientização Dos Clientes Contra O Desperdício De Alimentos Em Um Serviço De Alimentação Hospitalar. *Rev. Simbio-Logias* **2010**, 1–3. Available online: https://www.ibb.unesp.br/Home/ensino/departamentos/educacao/avaliacao_indice_de_resto_ingesta_apos_campanha_conscienti.pdf (accessed on 22 April 2024).
53. Silvennoinen, K.; Heikkilä, L.; Katajajuuri, J.-M.; Reinikainen, A. Food waste volume and origin: Case studies in the Finnish food service sector. *Waste Manag.* **2015**, *46*, 140–145. [CrossRef]
54. Strapazzon, J.; Aralde, Q.M.; Dos Anjos, M.B.; Cozer, M.; França, V.F. Sobras e resto ingesta: Uma avaliação do desperdício. *Nutr. Bras.* **2015**, *14*, 127–131. [CrossRef]
55. de Sousa, B.J.; Monteiro, C.C.; Costa, V.P.G.; Borges, T.A.d.M.; de Oliva, P.A.B.F. Food consumption and plate waste study in a public hospital food service in Natal, RN, Brazil. *GSC Adv. Res. Rev.* **2022**, *11*, 56–65. [CrossRef]
56. Thiagarajah, K.; Getty, V.M. Impact on Plate Waste of Switching from a Tray to a Trayless Delivery System in a University Dining Hall and Employee Response to the Switch. *J. Acad. Nutr. Diet.* **2013**, *113*, 141–145. [CrossRef] [PubMed]
57. Viana, K.L.S.; de Souza, A.L.M. Avaliação Do Indice De Resto Ingestão, Antes E Durante Uma Campanha Educativa, Em Unidade De Alimentação E Nutrição (Uan), Porto Velho-Ro. *Rev. Eletrônica UNIVAG* **2016**. [CrossRef]
58. Viana, R.M.; Ferreira, L.C. Avaliação Do Desperdício De Alimentos Em Unidade De Alimentação E Nutrição Cidade De Januária. MG. *Hig. Aliment.* **2017**, *31*, 22–26.
59. Zandonadi, H.S.; Maurício, A.A. Avaliação Do Índice De Resto-Ingesta. De Refeições Consumidas Por Trabalhadores Da Construção Civil No Município De Cuiabá. *Hig. Aliment.* **2012**, *26*, 64–70.
60. Zeineddine, M.; Kharroubi, S.; Chalak, A.; Hassan, H.; Abiad, M.G. Post-Consumer Food Waste Generation While Dining Out: A Close-Up View. *PLoS ONE* **2021**, *16*, e0251947. [CrossRef]
61. Wang, L.-E.; Liu, G.; Liu, X.; Liu, Y.; Gao, J.; Zhou, B.; Gao, S.; Cheng, S. The Weight of Unfinished Plate: A Survey Based Characterization of Restaurant Food Waste in Chinese Cities. *Waste Manag.* **2017**, *66*, 3–12. [CrossRef]
62. Carrijo, A.D.P.; Botelho, R.B.A.; de Almeida Akutsu, R.D.C.C.; Zandonadi, R.P. Is What Low-Income Brazilians Are Eating in Popular Restaurants Contributing to Promote Their Health? *Nutrients* **2018**, *10*, 414. [CrossRef]
63. Lafraire, J.; Rioux, C.; Giboreau, A.; Picard, D. Food Rejections in Children: Cognitive and Social/Environmental Factors Involved in Food Neophobia and Picky/Fussy Eating Behavior. *Appetite* **2016**, *96*, 347–357. [CrossRef]
64. Juvan, E.; Grün, B.; Baruca, P.Z.; Dolnicar, S. Drivers of Plate Waste at Buffets: A Comprehensive Conceptual Model Based on Observational Data and Staff Insights. *Ann. Tour. Res. Empir. Insights* **2021**, *2*, 100010. [CrossRef]

Disclaimer/Publisher's Note: The statements, opinions and data contained in all publications are solely those of the individual author(s) and contributor(s) and not of MDPI and/or the editor(s). MDPI and/or the editor(s) disclaim responsibility for any injury to people or property resulting from any ideas, methods, instructions or products referred to in the content.

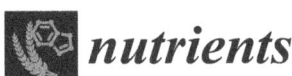 *nutrients*

Systematic Review

Combined Effects of Physical Activity and Diet on Cancer Patients: A Systematic Review and Meta-Analysis

Petros C. Dinas [1,2,*], on behalf of the Students of Module 5104 (Introduction to Systematic Reviews) [1,†], Marianthi Karaventza [1], Christina Liakou [3], Kalliopi Georgakouli [1], Dimitrios Bogdanos [4] and George S. Metsios [1]

1. Department of Nutrition and Dietetics, School of Physical Education, Sport Science and Dietetics, University of Thessaly, 42130 Trikala, Greece; aikmakri@uth.gr (on behalf of the Students of Module 5104 (Introduction to Systematic Reviews)); markaraventza@gmail.com (M.K.); kgeorgakouli@uth.gr (K.G.); g.metsios@uth.gr (G.S.M.)
2. FAME Laboratory, School of Physical Education, Sport Science and Dietetics, University of Thessaly, 42131 Trikala, Greece
3. School of Physical Education, Sport Science and Dietetics, University of Thessaly, 42131 Trikala, Greece; cliakou@uth.gr
4. Department of Internal Medicine, University Hospital of Larissa, Faculty of Medicine, School of Health Sciences, University of Thessaly, 41110 Larissa, Greece; bogdanos@uth.gr
* Correspondence: petros.cd@gmail.com
† A full list of the co-authors is provided in Appendix A.

Abstract: Background: The purpose of our systematic review was to examine the effects of any physical activity/exercise intervention combined with any diet/nutrition intervention on any biological/biochemical index, quality of life (QoL), and depression in breast, lung, colon and rectum, prostate, stomach, and liver cancer patients and/or cancer survivors. Methods: A systematic review and meta-analysis were undertaken, using PRISMA guidelines and the Cochrane Handbook. The systematic review protocol can be found in the PROSPERO database; registration number: CRD42023481429. Results: We found moderate-quality evidence that a combined intervention of physical activity/exercise and nutrition/diet reduced body mass index, body weight, fat mass, insulin, homeostatic model assessment for insulin resistance, C-reactive protein, triglycerides, and depression, while it increased high-density lipoprotein, the physical component of QoL, and general functional assessment of cancer therapy. Conclusions: We conclude that a combined intervention of physical activity/exercise and diet/nutrition may decrease body weight, fat mass, insulin levels, and inflammation, and improve lipidemic profile, the physical component of QoL, and depression in cancer patients and survivors. These outcomes indicate a lower risk for carcinogenesis; however, their applicability depends on the heterogeneity of the population and interventions, as well as the potential medical treatment of cancer patients and survivors.

Keywords: nutrition; exercise; cancer indices

1. Introduction

Cancer is a group of diseases that can affect almost all organs and tissues in the human body. It is characterized by the rapid creation of abnormal cells that grow unusually and spread around the body, which causes a cascade of unfavorable health effects [1]. Potential reasons for the development of cancer cells include exposure to ultraviolet and ionizing radiation, certain chemicals (e.g., asbestos, tobacco smoke, and alcohol), nutritional contaminants, and certain infections [1]. The most common types of cancers that appear in humans are breast, lung, colorectal, prostate, skin, and stomach cancers [1]. Cancer is a leading cause of human deaths worldwide, with approximately 10 million deaths in 2020; the most lethal cancers are lung, colon and rectum, liver, stomach, and breast cancer [1].

Cancer is also a major health burden, given its remarkable physical, emotional, and financial stress on patients, communities, and national health systems, especially those in low-income countries [1]. Recent evidence from 29 types of cancers and 204 countries and territories shows that the economic cost of cancers between 2020 and 2050 will be USD 25.2 trillion [2]. This is a substantial burden for national health systems, indicating the need for countermeasures to prevent and treat cancer. To date, several initiatives have been undertaken to reduce the cancer health burden and subsequently economic cost, such as the United Nations Sustainable Development Goal target 3.4 [3], the European Code Against Cancer [4], and the World Health Organization (WHO) Global Action Plan for the Prevention and Control of Noncommunicable Diseases [5].

The main pillars to consider for cancer prevention are as follows: (i) factors of cancer risk, namely smoking and tobacco use, infections, radiation, immunosuppressive medicines, and organ transplant; and (ii) factors that may pose a risk of cancer, namely nutrition, alcohol, physical inactivity, obesity, diabetes, and environmental factors [6]. Evidence on the contribution of several diets to cancer development is controversial, given that there are foods that reduce the risk of cancer and foods that increase the risk of cancer [7]. For instance, consumption of >1 sugar-sweetened beverage per day increases the incidence of liver cancer [8], while consumption of green-yellow and cruciferous vegetables reduces cancer risk [9]. Furthermore, evidence from systematic reviews [10–12] showed small or uncertain effects of red meat consumption, or a reduction in its consumption, on cancer prevalence and mortality. Also, there is no association between animal protein or plant protein consumption and cancer mortality [13]. Alcohol consumption is associated with an increased risk of breast cancer, whereas consumption of fruits and vegetables is inversely associated with lung cancer [7]. Regarding physical activity, there is solid evidence that increased levels are associated with a 20% reduced risk of breast cancer and a 40–50% reduced risk of colorectal cancer [7]. This evidence suggests that physical activity is a very promising intervention to reduce cancer incidence. Cancer patients also have a poor quality of life (QoL) [14] and depression [15]. It was found that only 5.02% of cancer patients displayed high QoL and 12.54% displayed average QoL [14]. Evidence has shown that increased physical activity reduces depression levels, whereas high intensities of physical activity cause euphoria due to increased production of β-endorphin in the brain, indicating decreased levels of anxiety and depression [16].

There is a growing interest in exploring the effects of combined dietary and physical activity interventions on cancer patients. Indeed, several randomized controlled trials explored this issue [17–20]. To the best of our knowledge, there is no relevant systematic review that has summarized this evidence. Therefore, the purpose of our systematic review was to examine the effects of any physical activity/exercise intervention combined with any diet/nutrition intervention on any biological/biochemical index, quality of life (QoL), and depression in breast, lung, colon and rectum, prostate, stomach, and liver cancer patients and/or cancer survivors.

2. Materials and Methods

A systematic review and meta-analysis were undertaken, using the Preferred Reporting Items for Systematic Reviews and Meta-analyses (PRISMA) guidelines [21] and the Cochrane Handbook [22]. We registered a systematic review in the International Prospective Register of Systematic Reviews (PROSPERO) database; registration number: CRD42023481429 [23].

2.1. Searching and Selection Processes

PubMed, EMBASE, and SportDiscus were explored from their inception to November 2023. We applied no limitations in the search for the date, language of publication, and study design. The search algorithm for PubMed is shown in Supplement S1 (pages 1–2). The co-authors shaped the keyword algorithm, and the search was completed by PCD and tested by GSM. Seven teams of co-authors were created to execute the selection procedure.

Each team assessed an equal number of retrieved publications according to the eligibility criteria. The results of the selection procedure were tested by PCD, and any disagreements were resolved by a referee (GSM). Finally, PCD screened the reference lists of eligible publications to identify any additional eligible publications.

2.2. Inclusion and Exclusion Criteria

The eligible studies included the following:

1. Population: Adult human (>18 years) breast, lung, colon and rectum, prostate, stomach, and liver cancer patients, and/or cancer survivors. Patients at any cancer stage, with any comorbidity, at any body mass index (BMI), or under any pharmacological treatment were included.
2. Intervention: Any physical activity/exercise intervention combined with any diet/nutrition intervention, as well as physical and/or remote counseling, behavioral models, education as a combined physical activity/exercise, and diet/nutrition intervention, as long as this intervention was specific and measurable. Interventions took place for at least two weeks.
3. Comparator: As a control condition, we included randomized controlled trials (RCT) with a control group (i.e., usual care) and RCT with a cross-over design control condition.
4. Outcome: Measurement of biological/biochemical indices, QoL, and depression.
5. Study design: RCTs with parallel or cross-over design.
6. We rejected studies that involved animals, reviews, letters, congress papers, magazines, and gray literature.

2.3. Risk of Bias Assessment

The Risk of Bias 2 (RoB2) Cochrane library tool was incorporated to assess the eligible RCTs [24]. Each team of co-authors evaluated an equal number of eligible papers. PCD coordinated the process, and GSM acted as a referee in the case of conflicts.

2.4. Data Extraction

The following data were extracted: (a) first author name and year of publication, (b) participants' anthropometric characteristics (i.e., age, gender, and BMI), (c) cancer type and cancer stage, (d) physical activity/exercise interventions/measurements, (e) diet/nutrition interventions/measurements, and (f) outcomes. The study characteristics are displayed in Supplement S1 (Table S1, pages 3–17). An initial data extraction calibration was performed to determine the type of data and format that should be extracted. Each team of co-authors extracted data from an equal number of eligible publications. PCD coordinated the data extraction procedure, and GSM acted as a referee in the case of conflicts.

2.5. Data Synthesis

We incorporated a narrative data synthesis for eligible studies that offered no data for meta-analyses. To conduct our meta-analyses, we used a random-effect model due to the heterogeneity of the eligible studies in characteristics, such as populations, type of cancer, physical activity/exercise, and diet/nutrition interventions and duration. We used the RevMan 5.4.1, 2020 software (The Cochrane Collaboration, London, UK) [25] to perform the meta-analyses. An inverse variance continuous method was incorporated to test the mean differences (MD) between a combined intervention of physical activity/exercise and diet/nutrition and a control group/condition. A standardized mean difference (SMD) method was used for different units of the variables included in the meta-analysis [22]. The following variables were used in our meta-analyses: BMI, body weight (kg), fat mass (kg), fat-free mass (kg), insulin levels, homeostatic model assessment for insulin resistance (HOMA-IR), glucose, C-reactive protein, high-density lipoprotein (HDL), low-density lipoprotein (LDL), triglycerides, bone mineral density, components of QoL (physical, mental, social, and bodily pain), and depression. Standard errors were converted into standard deviations (SD) using the equation: SD = $standard\ error * \sqrt{n}$ [22]. Similarly, in the case of medians and if the 1st–3rd quartiles were provided, we calculated the mean and SD using the following equation: $mean = (q1 + m + q3)/3$; SD = $(q3 - q1)/1.35$ [22,26]. Overall, from the 38 eligible RCTs, 30 offered data for a meta-analysis [17–20,27–52]. For all meta-analyses, we created forest plots, but we produced funnel plots when a meta-analysis included >10 studies [22].

2.6. Quality of Evidence

We evaluated the quality of evidence for each meta-analysis using the Grading of Recommendations Assessment, Development, and Evaluation (GRADE) analysis [22,53].

3. Results

3.1. Searching and Selection Processes Results

The search procedure yielded 4337 publications. We removed 306 duplicate publications, and 848 were ineligible by screening their titles. The remaining 3183 publications were screened for eligibility (titles, abstract, and full texts), and 2037 of them were excluded, given that they were reviews, editorials, case reports, consensus papers, and conference proceedings. We also excluded 1113 publications that did not fulfill the eligibility criteria. Thus, 33 publications were included as eligible. We then screened the reference lists of these 33 publications (overall 1594 citations) and we identified five more eligible publications that did not appear in the initial search procedure. In total, 38 publications were finally included as eligible for our systematic review. A PRISMA flow diagram can be found in Supplement S1 (Figure S1, page 18).

3.2. Risk of Bias Assessment Results

In total, 30 (79%) out of 38 eligible studies displayed an overall high risk of bias, mainly due to a high risk of bias in the "measurement of the outcome" (55% of the studies) and the "selection of the reported results" (37% of the studies). Two (5%) eligible studies [27,31] showed an overall low risk, and six (16%) eligible studies [18,30,38,45,48,54] overall displayed some concerns of bias. The detailed risk of bias assessment results can be found in Table S2 in Supplement S1 (pages 19–20), and a summary of the risk of bias can be found in Figure 1.

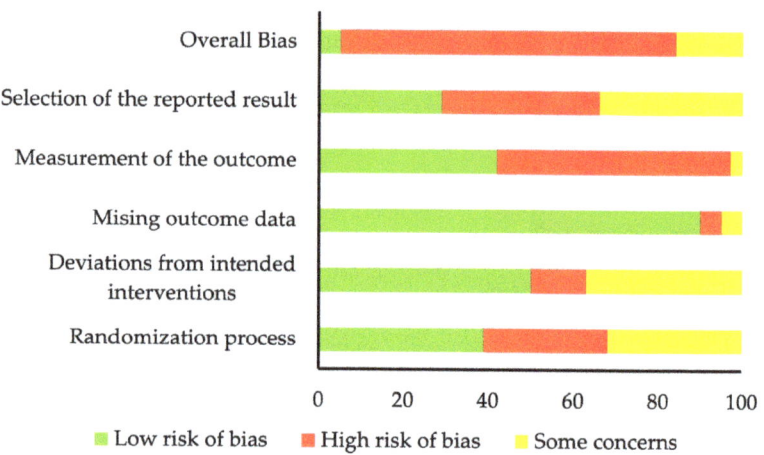

Figure 1. Summary of risk of bias assessment.

3.3. Narrative Data Synthesis Results

Eight eligible studies [54–61] did not offer data for a meta-analysis; therefore, a narrative data synthesis approach was used. The results of this synthesis can be found in Table 1.

Table 1. Narrative data synthesis results. Green color represents a positive effect of the intervention; orange color represents no effect of the intervention; QoL = quality of life; BMI = body mass index; WCRF = World Cancer Research Fund.

Study	Aim	Type of Exercise/Physical Activity and Diet/Nutrition	Outcome
Brown 2022 (Breast cancer) [55]	To examine the effects of the intervention (physical activity and diet) on sex steroid hormones.	Duration: 52 weeks. Exercise Type: Resistance + aerobic. Exercise Content: 9 exercises twice weekly, 2–3 sets, weight permitted 10 repetitions. Moderate-intensity aerobic exercise, 180 min 3–6 days/week. Diet Type: Hypocaloric diet 10% loss of body weight. Diet Content: 7 daily servings of fruits and vegetables; behavioral techniques to prepare food.	No effect of the intervention on sex steroid hormones.
Schmitz 2019 (Breast cancer) [59]	To examine the effects of the intervention (physical activity and diet) on breast cancer-related lymphedema.	Duration: 52 weeks. Exercise Type: Walking + resistance exercises Exercise Content: Walking goals/week were 90 min for weeks 1–3, 120 min for week 4, 150 min for weeks 5–6, and 180 min thereafter. Intensity was limited by 0.45–0.90 kg per 2 weeks, up to 9.45 kg, twice/session during weeks 1–6 and 3 times/session thereafter. Diet Type: Weight loss. Diet Content: Weeks 1–20: 7 servings of fruits and vegetables per day. Weeks 21–24 lessons for preparing food. Weeks 25–52, monthly meetings for weigh-ins and weight maintenance instructions, to achieve 10% weight reduction in comparison to baseline.	The intervention did not improve breast cancer-related lymphedema.
Brown 2023 (Breast cancer) [56]	To examine the effects of the intervention (physical activity and diet) on oxidative stress and telomere length.	Duration: 52 weeks. Exercise Type: Resistance + aerobic. Exercise Content: 9 exercises twice weekly, 2–3 sets, weight permitted 10 repetitions. Moderate-intensity aerobic exercise, 180 min 3–6 days/week. Diet Type: Hypocaloric diet 10% loss of body weight. Diet Content: 7 portions of fruits and vegetables per day; behavioral techniques to prepare food.	The intervention was associated with reduced oxidative stress. No effect of the intervention on telomere length.
Carayol 2019 (Breast cancer) [57]	To examine the effects of the intervention (physical activity and diet) on cancer-related fatigue, QoL, anxiety, depression, BMI, and body composition.	Duration: 26 weeks. Exercise Type: Resistance + aerobic. Exercise Content: 1 resistance session/week, 2–5 sets, 6–12 repetitions. Two moderate-intensity 30–45 min aerobic sessions/week, 50–75% maximum heart rate. Diet Type: Balanced dietary intake. Diet Content: Diet prepared according to WCRF.	The intervention had positive changes in terms of psychological, physiological, and behavioral outcomes.

Table 1. Cont.

Study	Aim	Type of Exercise/Physical Activity and Diet/Nutrition	Outcome
Karimi 2013 (Breast cancer) [54]	To examine the effects of the intervention (physical activity and diet) on adiponectin and oxidative stress.	Duration: 6 weeks. Exercise Type: Water-based exercise. Exercise Content: 50–75% of heart rate reserve, in a pool, 4 times/week. Diet Type: Oral ginger supplement. Diet Content: Ginger rhizome powder (750 mg) in 250 mL of water, 4 times/day, during all main meals and in the afternoon.	The intervention had an antioxidant and anti-dysmetabolism effect.
Sanft 2018 (Breast cancer) [58]	To examine the effects of the intervention (physical activity and diet) on telomere length.	Duration: 6 months. Exercise Type: Home-based exercise (walking). Exercise Content: 150 min/week of moderate-intensity activity and 10,000 steps/day. Diet Type: Reduced caloric intake. Diet Content: Reduction of 1200–2000 kcal/day, based on baseline weight, and decreasing fat to <25% of total energy intake.	The intervention led to telomere lengthening.
Frattaroli 2008 (Prostate cancer) [60]	To examine the effects of the intervention (physical activity and diet) on prostate-specific antigen.	Duration: 2 years. Exercise Type: Moderate aerobic exercise. Exercise Content: Walking 30 min/day, 6 days/week. Diet Type: Vegan diet. Diet Content: Fruits, vegetables, whole grains, legumes, and soy products, low in carbohydrates, and 10% of calorie intake from fat.	The intervention allowed active surveillance to delay conventional treatment.
Lee 2018 (Colorectal cancer) [61]	To examine the effects of the intervention (physical activity and diet) on consumption of red and processed meat.	Duration: 12 months. Exercise Type: Moderate to vigorous physical activity. Exercise Content: 60 min of moderate-vigorous physical activity, 5 days/week. Diet Type: Consultation using interviews and phone calls. Diet Content: High dietary fiber, low red and processed meat, and refined grain.	The intervention showed potential for the cancer survivors to modify their dietary habits.

3.4. Meta-Analysis Outcomes

3.4.1. Biological/Biochemical Indices

We found that the intervention reduced BMI [(MD = −0.67, confidence interval (CI) = (−1.09)–(−0.25), Z = 3.14, I^2 = 38%, and p = 0.002; Figure 2, Figure S2 in Supplement S1, page 20]. Subgroup analysis revealed no differences between cancer types (p > 0.05; Figure S3 in Supplement S1, page 20.

Study or Subgroup	Exercise+Diet Mean	SD	Total	Control Mean	SD	Total	Weight	Mean Difference IV, Random, 95% CI
Freedland 2019 (prostate)	23.66	14.44	11	31.2	6.75	18	0.2%	−7.54 [−16.63, 1.55]
Mefferd 2007 (breast)	28.7	4.2	47	31.2	5.1	29	3.3%	−2.50 [−4.71, −0.29]
Pakiz 2011 (breast)	28.7	2.5	44	31.2	3.7	24	5.4%	−2.50 [−4.15, −0.85]
Puklin 2023 (breast)	30.2	4.09	45	31.72	3.26	41	6.0%	−1.52 [−3.08, 0.04]
O'Neil 2015 (prostate)	29	4.5	47	30	4.5	47	4.6%	−1.00 [−2.82, 0.82]
Fruge 2018 (prostate)	29.03	3.78	11	30	4	11	1.6%	−0.97 [−4.22, 2.28]
Hebert 2012 (prostate)	28.5	5.33	26	29.2	5.38	21	1.8%	−0.70 [−3.78, 2.38]
Demark-Wahnefried 2012 (multiple)	28.2	3.28	269	28.8	3.4	289	21.4%	−0.60 [−1.15, −0.05]
Morey 2009 (multiple)	28.42	1.25	319	28.89	1.44	322	31.4%	−0.47 [−0.68, −0.26]
Bourke 2014 (prostate)	27.9	1.96	35	28.2	1.9	33	13.0%	−0.30 [−1.22, 0.62]
Jacot 2020 (breast)	25.29	4.79	180	24.95	5.01	180	11.4%	0.34 [−0.67, 1.35]
Total (95% CI)			1034			1015	100.0%	−0.67 [−1.09, −0.25]

Heterogeneity: Tau^2 = 0.13; Chi^2 = 16.11, df = 10 (P = 0.10); I^2 = 38%
Test for overall effect: Z = 3.14 (P = 0.002)

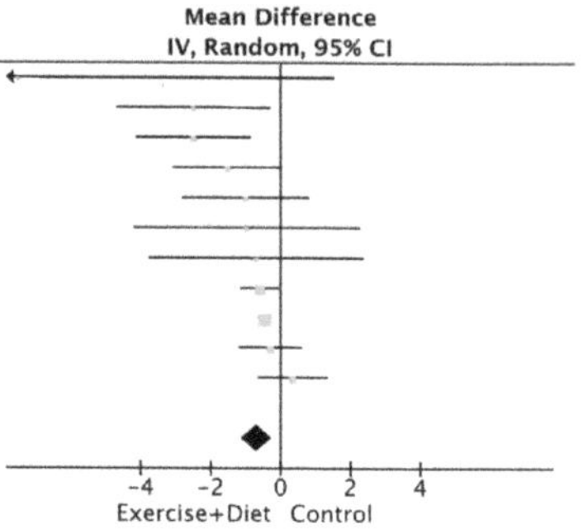

Figure 2. Forest plot of the effects of physical activity/exercise and diet/nutrition intervention on body mass index. SD: standard deviation; CI: confidence interval.

We also found that the intervention decreased body weight [(MD = −2.88, CI = (−4.30)–(−1.45), Z = 3.95, I^2 = 86%, and p < 0.0001; Figure 3, Figure S4 in Supplement S1, page 21]. Subgroup analysis (p = 0.001) revealed that the intervention was more effective in breast cancer (MD = −3.50) than in prostate cancer (MD = −3.19) and in patients with multiple cancers (MD = 0.07); Figure 3.

The fat mass of cancer patients and survivors was also reduced due to the intervention [(MD = −2.85, CI = (−4.45)–(−1.25), Z = 3.49, I^2 = 79%, and p = 0.0005; Figure 4, Figure S5 in Supplement S1, page 21]. Subgroup analysis showed no differences between cancer types (Figure S6 in Supplement S1, page 22).

A meta-analysis of the effects of the intervention on fat-free mass showed that this was reduced in the control group [(MD = −1.04, CI = (−1.84)–(−0.23), Z = 2.53, I^2 = 74%, and p = 0.01; Figure 5, Figure S7 in Supplement S1, page 22], with no differences between cancer types (p > 0.05; Figure S8 in Supplement S1, page 23).

Six studies offered data for the meta-analysis of insulin levels. This revealed that the intervention decreased insulin levels compared to the control group [(SMD = −0.41, CI = (−0.74)–(−0.08), Z = 2.44, I^2 = 45%, p = 0.01; Figure 6], with no differences between cancer types (p > 0.05; Figure S9 in Supplement S1, page 23).

In line with insulin levels, a meta-analysis of HOMA-IR showed that the intervention reduced insulin levels [(SMD = −0.55, CI = (−0.77)–(−0.33), Z = 4.98, I^2 = 0%, and p < 0.00001; Figure 7], whereas there was no effect on glucose levels (p > 0.05; Figure S10 in Supplement S1, page 23).

Regarding the chronic inflammation indices of cancer patients and survivors, a meta-analysis of C-reactive protein showed that the intervention reduced this [(MD = −0.97, CI = (−1.88)–(−0.06), Z = 2.09, I^2 = 69%, and p = 0.01; Figure 8], whereas a subgroup analysis revealed that this occurs only in patients and survivors with breast cancer but not in those with prostate cancer (p = 0.02 and I^2 = 82.2%; Figure 8).

Study or Subgroup	Exercise+Diet Mean	Exercise+Diet SD	Exercise+Diet Total	Control Mean	Control SD	Control Total	Weight	Mean Difference IV, Random, 95% CI
1.5.1 Breast cancer								
Puklin 2021 (breast)	79.6	14.9	76	90.6	13.98	52	3.8%	-11.00 [-16.07, -5.93]
Harrigan 2016 (breast-in telephone)	75.23	15.04	15	85.1	18.67	19	1.3%	-9.87 [-21.20, 1.46]
Pakiz 2011 (breast)	78.2	8.3	44	87	10.6	24	4.0%	-8.80 [-13.70, -3.90]
Mefferd 2007 (breast)	78.2	12.6	47	85.8	15	29	2.9%	-7.60 [-14.14, -1.06]
Reeves 2016 (breast)	77.6	4.79	45	83.1	3.93	45	6.6%	-5.50 [-7.31, -3.69]
Brown 2021 (breast)	84.25	6.25	87	89.03	5.98	90	6.6%	-4.78 [-6.58, -2.98]
Reeves 2021 (breast)	80.87	5.49	68	83.04	5.35	60	6.6%	-2.17 [-4.05, -0.29]
Puklin 2023 (breast)	83.5	4.37	102	85.54	2.63	103	7.2%	-2.04 [-3.03, -1.05]
Harrigan 2016 (breast)	83.63	17.26	22	85.1	18.67	19	1.4%	-1.47 [-12.54, 9.60]
Sanft 2023 (breast)	78	24.5	87	78.2	22.8	86	2.6%	-0.20 [-7.25, 6.85]
Jacot 2020 (breast)	67.57	13.56	180	66.23	12.93	180	5.8%	1.34 [-1.40, 4.08]
Greenlee 2013 (breast)	83.34	3.21	21	81.66	3.77	17	6.2%	1.68 [-0.58, 3.94]
Subtotal (95% CI)			**794**			**724**	**55.0%**	**-3.50 [-5.41, -1.59]**
Heterogeneity: Tau² = 6.98; Chi² = 59.64, df = 11 (P < 0.00001); I² = 82%								
Test for overall effect: Z = 3.60 (P = 0.0003)								
1.5.2 Prostate cancer								
Chaplow 2020 (prostate)	92.1	2.91	16	99.48	1.7	14	6.7%	-7.38 [-9.06, -5.70]
Fruge 2018 (prostate)	89.63	8.52	11	95.23	6.15	11	3.1%	-5.60 [-11.81, 0.61]
Focht 2018 (prostate)	92.64	14.48	14	97.36	19.15	11	1.0%	-4.72 [-18.34, 8.90]
O'Neil 2015 (prostate)	85.9	10.5	47	90	14.3	47	3.8%	-4.10 [-9.17, 0.97]
Baguley 2022 (prostate)	88.7	1.94	11	91.6	1.94	10	6.7%	-2.90 [-4.56, -1.24]
Wilson 2021 (prostate)	95.5	14.1	14	98.3	14.7	14	1.4%	-2.80 [-13.47, 7.87]
Freedland 2019 (prostate)	88.23	26.07	11	88.33	15.78	18	0.6%	-0.10 [-17.14, 16.94]
Bourke 2011 (prostate)	81.8	10.2	25	81.5	8.2	25	3.8%	0.30 [-4.83, 5.43]
Bourke 2014 (prostate)	86.6	10.2	35	84.8	8.2	33	4.4%	1.80 [-2.59, 6.19]
Subtotal (95% CI)			**184**			**183**	**31.5%**	**-3.19 [-5.84, -0.54]**
Heterogeneity: Tau² = 8.17; Chi² = 26.59, df = 8 (P = 0.0008); I² = 70%								
Test for overall effect: Z = 2.36 (P = 0.02)								
1.5.3 Multiple cancers								
Morey 2009 (multiple)	83.64	3.39	319	83.78	3.59	322	7.3%	-0.14 [-0.68, 0.40]
Demark-Wahnefried 2012 (multiple)	83.31	13.56	243	82.03	13.46	245	6.1%	1.28 [-1.12, 3.68]
Subtotal (95% CI)			**562**			**567**	**13.5%**	**0.07 [-0.92, 1.06]**
Heterogeneity: Tau² = 0.22; Chi² = 1.28, df = 1 (P = 0.26); I² = 22%								
Test for overall effect: Z = 0.14 (P = 0.89)								
Total (95% CI)			**1540**			**1474**	**100.0%**	**-2.88 [-4.30, -1.45]**
Heterogeneity: Tau² = 7.15; Chi² = 157.27, df = 22 (P < 0.00001); I² = 86%								
Test for overall effect: Z = 3.95 (P < 0.0001)								
Test for subgroup differences: Chi² = 13.70, df = 2 (P = 0.001), I² = 85.4%								

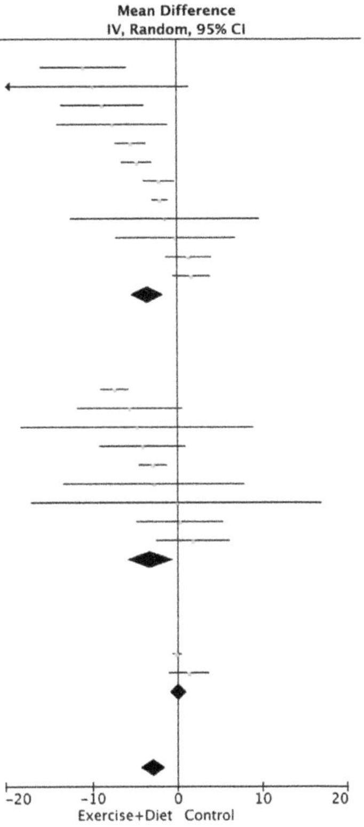

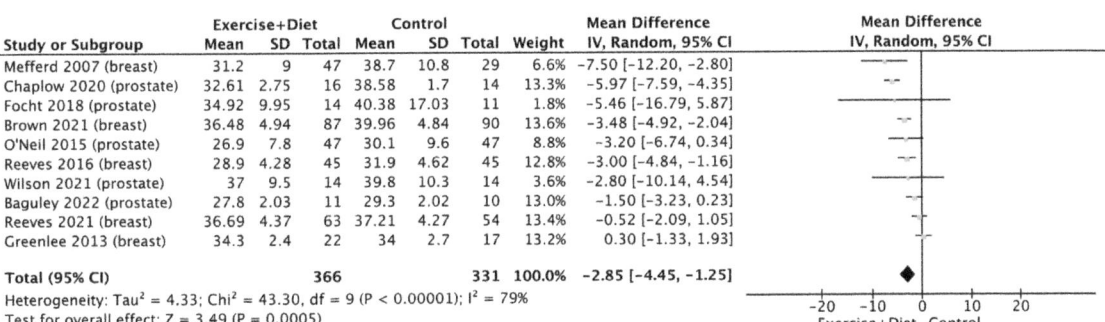

Figure 3. Forest plot of the effects of physical activity/exercise and diet/nutrition intervention on body weight. SD: standard deviation; CI: confidence interval.

Study or Subgroup	Exercise+Diet Mean	Exercise+Diet SD	Exercise+Diet Total	Control Mean	Control SD	Control Total	Weight	Mean Difference IV, Random, 95% CI
Mefferd 2007 (breast)	31.2	9	47	38.7	10.8	29	6.6%	-7.50 [-12.20, -2.80]
Chaplow 2020 (prostate)	32.61	2.75	16	38.58	1.7	14	13.3%	-5.97 [-7.59, -4.35]
Focht 2018 (prostate)	34.92	9.95	14	40.38	17.03	11	1.8%	-5.46 [-16.79, 5.87]
Brown 2021 (breast)	36.48	4.94	87	39.96	4.84	90	13.6%	-3.48 [-4.92, -2.04]
O'Neil 2015 (prostate)	26.9	7.8	47	30.1	9.6	47	8.8%	-3.20 [-6.74, 0.34]
Reeves 2016 (breast)	28.9	4.28	45	31.9	4.62	45	12.8%	-3.00 [-4.84, -1.16]
Wilson 2021 (prostate)	37	9.5	14	39.8	10.3	14	3.6%	-2.80 [-10.14, 4.54]
Baguley 2022 (prostate)	27.8	2.03	11	29.3	2.02	10	13.0%	-1.50 [-3.23, 0.23]
Reeves 2021 (breast)	36.69	4.37	63	37.21	4.27	54	13.4%	-0.52 [-2.09, 1.05]
Greenlee 2013 (breast)	34.3	2.4	22	34	2.7	17	13.2%	0.30 [-1.33, 1.93]
Total (95% CI)			**366**			**331**	**100.0%**	**-2.85 [-4.45, -1.25]**
Heterogeneity: Tau² = 4.33; Chi² = 43.30, df = 9 (P < 0.00001); I² = 79%								
Test for overall effect: Z = 3.49 (P = 0.0005)								

Figure 4. Forest plot of the effects of physical activity/exercise and diet/nutrition intervention on fat mass. SD: standard deviation; CI: confidence interval.

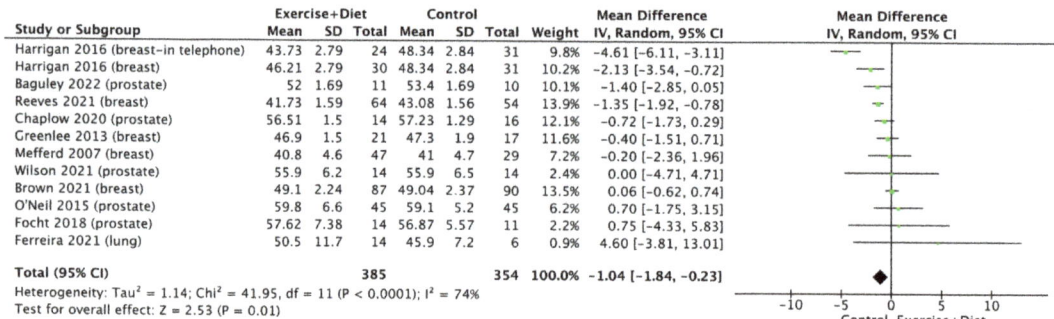

Figure 5. Forest plot of the effects of physical activity/exercise and diet/nutrition intervention on fat-free mass. SD: standard deviation; CI: confidence interval.

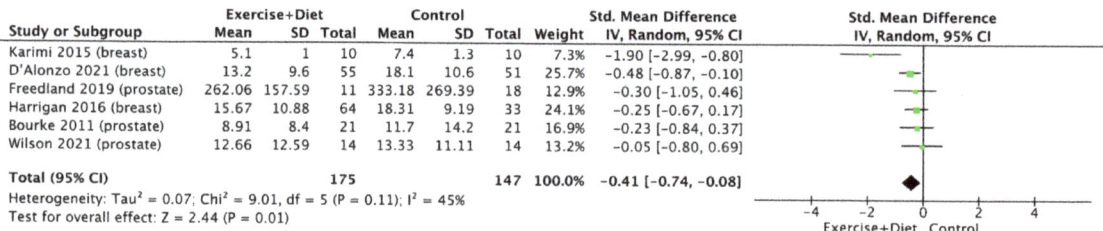

Figure 6. Forest plot of the effects of physical activity/exercise and diet/nutrition intervention on insulin levels. SD: standard deviation; CI: confidence interval.

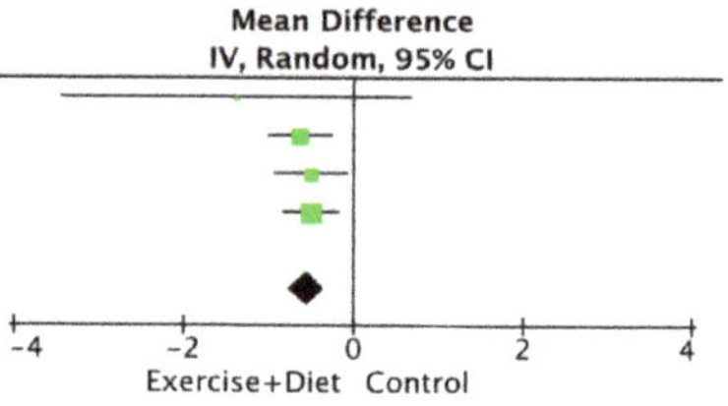

Figure 7. Forest plot of the effects of physical activity/exercise and diet/nutrition intervention on homeostatic assessment model for insulin resistance. SD: standard deviation; CI: confidence interval.

Regarding the lipidemic profile of the participants, HDL increased due to the intervention (SMD = 0.34, CI = 0.07–0.61, Z = 2.49, I^2 = 29%, and p = 0.01; Figure 9), whereas there were no differences between cancer types ($p > 0.05$; Figure S11 in Supplement S1, page 24). Additionally, the intervention had no effect on LDL ($p > 0.05$; Figure S12 in Supplement S1, page 24), whereas the intervention decreased triglycerides [(SMD = −0.38, CI = (−0.62)–(−0.14), Z = 3.09, I^2 = 0%, and p = 0.002; Figure 10], with no differences between cancer types ($p > 0.05$; Figure S13 in Supplement S1, page 24). Finally, no effect of the intervention was found in bone mineral density ($p > 0.05$; Figure S14 in Supplement S1, page 25).

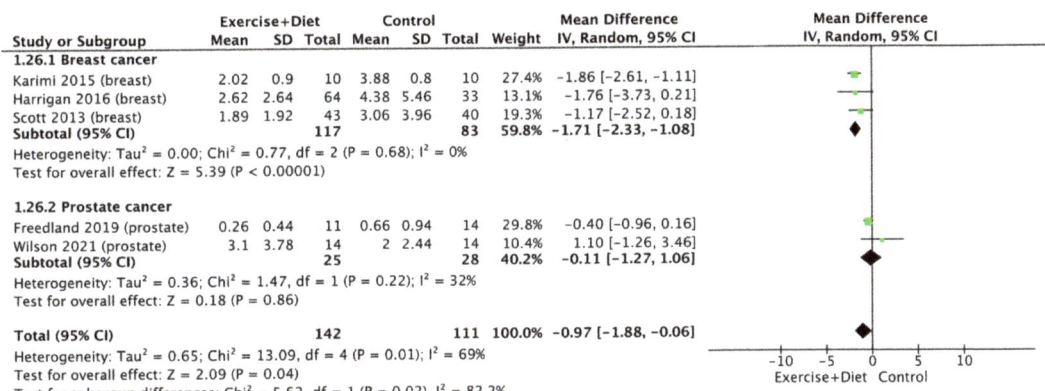

Figure 8. Forest plot of the effects of physical activity/exercise and diet/nutrition intervention on C-reactive protein. SD: standard deviation; CI: confidence interval.

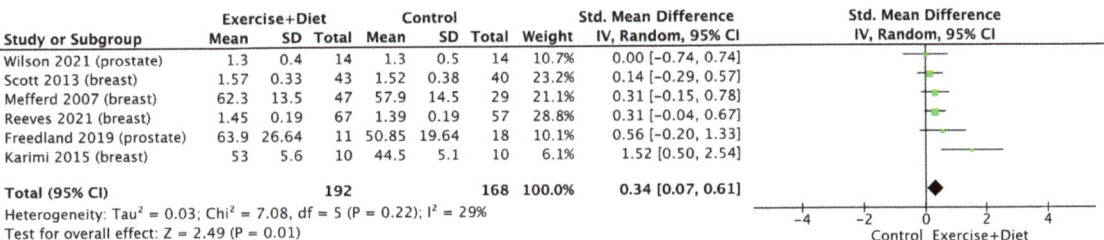

Figure 9. Forest plot of the effects of physical activity/exercise and diet/nutrition intervention on high-density lipoprotein. SD: standard deviation; CI: confidence interval.

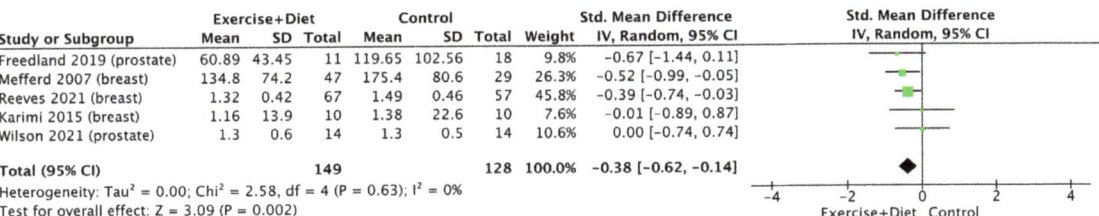

Figure 10. Forest plot of the effects of physical activity/exercise and diet/nutrition intervention on triglycerides. SD: standard deviation; CI: confidence interval.

3.4.2. Quality of Life Indices

Meta-analyses on QoL indices showed no effect of the intervention on the mental health summary score ($p > 0.05$; Figure S15 in Supplement S1, page 25), social functioning ($p > 0.05$; Figure S16 in Supplement S1, page 25), and bodily pain ($p > 0.05$; Figure S17 in Supplement S1, page 25). On the other hand, the intervention showed an increase in the physical component summary score (SMD = 0.20, CI = 0.09–0.31, Z = 3.70, $I^2 = 0\%$, and $p = 0.0002$; Figure 11), with no differences between cancer types ($p > 0.05$; Figure S18 in Supplement S1, page 26). Similarly, the intervention increased QoL physical functioning (SMD = 0.18, CI = 0.06–0.29, Z = 2.99, $I^2 = 0\%$, and $p = 0.003$; Figure 12), with no differences between cancer types ($p > 0.05$; Figure S19 in Supplement S1, page 26).

Study or Subgroup	Exercise+Diet Mean	SD	Total	Control Mean	SD	Total	Weight	Std. Mean Difference IV, Random, 95% CI
Baguley 2022 (prostate)	48.7	6.09	11	49.6	6.13	10	1.6%	−0.14 [−1.00, 0.72]
Reeves 2016 (breast)	49.5	88.8	43	49.1	10.5	44	6.5%	0.01 [−0.41, 0.43]
Morey 2009 (multiple)	73.75	16.07	319	70.76	16.15	322	47.4%	0.19 [0.03, 0.34]
O'Neil 2015 (prostate)	22.7	5.7	45	21.4	6.1	45	6.6%	0.22 [−0.20, 0.63]
Reeves 2021 (breast)	47.96	6.9	65	46.4	6.6	58	9.1%	0.23 [−0.13, 0.58]
Brown 2021a (breast)	69.49	15.86	87	65.6	16.41	90	13.1%	0.24 [−0.06, 0.54]
Ferreira 2021 (lung)	67	20.1	18	61.8	21.2	8	1.6%	0.25 [−0.59, 1.08]
Ho 2020 (colorectal)	50.1	5.1	55	48.3	7.3	56	8.2%	0.28 [−0.09, 0.66]
Daubenmier 2006 (prostate)	53.2	6.6	40	50.2	9.5	42	6.0%	0.36 [−0.07, 0.80]
Total (95% CI)			**683**			**675**	**100.0%**	**0.20 [0.09, 0.31]**

Heterogeneity: Tau² = 0.00; Chi² = 2.29, df = 8 (P = 0.97); I² = 0%
Test for overall effect: Z = 3.70 (P = 0.0002)

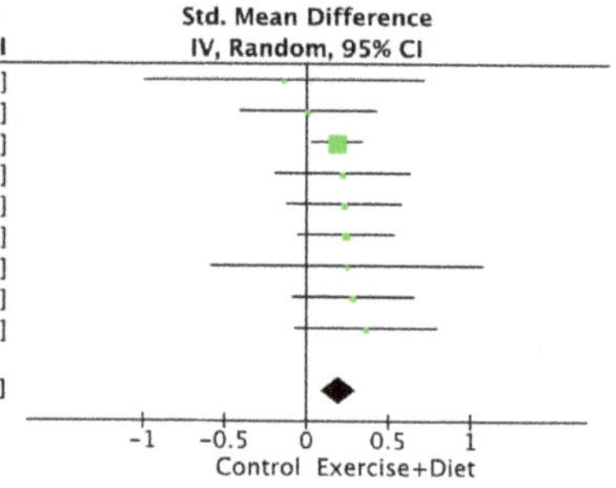

Figure 11. Forest plot of the effects of physical activity/exercise and diet/nutrition intervention on quality of life physical component summary score. SD: standard deviation; CI: confidence interval.

Study or Subgroup	Exercise+Diet Mean	SD	Total	Control Mean	SD	Total	Weight	Std. Mean Difference IV, Random, 95% CI
Ferreira 2021 (lung)	59.4	26.5	18	69.4	26	8	1.9%	−0.37 [−1.21, 0.47]
Baguley 2022 (prostate)	78.3	15.99	11	82.2	16.05	10	1.8%	−0.23 [−1.09, 0.63]
Jacot 2020 (breast)	86.49	17.11	180	84.4	15.38	180	31.8%	0.13 [−0.08, 0.34]
Demark-Wahnefried 2012 (multiple)	74.4	17.88	269	70.5	18.7	289	49.0%	0.21 [0.05, 0.38]
Brown 2021a (breast)	74.03	16.04	87	69.36	16.41	90	15.5%	0.29 [−0.01, 0.58]
Total (95% CI)			**565**			**577**	**100.0%**	**0.18 [0.06, 0.29]**

Heterogeneity: Tau² = 0.00; Chi² = 3.41, df = 4 (P = 0.49); I² = 0%
Test for overall effect: Z = 2.99 (P = 0.003)

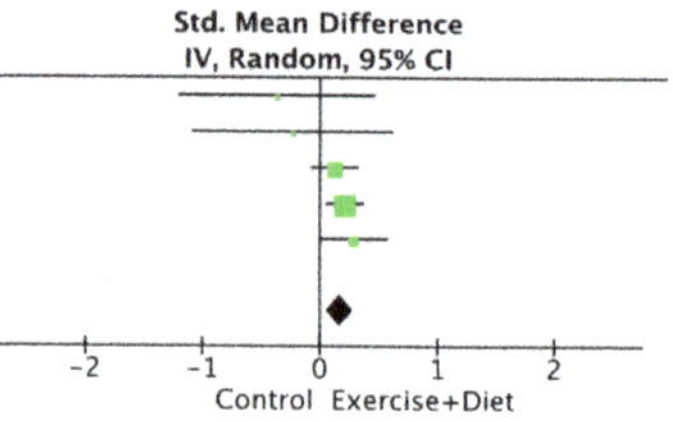

Figure 12. Forest plot of the effects of physical activity/exercise and diet/nutrition intervention on quality of life physical functioning. SD: standard deviation; CI: confidence interval.

Finally, the meta-analyses revealed that the intervention increased the general functional assessment of cancer therapy (FACT-general) (MD = 4.41, CI = 1.34–7.48, Z = 2.81, I² = 0%, and p = 0.005; Figure 13), as well as decreased depression (MD = −0.99, CI = (−1.92)–(−0.06), Z = 2.09, I² = 47%, and p = 0.04; Figure 14) in cancer patients and survivors.

Study or Subgroup	Exercise+Diet Mean	SD	Total	Control Mean	SD	Total	Weight	Mean Difference IV, Random, 95% CI
O'Neil 2015 (prostate)	83.9	15.2	45	83.4	16.6	45	21.8%	0.50 [−6.08, 7.08]
Bourke 2011 (prostate)	91	10	21	86	18	22	12.6%	5.00 [−3.65, 13.65]
Ho 2020 (colorectal)	95.8	7.6	55	90.2	12.3	56	65.5%	5.60 [1.80, 9.40]
Total (95% CI)			**121**			**123**	**100.0%**	**4.41 [1.34, 7.48]**

Heterogeneity: Tau² = 0.00; Chi² = 1.75, df = 2 (P = 0.42); I² = 0%
Test for overall effect: Z = 2.81 (P = 0.005)

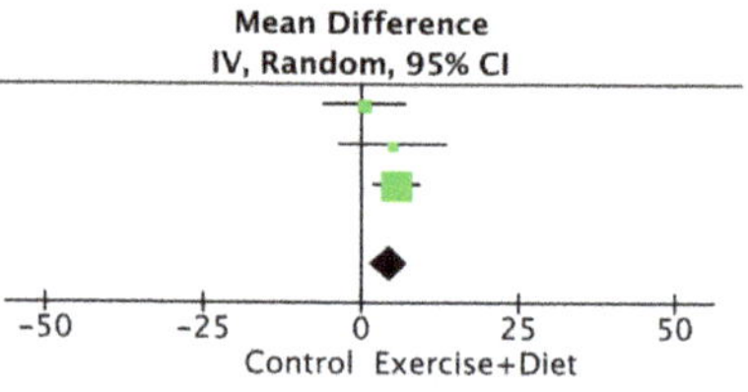

Figure 13. Forest plot of the effects of physical activity/exercise and diet/nutrition intervention on the general functional assessment of cancer therapy. SD: standard deviation; CI: confidence interval.

Study or Subgroup	Exercise+Diet Mean	SD	Total	Control Mean	SD	Total	Weight	Mean Difference IV, Random, 95% CI
Ho 2020 (colorectal)	8.5	1.8	55	10.1	3	56	42.5%	−1.60 [−2.52, −0.68]
Ferreira 2021 (lung)	3.7	2.7	18	4.9	3.4	8	10.4%	−1.20 [−3.87, 1.47]
Jacot 2020 (breast)	19.87	3.62	124	20.26	2.87	130	47.1%	−0.39 [−1.20, 0.42]
Total (95% CI)			**197**			**194**	**100.0%**	**−0.99 [−1.92, −0.06]**

Heterogeneity: Tau² = 0.31; Chi² = 3.81, df = 2 (P = 0.15); I² = 47%
Test for overall effect: Z = 2.09 (P = 0.04)

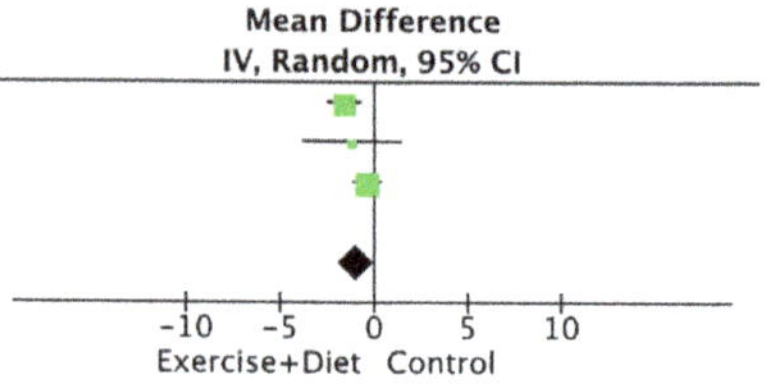

Figure 14. Forest plot of the effects of physical activity/exercise and diet/nutrition intervention on depression. SD: standard deviation; CI: confidence interval.

3.5. Quality of Evidence Results

The GRADE analysis revealed 2 out of 13 meta-analyses as low-quality evidence, while 11 meta-analyses were rated as moderate quality, mainly because of the high risk of bias that the eligible studies displayed. The outcomes of the GRADE analysis can be found in Table 2, and the detailed GRADE analysis for each meta-analysis can be found in Supplement S2.

Table 2. GRADE analysis outcomes: CI: confidence interval; BMI: body mass index; MD: mean difference; SMD: standardized mean difference; HOMA-IR: homeostatic assessment mode for insulin resistance; HDL: high-density lipoprotein; FACT: functional assessment of cancer therapy.

Outcomes	No of Participants (Studies/Entries)	Quality of the Evidence (GRADE)	Relative Effect (95% CI)
Exercise+Diet vs. Control BMI	2049 (11 studies/entries)	Moderate ⊕⊕⊕◯ due risk of bias	MD: −0.67, CI: −1.09, −0.25
Exercise+Diet vs. Control Body weight	3014 (23 studies/entries)	Low ⊕⊕◯◯ due to risk of bias and inconsistency of results	MD: −2.88, CI: −4.30, −1.25
Exercise+Diet vs. Control Fat mass	697 (10 studies/entries)	Low ⊕⊕◯◯ due to risk of bias and inconsistency of results	MD: −2.85, CI: −4.45, −1.25
Exercise+Diet vs. Control Fat-Free mmass	739 (12 studies/entries)	Moderate ⊕⊕⊕◯ due risk of bias	MD: −1.04, CI: −1.84, −0.23
Exercise+Diet vs. Control Insulin	322 (6 studies/entries)	Moderate ⊕⊕⊕◯ due risk of bias	SMD: −0.41, CI: −0.74, −0.08
Exercise+Diet vs. Control HOMA-IR	238 (4 studies/entries)	Moderate ⊕⊕⊕◯ due risk of bias	MD: −0.55, CI: −0.77, −0.33
Exercise+Diet vs. Control C-reactive protein	253 (5 studies/entries)	Moderate ⊕⊕⊕◯ due risk of bias	MD: −0.97, CI: −1.88, −0.06
Exercise+Diet vs. Control HDL	360 (6 studies/entries)	Moderate ⊕⊕⊕◯ due risk of bias	SMD: 0.34, CI: 0.07, 0.61
Exercise+Diet vs. Control Triglycerides	297 (5 studies/entries)	Moderate ⊕⊕⊕◯ due risk of bias	SMD: −0.38, CI: −0.62, −0.14
Exercise+Diet vs. Control QoL physical component summary score	1358 (9 studies/entries)	Moderate ⊕⊕⊕◯ due risk of bias	SMD: 0.20, CI: 0.09, 0.31
Exercise+Diet vs. Control QoL physical functioning	1142 (5 studies/entries)	Moderate ⊕⊕⊕◯ due risk of bias	SMD: 0.18, CI: 0.06, 0.29
Exercise+Diet vs. Control FACT general	244 (3 studies/entries)	Moderate ⊕⊕⊕◯ due risk of bias	MD: 4.41, CI: 1.34, 7.48
Exercise+Diet vs. Control Depression	391 (3 studies/entries)	Moderate ⊕⊕⊕◯ due risk of bias	MD: −0.99, CI: −1.92, −0.06

4. Discussion

4.1. Summary of Main Findings

The current systematic review and meta-analysis revealed moderate-quality evidence that combined intervention of physical activity/exercise and diet/nutrition reduced BMI, insulin, HOMA-IR, C-reactive protein, triglycerides, and depression in the intervention group, while it reduced fat-free mass in the control group. The meta-analysis also revealed low-quality evidence that the intervention reduced body weight and fat mass, while moderate-quality evidence showed that it increased HDL, QoL physical component summary score, QoL physical functioning, and FACT general.

The narrative data synthesis showed that combined intervention of physical activity/exercise and diet/nutrition had no effect on sex steroid hormones and breast cancer-related lymphedema. On the other hand, the intervention reduced oxidative stress and improved psychological, physiological, and behavioral outcomes, while it had an antidysmetabolism effect, leading to telomere lengthening, delayed conventional treatment, and modified dietary habits.

4.2. Completeness and Applicability of Evidence

We found an adequate number of studies with an adequate sample size (n > 5000) to test whether the combined intervention of physical activity/exercise and diet/nutrition can affect the body weight and body composition of cancer patients and survivors. Our results showed that the intervention reduced BMI, body weight, and fat mass by 0.67 kg/m^2, 2.88 kg, and 2.85 kg, respectively, within a period of 3–12 months. Considering that there is a positive association between BMI, body weight, and fat mass [62], our findings are particularly important given that excessive body weight and adiposity can enhance cancer development [63]. Also, a reduction in fat mass is associated with a generally favorable metabolic profile (e.g., reduced circulating insulin levels) [64] and an inflammatory profile [65]. Indeed, excessive adipose tissue is associated with higher levels of insulin, which may enhance the proliferation of cancer cells [64]. Our meta-analysis showed that a combined intervention of physical activity/exercise and diet/nutrition reduced the insulin and HOMA-IR levels. A potential explanation is that physical activity/exercise can increase insulin sensitivity through increased expression of Glucose transporter-4 in the plasma membrane of skeletal muscle cells [66], while a reduction in sweet drinks, sweets, and consumption of low glycemic index food, as well as diets rich in fibers, may improve insulin sensitivity [67]. Regarding inflammation, we found that a combined intervention of physical activity/exercise and diet/nutrition reduced C-reactive protein, indicating a reduction in chronic inflammation, and thus, a reduction in carcinogenesis risk [63]. Collectively, a combined intervention of physical activity/exercise and diet/nutrition has the potential to reduce cancer development, which is particularly important in cancer survivors.

A previous systematic review showed that a combination of exercise and weight loss through energy-restricted diets can effectively reduce fat mass in overweight and obese individuals without posing a risk for sarcopenia [68]. In our meta-analysis, we found moderate-quality evidence that the control group of cancer patients and survivors reduced their fat-free mass during the period of the intervention. This is not a favorable effect, given that fat-free mass, particularly muscle mass, may produce a number of myokines with anti-inflammatory effects and increased insulin sensitivity, which is consequently associated with a reduced risk of cancer development [65]. A possible explanation for our finding is that cancer mortality is associated with decreased lean mass [69], indicating that cancer patients display relatively low levels of lean mass, including muscle mass. The extent to which we apply a combined intervention of physical activity/exercise and diet/nutrition to cancer patients and survivors should be approached with caution to avoid muscle mass reduction. One suggestion is to use a combination of resistance exercise and diets rich in protein, known to increase muscle mass [70].

We also detected moderate-quality evidence that a combined intervention of physical activity/exercise and diet/nutrition reduced triglycerides and increased HDL levels. Physical activity/exercise is associated with decreased levels of triglycerides and increased levels of HDL [71], whereas several nutrient consumption and/or diets have decreased triglycerides and increased HDL [72]. This beneficial effect may reduce cancer risk due to the involvement of triglycerides in the pathogenesis of several cancers, including lung, prostate, and rectal cancer [73]. We also detected moderate-quality evidence that a combined intervention of physical activity/exercise and diet/nutrition reduced depression in cancer patients and survivors. Depression results in higher rates of mortality among cancer patients [15,74] and poor QoL [15]. Physical activity/exercise reduces depression levels, while high intensities of physical activity/exercise cause euphoria due to increased production of β-endorphin in the brain, indicating decreased levels of depression [16]. Furthermore, a 12-week aerobic exercise program decreased depression levels [75], whereas a Cochrane systematic review showed that yoga exercise can reduce short-term symptoms of depression, anxiety, and fatigue in breast cancer patients [76]. Also, certain fatty acids (i.e., n-3 long-chain polyunsaturated, omega-3) consumption may improve depressive symptoms [77,78]. Depression is closely associated with poor QoL [15]. We found moderate-quality evidence that a combined intervention of physical activity/exercise and diet/nutrition improved both general physical functioning and functional assessment of cancer therapy in cancer patients and survivors. This outcome shows the already reported beneficial effect of physical activity/exercise on QoL in clinical populations [79], whereas the effect of dietary interventions on QoL is not well documented [80].

The narrative data synthesis offered limited data to answer our research question. There was an opposite outcome between the two studies [56,58] regarding the effects of a combined intervention of physical activity/exercise and diet/nutrition on telomere length. A previous systematic review showed that higher adherence to the Mediterranean diet is related to longer telomere length [81], whereas another systematic review showed that various dietary interventions are not associated with telomere length [82]. This evidence may partly explain the opposite outcome we observed in our systematic review, given that the diet interventions in the included studies were not entirely related to the Mediterranean diet (Table 1). Regarding exercise, the opposite outcome may be explained by the fact that the study that found no effect of the combined intervention on telomere length [56] used resistance along with aerobic exercise intervention. A previous systematic review showed that only aerobic exercise may improve telomere length [83], which was used in our included study [58] and showed a positive effect on telomere length. The rest of the narrative data synthesis outcomes are general and disparate.

The overall applicability of the evidence is moderate, based on the quality of the available evidence in the current systematic review and meta-analysis. However, given the heterogeneity of the interventions included in our meta-analysis (i.e., different physical activity/exercise types and modes and various diets and supplements), the outcomes of our systematic review should be treated with specific analysis. For instance, considering the specific characteristics of the populations and interventions involved in our systematic review, to apply interventions in practice.

4.3. Strengths and Limitations

The strengths of our systematic review include the development of a search algorithm using standardized indexing terms, which may capture papers that use another keyword to describe the same term [22]. Screening of eligible studies, risk of bias assessment, and data extraction were performed by two independent investigators. We accepted studies in any language and from any time of publication. Finally, we evaluated the quality of the meta-analyses using the GRADE analysis, which added value to their interpretation.

Limitations of our systematic review include the large heterogeneity of the populations, especially in the type of measurements, physical activity/exercise, and diet/nutrition schemes, which may have affected the interpretation of the results. Also, it was not possible to consider potential medicine schemes that were received by the participants due to missing information in the eligible publications. This may have affected the results of the eligible studies and, consequently, our systematic review results.

4.4. Important Deviations from the Published Protocol

We report no significant deviations from the published protocol [23].

5. Conclusions

We conclude that a combined intervention of physical activity/exercise and diet/nutrition may decrease body weight, fat mass, insulin levels, and inflammation and improve lipidemic profiles in cancer patients and survivors. We also conclude that a combined intervention of physical activity/exercise and diet/nutrition may improve the physical component of QoL, as well as depression levels, in cancer patients and survivors. These outcomes indicate a lower risk for carcinogenesis; however, their applicability depends on the heterogeneity of the population and interventions, as well as the potential medical treatment of cancer patients and survivors.

Supplementary Materials: The following supporting information can be downloaded at: https://www.mdpi.com/article/10.3390/nu16111749/s1, Figure S1. PRISMA flow diagram; Figure S2. Funnel plot on the effects of diet/nutrition and physical activity/exercise intervention on body mass index; Figure S3. Subgroup analysis of the effects of diet/nutrition and physical activity/exercise intervention on body mass index; Figure S4. Funnel plot on the effects of diet/nutrition and physical activity/exercise intervention on body weight; Figure S5. Funnel plot of the effects of diet/nutrition and physical activity/exercise intervention on fat mass; Figure S6. Subgroup analysis of the effects of diet/nutrition and physical activity/exercise intervention on fat mass; Figure S7. Funnel plot of the effects of diet/nutrition and physical activity/exercise intervention on fat free mass; Figure S8. Subgroup analysis of the effects of diet/nutrition and physical activity/exercise intervention on fat free mass; Figure S9. Subgroup analysis of the effects of diet/nutrition and physical activity/exercise intervention on insulin levels; Figure S10. Subgroup analysis of the effects of diet/nutrition and physical activity/exercise intervention on glucose levels; Figure S11. Subgroup analysis of the effects of diet/nutrition and physical activity/exercise intervention on HDL; Figure S12. Forest plot of the effects of diet/nutrition and physical activity/exercise intervention on LDL; Figure S13. Subgroup analysis of the effects of diet/nutrition and physical activity/exercise intervention on triglycerides; Figure S14. Forest plot of the effects of diet/nutrition and physical activity/exercise intervention on bone mineral density; Figure S15. Forest plot of the effects of diet/nutrition and physical activity/exercise intervention on QoL mental health summary score; Figure S16. Forest plot of the effects of diet/nutrition and physical activity/exercise intervention on QoL social functioning; Figure S17. Forest plot of the effects of diet/nutrition and physical activity/exercise intervention on QoL bodily pain; Figure S18. Subgroup analysis of the effects of diet/nutrition and physical activity/exercise intervention on QoL physical component summary score; Figure S19. Subgroup analysis of the effects of diet/nutrition and physical activity/exercise intervention on QoL physical functioning; Table S1. Characteristics of eligible studies. BMI: body mass index; QoL: quality of life; WCRF: world cancer research fund; HIIT: high intensity interval training; NR: not reported; HR: heart rate; RM: repetition maximum; CI: confidence interval; IQR: interquartile range; CDC: centre for disease control; ACSM: American college of sport medicine; HOMA-IR: homeostatic model assessment-insulin resistance. Table S2. Risk of bias assessment results.

Author Contributions: P.C.D.: Conceptualization, methodology, software, formal analysis, data curation, writing—original draft preparation, writing—review and editing, and supervision. Students of Module 5104 (Introduction to Systematic Reviews) (see Appendix A): Conceptualization, methodology, searching, risk of bias and data extraction, and review and editing. G.S.M. and D.B.: Conceptualization, methodology, writing—review and editing, and supervision. M.K., C.L. and K.G.: Conceptualization, searching, risk of bias assessment, data extraction, and checking the extracted data to be used for meta-analyses. All authors have read and agreed to the published version of the manuscript.

Funding: This research received no external funding.

Data Availability Statement: Extracted data used in the meta-analyses are available upon reasonable request.

Conflicts of Interest: The authors declare no conflicts of interest.

Appendix A

List of students who meet the criteria for co-authors (in alphabetical order)

	Full Name	Email
1	Apostolos Kamnitsas	akamnitsas@uth.gr
2	Aristoula Tzalidi	atzalidi@uth.gr
3	Aikaterini Pipertzi	apipertzi@uth.gr
4	Aikaterini Makedoniti	amakedoniti@uth.gr

	Full Name	Email
5	Aikaterini Makri	aikmakri@uth.gr
6	Asteria Skliri	askliri@uth.gr
7	Asteria Sideri Tsiami	asideri-tsami@uth.gr
8	Anastasia Riyinou	ariginou@uth.gr
9	Alkmini Rouchota	arouchota@uth.gr
10	Anastasia Kraniotaki	akraniotaki@uth.gr
11	Aggeliki Chalvatzi	anchalvantzi@uth.gr
12	Anastasia Kanaridou	akanaridou@uth.gr
13	Ariandi Marinou	armarinou@uth.gr
14	Angelos Chaniotakis	achaniotakis@uth.gr
15	Alexandros Foteinos	afoteinos@uth.gr
16	Apostolos Aggelos Patsatzis	apatsatzis@uth.gr
17	Argiro Diotima Tiktopoulou	atiktopoulou@uth.gr
18	Chariklia Fygka	cfygka@uth.gr
19	Chariklia Petropoulou	cpetropoulou@uth.gr
20	Chrisanthi Kyriazi Theodori	chkyriazi@uth.gr
21	Dimitris Grigoriou	dimgrigoriou@uth.gr
22	Eirini Mitou	emitou@uth.gr
23	Eirini Mpalampani	ebalampani@uth.gr
24	Eirini Pavlou	eirpavlou@uth.gr
25	Eugenia Anthi	eanthi@uth.gr
26	Evdokia Chatzimanoli	evchatzimanoli@uth.gr
27	Eleni Sofia Kapsokavadi	ekapsokavadi@uth.gr
28	Euaggelia Vordoni	evordoni@uth.gr
29	Eleni Papadima	elpapadima@uth.gr
30	Elisavet Pappa	elipappa@uth.gr
31	Ermioni Dimopoulou	erdimopoulou@uth.gr
32	Georgia Fafaliou	gfafaliou@uth.gr
33	Georgios Kalogiannakis	gkalogiannakis@uth.gr
34	Ioanna Apostolou	ioapostolou@uth.gr
35	Ioannis Manolarakis	imanolarakis@uth.gr
36	Konstantina Stamou	kstamou@uth.gr
37	Konstantina Michailidou	konmichailidou@uth.gr
38	Maria Gerostergiou	mgerostergiou@uth.gr
39	Maria Liveri	mliveri@uth.gr
40	Maria Mpoufikou	maboufikou@uth.gr
41	Maria Paschalidou	mapaschalidou@uth.gr
42	Marianthi Aristea Vasilopoulou	mvasilopoul@uth.gr
43	Marianthi Koropouli	vkotopouli@uth.gr
44	Nikolaos Gerasimos Efthimiadis	niefthymiadis@uth.gr
45	Niki Stathi	nstathi@uth.gr
46	Niki Ioanna Karanikola	nkaranikola@uth.gr

	Full Name	Email
47	Nektaria Dimitra Kotsiari	nkotsiari@uth.gr
48	Paoulina Maria Pietchoux	ppietsouch@uth.gr
49	Paraskevi Mpourda	pbourda@uth.gr
50	Petros Stefanidis	pstefanidis@uth.gr
51	Sevastiani Voulgaraki	svoulgaraki@uth.gr
52	Vasiliki Kotopouli	vkotopouli@uth.gr
53	Vasiliki Paraskevi Voutiritsa	voutyritsa@uth.gr
54	Vasiliki Alexaki	valexaki@uth.gr
55	Zoi Nona	znona@uth.gr
56	Zinovia Bermperi	zbermperi@uth.gr

References

1. World Health Organization. Cancer. Available online: https://www.who.int/news-room/fact-sheets/detail/cancer (accessed on 26 March 2024).
2. Chen, S.; Cao, Z.; Prettner, K.; Kuhn, M.; Yang, J.; Jiao, L.; Wang, Z.; Li, W.; Geldsetzer, P.; Bärnighausen, T.; et al. Estimates and Projections of the Global Economic Cost of 29 Cancers in 204 Countries and Territories from 2020 to 2050. *JAMA Oncol.* **2023**, *9*, 465–472. [CrossRef] [PubMed]
3. NCD Countdown 2030 collaborators. NCD Countdown 2030: Worldwide trends in non-communicable disease mortality and progress towards Sustainable Development Goal target 3.4. *Lancet* **2018**, *392*, 1072–1088. [CrossRef] [PubMed]
4. Schüz, J.; Espina, C.; Villain, P.; Herrero, R.; Leon, M.E.; Minozzi, S.; Romieu, I.; Segnan, N.; Wardle, J.; Wiseman, M.; et al. European Code against Cancer 4th Edition: 12 ways to reduce your cancer risk. *Cancer Epidemiol.* **2015**, *39* (Suppl. 1), S1–S10. [CrossRef] [PubMed]
5. World Health Organization. Global Action Plan for the Prevention and Control of Noncommunicable Diseases 2013–2020. Available online: https://apps.who.int/iris/handle/10665/94384 (accessed on 26 March 2024).
6. National Cancer Institute. Cancer Prevention Overview (PDQ®)–Patient Version. Available online: https://www.cancer.gov/about-cancer/causes-prevention/patient-prevention-overview-pdq (accessed on 26 March 2024).
7. National Cancer Institute. Cancer Prevention Overview (PDQ®)–Health Professional Version. Available online: https://www.cancer.gov/about-cancer/causes-prevention/hp-prevention-overview-pdq (accessed on 26 March 2024).
8. Zhao, L.; Zhang, X.; Coday, M.; Garcia, D.O.; Li, X.; Mossavar-Rahmani, Y.; Naughton, M.J.; Lopez-Pentecost, M.; Saquib, N.; Shadyab, A.H.; et al. Sugar-Sweetened and Artificially Sweetened Beverages and Risk of Liver Cancer and Chronic Liver Disease Mortality. *JAMA* **2023**, *330*, 537–546. [CrossRef] [PubMed]
9. Aune, D.; Giovannucci, E.; Boffetta, P.; Fadnes, L.T.; Keum, N.; Norat, T.; Greenwood, D.C.; Riboli, E.; Vatten, L.J.; Tonstad, S. Fruit and vegetable intake and the risk of cardiovascular disease, total cancer and all-cause mortality-a systematic review and dose-response meta-analysis of prospective studies. *Int. J. Epidemiol.* **2017**, *46*, 1029–1056. [CrossRef] [PubMed]
10. Han, M.A.; Zeraatkar, D.; Guyatt, G.H.; Vernooij, R.W.M.; El Dib, R.; Zhang, Y.; Algarni, A.; Leung, G.; Storman, D.; Valli, C.; et al. Reduction of Red and Processed Meat Intake and Cancer Mortality and Incidence: A Systematic Review and Meta-analysis of Cohort Studies. *Ann. Intern. Med.* **2019**, *171*, 711–720. [CrossRef] [PubMed]
11. Vernooij, R.W.M.; Zeraatkar, D.; Han, M.A.; El Dib, R.; Zworth, M.; Milio, K.; Sit, D.; Lee, Y.; Gomaa, H.; Valli, C.; et al. Patterns of Red and Processed Meat Consumption and Risk for Cardiometabolic and Cancer Outcomes: A Systematic Review and Meta-analysis of Cohort Studies. *Ann. Intern. Med.* **2019**, *171*, 732–741. [CrossRef] [PubMed]
12. Zeraatkar, D.; Johnston, B.C.; Bartoszko, J.; Cheung, K.; Bala, M.M.; Valli, C.; Rabassa, M.; Sit, D.; Milio, K.; Sadeghirad, B.; et al. Effect of Lower Versus Higher Red Meat Intake on Cardiometabolic and Cancer Outcomes: A Systematic Review of Randomized Trials. *Ann. Intern. Med.* **2019**, *171*, 721–731. [CrossRef] [PubMed]
13. Naghshi, S.; Sadeghi, O.; Willett, W.C.; Esmaillzadeh, A. Dietary intake of total, animal, and plant proteins and risk of all cause, cardiovascular, and cancer mortality: Systematic review and dose-response meta-analysis of prospective cohort studies. *BMJ* **2020**, *370*, m2412. [CrossRef]
14. Alam, M.M.; Rahman, T.; Afroz, Z.; Chakraborty, P.A.; Wahab, A.; Zaman, S.; Hawlader, M.D.H. Quality of Life (QoL) of cancer patients and its association with nutritional and performance status: A pilot study. *Heliyon* **2020**, *6*, e05250. [CrossRef]
15. Smith, H.R. Depression in cancer patients: Pathogenesis, implications and treatment (Review). *Oncol. Lett.* **2015**, *9*, 1509–1514. [CrossRef]
16. Dinas, P.C.; Koutedakis, Y.; Flouris, A.D. Effects of exercise and physical activity on depression. *Ir. J. Med. Sci.* **2011**, *180*, 319–325. [CrossRef] [PubMed]

17. Jacot, W.; Arnaud, A.; Jarlier, M.; Lefeuvre-Plesse, C.; Dalivoust, P.; Senesse, P.; Azzedine, A.; Tredan, O.; Sadot-Lebouvier, S.; Mas, S.; et al. Brief Hospital Supervision of Exercise and Diet During Adjuvant Breast Cancer Therapy Is Not Enough to Relieve Fatigue: A Multicenter Randomized Controlled Trial. *Nutrients* **2020**, *12*, 3081. [CrossRef] [PubMed]
18. Focht, B.C.; Lucas, A.R.; Grainger, E.; Simpson, C.; Fairman, C.M.; Thomas-Ahner, J.M.; Buell, J.; Monk, J.P.; Mortazavi, A.; Clinton, S.K. Effects of a Group-Mediated Exercise and Dietary Intervention in the Treatment of Prostate Cancer Patients Undergoing Androgen Deprivation Therapy: Results from the IDEA-P Trial. *Ann. Behav. Med.* **2018**, *52*, 412–428. [CrossRef] [PubMed]
19. O'Neill, R.F.; Haseen, F.; Murray, L.J.; O'Sullivan, J.M.; Cantwell, M.M. A randomised controlled trial to evaluate the efficacy of a 6-month dietary and physical activity intervention for patients receiving androgen deprivation therapy for prostate cancer. *J. Cancer Surviv.* **2015**, *9*, 431–440. [CrossRef] [PubMed]
20. Puklin, L.S.; Harrigan, M.; Cartmel, B.; Sanft, T.; Gottlieb, L.; Zhou, B.; Ferrucci, L.M.; Li, F.Y.; Spiegelman, D.; Sharifi, M.; et al. Randomized Trial Evaluating a Self-Guided Lifestyle Intervention Delivered via Evidence-Based Materials versus a Waitlist Group on Changes in Body Weight, Diet Quality, Physical Activity, and Quality of Life among Breast Cancer Survivors. *Cancers* **2023**, *15*, 4719. [CrossRef] [PubMed]
21. Page, M.J.; McKenzie, J.E.; Bossuyt, P.M.; Boutron, I.; Hoffmann, T.C.; Mulrow, C.D.; Shamseer, L.; Tetzlaff, J.M.; Akl, E.A.; Brennan, S.E.; et al. The PRISMA 2020 statement: An updated guideline for reporting systematic reviews. *BMJ* **2021**, *372*, n71. [CrossRef] [PubMed]
22. Higgins, J.P.T.; Thomas, J.; Chandler, J.; Cumpston, M.; Li, T.; MJ, P. *Cochrane Handbook for Systematic Review of Interventions Version 6.2*; Cochrane Collaboration: London, UK, 2021.
23. PROSPERO. Available online: https://www.crd.york.ac.uk/prospero/display_record.php?RecordID=481429 (accessed on 22 February 2024).
24. Sterne, J.A.C.; Savović, J.; Page, M.J.; Elbers, R.G.; Blencowe, N.S.; Boutron, I.; Cates, C.J.; Cheng, H.-Y.; Corbett, M.S.; Eldridge, S.M.; et al. RoB 2: A revised tool for assessing risk of bias in randomised trials. *BMJ* **2019**, *366*, l4898. [CrossRef] [PubMed]
25. Review Manager (RevMan) [Computer Program]. Version 5.4.1. The Cochrane Collaboration: London, UK, 2020. Available online: https://revman.cochrane.org (accessed on 22 February 2024).
26. Wan, X.; Wang, W.; Liu, J.; Tong, T. Estimating the sample mean and standard deviation from the sample size, median, range and/or interquartile range. *BMC Med. Res. Methodol.* **2014**, *14*, 135. [CrossRef]
27. Bourke, L.; Gilbert, S.; Hooper, R.; Steed, L.A.; Joshi, M.; Catto, J.W.; Saxton, J.M.; Rosario, D.J. Lifestyle changes for improving disease-specific quality of life in sedentary men on long-term androgen-deprivation therapy for advanced prostate cancer: A randomised controlled trial. *Eur. Urol.* **2014**, *65*, 865–872. [CrossRef]
28. Demark-Wahnefried, W.; Morey, M.C.; Sloane, R.; Snyder, D.C.; Miller, P.E.; Hartman, T.J.; Cohen, H.J. Reach out to enhance wellness home-based diet-exercise intervention promotes reproducible and sustainable long-term improvements in health behaviors, body weight, and physical functioning in older, overweight/obese cancer survivors. *J. Clin. Oncol.* **2012**, *30*, 2354–2361. [CrossRef]
29. Freedland, S.J.; Howard, L.; Allen, J.; Smith, J.; Stout, J.; Aronson, W.; Inman, B.A.; Armstrong, A.J.; George, D.; Westman, E.; et al. A lifestyle intervention of weight loss via a low-carbohydrate diet plus walking to reduce metabolic disturbances caused by androgen deprivation therapy among prostate cancer patients: Carbohydrate and prostate study 1 (CAPS1) randomized controlled trial. *Prostate Cancer Prostatic Dis.* **2019**, *22*, 428–437. [CrossRef]
30. Frugé, A.D.; Ptacek, T.; Tsuruta, Y.; Morrow, C.D.; Azrad, M.; Desmond, R.A.; Hunter, G.R.; Rais-Bahrami, S.; Demark-Wahnefried, W. Dietary Changes Impact the Gut Microbe Composition in Overweight and Obese Men with Prostate Cancer Undergoing Radical Prostatectomy. *J. Acad. Nutr. Diet.* **2018**, *118*, 714–723.e1. [CrossRef]
31. Hébert, J.R.; Hurley, T.G.; Harmon, B.E.; Heiney, S.; Hebert, C.J.; Steck, S.E. A diet, physical activity, and stress reduction intervention in men with rising prostate-specific antigen after treatment for prostate cancer. *Cancer Epidemiol.* **2012**, *36*, e128–e136. [CrossRef]
32. Mefferd, K.; Nichols, J.F.; Pakiz, B.; Rock, C.L. A cognitive behavioral therapy intervention to promote weight loss improves body composition and blood lipid profiles among overweight breast cancer survivors. *Breast Cancer Res. Treat* **2007**, *104*, 145–152. [CrossRef] [PubMed]
33. Morey, M.C.; Snyder, D.C.; Sloane, R.; Cohen, H.J.; Peterson, B.; Hartman, T.J.; Miller, P.; Mitchell, D.C.; Demark-Wahnefried, W. Effects of home-based diet and exercise on functional outcomes among older, overweight long-term cancer survivors: RENEW: A randomized controlled trial. *JAMA* **2009**, *301*, 1883–1891. [CrossRef]
34. Pakiz, B.; Flatt, S.W.; Bardwell, W.A.; Rock, C.L.; Mills, P.J. Effects of a weight loss intervention on body mass, fitness, and inflammatory biomarkers in overweight or obese breast cancer survivors. *Int. J. Behav. Med.* **2011**, *18*, 333–341. [CrossRef] [PubMed]
35. Brown, J.C.; Sarwer, D.B.; Troxel, A.B.; Sturgeon, K.; DeMichele, A.M.; Denlinger, C.S.; Schmitz, K.H. A randomized trial of exercise and diet on body composition in survivors of breast cancer with overweight or obesity. *Breast Cancer Res. Treat.* **2021**, *189*, 145–154. [CrossRef] [PubMed]
36. Brown, J.C.; Sarwer, D.B.; Troxel, A.B.; Sturgeon, K.; DeMichele, A.M.; Denlinger, C.S.; Schmitz, K.H. A randomized trial of exercise and diet on health-related quality of life in survivors of breast cancer with overweight or obesity. *Cancer* **2021**, *127*, 3856–3864. [CrossRef]

37. Chaplow, Z.L.; Focht, B.C.; Lucas, A.R.; Grainger, E.; Simpson, C.; Buell, J.; Fairman, C.M.; Thomas-Ahner, J.M.; Bowman, J.; DeScenza, V.R.; et al. Effects of a lifestyle intervention on body composition in prostate cancer patients on androgen deprivation therapy. *JCSM Clin. Rep.* **2020**, *5*, 52–60. [CrossRef]
38. Greenlee, H.A.; Crew, K.D.; Mata, J.M.; McKinley, P.S.; Rundle, A.G.; Zhang, W.; Liao, Y.; Tsai, W.Y.; Hershman, D.L. A pilot randomized controlled trial of a commercial diet and exercise weight loss program in minority breast cancer survivors. *Obesity* **2013**, *21*, 65–76. [CrossRef]
39. Harrigan, M.; Cartmel, B.; Loftfield, E.; Sanft, T.; Chagpar, A.B.; Zhou, Y.; Playdon, M.; Li, F.; Irwin, M.L. Randomized Trial Comparing Telephone Versus In-Person Weight Loss Counseling on Body Composition and Circulating Biomarkers in Women Treated for Breast Cancer: The Lifestyle, Exercise, and Nutrition (LEAN) Study. *J. Clin. Oncol.* **2016**, *34*, 669–676. [CrossRef]
40. Puklin, L.; Cartmel, B.; Harrigan, M.; Lu, L.; Li, F.Y.; Sanft, T.; Irwin, M.L. Randomized trial of weight loss on circulating ghrelin levels among breast cancer survivors. *npj Breast Cancer* **2021**, *7*, 49. [CrossRef] [PubMed]
41. Reeves, M.; Winkler, E.; McCarthy, N.; Lawler, S.; Terranova, C.; Hayes, S.; Janda, M.; Demark-Wahnefried, W.; Eakin, E. The Living Well after Breast Cancer™ Pilot Trial: A weight loss intervention for women following treatment for breast cancer. *Asia-Pac. J. Clin. Oncol.* **2017**, *13*, 125–136. [CrossRef] [PubMed]
42. Sanft, T.; Harrigan, M.; McGowan, C.; Cartmel, B.; Zupa, M.; Li, F.Y.; Ferrucci, L.M.; Puklin, L.; Cao, A.; Nguyen, T.H.; et al. Randomized Trial of Exercise and Nutrition on Chemotherapy Completion and Pathologic Complete Response in Women With Breast Cancer: The Lifestyle, Exercise, and Nutrition Early After Diagnosis Study. *J. Clin. Oncol.* **2023**, *41*, Jco2300871. [CrossRef]
43. Wilson, R.L.; Taaffe, D.R.; Newton, R.U.; Hart, N.H.; Lyons-Wall, P.; Galvao, D.A. Maintaining weight loss in obese men with prostate cancer following a supervised exercise and nutrition program—A pilot study. *Cancers* **2021**, *13*, 3411. [CrossRef]
44. Reeves, M.M.; Terranova, C.O.; Winkler, E.A.H.; McCarthy, N.; Hickman, I.J.; Ware, R.S.; Lawler, S.P.; Eakin, E.G.; Demark-Wahnefried, W. Effect of a Remotely Delivered Weight Loss Intervention in Early-Stage Breast Cancer: Randomized Controlled Trial. *Nutrients* **2021**, *13*, 4091. [CrossRef] [PubMed]
45. Daubenmier, J.J.; Weidner, G.; Marlin, R.; Crutchfield, L.; Dunn-Emke, S.; Chi, C.; Gao, B.; Carroll, P.; Ornish, D. Lifestyle and health-related quality of life of men with prostate cancer managed with active surveillance. *Urology* **2006**, *67*, 125–130. [CrossRef]
46. Ferreira, V.; Lawson, C.; Carli, F.; Scheede-Bergdahl, C.; Chevalier, S. Feasibility of a novel mixed-nutrient supplement in a multimodal prehabilitation intervention for lung cancer patients awaiting surgery: A randomized controlled pilot trial. *Int. J. Surg.* **2021**, *93*, 106079. [CrossRef]
47. Ho, M.; Ho, J.W.C.; Fong, D.Y.T.; Lee, C.F.; Macfarlane, D.J.; Cerin, E.; Lee, A.M.; Leung, S.; Chan, W.Y.Y.; Leung, I.P.F.; et al. Effects of dietary and physical activity interventions on generic and cancer-specific health-related quality of life, anxiety, and depression in colorectal cancer survivors: A randomized controlled trial. *J. Cancer Surviv.* **2020**, *14*, 424–433. [CrossRef]
48. Karimi, N.; Dabidi Roshan, V.; Fathi Bayatiyani, Z. Individually and Combined Water-Based Exercise with Ginger Supplement, on Systemic Inflammation and Metabolic Syndrome Indices, Among the Obese Women with Breast Neoplasms. *Iran J. Cancer Prev.* **2015**, *8*, e3856. [CrossRef] [PubMed]
49. Scott, E.; Daley, A.J.; Doll, H.; Woodroofe, N.; Coleman, R.E.; Mutrie, N.; Crank, H.; Powers, H.J.; Saxton, J.M. Effects of an exercise and hypocaloric healthy eating program on biomarkers associated with long-term prognosis after early-stage breast cancer: A randomized controlled trial. *Cancer Causes Control* **2013**, *24*, 181–191. [CrossRef] [PubMed]
50. Bourke, L.; Doll, H.; Crank, H.; Daley, A.; Rosario, D.; Saxton, J.M. Lifestyle intervention in men with advanced prostate cancer receiving androgen suppression therapy: A feasibility study. *Cancer Epidemiol. Biomark. Prev.* **2011**, *20*, 647–657. [CrossRef] [PubMed]
51. Baguley, B.J.; Adlard, K.; Jenkins, D.; Wright, O.R.L.; Skinner, T.L. Mediterranean Style Dietary Pattern with High Intensity Interval Training in Men with Prostate Cancer Treated with Androgen Deprivation Therapy: A Pilot Randomised Control Trial. *Int. J. Environ. Res. Public Health* **2022**, *19*, 5709. [CrossRef] [PubMed]
52. D'Alonzo, N.J.; Qiu, L.; Sears, D.D.; Chinchilli, V.; Brown, J.C.; Sarwer, D.B.; Schmitz, K.H.; Sturgeon, K.M. WISER Survivor Trial: Combined Effect of Exercise and Weight Loss Interventions on Insulin and Insulin Resistance in Breast Cancer Survivors. *Nutrients* **2021**, *13*, 3108. [CrossRef]
53. Schünemann, H.; Brożek, J.; Guyatt, G.; Oxman, A. Handbook for grading the quality of evidence and the strength of recommendations using the GRADE approach. *Updat. Oct.* **2013**, *2013*, 15.
54. Karimi, N.; Roshan, V.D. Change in adiponectin and oxidative stress after modifiable lifestyle interventions in breast cancer cases. *Asian Pac. J. Cancer Prev.* **2013**, *14*, 2845–2850. [CrossRef] [PubMed]
55. Brown, J.C.; Sturgeon, K.; Sarwer, D.B.; Troxel, A.B.; DeMichele, A.M.; Denlinger, C.S.; Schmitz, K.H. The effects of exercise and diet on sex steroids in breast cancer survivors. *Endocr. Relat. Cancer* **2022**, *29*, 485–493. [CrossRef] [PubMed]
56. Brown, J.C.; Sturgeon, K.; Sarwer, D.B.; Troxel, A.B.; DeMichele, A.M.; Denlinger, C.S.; Schmitz, K.H. The effects of exercise and diet on oxidative stress and telomere length in breast cancer survivors. *Breast Cancer Res. Treat.* **2023**, *199*, 109–117. [CrossRef]
57. Carayol, M.; Ninot, G.; Senesse, P.; Bleuse, J.P.; Gourgou, S.; Sancho-Garnier, H.; Sari, C.; Romieu, I.; Romieu, G.; Jacot, W. Short- and long-term impact of adapted physical activity and diet counseling during adjuvant breast cancer therapy: The "APAD1" randomized controlled trial. *BMC Cancer* **2019**, *19*, 737. [CrossRef]

58. Sanft, T.; Usiskin, I.; Harrigan, M.; Cartmel, B.; Lu, L.; Li, F.Y.; Zhou, Y.; Chagpar, A.; Ferrucci, L.M.; Pusztai, L.; et al. Randomized controlled trial of weight loss versus usual care on telomere length in women with breast cancer: The lifestyle, exercise, and nutrition (LEAN) study. *Breast Cancer Res. Treat* **2018**, *172*, 105–112. [CrossRef] [PubMed]
59. Schmitz, K.H.; Troxel, A.B.; Dean, L.T.; DeMichele, A.; Brown, J.C.; Sturgeon, K.; Zhang, Z.; Evangelisti, M.; Spinelli, B.; Kallan, M.J.; et al. Effect of Home-Based Exercise and Weight Loss Programs on Breast Cancer-Related Lymphedema Outcomes Among Overweight Breast Cancer Survivors: The WISER Survivor Randomized Clinical Trial. *JAMA Oncol.* **2019**, *5*, 1605–1613. [CrossRef] [PubMed]
60. Frattaroli, J.; Weidner, G.; Dnistrian, A.M.; Kemp, C.; Daubenmier, J.J.; Marlin, R.O.; Crutchfield, L.; Yglecias, L.; Carroll, P.R.; Ornish, D. Clinical events in prostate cancer lifestyle trial: Results from two years of follow-up. *Urology* **2008**, *72*, 1319–1323. [CrossRef] [PubMed]
61. Lee, C.F.; Ho, J.W.C.; Fong, D.Y.T.; Macfarlane, D.J.; Cerin, E.; Lee, A.M.; Leung, S.; Chan, W.Y.Y.; Leung, I.P.F.; Lam, S.H.S.; et al. Dietary and Physical Activity Interventions for Colorectal Cancer Survivors: A Randomized Controlled Trial. *Sci. Rep.* **2018**, *8*, 5731. [CrossRef] [PubMed]
62. Okorodudu, D.O.; Jumean, M.F.; Montori, V.M.; Romero-Corral, A.; Somers, V.K.; Erwin, P.J.; Lopez-Jimenez, F. Diagnostic performance of body mass index to identify obesity as defined by body adiposity: A systematic review and meta-analysis. *Int. J. Obes.* **2010**, *34*, 791–799. [CrossRef] [PubMed]
63. Iyengar, N.M.; Hudis, C.A.; Dannenberg, A.J. Obesity and cancer: Local and systemic mechanisms. *Annu. Rev. Med.* **2015**, *66*, 297–309. [CrossRef] [PubMed]
64. Zimmet, P.Z. Hyperinsulinemia--how innocent a bystander? *Diabetes Care* **1993**, *16* (Suppl. 3), 56–70. [CrossRef]
65. Kirk, B.; Feehan, J.; Lombardi, G.; Duque, G. Muscle, Bone, and Fat Crosstalk: The Biological Role of Myokines, Osteokines, and Adipokines. *Curr. Osteoporos. Rep.* **2020**, *18*, 388–400. [CrossRef] [PubMed]
66. Borghouts, L.B.; Keizer, H.A. Exercise and insulin sensitivity: A review. *Int. J. Sports Med.* **2000**, *21*, 1–12. [CrossRef]
67. Gołąbek, K.D.; Regulska-Ilow, B. Dietary support in insulin resistance: An overview of current scientific reports. *Adv. Clin. Exp. Med.* **2019**, *28*, 1577–1585. [CrossRef]
68. Eglseer, D.; Traxler, M.; Embacher, S.; Reiter, L.; Schoufour, J.D.; Weijs, P.J.M.; Voortman, T.; Boirie, Y.; Cruz-Jentoft, A.; Bauer, S. Nutrition and Exercise Interventions to Improve Body Composition for Persons with Overweight or Obesity Near Retirement Age: A Systematic Review and Network Meta-Analysis of Randomized Controlled Trials. *Adv. Nutr.* **2023**, *14*, 516–538. [CrossRef]
69. Au, P.C.; Li, H.L.; Lee, G.K.; Li, G.H.; Chan, M.; Cheung, B.M.; Wong, I.C.; Lee, V.H.; Mok, J.; Yip, B.H.; et al. Sarcopenia and mortality in cancer: A meta-analysis. *Osteoporos. Sarcopenia* **2021**, *7*, S28–S33. [CrossRef] [PubMed]
70. Kim, C.B.; Park, J.H.; Park, H.S.; Kim, H.J.; Park, J.J. Effects of Whey Protein Supplement on 4-Week Resistance Exercise-Induced Improvements in Muscle Mass and Isokinetic Muscular Function under Dietary Control. *Nutrients* **2023**, *15*, 1003. [CrossRef] [PubMed]
71. Franczyk, B.; Gluba-Brzózka, A.; Ciałkowska-Rysz, A.; Ławiński, J.; Rysz, J. The Impact of Aerobic Exercise on HDL Quantity and Quality: A Narrative Review. *Int. J. Mol. Sci.* **2023**, *24*, 4653. [CrossRef] [PubMed]
72. Luna-Castillo, K.P.; Olivares-Ochoa, X.C.; Hernández-Ruiz, R.G.; Llamas-Covarrubias, I.M.; Rodríguez-Reyes, S.C.; Betancourt-Núñez, A.; Vizmanos, B.; Martínez-López, E.; Muñoz-Valle, J.F.; Márquez-Sandoval, F.; et al. The Effect of Dietary Interventions on Hypertriglyceridemia: From Public Health to Molecular Nutrition Evidence. *Nutrients* **2022**, *14*, 1104. [CrossRef] [PubMed]
73. Ulmer, H.; Borena, W.; Rapp, K.; Klenk, J.; Strasak, A.; Diem, G.; Concin, H.; Nagel, G. Serum triglyceride concentrations and cancer risk in a large cohort study in Austria. *Br. J. Cancer* **2009**, *101*, 1202–1206. [CrossRef]
74. Colleoni, M.; Mandala, M.; Peruzzotti, G.; Robertson, C.; Bredart, A.; Goldhirsch, A. Depression and degree of acceptance of adjuvant cytotoxic drugs. *Lancet* **2000**, *356*, 1326–1327. [CrossRef]
75. Aydin, M.; Kose, E.; Odabas, I.; Meric Bingul, B.; Demirci, D.; Aydin, Z. The Effect of Exercise on Life Quality and Depression Levels of Breast Cancer Patients. *Asian Pac. J. Cancer Prev.* **2021**, *22*, 725–732. [CrossRef]
76. Cramer, H.; Lauche, R.; Klose, P.; Lange, S.; Langhorst, J.; Dobos, G.J. Yoga for improving health-related quality of life, mental health and cancer-related symptoms in women diagnosed with breast cancer. *Cochrane Database Syst. Rev.* **2017**, *1*, Cd010802. [CrossRef]
77. Appleton, K.M.; Rogers, P.J.; Ness, A.R. Updated systematic review and meta-analysis of the effects of n-3 long-chain polyunsaturated fatty acids on depressed mood. *Am. J. Clin. Nutr.* **2010**, *91*, 757–770. [CrossRef]
78. Kraguljac, N.V.; Montori, V.M.; Pavuluri, M.; Chai, H.S.; Wilson, B.S.; Unal, S.S. Efficacy of omega-3 fatty acids in mood disorders—A systematic review and metaanalysis. *Psychopharmacol. Bull.* **2009**, *42*, 39–54. [PubMed]
79. Marquez, D.X.; Aguiñaga, S.; Vásquez, P.M.; Conroy, D.E.; Erickson, K.I.; Hillman, C.; Stillman, C.M.; Ballard, R.M.; Sheppard, B.B.; Petruzzello, S.J.; et al. A systematic review of physical activity and quality of life and well-being. *Transl. Behav. Med.* **2020**, *10*, 1098–1109. [CrossRef] [PubMed]
80. Carson, T.L.; Hidalgo, B.; Ard, J.D.; Affuso, O. Dietary interventions and quality of life: A systematic review of the literature. *J. Nutr. Educ. Behav.* **2014**, *46*, 90–101. [CrossRef] [PubMed]
81. Canudas, S.; Becerra-Tomás, N.; Hernández-Alonso, P.; Galié, S.; Leung, C.; Crous-Bou, M.; De Vivo, I.; Gao, Y.; Gu, Y.; Meinilä, J.; et al. Mediterranean Diet and Telomere Length: A Systematic Review and Meta-Analysis. *Adv. Nutr.* **2020**, *11*, 1544–1554. [CrossRef]

82. Pérez, L.M.; Amaral, M.A.; Mundstock, E.; Barbé-Tuana, F.M.; Guma, F.; Jones, M.H.; Machado, D.C.; Sarria, E.E.; Marques, E.M.M.; Preto, L.T.; et al. Effects of Diet on Telomere Length: Systematic Review and Meta-Analysis. *Public Health Genom.* **2017**, *20*, 286–292. [CrossRef]
83. Song, S.; Lee, E.; Kim, H. Does Exercise Affect Telomere Length? A Systematic Review and Meta-Analysis of Randomized Controlled Trials. *Medicina* **2022**, *58*, 242. [CrossRef]

Disclaimer/Publisher's Note: The statements, opinions and data contained in all publications are solely those of the individual author(s) and contributor(s) and not of MDPI and/or the editor(s). MDPI and/or the editor(s) disclaim responsibility for any injury to people or property resulting from any ideas, methods, instructions or products referred to in the content.

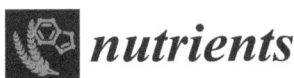

Review

Gluten-Free Diet Adherence Tools for Individuals with Celiac Disease: A Systematic Review and Meta-Analysis of Tools Compared to Laboratory Tests

Camila dos Santos Ribeiro [1,*], Rosa Harumi Uenishi [1,2], Alessandra dos Santos Domingues [2], Eduardo Yoshio Nakano [3], Raquel Braz Assunção Botelho [1], António Raposo [4,*] and Renata Puppin Zandonadi [1,*]

1. Department of Nutrition, University of Brasília, Brasília 70910-900, Brazil; rosa.uenishi@gmail.com (R.H.U.); raquelbotelho@unb.br (R.B.A.B.)
2. Brasilia University Hospital, University of Brasília, Brasília 70840-901, Brazil; alessandra_gastro@hotmail.com
3. Department of Statistics, University of Brasília, Brasilia 70910-900, Brazil; nakano@unb.br
4. CBIOS (Research Center for Biosciences and Health Technologies), Universidade Lusófona de Humanidades e Tecnologias, Campo Grande 376, 1749-024 Lisboa, Portugal
* Correspondence: camilasribeiro15@gmail.com (C.d.S.R.); antonio.raposo@ulusofona.pt (A.R.); renatapz@unb.br (R.P.Z.)

Abstract: This systematic review aimed to find the tool that best predicts celiac individuals' adherence to a gluten-free diet (GFD). The Transparent Reporting of Multivariable Prediction Models for Individual Prognosis or Diagnosis (TRIPOD-SRMA) guideline was used for the construction and collection of data from eight scientific databases (PubMed, EMBASE, LILACS, Web of Science, LIVIVO, SCOPUS, Google Scholar, and Proquest) on 16 November 2023. The inclusion criteria were studies involving individuals with celiac disease (CD) who were over 18 years old and on a GFD for at least six months, using a questionnaire to predict adherence to a GFD, and comparing it with laboratory tests (serological tests, gluten immunogenic peptide—GIP, or biopsy). Review articles, book chapters, and studies without sufficient data were excluded. The Checklist for Critical Appraisal and Data Extraction for Systematic Reviews of Prediction Modeling Studies (CHARMS) was used for data collection from the selected primary studies, and their risk of bias and quality was assessed using the Prediction Risk of Bias Assessment Tool (PROBAST). The association between the GFD adherence determined by the tool and laboratory test was assessed using the phi contingency coefficient. The studies included in this review used four different tools to evaluate GFD adherence: BIAGI score, Coeliac Dietary Adherence Test (CDAT), self-report questions, and interviews. The comparison method most often used was biopsy (n = 19; 59.3%), followed by serology (n = 14; 43.7%) and gluten immunogenic peptides (GIPs) (n = 4; 12.5%). There were no significant differences between the interview, self-report, and BIAGI tools used to evaluate GFD adherence. These tools were better associated with GFD adherence than the CDAT. Considering their cost, application time, and prediction capacity, the self-report and BIAGI were the preferred tools for evaluating GFD adherence.

Keywords: gluten-free diet; celiac disease; treatment adherence; laboratory test

Citation: Ribeiro, C.d.S.; Uenishi, R.H.; Domingues, A.d.S.; Nakano, E.Y.; Botelho, R.B.A.; Raposo, A.; Zandonadi, R.P. Gluten-Free Diet Adherence Tools for Individuals with Celiac Disease: A Systematic Review and Meta-Analysis of Tools Compared to Laboratory Tests. *Nutrients* 2024, *16*, 2428. https://doi.org/10.3390/nu16152428

Academic Editor: Fabiana Zingone

Received: 22 June 2024
Revised: 18 July 2024
Accepted: 23 July 2024
Published: 26 July 2024

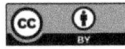

Copyright: © 2024 by the authors. Licensee MDPI, Basel, Switzerland. This article is an open access article distributed under the terms and conditions of the Creative Commons Attribution (CC BY) license (https://creativecommons.org/licenses/by/4.0/).

1. Introduction

Celiac disease (CD) is a chronic autoimmune condition that affects the small intestine with villous atrophy, causing intestinal and extraintestinal symptoms, and is triggered by the ingestion of gluten in genetically predisposed individuals [1,2]. It can trigger severe symptoms of malabsorption and nutritional deficiencies, such as anemia, diarrhea, constipation, short stature, muscular atrophy, and dermatitis herpetiformis, among others [1,3–5]. It is estimated that CD affects between 0.7% and 1.4% of the world population and is predominant in females; however, it is considered a neglected and underdiagnosed condition [5–7].

A gluten-free diet (GFD) is the only current treatment for the disease [8–10]. It can reverse the damage caused to the intestinal mucosa, primarily reducing morbidity and improving the quality of life of individuals with CD. GFDs entail completely restricting the consumption of gluten, a protein complex in wheat, rye, and barley, and its derivatives. Given the widespread presence of gluten in confectionery, bakery, pasta, and other industrialized products, adherence to a GFD can become a critical challenge for people affected by CD [11].

Several factors are involved in GFD adherence, such as the level of education received, the patient's own perception and self-efficacy regarding the diet, knowledge, the duration of the GFD, instruction from qualified professionals, social restrictions, and even food labeling. The main reasons for GFD transgression are social events and changes in the food consumption environment [12,13]. However, assessing GFD adherence in individuals with CD is still challenging for researchers and health professionals, and how to monitor patients with CD is not well defined [11].

The methods for assessing GFD adherence are diverse and may have advantages and disadvantages. Despite being essential for adult diagnoses and the gold standard for evaluating mucosal recovery, biopsy is an invasive and high-cost method for monitoring the disease [14]. It is believed that it is possible to use alternative and less invasive methods to assess GFD adherence, such as interviews conducted by qualified professionals, the use of questionnaires, serological tests, or screening for gluten-derived peptides (GIPs) in feces or urine [9,15,16]. The serological tests recommended for predicting GFD adherence are tTG antibodies (tissue anti-transglutaminase), EMA (anti endomysium), and anti-DGPs (anti-deamidated gliadin peptides) of the IgA and IgG classes. Their high levels indicate low adherence, but negative values may not confirm strict adherence to the GFD and may be inaccessible in practice due to the lack of testing in healthcare services, patients refusing to have blood samples collected, and the cost [1,11,17]. The measurement of GIPs in feces and urine is the most recently established method; therefore, it is not yet widely available. It is expensive and has been rejected by patients [11].

GFD adherence must be guided and evaluated by health professionals with experience in CD, especially dietitians, through dietary interviews, food diaries, and questionnaires [11]. Questionnaires are simple, quick, and easy instruments that can be applied in clinical practice. Some of them are validated and widely used in studies, with good reliability [11,18–20]. However, there is no study that recommends the best tool to assess adherence to the DSG or which tool best predicts the GFD adherence of CD individuals, which is why this work is essential for contributing to the scientific literature and monitoring people with CD.

GFD adherence is essential in preventing symptoms, improving the quality of life of individuals with CD, and reducing health costs related to this condition [14]. However, confirming GFD adherence via an unreliable method may pose a risk to individuals with CD in terms of their diet [10]. Therefore, looking for a reliable, low-cost, and less invasive tool can benefit CD individuals, the health professionals who monitor their treatment, and researchers in the field. It is necessary to explore the literature on this topic better, expose the criteria used to evaluate GFD adherence in CD individuals, and, consequently, contribute to improving the monitoring of the dietary treatments used in CD and the quality of life of CD individuals. In this sense, this systematic review aimed to evaluate the non-invasive method that best predicts the adherence of individuals with celiac disease to a gluten-free diet.

2. Materials and Methods

2.1. Study Design

This systematic prediction review used the Transparent Reporting of Multivariable Prediction Models for Individual Prognosis or Diagnosis (TRI-POD-SRMA) guidelines for its construction. This type of review seeks to gather and summarize studies to predict health outcomes and inform prognoses or diagnoses [21]. The review was registered on the systematic review registration platform PROSPERO (International Prospective Register of Systematic Reviews) and is being analyzed by it under opinion number CRD42024518034.

The first stages consisted of general research on the topic, a search for previous systematic reviews, and the study feasibility study. The search question was "In adults with celiac disease undergoing treatment (gluten-free diet) for more than six months, which tool best predicts treatment adherence, compared to laboratory tests?". A preliminary search strategy was carried out using the main keywords, following the acronym PICOT (P: person; I: intervention; C: comparison; O: outcome/result; and T: time), which is essential to guide the viability of a systematic review. A definitive search strategy was developed for each database, as well as the terms Mesh, DeCS, and Emtree (Table S1).

2.2. Eligibility Criteria

The following were included: (i) studies on adults older than 18 years old with a CD diagnosis and (ii) who have been undergoing treatment with a GFD for at least six months and (iii) studies which used questionnaires to predict adherence to the diet and compared it with a direct assessment method (tTG, EMA, DGP, GIP, or biopsy). The exclusion criteria were (i) studies carried out on people under 18 years old (ii) who had been on a GFD for less than six months (iii) and had no diagnosis of CD; (iv) review articles, book chapters, and conference proceedings; (v) studies without sufficient data for extraction; (vi) studies that did not evaluate adherence to a GFD.

2.3. Search and Data Extraction Strategy

Reviewers 1 and 2 (R1 and R2) collected the primary studies simultaneously and independently from eight scientific databases: PubMed, EMBASE, LILACS, Web of Science, LIVIVO, SCOPUS, Google Scholar, and Proquest. The search used the appropriate terms for each database (Table S1) without language or publication time restrictions.

2.4. Reference and Selection Manager

EndNote Web software was used to organize and remove 100% identical duplicates automatically. Then, the selected studies were exported to Rayyan software to organize the data and remove duplicates manually, before Phase 1 selection. The steps of organizing the data and duplicate removal were performed only by R1.

Two independent reviewers (R1 and R2) selected the articles to be included in two phases. Phase 1 selection involved independently reading the studies' titles and abstracts in Rayyan software and applying the eligibility criteria. After that, differences were discussed and judged. Phase 2 selection consisted of the complete reading of the articles selected in Phase 1 and an additional search within the reference lists of the articles read in full to find studies with potential eligibility for this review. If disagreements arose in either phase, a third reviewer (R3) evaluated them before making a final decision. During Phase 2 selection, the exclusion criteria were numbered in order of importance, and a numbered reason was assigned to each excluded study.

2.5. Data Collection and Risk of Bias Analysis

To collect data from the primary studies that were included in Phase 2 selection within this study, the CHARMS checklist (CHecklist for critical Appraisal and data extraction for systematic Reviews of prediction Modeling Studies) was used [22]. Missing studies were asked for directly by email to the authors, with a maximum of three attempts made. Data collection was also conducted independently by R1 and R2. After data collection, the two reviewers (R1 and R2) completed the PROBAST list (Prediction Risk Of Bias Assessment Tool), also independently [23].

To extract data and generate tables and graphs, a Microsoft Excel® (Office 365 version) model was independently used by the two reviewers and, at the end, a consensus meeting was held. R3 was consulted to solve divergencies. The file to be completed consisted of two spreadsheets, a template CHARMS and PROBAST, developed in previous studies [24].

2.6. Statistical Analysis and Meta-Analysis

The association between the GFD adherence calculated by the tool and laboratory test was assessed using the phi contingency coefficient. The phi coefficient measures the association between two binary variables and takes values between -1 and 1, with phi < 0 indicating a negative association, phi > 0 a positive association, and phi = 0 indicating no association. A meta-analysis of the studies that addressed the association between the GFD adherence calculated by the tool and laboratory tests was performed. Phi's meta-analytic measurement (grouped value) was obtained using a random effects model.

Point estimates of the grouped phi values and their respective 95% confidence intervals (95% CI) are presented. The estimates were obtained by considering a single grouping of all the studies and also by considering subgroups according to the instrument adopted. The association between the GFD adherence calculated by the tool and laboratory test was considered significant (at a significance level of 5%) when the 95% CI did not contain a zero value. Additionally, the associations between two subgroups were considered significantly different when their respective CIs did not intersect. The analyses were performed using the R program's metafor package, version 4.4.0 [25].

3. Results

3.1. Study Selection

The database search resulted in 4883 articles, of which 2444 were duplicates. After Phase 1 selection, 2439 articles remained for the reading of their titles and abstracts, 114 of which were read in full and had their bibliographic references consulted (Phase 2 selection). The excluded studies and the reasons for their exclusion are presented in Table S2. Finally, 32 studies were eligible for this systematic review and 31 for a meta-analysis, as shown in the PRISMA flowchart (Figure 1).

3.2. The Studies' Characteristics

The studies were performed from 1997 to 2024 and ranged from 18 to 694 (137.82 ± 145.24) participants. Thirty-one studies were characterized as cohort studies, and one was a randomized clinical trial study (Table 1). Most studies were performed in Italy [9,18,26–35] (n = 13; 40.6%), followed by Finland [36–39] (n = 4; 12.5%), the United Kingdom [35,40,41] and the United States [12,35,42] (n = 3, 9.3%), Argentina [43,44], Australia [45,46], Canada [47,48], Norway [49,50] (n = 2, 6.25%), while Paraguay, Poland, Romania, Spain, and Türkiye had one study each [20,35,51–53].

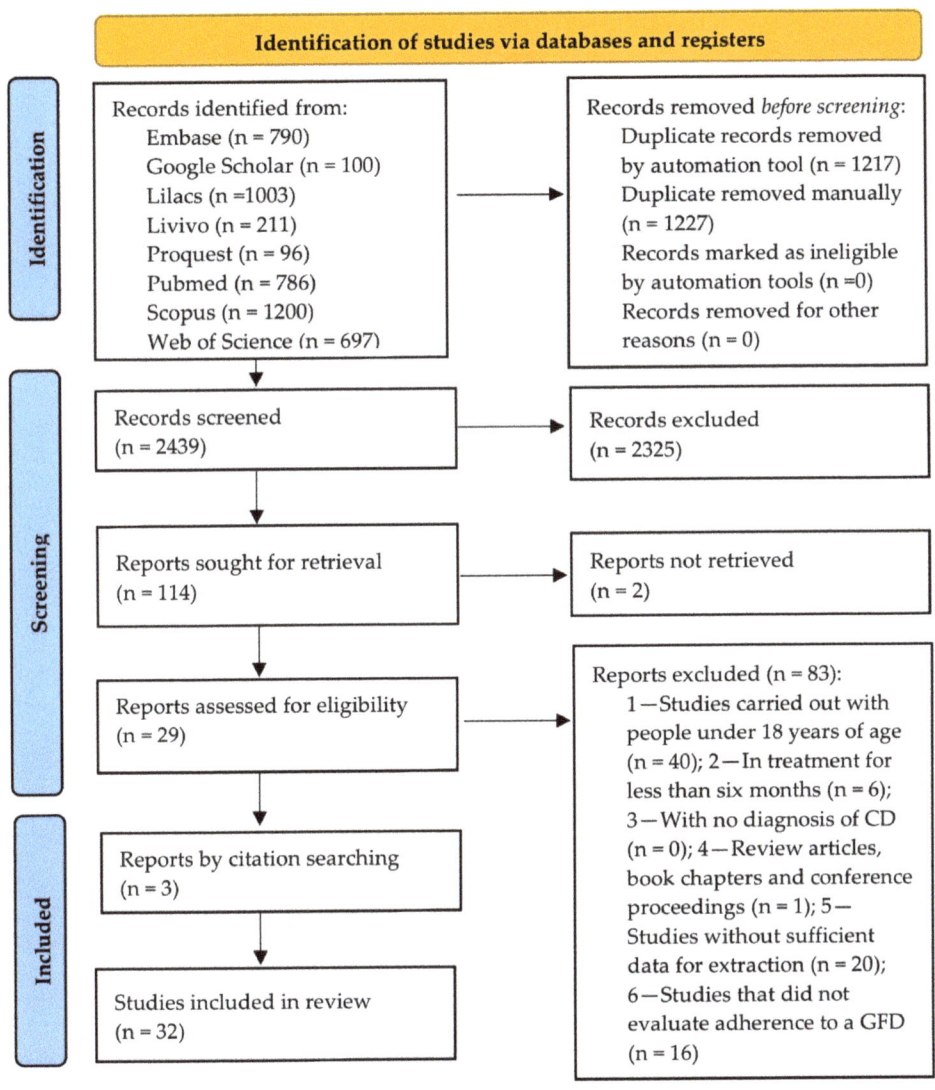

Figure 1. PRISMA flow diagram of literature search and selection criteria.

The studies included in this review used four different tools to evaluate GFDs: BIAGI scores [26], the Coeliac Dietary Adherence Test (CDAT) [19], self-report questionnaires, and interviews. Most of them used a biopsy [9,18,20,26,27,29,32,34–38,40–42,45,47,49,52] (n = 19; 59.3%), followed by serology [12,18,26–28,30,31,33,36,39,43,44,51,53] (n = 14; 43.7%) and GIPs [9,46,48,50] (n = 4; 12.5%). Of the 32 studies, most (n = 45; 46.8%) used the self-report method to evaluate GFD adherence [27,30,32,34,36,38,39,41,43–45,47,51–53], followed by the CDAT [9,12,20,40,46,48–50] (n = 8; 25%), BIAGI [18,26,31,33,40] (n = 5; 15.6%), and interviews [28,29,37,42] (n = 4; 12.5%), while only one used the Standardized Dietitian Evaluation (SDE) [20] and one of the studies used both the BIAGI and CDAT tools [35].

Table 1. Baseline characteristics of the studies included.

Author, Year	Study Design	Enrolment Period	Country	n	Females (n)	Age	GFD Period (Month)	GFD Adherence Tool	%Adherence Using the Tool	Laboratory Test	%Adherence Using the Laboratory Test
Biagi et al., 2009 [26]	Cohort	NI	Italy	168 162	126 NI	42.4 ± 13.9	82 (15–389)	BIAGI	79.7	Biopsy EMA	91 70.3
Biagi et al., 2012 [18]	Cohort	2008–2011	Italy	141	108	34 ± 15	27 (6–298)	BIAGI	82.2	Biopsy EMA	85.8 73
Galli et al., 2014 [31]	Cohort	2009–2012	Italy	65 57	47 NI	38 (18–70)	12	BIAGI	81.5	Biopsy EMA/tTG	67.6 70
Marsilio et al., 2020 [33]	Cohort	2020	Italy	100	86	39.73 ± 13.51	79.68 ± 76.68	BIAGI	90	tTG	85
Coleman et al., 2021 [40]	Cohort	2013–2019	UK	201	136	50.3	>30	BIAGI	91	Biopsy	68.6
Villafuerte-Galvez et al., 2015 [12]	Cohort	2011–2012	USA	118	NI	53.6 ± 15.4	118.8 ± 76.8	CDAT	73.7	tTG	82
Haere et al., 2016 [49]	Cohort	NI	Norway	127	79	55 ± 14	111.6 ± 60	CDAT	46.4	Biopsy	94.4
Gladys et al., 2020 [20]	Cohort	2015–2018	Poland	44	38	40.8	78 ± 86.4	CDAT	47.7	Biopsy	56.8
Silvester et al., 2020 [48]	Cohort	NI	Canada	18	12	41 (21–77)	24	CDAT	77.7	uGIPs fGIPs	33.3
Coleman et al., 2021 [40]	Cohort	2013–2019	England	201	136	50.3	>30	CDAT	49.7	Biopsy	68.6
Skodje et al., 2022 [50]	Cohort	NI	Norway	70	59	45	12	CDAT	53	fGIPs	91.4
Lombardo et al., 2023 [9]	Cohort	2019–2020	Italy	280	232	42.9	133.2 ± 122.4	CDAT	69.2	uGIPs	88.5
Russell et al., 2024 [46]	RCT	2020–2021	Australia	51	36	55 (44–62)	120 (60–168)	CDAT	72.5	fGIPs	23.5
Schiepatti et al., 2023 [35]	Cohort	2020–2022	Italy, Spain, UK, USA	694	491	>18	32 (15–61)	CDAT/BIAGI	83.5	Biopsy	77.3
Ciacci et al., 2002 [29]	Cohort	2002	Italy	390	299	27.9 ± 10.9	82.8 ± 90	Interview	42.5	Biopsy	76
Usai et al., 2002 [28]	Cohort	2002	Italy	66	66	46 (18–74)	>24	Interview	59	EMA/AGA	57.5
Metso et al., 2012 [37]	Cohort	2003–2006	Finland	26	22	>45	>12 meses	Interview	92.3	Biopsy	100
Gong et al., 2023 [42]	Cohort	2008–2019	USA	106	66	43.9	84	Interview	74.5	Biopsy	54.7
Gladys et al., 2020 [20]	Cohort	2020	Italy	44	38	40.8	78 ± 86.4	SDE	75	Biopsy	56.8

Table 1. Cont.

Author, Year	Study Design	Enrolment Period	Country	n	Females (n)	Age	GFD Period (Month)	GFD Adherence Tool	%Adherence Using the Tool	Laboratory Test	%Adherence Using the Laboratory Test
Bai et al., 1997 [43]	Cohort	1997	Argentina	22	NI	44 (21–73)	47 (23–75)	Self-reported	59	EMA/tTG	95.4
Kaukinen et al., 2002 [36]	Cohort	2002	Finland	57 87 87	NI 63 63	49 (22–73)	12 (12–216)	Self-reported	80.7 87.3 87.3	Biopsy EMA tTG	52.6 87.3 73.3
Viljamaa et al., 2005 [39]	Cohort	NI	Finland	97	51	51	144	Self-reported	83	tTG	91.7
Lanzini et al., 2009 [32]	Cohort	2009	Italy	465	356	31 (18–81)	16 (13–222)	Self-reported	85.8	Biopsy	79.5
Duerksen et al., 2010 [47]	Cohort	NI	Canada	21	19	50.5	116.4	Self-reported	71.4	Biopsy	71.4
Hutchinson et al., 2010 [41]	Cohort	2009	UK	234	202	>18	34.8	Self-reported	88	Biopsy	35
Nachman et al., 2011 [44]	Cohort	2004–2005	Argentina	53	48	18–66	12 48 12 48	Self-reported	60.3 52.8 60.3 52.8	TTG TTG tTG/DGP tTG/DGP	62.2 49 79.2 71.7
Newnham et al., 2016 [45]	Cohort	NI	Australia	44	NI	40 (18–71)	60	Self-reported	97.7	Biopsy	16
Stasi et al., 2016 [27]	Cohort	NI	Italy	39 52	NI	40	66 (13–261)	Self-reported	53.8 86.5	Biopsy EMA	84.6 75
Pekki et al., 2017 [38]	Cohort	NI	Finland	476	NI	55	96	Self-reported	98.7	Biopsy	58
Ferreira et al., 2018 [51]	Cohort	2015–2017	Paraguay	72	55	35.6 ± 12.4	294	Self-reported	68	tTG	44.4
Norsa et al., 2018 [34]	Cohort	2014–2015	Italy	63	NI	31.34	320 (1–432)	Self-reported	46	Biopsy	74.6
Elli et al., 2020 [30]	Cohort	2017–2018	Italy	197	159	44.6	87 ± 74	Self-reported	75.6	tTG	94.4
Sayar et al., 2021 [53]	Cohort	2010	Türkiye	78	68	36.8 ± 7.7	31	Self-reported	78.2	EMA/tTG	59
Nemteanu et al., 2023 [52]	Cohort	2016–2021	Romania	102	79	39.54 ± 12.70	22.6	Self-reported	27.4	tTG	71.5

Abbreviation: BIAGI = Biagi score; CDAT = Coeliac Dietary Adherence Test; GFD = gluten-free diet; SDE = Standardized Dietician Evaluation; AGA = gliadin antibody; tTG = tissue anti-transglutaminase antibody; EMA = anti-endomysium antibody; DGP = anti-deamidated gliadin peptide; fGIPs = gluten-derived peptides in feces; uGIPs = gluten-derived peptides in urine; RCT = randomized clinical trial; NI = no information.

3.3. Meta-Analysis

The results of the meta-analysis of the association between the GFD adherence calculated by the tool and laboratory tests are shown in Table 2 and Figure 2.

One study was excluded from the subgroup analysis because it used two instruments simultaneously (CDAT and BIAGI) and it was impossible to separate the data [35]. There were no significant differences between the interview, self-report, and BIAGI tools used to evaluate GFD adherence. These tools were better associated with GFD adherence than the CDAT. The Standardized Assessment of Dietitians (SDE) did not demonstrate an association with adherence to a GFD. However, it was evaluated in only one study and did not show statistically significant differences from any other instrument.

Table 2. Meta-analysis results for the association between the GFD adherence calculated by tools and laboratory tests.

	Number of Studies	Grouped Estimation Phi (CI 95%)
TOTAL	42	0.297 (0.220; 0.372)
Tool used to evaluate GFD adherence *		
CDAT	8	0.112 (0.032; 0.192) [A]
SDE	1	0.238 (−0.051; 0.528) [AB]
BIAGI	8	0.242 (0.073; 0.410) [AB]
Self-report	21	0.308 (0.209; 0.406) [B]
Interview	3	0.641 (0.380; 0.903) [B]
Laboratory test used to evaluate GFD adherence		
GIP	4	0.088 (−0.031; 0.207) [A]
Biopsy	20	0.264 (0.163; 0.365) [AB]
Serological (TTG, EMA, AGA)	18	0.378 (0.256; 0.501) [B]
Tool X laboratory test *		
BIAGI and Serological	4	0.066 (−0.126; 0.258) [A]
CDAT and GIP	4	0.088 (−0.031; 0.207) [A]
Self-report and Biopsy	9	0.116 (0.016; 0.216) [A]
CDAT and Biopsy	3	0.126 (−0.053; 0.304) [AB]
CDAT and Serological	1	0.226 (0.027; 0.425) [ABC]
SDE and Biopsy	1	0.238 (−0.051; 0.528) [ABC]
BIAGI and Biopsy	4	0.410 (0.268; 0.551) [BC]
Self-report and Serological	12	0.467 (0.384; 0.551) [C]
Interview and Biopsy	2	0.489 (0.419; 0.559) [C]
Interview and Serological	1	0.903 (0.796; 1.000) [D]

* The study by Schiepatti et al. (2023) [35] adopted the CDAT/BIAGI questionnaires; therefore, it does not fit (in isolation) into either instrument. Groups with the same letters do not differ significantly. Abbreviations: BIAGI = Biagi score; CDAT = Coeliac Dietary Adherence Test; GFD = gluten-free diet; SDE = Standardized Dietician Evaluation; AGA = gliadin antibody; TTG = tissue anti-transglutaminase antibody; EMA = anti-endomysium antibody; GIP = gluten-derived peptide; CI = confidence interval.

3.4. Risk of Bias and Concern

Figures 3 and 4 present the analysis of the risk of bias and concern in the included studies, classified according to PROBAST [23]. In total, 50% (n = 16) of the included studies demonstrated a low risk of bias [9,12,18,20,30,32,34,40,43,44,46,49,51,52,54]. A high risk of bias was identified in four studies [27,28,37,48], one of which used the self-report method [27], another an interview [28], and another the CDAT [48].

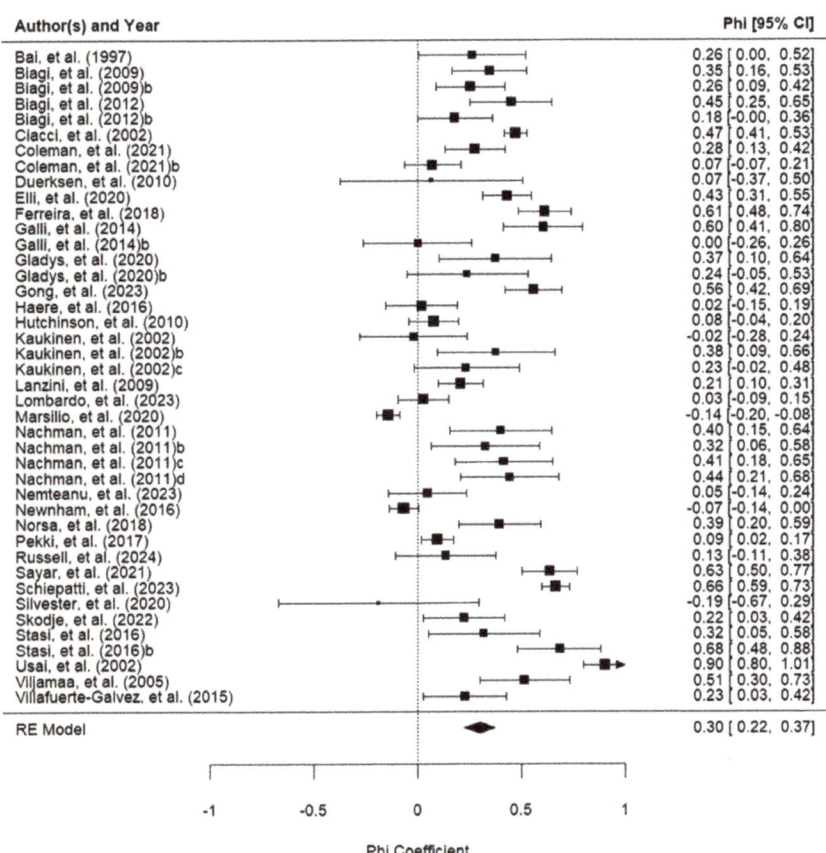

Figure 2. Forest plot of the phi coefficients of the association between the adherence measured with the tools and the adherence measured with the laboratory tests (42 studies) [9,12,18,20,26–36,38–51,53].

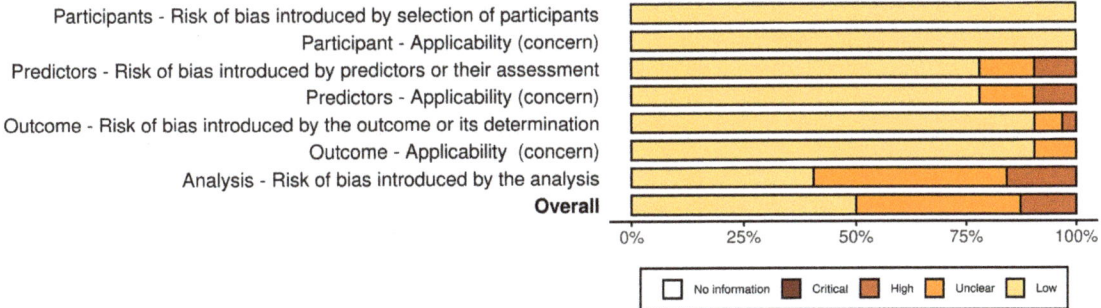

Figure 3. Risk of bias and concern in the included studies by domain, classified according to PROBAST.

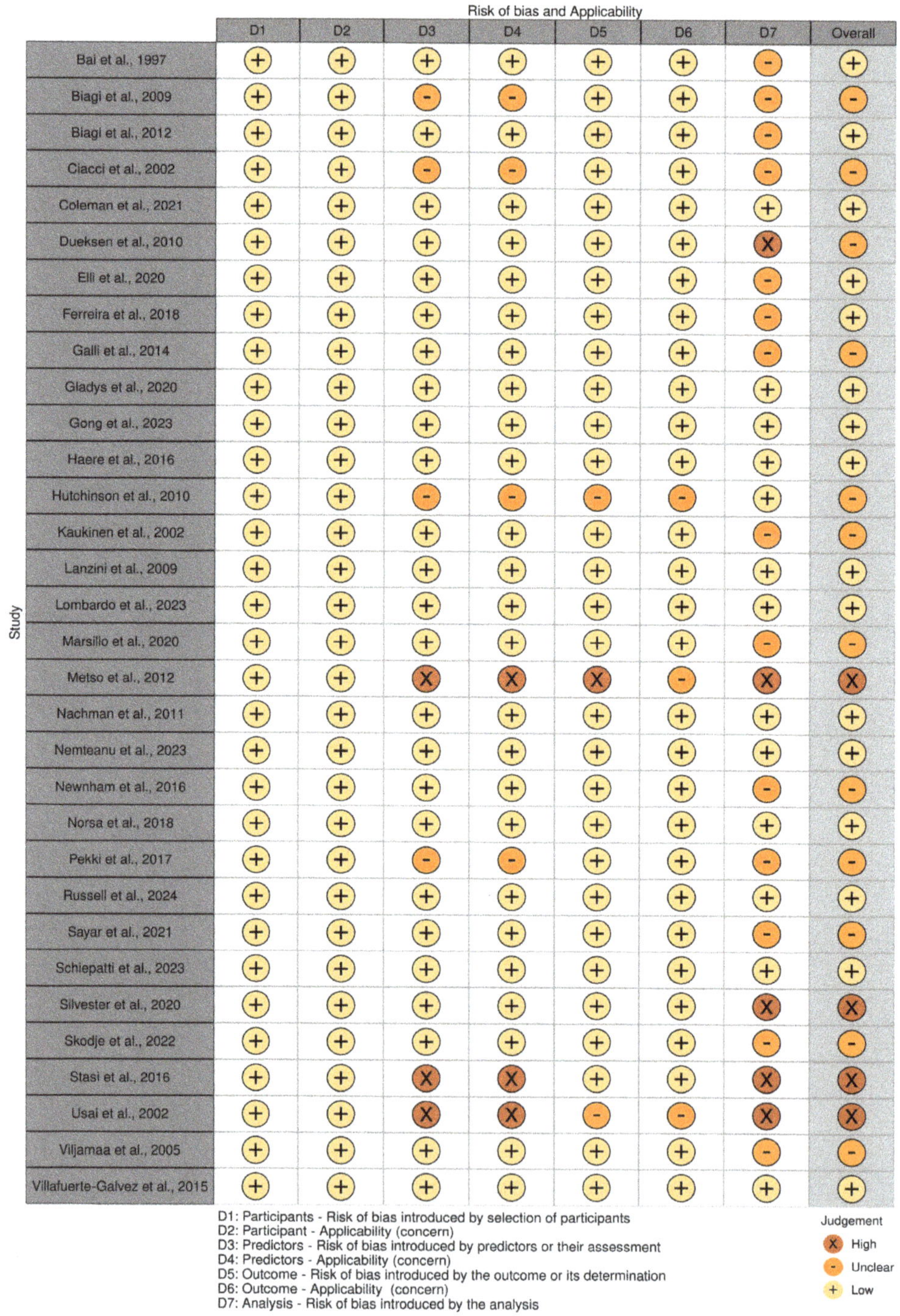

Study	D1	D2	D3	D4	D5	D6	D7	Overall
Bai et al., 1997	+	+	+	+	+	+	−	+
Biagi et al., 2009	+	+	−	−	+	+	−	−
Biagi et al., 2012	+	+	+	+	+	+	−	+
Ciacci et al., 2002	+	+	−	−	+	+	−	−
Coleman et al., 2021	+	+	+	+	+	+	+	+
Dueksen et al., 2010	+	+	+	+	+	+	X	−
Elli et al., 2020	+	+	+	+	+	+	+	+
Ferreira et al., 2018	+	+	+	+	+	+	−	+
Galli et al., 2014	+	+	+	+	+	+	−	−
Gladys et al., 2020	+	+	+	+	+	+	+	+
Gong et al., 2023	+	+	+	+	+	+	+	+
Haere et al., 2016	+	+	+	+	+	+	+	+
Hutchinson et al., 2010	+	+	−	−	−	−	+	−
Kaukinen et al., 2002	+	+	+	+	+	+	−	−
Lanzini et al., 2009	+	+	+	+	+	+	+	+
Lombardo et al., 2023	+	+	+	+	+	+	+	+
Marsilio et al., 2020	+	+	+	+	+	+	−	−
Metso et al., 2012	+	+	X	X	X	−	X	X
Nachman et al., 2011	+	+	+	+	+	+	+	+
Nemteanu et al., 2023	+	+	+	+	+	+	+	+
Newnham et al., 2016	+	+	+	+	+	+	−	−
Norsa et al., 2018	+	+	+	+	+	+	+	+
Pekki et al., 2017	+	+	−	−	+	+	−	−
Russell et al., 2024	+	+	+	+	+	+	+	+
Sayar et al., 2021	+	+	+	+	+	+	−	−
Schiepatti et al., 2023	+	+	+	+	+	+	+	+
Silvester et al., 2020	+	+	+	+	+	+	X	X
Skodje et al., 2022	+	+	+	+	+	+	−	−
Stasi et al., 2016	+	+	X	X	+	+	X	X
Usai et al., 2002	+	+	X	X	−	−	X	X
Viljamaa et al., 2005	+	+	+	+	+	+	−	−
Villafuerte-Galvez et al., 2015	+	+	+	+	+	+	+	+

D1: Participants - Risk of bias introduced by selection of participants
D2: Participant - Applicability (concern)
D3: Predictors - Risk of bias introduced by predictors or their assessment
D4: Predictors - Applicability (concern)
D5: Outcome - Risk of bias introduced by the outcome or its determination
D6: Outcome - Applicability (concern)
D7: Analysis - Risk of bias introduced by the analysis

Judgement
X High
− Unclear
+ Low

Figure 4. Risk of bias and applicability of the included studies, classified according to PROBAST [9,12,18,20,26–53].

4. Discussion

This is the first systematic review with a meta-analysis to evaluate which non-invasive method best predicts the gluten-free diet adherence of individuals with celiac disease. Most studies were performed (n = 25; 78%) in Europe, and mainly in Italy (n = 12; 37.5%). Even though CD is considered a major worldwide public health problem and its prevalence varies by sex, age, and geographic location, the global estimates show that most of the population with CD is found in European countries [5,6], which justifies the large number of studies in Europe. In addition, about twenty years ago, Italy was considered the birthland of CD epidemiology due to the serological screening of its population; therefore, several studies on CD have been performed in this country [55,56].

Four methods were used in the studies and compared to laboratory tests: the CDAT, BIAGI, self-reports, and interviews. The self-report method was the most used tool to evaluate GFD adherence [27,30,32,34,36,38,39,41,43–45,47,51–53]. This method is characterized by an individual reporting whether or not they adhere to a GFD, in a dichotomous way (yes or no) or using a Likert scale (from never to always), or reporting their food intake through three-, four-, or seven-day food records to be analyzed or a dietary history. The dichotomous and Likert-scale methods used to evaluate GFD adherence are related to perceived adherence to the GFD, and their advantages are accessibility, quickness, and simplicity. However, records or dietary histories may take more time and be more complex, despite being helpful in evaluating food quality [57]. Although a food diary with a dietary interview was indicated by a study to adequately assess GFD adherence [11], the lack of classification standardization, the need for an expert, and memory bias can become barriers in practice. Self-reported adherence was positively correlated with dietitian assessments but not with the CDAT, according to authors [58]. However, some authors consider a self-report method for assessing GFD adherence problematic, since individuals with CD can incorrectly report (intentionally or not) their level of GFD adherence, leading to an over- or underestimation of their adherence to a GFD [59]. A prospective comparative study comparing the predictive value of self-reported GFD adherence to serological tests and expert dietitian evaluations showed that self-reporting is less reliable than serological tests, biopsies, and dietitian evaluations [60]. Despite this, our systematic review showed that self-reported GFD adherence did not differ from the BIAGI score and interviews and presented better accuracy than the CDAT tool. A structured interview conducted by a qualified professional can be a sensitive method for assessing GFD adherence, either through an SDE or through the self-reporting of diet by individuals with CD [1,10], as confirmed by our results. The SDE consists of a tool composed of structured questions, with food records lasting up to three days, assessing the patient's ability to identify gluten in foods or other products, such as medicines and cosmetics. The disadvantages are that the SDE is subjective, takes more time, and a specialist is not always available in health services.

The BIAGI score was developed and validated in Italy in 2012 by a multicenter study [18,26]. Five studies included in this review used the BIAGI tool [18,26,31,33,40]. Four simple questions were developed based on the researchers' clinical experience. One of the advantages is that the instrument can be applied even by those with no experience in CD and GFDs [18]. Studies have been using this tool with satisfactory reproducibility results [14,61,62]. Its classification varies from 0 to 4, with 0–1 points for those who do not follow a strict GFD; 2 points for those following a GFD but with important errors that require correction, and 3–4 points for those following a strict GFD. The authors state that it is possible to apply this to different ethnicities, with the last question (Do you only eat packaged foods guaranteed by the Celiac Association?) able to be omitted without affecting the final result in some countries, as local celiac societies may not provide lists of gluten-free packaged foods. Therefore, when validating the BIAGI tool in each country it will be applied as necessary.

The CDAT was created in 2009 in the USA from a meeting of specialists (gastroenterologists, dietitians, psychologists, and CD individuals) to assess GFD adherence specifically [19]. After the meeting, they chose the five most important domains for evaluating GFD adherence: (1) symptoms related to CD, (2) specific knowledge of the disease, (3) self-efficacy, (4) reasons for maintaining a GFD, and (5) perceived adherence to the GFD. The CDAT consists of a seven-item questionnaire on a scale of 1 to 5. The minimum score is seven, and the maximum score is 35 points, with less than 13 points indicating good adherence [19]. This instrument has been translated into Spanish, Polish, and Norwegian [20,49,63,64], which are important for comparing different populations. However, its application takes time due to the number of items it contains and, in this systematic review, the CDAT presented the lowest association with laboratory tests.

The guidelines for celiac disease highlight that monitoring must be carried out through clinical evaluation, laboratory tests, and serology [1,65,66]. The normalization of laboratory tests indicates the remission of the disease, but the negativation of the tests is not immediate, and each test also has disadvantages that can limit its results. The quantification of antibodies, such as tTG, EMA, and DGP, is strongly recommended due to their high specificity and sensitivity [11,67]. Even though negative values cannot confirm a lack of exposure to gluten [11], it is evident that antibody values gradually decrease after months of a GFD [44]. Therefore, serology alone is not indicated to determine strict adherence to a gluten-free diet, and normalization does not indicate mucosal recovery [11,16].

Biopsy is considered the gold standard for evaluating mucosal healing; however, its invasive and high-cost nature means that the exam is not mandatory in monitoring CD, and the mucosal recovery time after a GFD is slow. Moreover, it varies for each individual. Studies differ on the indication period for biopsy, varying between repeating the biopsy after two years on a gluten-free diet or when symptoms and serological levels are altered [11,65,66,68]. In this systematic review, most of the studies performed a biopsy after a gluten-free diet was maintained for more than two years [20,29,38,40–42,45,47,49], which minimized the bias in the results.

Quantifying GIPs in feces and urine is a promising test that has also detected involuntary gluten consumption [46,69,70] and is recommended as a good direct approach to assessing adherence to a gluten-free diet and is helpful when available [1,11]; however, few studies used this comparator [9,46,48,50]. More studies are needed due to the individual variability in gluten metabolization and as their detectable time after ingestion is short (up to seven days) [11]. The consensus is that monitoring should be carried out frequently to assess the response to treatment and the adherence to a gluten-free diet [1,44,65,66]. Therefore, searching for less invasive, low-cost, and fast instruments to evaluate GFD adherence is essential.

This systematic review also has limitations. By including only studies on individuals over 18 years of age with celiac disease, many studies with the potential for analyzing the prediction of these instruments may have been excluded. Although biopsy is the gold standard for visualizing mucosal recovery, it can take up to five years for complete recovery in adults [10,17], which may have been a barrier in articles that used biopsy as a comparator over a short period for adherence assessments. In addition, the use of different methods (biopsy, serological, and GIP tests) may be a potential limitation, since the studies did not use the same method to evaluate GFD adherence. In order to minimize this, the tests were analyzed separately (Table 2).

A high risk of bias was only identified in four studies [27,28,37,48], and the concern was relatively low among the included studies. Accurately determining adherence to a GFD remains a challenge, particularly with respect to unintentional consumption. Both self-reports and tools rely on prior knowledge about the presence of gluten in foods, and this knowledge is not always accurate [59]. However, a standardized and straightforward tool facilitates the monitoring of individuals with celiac disease and guides professionals toward better management practices. Therefore, through this systematic review and meta-analysis, it is possible to emphasize the importance of using practical tools capable of predicting adherence to a GFD, thereby ensuring the effective monitoring of individuals with celiac disease.

5. Conclusions

There were no significant differences between the interview, self-report, and BIAGI tools used to evaluate GFD adherence. These tools were better associated with GFD adherence than the CDAT. Considering their cost, application time, potential accuracy of the level of GFD adherence, and prediction capacity, the self-report and BIAGI tools were considered the preferred tools to evaluate GFD adherence. These instruments are questionnaires completed by individuals. The evaluated tools depend on the CD patient's responses in interviews or to questionnaires; therefore, it is necessary to raise awareness about the importance of accurately filling out these questionnaires and to expand patients' knowledge about foods and the gluten-free diet to obtain the most accurate responses. Furthermore, additional studies are required to create standardized methods for evaluating diet adherence in various regions. These methods should be easily translatable and validated in multiple languages. They should also be simple to implement and highly accurate.

Supplementary Materials: The following supporting information can be downloaded at https://www.mdpi.com/article/10.3390/nu16152428/s1, Table S1: Database search strategy; Table S2: Excluded references and reasons.

Author Contributions: Conceptualization, C.d.S.R., R.H.U., A.d.S.D. and R.P.Z.; methodology, C.d.S.R., R.H.U., E.Y.N., A.d.S.D. and R.P.Z.; formal analysis, C.d.S.R., R.H.U., E.Y.N. and R.P.Z.; resources, R.P.Z., R.B.A.B. and A.R.; data curation, C.d.S.R., R.H.U., E.Y.N. and R.P.Z.; writing—original draft preparation, C.d.S.R., R.H.U., E.Y.N. and R.P.Z.; writing—review and editing, C.d.S.R., R.H.U., E.Y.N., R.B.A.B., A.d.S.D., A.R. and R.P.Z.; visualization, C.d.S.R., R.H.U., E.Y.N. and R.P.Z.; supervision, R.H.U. and R.P.Z.; project administration, R.H.U., A.R. and R.P.Z. All authors have read and agreed to the published version of the manuscript.

Funding: The study was partially supported by FAPDF N° 539/2022; and the Brazilian National Council for Scientific and Technological Development (CNPq—N° 302602/2021-6).

Acknowledgments: Renata Puppin Zandonadi acknowledges the *Fundação de Apoio à Pesquisa do Distrito Federal* (FAP-DF) and the Brazilian National Council for Scientific and Technological Development (CNPq) for their scientific support.

Conflicts of Interest: The authors declare no conflicts of interest.

References

1. Al-Toma, A.; Volta, U.; Auricchio, R.; Castillejo, G.; Sanders, D.S.; Cellier, C.; Mulder, C.J.; Lundin, K.E.A. European Society for the Study of Coeliac Disease (ESsCD) Guideline for Coeliac Disease and Other Gluten-Related Disorders. *United Eur. Gastroenterol. J.* **2019**, *7*, 583–613. [CrossRef] [PubMed]
2. Fasano, A.; Catassi, C. Celiac Disease. *N. Engl. J. Med.* **2012**, *367*, 2419–2426. [CrossRef] [PubMed]
3. Itzlinger, A.; Branchi, F.; Elli, L.; Schumann, M. Gluten-Free Diet in Celiac Disease—Forever and for All? *Nutrients* **2018**, *10*, 1796. [CrossRef] [PubMed]
4. Ludvigsson, J.F.; Leffler, D.A.; Bai, J.C.; Biagi, F.; Fasano, A.; Green, P.H.R.; Hadjivassiliou, M.; Kaukinen, K.; Kelly, C.P.; Leonard, J.N.; et al. The Oslo Definitions for Coeliac Disease and Related Terms. *Gut* **2013**, *62*, 43–52. [CrossRef] [PubMed]
5. Sahin, Y. Celiac Disease in Children: A Review of the Literature. *World J. Clin. Pediatr.* **2021**, *10*, 53–71. [CrossRef] [PubMed]
6. Singh, P.; Arora, A.; Strand, T.A.; Leffler, D.A.; Catassi, C.; Green, P.H.; Kelly, C.P.; Ahuja, V.; Makharia, G.K. Global Prevalence of Celiac Disease: Systematic Review and Meta-Analysis. *Clin. Gastroenterol. Hepatol.* **2018**, *16*, 823–836. [CrossRef] [PubMed]
7. Taraghikhah, N.; Ashtari, S.; Asri, N.; Shahbazkhani, B.; Al-Dulaimi, D.; Rostami-Nejad, M.; Rezaei-Tavirani, M.; Razzaghi, M.R.; Zali, M.R. An Updated Overview of Spectrum of Gluten-Related Disorders: Clinical and Diagnostic Aspects. *BMC Gastroenterol.* **2020**, *20*, 258. [CrossRef]
8. Bernardo, D.; Peña, A.S. Developing Strategies to Improve the Quality of Life of Patients with Gluten Intolerance in Patients with and without Coeliac Disease. *Eur. J. Intern. Med.* **2012**, *23*, 6–8. [CrossRef] [PubMed]
9. Galli, G.; Esposito, G.; Lahner, E.; Pilozzi, E.; Corleto, V.D.; Di Giulio, E.; Aloe Spiriti, M.A.; Annibale, B. Histological Recovery and Gluten-Free Diet Adherence: A Prospective 1-Year Follow-up Study of Adult Patients with Coeliac Disease. *Aliment. Pharmacol. Ther.* **2014**, *40*, 639–647. [CrossRef]
10. Wieser, H.; Ruiz-Carnicer, Á.; Segura, V.; Comino, I.; Sousa, C. Challenges of Monitoring the Gluten-Free Diet Adherence in the Management and Follow-Up of Patients with Celiac Disease. *Nutrients* **2021**, *13*, 2274. [CrossRef]

11. Elli, L.; Leffler, D.; Cellier, C.; Lebwohl, B.; Ciacci, C.; Schumann, M.; Lundin, K.E.A.; Chetcuti Zammit, S.; Sidhu, R.; Roncoroni, L.; et al. Guidelines for Best Practices in Monitoring Established Coeliac Disease in Adult Patients. *Nat. Rev. Gastroenterol. Hepatol.* **2024**, *21*, 198–215. [CrossRef] [PubMed]
12. Villafuerte-Galvez, J.; Vanga, R.R.; Dennis, M.; Hansen, J.; Leffler, D.A.; Kelly, C.P.; Mukherjee, R. Factors Governing Long-Term Adherence to a Gluten-Free Diet in Adult Patients with Coeliac Disease. *Aliment. Pharmacol. Ther.* **2015**, *42*, 753–760. [CrossRef] [PubMed]
13. Fernández Miaja, M.; José, J.; Martín, D.; Treviño, S.J.; Suárez González, M.; Bousoño García, C. Study of Adherence to the Gluten-Free Diet in Coeliac Patients. *An. Pediatría* **2021**, *94*, 377–384. [CrossRef]
14. Paganizza, S.; Zanotti, R.; D'Odorico, A.; Scapolo, P.; Canova, C. Is Adherence to a Gluten-Free Diet by Adult Patients with Celiac Disease Influenced by Their Knowledge of the Gluten Content of Foods? *Gastroenterol. Nurs.* **2019**, *42*, 55–64. [CrossRef] [PubMed]
15. Muhammad, H.; Reeves, S.; Jeanes, Y.M. Identifying and Improving Adherence to the Gluten-Free Diet in People with Coeliac Disease. *Proc. Nutr. Soc.* **2019**, *78*, 418–425. [CrossRef] [PubMed]
16. Silvester, J.A.; Kurada, S.; Szwajcer, A.; Kelly, C.P.; Leffer, D.A.; Duerksen, D. Tests for Serum Transglutaminase and Endomysial Antibodies Do Not Detect Most Patients With Celiac Disease and Persistent Villous Atrophy on Gluten-Free Diets: A Meta-Analysis. *Gastroenterology* **2017**, *153*, 689–701. [CrossRef] [PubMed]
17. Rodrigo, L.; Pérez-Martinez, I.; Lauret-Braña, E.; Suárez-González, A. Descriptive Study of the Diffe:.Rent Tools Used to Evaluate the Adherence to a Gluten-Free Diet in Celiac Disease Patients. *Nutrients* **2018**, *10*, 1777. [CrossRef] [PubMed]
18. Biagi, F.; Bianchi, P.I.; Marchese, A.; Trotta, L.; Vattiato, C.; Balduzzi, D.; Brusco, G.; Andrealli, A.; Cisarò, F.; Astegiano, M.; et al. A Score That Verifies Adherence to a Gluten-Free Diet: A Cross-Sectional, Multicentre Validation in Real Clinical Life. *Br. J. Nutr.* **2012**, *108*, 1884–1888. [CrossRef] [PubMed]
19. Leffler, D.A.; Dennis, M.; Edwards George, J.B.; Jamma, S.; Magge, S.; Cook, E.F.; Schuppan, D.; Kelly, C.P. A Simple Validated Gluten-Free Diet Adherence Survey for Adults With Celiac Disease. *Clin. Gastroenterol. Hepatol.* **2009**, *7*, 530–536. [CrossRef]
20. Gładyś, K.; Dardzińska, J.; Guzek, M.; Adrych, K.; Małgorzewicz, S. Celiac Dietary Adherence Test and Standardized Dietician Evaluation in Assessment of Adherence to a Gluten-Free Diet in Patients with Celiac Disease. *Nutrients* **2020**, *12*, 2300. [CrossRef]
21. Snell, K.I.E.; Levis, B.; Damen, J.A.A.; Dhiman, P.; Debray, T.P.A.; Hooft, L.; Reitsma, J.B.; Moons, K.G.M.; Collins, G.S.; Riley, R.D. Transparent Reporting of Multivariable Prediction Models for Individual Prognosis or Diagnosis: Checklist for Systematic Reviews and Meta-Analyses (TRIPOD-SRMA). *BMJ* **2023**, *381*, e073538. [CrossRef]
22. Moons, K.G.M.; de Groot, J.A.H.; Bouwmeester, W.; Vergouwe, Y.; Mallett, S.; Altman, D.G.; Reitsma, J.B.; Collins, G.S. Critical Appraisal and Data Extraction for Systematic Reviews of Prediction Modelling Studies: The CHARMS Checklist. *PLoS Med.* **2014**, *11*, e1001744. [CrossRef]
23. Wolff, R.F.; Moons, K.G.M.; Riley, R.D.; Whiting, P.F.; Westwood, M.; Collins, G.S.; Reitsma, J.B.; Kleijnen, J.; Mallett, S. PROBAST: A Tool to Assess the Risk of Bias and Applicability of Prediction Model Studies. *Ann. Intern. Med.* **2019**, *170*, 51–58. [CrossRef] [PubMed]
24. Fernandez-Felix, B.M.; López-Alcalde, J.; Roqué, M.; Muriel, A.; Zamora, J. CHARMS and PROBAST at Your Fingertips: A Template for Data Extraction and Risk of Bias Assessment in Systematic Reviews of Predictive Models. *BMC Med. Res. Methodol.* **2023**, *23*, 44. [CrossRef] [PubMed]
25. R Core Team. *R: A Language and Environment for Statistical Computing*; R Foundation for Statistical Computing: Vienna, Austria, 2018; Available online: https://www.R-project.org/ (accessed on 14 June 2024).
26. Biagi, F.; Andrealli, A.; Bianchi, P.I.; Marchese, A.; Klersy, C.; Corazza, G.R. A Gluten-Free Diet Score to Evaluate Dietary Compliance in Patients with Coeliac Disease. *Br. J. Nutr.* **2009**, *102*, 882–887. [CrossRef]
27. Norsa, L.; Branchi, F.; Bravo, M.; Ferretti, F.; Roncoroni, L.; Somalvico, F.; Conte, D.; Bardella, M.T.; Barigelletti, G.; Elli, L. Celiac Disease 30 Years after Diagnosis: Struggling with Gluten-Free Adherence or Gaining Gluten Tolerance? *J. Pediatr. Gastroenterol. Nutr.* **2018**, *67*, 361–366. [CrossRef]
28. Schiepatti, A.; Maimaris, S.; Raju, S.A.; Green, O.L.; Linden, J.; Mantica, G.; Therrien, A.; Flores-, D.; Bañares, F.F.-; Esteve, M.; et al. Persistent Villous Atrophy Predicts Development of Complications and Mortality in Adult Patients with Coeliac Disease: A Multicentre Longitudinal Cohort Study and Development of a Score to Identify High-Risk Patients. *Gut* **2023**, *72*, 2095–2102. [CrossRef] [PubMed]
29. Stasi, E.; Marafini, I.; Caruso, R.; Soderino, F.; Angelucci, E.; Del Vecchio Blanco, G.; Paoluzi, O.A.; Calabrese, E.; Sedda, S.; Zorzi, F.; et al. Frequency and Cause of Persistent Symptoms in Celiac Disease Patients on a Long-Term Gluten-Free Diet. *J. Clin. Gastroenterol.* **2016**, *50*, 239–243. [CrossRef]
30. Usai, P.; Minerba, L.; Marini, B.; Cossu, R.; Spada, S.; Carpiniello, B.; Cuomo, R.; Boy, M.F. Case Control Study on Health-Related Quality of Life in Adult Coeliac Disease. *Dig. Liver Dis.* **2002**, *34*, 547–552. [CrossRef]
31. Ciacci, C.; Cirillo, M.; Cavallaro, R.; Mazzacca, G. Long-Term Follow-up of Celiac Adults on Gluten-Free Diet: Prevalence and Correlates of Intestinal Damage. *Digestion* **2002**, *66*, 178–185. [CrossRef]
32. Elli, L.; Bascuñán, K.; Di Lernia, L.; Bardella, M.T.; Doneda, L.; Soldati, L.; Orlando, S.; Ferretti, F.; Lombardo, V.; Barigelletti, G.; et al. Safety of Occasional Ingestion of Gluten in Patients with Celiac Disease: A Real-Life Study. *BMC Med.* **2020**, *18*, 42. [CrossRef] [PubMed]

33. Lanzini, A.; Lanzarotto, F.; Villanacci, V.; Mora, A.; Bertolazzi, S.; Turini, D.; Carella, G.; Malagoli, A.; Ferrante, G.; Cesana, B.M.; et al. Complete Recovery of Intestinal Mucosa Occurs Very Rarely in Adult Coeliac Patients despite Adherence to Gluten-Free Diet. *Aliment. Pharmacol. Ther.* **2009**, *29*, 1299–1308. [CrossRef] [PubMed]
34. Lombardo, V.; Scricciolo, A.; Costantino, A.; Elli, L.; Legnani, G.; Cebolla, Á.; Doneda, L.; Mascaretti, F.; Vecchi, M.; Roncoroni, L. Evaluation of a Single Determination of Gluten Immunogenic Peptides in Urine from Unaware Celiac Patients to Monitor Gluten-Free Diet Adherence. *Nutrients* **2023**, *15*, 1259. [CrossRef] [PubMed]
35. Marsilio, I.; Canova, C.; D'odorico, A.; Ghisa, M.; Zingone, L.; Lorenzon, G.; Savarino, E.V.; Zingone, F. Quality-of-Life Evaluation in Coeliac Patients on a Gluten-Free Diet. *Nutrients* **2020**, *12*, 2981. [CrossRef]
36. Kaukinen, K.; Sulkanen, S.; Mäki, M.; Collin, P. IgA-Class Transglutaminase Antibodies in Evaluating the Efficacy of Gluten-Free Diet in Coeliac Disease. *Eur. J. Gastroenterol. Hepatol.* **2002**, *14*, 311–315. [CrossRef] [PubMed]
37. Metso, S.; Hyytiä-Ilmonen, H.; Kaukinen, K.; Huhtala, H.; Jaatinen, P.; Salmi, J.; Taurio, J.; Collin, P. Gluten-Free Diet and Autoimmune Thyroiditis in Patients with Celiac Disease. A Prospective Controlled Study. *Scand. J. Gastroenterol.* **2012**, *47*, 43–48. [CrossRef] [PubMed]
38. Pekki, H.; Kurppa, K.; Mäki, M.; Huhtala, H.; Laurila, K.; Ilus, T.; Kaukinen, K. Performing Routine Follow-up Biopsy 1 Year after Diagnosis Does Not Affect Long-Term Outcomes in Coeliac Disease. *Aliment. Pharmacol. Ther.* **2017**, *45*, 1459–1468. [CrossRef] [PubMed]
39. Viljamaa, M.; Collin, P.; Huhtala, H.; Sievänen, H.; Mäki, M.; Kaukinen, K. Is Coeliac Disease Screening in Risk Groups Justified? A Fourteen-Year Follow-up with Special Focus on Compliance and Quality of Life. *Aliment. Pharmacol. Ther.* **2005**, *22*, 317–324. [CrossRef] [PubMed]
40. Coleman, S.H.; Rej, A.; Baggus, E.M.R.; Lau, M.S.; Marks, L.J.; Hadjivassiliou, M.; Cross, S.S.; Leffler, D.A.; Elli, L.; Sanders, D.S. What Is the Optimal Method Assessing for Persistent Villous Atrophy in Adult Coeliac Disease? *J. Gastrointest. Liver Dis.* **2021**, *30*, 205–212. [CrossRef]
41. Hutchinson, J.M.; West, N.P.; Robins, G.G.; Howdle, P.D. Long-Term Histological Follow-up of People with Coeliac Disease in a UK Teaching Hospital. *QJM Int. J. Med.* **2010**, *103*, 511–517. [CrossRef]
42. Gong, C.; Saborit, C.; Long, X.; Wang, A.; Zheng, B.; Chung, H.; Lewis, S.K.; Krishnareddy, S.; Bhagat, G.; Green, P.H.R.; et al. Serological Investigation of Persistent Villous Atrophy in Celiac Disease. *Clin. Transl. Gastroenterol.* **2023**, *14*, e00639. [CrossRef]
43. Bai, J.C.; Gonzalez, D.; Mautalen, C.; Mazure, R.; Pedreira, S.; Vazquez, H.; Smecuol, E.; Siccardi, A.; Cataldi, M.; Niveloni, S.; et al. Long-Term Effect of Gluten Restriction on Bone Mineral Density of Patients with Coeliac Disease. *Aliment. Pharmacol. Ther.* **1997**, *11*, 157–164. [CrossRef]
44. Nachman, F.; Sugai, E.; Vázquez, H.; González, A.; Andrenacci, P.; Niveloni, S.; Mazure, R.; Smecuol, E.; Moreno, M.L.; Hwang, H.J.; et al. Serological Tests for Celiac Disease as Indicators of Long-Term Compliance with the Gluten-Free Diet. *Eur. J. Gastroenterol. Hepatol.* **2011**, *23*, 473–480. [CrossRef] [PubMed]
45. Newnham, E.D.; Shepherd, S.J.; Strauss, B.J.; Hosking, P.; Gibson, P.R. Adherence to the Gluten-Free Diet Can Achieve the Therapeutic Goals in Almost All Patients with Coeliac Disease: A 5-Year Longitudinal Study from Diagnosis. *J. Gastroenterol. Hepatol.* **2016**, *31*, 342–349. [CrossRef] [PubMed]
46. Russell, A.K.; Lucas, E.C.; Henneken, L.M.; Pizzey, C.J.; Clarke, D.; Myleus, A.; Tye-Din, J.A. Stool Gluten Peptide Detection Is Superior to Urinary Analysis, Coeliac Serology, Dietary Adherence Scores and Symptoms in the Detection of Intermittent Gluten Exposure in Coeliac Disease: A Randomised, Placebo-Controlled, Low-Dose Gluten Challenge Study. *Nutrients* **2024**, *16*, 279. [CrossRef] [PubMed]
47. Duerksen, D.R.; Wilhelm-Boyles, C.; Veitch, R.; Kryszak, D.; Parry, D.M. A Comparison of Antibody Testing, Permeability Testing, and Zonulin Levels with Small-Bowel Biopsy in Celiac Disease Patients on a Gluten-Free Diet. *Dig. Dis. Sci.* **2010**, *55*, 1026–1031. [CrossRef] [PubMed]
48. Silvester, J.A.; Comino, I.; Kelly, C.P.; Sousa, C.; Duerksen, D.R. Most Patients With Celiac Disease on Gluten-Free Diets Consume Measurable Amounts of Gluten. *Gastroenterology* **2020**, *158*, 1497–1499. [CrossRef] [PubMed]
49. Hære, P.; Høie, O.; Schulz, T.; Schönhardt, I.; Raki, M.; Lundin, K.E.A. Long-Term Mucosal Recovery and Healing in Celiac Disease Is the Rule—Not the Exception. *Scand. J. Gastroenterol.* **2016**, *51*, 1439–1446. [CrossRef]
50. Skodje, G.I.; van Megen, F.; Stendahl, M.; Henriksen, C.; Lundin, K.E.A.; Veierød, M.B. Detection of Gluten Immunogenic Peptides and the Celiac Disease Adherence Test to Monitor Gluten-Free Diet: A Pilot Study. *Eur. J. Clin. Nutr.* **2022**, *76*, 902–903. [CrossRef] [PubMed]
51. Ferreira, S.; Chamorro, M.E.; Ortíz, J.; Carpinelli, M.M.; Giménez, V.; Langjahr, P. Anti-Transglutaminase Antibody in Adults with Celiac Disease and Their Relation to the Presence and Duration of Gluten-Free Diet. *Rev. Gastroenterol. Peru* **2018**, *38*, 228–233.
52. Nemteanu, R.; Danciu, M.; Girleanu, I.; Ciortescu, I.; Gheorghe, L.; Trifan, A.; Plesa, A. Predictors of Slow Responsiveness and Partial Mucosal Recovery in Adult Patients with Celiac Disease. *Gastroenterol. Hepatol. Bed Bench* **2023**, *16*, 194–202. [PubMed]
53. Sayar, S.; Aykut, H.; Kaya, Ö.; Kürbüz, K.; Ak, Ç.; Gökçen, P.; Bilgiç, N.M.; Adalı, G.; Kahraman, R.; Doganay, L.; et al. Bone Mineral Density Screening and the Frequency of Osteopenia/Osteoporosis in Turkish Adult Patients with Celiac Disease. *Turk. J. Gastroenterol.* **2021**, *32*, 600–607. [CrossRef] [PubMed]
54. Schiepatti, A.; Maimaris, S.; Lusetti, F.; Scalvini, D.; Minerba, P.; Cincotta, M.; Fazzino, E.; Biagi, F. High Prevalence of Functional Gastrointestinal Disorders in Celiac Patients with Persistent Symptoms on a Gluten-Free Diet: A 20-Year Follow-Up Study. *Dig. Dis. Sci.* **2023**, *68*, 3374–3382. [CrossRef] [PubMed]

55. Lionetti, E.; Pjetraj, D.; Gatti, S.; Catassi, G.; Bellantoni, A.; Boffardi, M.; Cananzi, M.; Cinquetti, M.; Francavilla, R.; Malamisura, B.; et al. Prevalence and Detection Rate of Celiac Disease in Italy: Results of a SIGENP Multicenter Screening in School-Age Children. *Dig. Liver Dis.* **2023**, *55*, 608–613. [CrossRef] [PubMed]
56. Volta, U.; Bellentani, S.; Bianchi, F.B.; Brandi, G.; De Franceschi, L.; Miglioli, L.; Granito, A.; Balli, F.; Tiribelli, C. High Prevalence of Celiac Disease in Italian General Population. *Dig. Dis. Sci.* **2001**, *46*, 1500–1505. [CrossRef] [PubMed]
57. Barone, M.; Della Valle, N.; Rosania, R.; Facciorusso, A.; Trotta, A.; Cantatore, F.P.; Falco, S.; Pignatiello, S.; Viggiani, M.T.; Amoruso, A.; et al. A Comparison of the Nutritional Status between Adult Celiac Patients on a Long-Term, Strictly Gluten-Free Diet and Healthy Subjects. *Eur. J. Clin. Nutr.* **2016**, *70*, 23–27. [CrossRef] [PubMed]
58. Atsawarungruangkit, A.; Silvester, J.A.; Weiten, D.; Green, K.L.; Wilkey, K.E.; Rigaux, L.N.; Bernstein, C.N.; Graff, L.A.; Walker, J.R.; Duerksen, D.R. Development of the Dietitian Integrated Evaluation Tool for Gluten-Free Diets (DIET-GFD). *Nutrition* **2020**, *78*, 110819. [CrossRef] [PubMed]
59. Silvester, J.A.; Weiten, D.; Graff, L.A.; Walker, J.R.; Duerksen, D.R. Is It Gluten-Free? Relationship between Self-Reported Gluten-Free Diet Adherence and Knowledge of Gluten Content of Foods. *Nutrition* **2016**, *32*, 777–783. [CrossRef]
60. Leffler, D.A.; George, J.B.E.; Dennis, M.; Cook, E.F.; Schuppan, D.; Kelly, C.P. A Prospective Comparative Study of Five Measures of Gluten-Free Diet Adherence in Adults with Coeliac Disease. *Aliment. Pharmacol. Ther.* **2007**, *26*, 1227–1235. [CrossRef]
61. De Moreno, M.L.; Rodríguez-Herrera, A.; Sousa, C.; Comino, I. Biomarkers to Monitor Gluten-Free Diet Compliance in Celiac Patients. *Nutrients* **2017**, *9*, 46. [CrossRef]
62. Sbravati, F.; Pagano, S.; Retetangos, C.; Spisni, E.; Bolasco, G.; Labriola, F.; Filardi, M.C.; Grondona, A.G.; Alvisi, P. Adherence to Gluten-Free Diet in a Celiac Pediatric Population Referred to the General Pediatrician After Remission. *J. Pediatr. Gastroenterol. Nutr.* **2020**, *71*, 78–82. [CrossRef] [PubMed]
63. Fueyo Díaz, R.; Santos, S.G.; Asensio Martínez, Á.; Antonia, M.; Calavera, S.; Magallón Botaya, R.; Díaz, F.; Santos, G.; Martínez, A.; Sánchez Cala-Vera, M.A.; et al. Adaptación Transcultural y Validación Del Celiac Dietary Adherence Test. Un Cuestionario Sencillo Para Determinar La Adherencia a La Dieta Sin Gluten. *Rev. Esp. Enfermedades Dig.* **2016**, *108*, 138–144.
64. Johansson, K.; Norström, F.; Nordyke, K.; Myleus, A. Celiac Dietary Adherence Test Simplifies Determining Adherence to a Gluten-Free Diet in Swedish Adolescents. *J. Pediatr. Gastroenterol. Nutr.* **2019**, *69*, 575–580. [CrossRef] [PubMed]
65. Rubio-Tapia, A.; Hill, I.D.; Semrad, C.; Ciar, C.; Kelly, C.P.; Lebwohl, B. American College of Gastroenterology Guidelines Update: Diagnosis and Management of Celiac Disease. *Am. J. Gastroenterol.* **2023**, *118*, 59–76. [CrossRef]
66. Raiteri, A.; Granito, A.; Giamperoli, A.; Catenaro, T.; Negrini, G.; Tovoli, F. Current Guidelines for the Management of Celiac Disease: A Systematic Review with Comparative Analysis. *World J. Gastroenterol.* **2022**, *28*, 154–175. [CrossRef] [PubMed]
67. Leffler, D.A.; Schuppan, D. Update on Serologic Testing in Celiac Disease. *Am. J. Gastroenterol.* **2010**, *105*, 2520–2524. [CrossRef] [PubMed]
68. Ludvigsson, J.F.; Bai, J.C.; Biagi, F.; Card, T.R.; Ciacci, C.; Ciclitira, P.J.; Green, P.H.R.; Hadjivassiliou, M.; Holdoway, A.; Van Heel, D.A.; et al. Diagnosis and Management of Adult Coeliac Disease: Guidelines from the British Society of Gastroenterology. *Gut* **2014**, *63*, 1210–1228. [CrossRef] [PubMed]
69. Comino, I.; Fernández-Bañares, F.; Esteve, M.; Ortigosa, L.; Castillejo, G.; Fambuena, B.; Ribes-Koninckx, C.; Sierra, C.; Rodríguez-Herrera, A.; Salazar, J.C.; et al. Fecal Gluten Peptides Reveal Limitations of Serological Tests and Food Questionnaires for Monitoring Gluten-Free Diet in Celiac Disease Patients. *Am. J. Gastroenterol.* **2016**, *111*, 1456–1465. [CrossRef]
70. Monachesi, C.; Verma, A.K.; Catassi, G.N.; Franceschini, E.; Gatti, S.; Gesuita, R.; Lionetti, E.; Catassi, C. Determination of Urinary Gluten Immunogenic Peptides to Assess Adherence to the Gluten-Free Diet: A Randomized, Double-Blind, Controlled Study. *Clin. Transl. Gastroenterol.* **2021**, *12*, E00411. [CrossRef]

Disclaimer/Publisher's Note: The statements, opinions and data contained in all publications are solely those of the individual author(s) and contributor(s) and not of MDPI and/or the editor(s). MDPI and/or the editor(s) disclaim responsibility for any injury to people or property resulting from any ideas, methods, instructions or products referred to in the content.

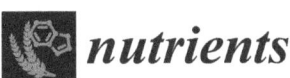

Article

New Food Frequency Questionnaire to Estimate Vitamin K Intake in a Mediterranean Population

Ezequiel Pinto [1,2], Carla Viegas [3,4], Paula Ventura Martins [5], Tânia Nascimento [1,2], Leon Schurgers [6] and Dina Simes [3,4,*]

[1] Centro de Estudos e Desenvolvimento em Saúde, Campus de Gambelas, Universidade do Algarve, 8005-139 Faro, Portugal; epinto@ualg.pt (E.P.); tinascimento@ualg.pt (T.N.)
[2] Algarve Biomedical Center Research Institute (ABC-RI), Campus de Gambelas, Universidade do Algarve, 8005-139 Faro, Portugal
[3] Centre of Marine Sciences (CCMAR), Campus de Gambelas, Universidade do Algarve, 8005-139 Faro, Portugal; caviegas@ualg.pt
[4] GenoGla Diagnostics, Centre of Marine Sciences (CCMAR), Campus de Gambelas, Universidade do Algarve, 8005-139 Faro, Portugal
[5] Research Centre for Tourism, Sustainability and Well-Being, CinTurs, Campus de Gambelas, Universidade do Algarve, 8005-139 Faro, Portugal; pventura@ualg.pt
[6] Department of Biochemistry, Cardiovascular Research Institute Maastricht, 6200 MD Maastricht, The Netherlands; l.schurgers@maastrichtuniversity.nl
* Correspondence: dsimes@ualg.pt; Tel.: +351-289-800100

Abstract: Vitamin K is a multifunctional micronutrient essential for human health, and deficiency has been linked to multiple pathological conditions. In this study, we aimed to develop and validate a new food frequency questionnaire (FFQ) to estimate total vitamin K intake, over the course of a 30-day interval, in a Portuguese, Mediterranean-based, population. We conducted a prospective study in a non-random sample of 38 healthy adult volunteers. The FFQ was designed based on a validated Portuguese FFQ used in nationally representative studies and on literature reviews, to include foods containing ≥5 μg of vitamin K/100 g and foods with a lower vitamin K content, yet commonly included in a Mediterranean diet. Vitamin K intake was estimated from 24 h recalls and six days of food records. The final FFQ included 54 food items which, according to regression analyses, explains 90% of vitamin K intake. Mean differences in vitamin K intake based on food records (80 ± 47.7 μg/day) and on FFQ (96.5 ± 64.3 μg/day) were statistically non-significant. Further, we found a strong correlation between both methods (r = 0.7; p = 0.003). Our results suggest that our new FFQ is a valid instrument to assess the last 30 days of vitamin K intake in the Portuguese Mediterranean population.

Keywords: vitamin K; food frequency questionnaire; dietary intake; Mediterranean diet

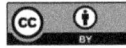

1. Introduction

Vitamin K is a liposoluble vitamin essential for maintaining proper human health, and its deficiency has been linked to age-related diseases, such as cardiovascular disease, osteoarthritis, dementia, cognitive impairment, mobility disability, and frailty [1,2]. Vitamin K has been historically described as a co-factor for the gamma-glutamylcarboxylation of vitamin K-dependent proteins (VKDPs) with a multitude of functions in multiple body tissues and molecular processes. Vitamin K is considered an essential nutrient for blood coagulation and cardiovascular and bone health. In addition, vitamin K has been shown to exert novel roles independent of VKDPs carboxylation, such as anti-inflammatory, antioxidant, antiferroptosis, transcriptional regulator of osteoblastic genes, inhibition of tumor progression, and cognition promoter [1–3].

Naturally occurring vitamin K includes phylloquinone (vitamin K1) and several forms of menaquinones (MKn or vitamin K2). Vitamin K1 (VK1) is mostly found in photosynthetic organisms, including green leafy vegetables, herbs, algae, and vegetable oils. Vitamin K2 (VK2) is primarily produced by bacteria and is obtained through the consumption of meat, fermented foods, and dairy products [1,4]. Although, collectively, VK1 and VK2 comprise the generally described vitamin K, these isoforms differ not only in the source, but also in absorption rates, tissue distribution, bioavailability, and target activity [1]. Despite the fact that vitamin K can be recycled, that microbiota can produce VK2, and that MK-4 is a product of conversion from vitamin K at tissue level, vitamin K1 and K2 sources are mainly dietary [5,6]. According to the estimated dietary consumption, vitamin K1 accounts for 90% of the total vitamin K in the diet [7], but evidence from basic research and clinical studies has highlighted the importance of VK2. In fact, it was suggested that VK2 might account for 70% of total extrahepatic activity, while VK1 contributes only 5% [8]. Vitamin K has a recommended daily intake (RDI) based on the median intake of VK1 in American adults, and an adequate intake recommendation (adequate intake—AI) set at 120 µg/day for men and 90 µg/day for women [9]. In Europe, 75 µg vitamin K has been recommended as daily allowance (Commission Directive 2008/100/EC). Additionally, VK2 has been suggested to be suitable for consideration for a specific dietary recommendation intake [8].

While most diets are considered to contain an adequate amount of vitamin K, further research is needed, especially because the intake estimates of vitamin K are not consistent and mostly focused on VK1. Additionally, habitual intake is influenced by factors including food diversity, eating patterns, and different contents of vitamin K, which may vary with soil, climate, and agricultural conditions [10].

Food frequency questionnaires (FFQ) are commonly used to assess dietary intake in epidemiological studies because they are relatively easy to administer, are cost-effective, and are able to capture long-term habitual intake [11]. However, the validity of FFQ is dependent on the accuracy of the food composition database and the ability of participants to recall their intake over a specific period [12].

Validated FFQ to assess vitamin K intake exists, constructed using American populations, but these tools cannot be directly applied to a Mediterranean population, which traditionally follows an eating pattern where vitamin K-rich foods, such are leafy green vegetables and different types of cheeses, are frequently consumed.

The aim of this study was to develop and validate a new FFQ for assessing vitamin K intake, including VK1 and VK2, in a Mediterranean-based sample. To our knowledge, this is the first study to evaluate the validity of a FFQ specifically designed to assess vitamin K intake in this setting.

2. Materials and Methods

2.1. Study Design and Participants

We conducted a prospective study in a non-random sample of healthy adult volunteers, recruited by direct contact and through social media. Inclusion criteria were: (i) age $\geq$ 18 years and (ii) cognitive ability to fulfil the data collection tools. Exclusion criteria were: (i) currently under treatment for serious chronic illness, such as cancer or autoimmune diseases; (ii) diagnosis of a disease that impairs nutrition or food choice, such as Crohn's disease, other malabsorption syndromes or food allergies; and (iii) on anticoagulant therapy.

Sample size calculation, according to methods proposed by Huley et al. [11], considering 90% power, 5% statistical significance, and a minimum predicted correlation coefficient of 0.55 between vitamin K intake estimated by FFQ and estimated by dietary recalls, yielded a minimum sample size of 30 individuals. Accounting for a 10% dropout rate, we set the minimum sample size at 35 individuals. On recruitment, 38 participants were eligible, and all proceeded to be a part of the study and concluded data collection.

All participants signed informed consent forms and this study was approved by the Ethics Committee of the University of Algarve, Portugal.

2.2. Data Collection

To apply the inclusion criteria, participants were recruited in a face-to-face interview and all details of the study were explained. Intake of vitamin K was assessed by one 24 h recall, conducted by a trained dietitian at the day of recruitment, and two self-fulfillment dietary records, comprising three, consecutive, complete days each. The first dietary record was completed in the days following recruitment, and the final record was completed one month later. One of the records was relative to weekend days (Friday, Saturday, and Sunday), and researchers contacted participants by e-mail to encourage them to fulfil the dietary records on the set dates.

Participants were asked to report the brand and type of each food item whenever possible. In the recruitment interview, participants were provided with forms to record their dietary intake, and any questions regarding this stage were addressed. Forms for the study were based on the EPIC-Norfolk dietary records forms [12] and in the Portuguese National Health and Physical Activity Survey [13] forms, which include detailed instructions and images showing portion sizes and common measurement cups and spoons. Researchers were available by phone at any time to address any additional questions during data collection.

After fulfilling the second dietary record, participants were also asked to complete the FFQ created for this study as detailed below. Participants were also asked to report their height, weight, education level, age, and gender.

2.3. Food Frequency Questionnaire (FFQ)

To construct the FFQ for this study, we based our food list on a validated Portuguese FFQ used in nationally representative studies [13]. Based on previous research [14–16] and on published food composition tables for vitamin K [7,17], we identified and selected foods with ≥ 5 µg of vitamin K/100 g of food and included them in the FFQ. Additionally, we identified foods that, despite having <5 µg of vitamin K/100 g of food, are commonly included in a Mediterranean diet, such as some types of soft cheese, boiled chickpeas, pumpkin, bell pepper, mackerel, sardines, almonds, walnuts, and coffee [18,19]. The initial FFQ included a total of 103 food items. Statistical analysis for this validation study, detailed in the results, allowed us to propose a final FFQ with 54 food items.

Participants were asked to report the frequency of intake in the last month of all listed food items by choosing one of eight frequency options: never or less than once per month, 1–3 per month, 1 per week, 2–4 per week, 5–6 per week, 1 per day, 2–3 per day, 4+ per day.

All food items were presented with a photograph with a recommended portion weight, also used in the Portuguese National Health and Physical Activity Survey [13], and participants reported if their average portion was the same, smaller (defined as 0.5 times smaller), or larger (1.5 times larger) than the recommended size.

Vitamin K intake for each food item was computed based on the following formula: nutrient content in portion × average portion size × frequency conversion factor. The conversion factors were those proposed in previous research on this subject [20–22] and are presented in Table 1.

Table 1. Frequency intake and conversion factors.

Intake Frequency	Conversion Factor
Never or less than once per month	0.02
1–3 per month	0.07
1 per week	0.14
2–4 per week	0.43
5–6 per week	0.79
1 per day	1
2–3 per day	2.5
4+ per day	4

Vitamin K intake was calculated using a food composition database constructed for this study in Microsoft Excel, which included data on vitamin K content of foods from previous research [7] and data from both McCance and Widdowson's and the United States Department of Agriculture's food composition databases [17,23].

2.4. Statistical Analysis

Data were analyzed using IBM SPSS for Windows (version 29.0, 2022, IBM Corporation). Mean, median, standard deviation (SD), and interquartile range (IQR) were computed whenever appropriate, and we used the Shapiro–Wilk test to assess adherence to the normal distribution of variables regarding vitamin K intake. As the distribution of these variables was non-Gaussian for both food records and FFQ, data were log-transformed for some statistical inference tests.

Agreement was analyzed using Student's t-tests and plotted according to the Bland–Altman method [24]. We also computed Pearson's correlation coefficient on the log transformed data.

Statistical significance for all procedures was set at 0.05.

3. Results

3.1. Participants

All participants (n = 38) followed the data collection procedures for the study and completed the food records and the FFQ.

Participants were predominantly females (n = 23; 60.5%). All of the men (n = 15; 100%) and 48% of the women (n = 11) had a college level degree. Mean body mass index (BMI) was 24.6 ± 0.6 kg/m^2 and ages ranged between 18 and 65 years old. Female participants were significantly older (p = 0.004) and with a lower educational level than males (p = 0.002). Table 2 summarizes the characteristics of participants.

Table 2. Characteristics for all participants by gender.

Characteristics		All (n = 38)		Males (n = 15)		Females (n = 23)		p-Value
Age (years)	Mean (±SD)	37	(±12.2)	31	(±4.5)	41	(±14)	0.004 [a]
	Median (IQR)	36.5	(19)	31	(8)	44	(27)	
BMI (kg/m^2)	Mean (±SD)	24.6	(±0.6)	24.8	(±0.3)	24.5	(±0.7)	
	Median (IQR)	24.6	(0.5)	24.7	(0.6)	24.6	(0.6)	0.051 [b]
Education (level):								
Primary school (4 years); n (%)		2	(5%)	-		2	(9%)	0.002 [c]
Middle school (5–9 years); n (%)		2	(5%)	-		2	(9%)	
High school (10–12 years); n (%)		8	(21%)	-		8	(35%)	
College level degree; n (%)		26	(69%)	15	(100%)	11	(48%)	

BMI—Body mass index; SD—standard deviation; IQR—interquartile range. Gender differences computed with: [a]—Student's t-test; [b]—Mann–Whitney's test; [c]—Fisher–Freeman–Halton exact test; Statistical significance (p < 0.05) is **boldfaced**.

3.2. Food Frequency Questionnaire Items

To analyze the adequacy of the food item list in the FFQ, we conducted multiple regression analyses, with a stepwise method, using vitamin K intake as the dependent variable and all other food items as independent variables. The food items that contributed cumulatively up to 90% of vitamin K intake in a statistically significant model (F = 7.5, p = 0.004) were retained for the final version of the FFQ. From the initial list of 103 food items, we eliminated 43, and thus included 54 food items in our FFQ. The included food items are shown in Table 3.

Table 3. Food items in the final food frequency questionnaire.

Category	Food Item
Meat, fish, and eggs	Tuna in oil, drained; Beef, minced meat or hamburger; Cold cuts (ham, mortadella, chorizo, etc.); Mackerel, horse mackerel or small fish; Scrambled or fried egg
Grains and tubers	Homemade or restaurant French fries; Packaged potato chips or corn snacks; Homemade bread
Desserts and sweets	Cookies, biscuits; Cake, tart or other pastry product (croissant, etc.); Milk chocolate
Fruits	Plum, cherry; Almond, walnut, hazelnut; Peanut, cashew; Dried figs; Apple, pear; Strawberry; Nectarines; Peach; Grapes; Avocado
Vegetables and pulses	Pumpkin; Watercress, arugula; Lettuce or mixed green salad; Leek; Eggplant; Broccoli; Carrot; Coriander or parsley; Kale; Cabbage, collard greens, brussels sprouts; Cauliflower; Zucchini; Peas; Asparagus, green beans; Spinach; Cooked beans; Cooked chickpeas; Greens, creamed spinach, green vegetable puree; Cucumber; Green pepper; Red pepper; Tomato
Fats and oils	Olive oil; Butter, margarine or vegetable spread, mayonnaise; Cooking oil
Other	Espresso coffee
Meals	Lasagna or pasta; Stir-fry or stew with vegetables and/or pasta
Dairy products	Creamy cheese (Brie, Camembert) or Serra da Estrela cheese; Cream cheese, spreadable; Cured cow or sheep cheese, Edam cheese; Goat cheese; Cottage or fresh cheese

3.3. Comparison between Food Records and Food Frequency Questionnaire

Mean vitamin K intake was 80 µg (±47.7) according to food records and 96.5 µg (±64.3) according to the FFQ. Vitamin K estimates from the FFQ were, on average, 16.5 µg (±82.57) higher than estimates from food records. This difference is statistically non-significant ($p = 0.226$), supporting the existence of proper absolute agreement between both methods. The same results are observed in a paired Student's t-test on log-transformed vitamin K intake data ($p = 0.293$). We also found a strong and statistically significant correlation ($r = 0.697$; $p = 0.003$) between the FFQ and diet records, which suggests a good relative agreement and that the FFQ is a valid instrument to assess vitamin K intake in this population. Table 4 summarizes the results from the comparison between FFQ and food records.

Table 4. Vitamin K intake according to food records and food frequency questionnaire.

		Food Records		FFQ		p-Value
Vitamin K intake (µg)	Mean (±SD)	80	(±47.7)	96.5	(±64.3)	0.293 [a,b]
	Median (IQR)	77.4	(84.5)	80.9	(89.4)	
	Minimum	16.1		17		
	Maximum	173.8		319		
Difference between FFQ and food records: Mean (±SD); (95% CI)		16.5 (±82.57); (−10.7, 43.6)				0.226 [b]
Correlation between FFQ and food:		0.697				0.003 [a]

SD—Standard deviation; IQR—interquartile range; CI—confidence interval; FFQ—food frequency questionnaire. [a]—p-values corresponding to analysis on log-transformed variables; [b]—Student's t-test.

We constructed a Bland–Altman plot to assess agreement by computing mean vitamin K intake from FFQ data and six days of food records, and plotting this with the difference in mean intake obtained with these two methods. The plot shows that most participants fall in the acceptable limits of agreement in individual differences between both dietary estimate methods (Figure 1).

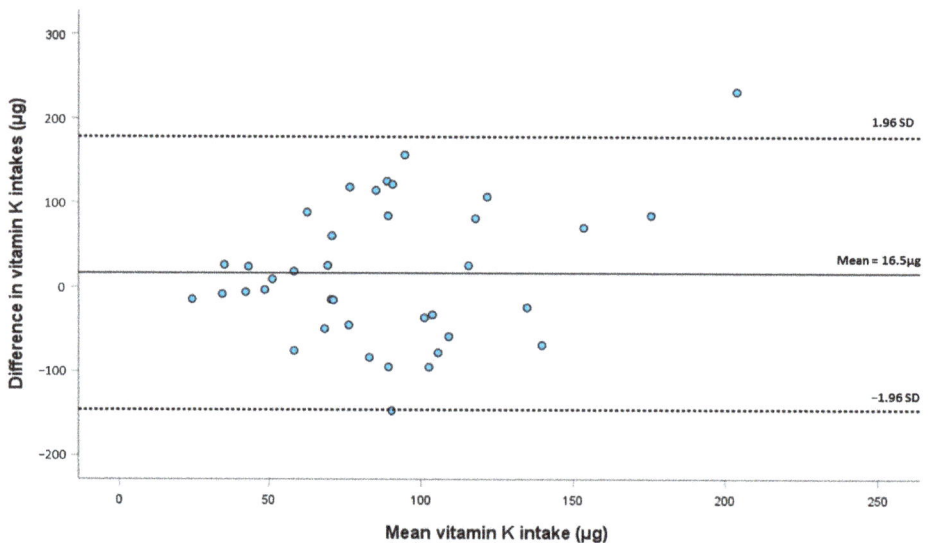

Figure 1. Bland–Altman plot to assess agreement in vitamin K intake between food records and the food frequency questionnaire.

Following the methods proposed by Doğan [25] and Ludbrook [26], we conducted a simple linear regression analysis using the Bland–Altman plot data, considering the difference in mean vitamin K intake as the dependent variable and mean vitamin K intake as independent variable. This analysis showed a regression where mean differences are not significantly different than zero (F = 0.004; p = 0.959) and a statistically non-significant (p = 0.949) $β_1$ coefficient, very close to the null value ($β_1$ = −0.024), suggesting that there is no proportional bias. This shows that the difference in values resulting from the two methods does not increase or decrease in proportion to the average values.

4. Discussion

The literature suggests that FFQ are valid, reliable, and easy-to-use tools in populational studies, but their accuracy in estimating some nutrients, particularly micronutrients, is still the subject of ongoing research [22,27–29]. Thus, the development of a valid FFQ for vitamin K that can be used in surveys, cohort studies, and other populational assessments can constitute worthwhile research, especially if the FFQ is aimed at populations that are associated with a specific dietary pattern, which includes vitamin K-rich foods.

Our study allowed the development of a valid FFQ for the assessment of vitamin K intake in a sample of Portuguese adults, with a very low cost of administration and processing, and with low respondent burden. Moreover, this FFQ is directed to estimate VK1 and VK2 intake as a more representative measurement of vitamin K status. Most FFQs developed to estimate the dietary consumption of vitamin K have specifically focused on VK1 mainly because, in the Western diet, it accounts for nearly 90% of total vitamin K intake [7]. However, accumulating evidence from basic research and clinical studies has highlighted the health beneficial effects of VK2, particularly due to its long half-life and extrahepatic distribution. While VK1 is preferentially accumulated in the liver and is poorly retained in the organism with a half-life time of 1–2 h, VK2 with a half-life time of 68 h is available to extrahepatic tissues through circulation, resulting in an increased bioavailability of the whole body [1,2]. Additionally, in terms of functionality, VK2 (particularly MK-7 and MK-4) has been shown to have a higher bioactivity than VK1 in different molecular processes, such as gamma-glutamylcarboxylation cofactor, inhibitory effect on bone resorption, antioxidant, activator of sphingolipid metabolism, and anticancer [30–35]. In fact, it was suggested that VK2 is the major active form of vitamin K, accounting for 70% of total extrahepatic activity, while VK1 contributes only 5%, and that the beneficial effects of VK2 are not covered by current RDI guidelines [8]. However, it should be noted that MK-4 is a result of vitamin K conversion and is dependent from VK1 intake, and that MK-4 is present in most extrahepatic tissues [5,6,36,37]. In this context, more attention should be given to the dietary intake of both VK1 and VK2.

Although we recorded some overestimation (16.5 ± 82.57 μg) of vitamin K intake when compared with food records, this overestimation was statistically non-significant and on par with the variability which, according to previous research, is to be expected [38–41]. Our FFQ showed an adequate relative agreement with food records, with a correlation coefficient of 0.697, which is above the minimum threshold of 0.4 proposed for FFQ validation studies [22,42]. Previous FFQ studies regarding vitamin K intake report correlations from 0.5 to 0.8 [15,16,40,43–45]. The Bland–Altman method of analysis also indicates good relative agreement, with one outlier participant above the 95% agreement limit, and one participant in the borderline of the lower agreement limit. Although this study is not intended to evaluate vitamin K intake in our population, the mean vitamin K of 96.5 ± 64.3 μg/day in our sample is within the RDI established for the American population and above the 75 μg/day recommended by the European Commission.

We identified several limitations of this study and propose future research directions in this topic. Although VK1 intake has been suggested to not vary significantly with season [46], we cannot rule out the interference of the seasonal nature of dietary patterns, particularly when considering a Mediterranean-based diet. We included items in the FFQ food list that cover the wide variety of products that are common in all harvesting seasons, but data were collected in springtime. This can imply that the final food list that derived from the regression analysis may not include items that provide an important intake of vitamin K, because these are mainly consumed during winter. We believe that wintertime products are represented in the final list, but additional studies to confirm this, conducted during colder months, are needed. Some research suggests that there is a high within-person variation in the intake of vitamin K [41] and green vegetables [42,43]. Therefore, additional studies assessing the reproducibility of our FFQ should also be undertaken, as we did not assess this parameter. Although the sample size of our study is adequate to compare methods of assessing dietary intake, our participants constituted a non-probabilistic, convenience sample, mainly composed of adults with a high educational level. Ages ranged from 18 to 65 years of age and, therefore, our data do not allow us to assess the validity of our FFQ in older adults, or in individuals with different sociodemographic characteristics, thereby compromising the generalization of our results.

It is also important to note that we focused on collecting vitamin K intake during a period of one month. The initial 24 h recall and the food records that were used to establish usual intake were collected during a 30-day interval and the FFQ was specifically constructed in such a way that participants recall their intake for an equivalent period. This limited timespan can favor recall, as participants' memory of recent food intake can contribute to the good agreement shown in the data. The aim of the FFQ we developed was to assess short-term intake and, thus, we cannot infer or extrapolate to longer periods of intake recall and propose this to be taken into account in future studies with this tool.

Overall, we constructed a valid, practical, and cost-effective tool to estimate vitamin K intake for a 30-day period. Our FFQ showed good absolute and relative agreement with food records and includes a list of food products that account for most of the VK1 and VK2 intake in a Mediterranean dietary pattern in the Portuguese population. Additional research is needed to assess the reproducibility of this tool to confirm that seasonality does not affect its validity, and to test its applicability to different populations.

Author Contributions: Conceptualization, E.P., C.V. and D.S.; methodology, E.P. and P.V.M.; software, P.V.M.; formal analysis, E.P. and T.N.; investigation, E.P., C.V. and D.S.; resources, L.S.; writing—original draft preparation, E.P., C.V. and D.S.; writing—review and editing, E.P., C.V., L.S. and D.S.; project administration, E.P. and D.S.; funding acquisition, E.P., C.V., P.V.M. and D.S. All authors have read and agreed to the published version of the manuscript.

Funding: This research was funded by the Portuguese National Funds from FCT—Foundation for Science and Technology, through transitional provision DL57/2016/CP1361/CT0006, projects EXPL/BTM-TEC/0990/2021, UIDB/04326/2020, UIDP/04326/2020 and LA/P/0101/2020 and AAC n° 41/ALG/2020—Project n° 072583—NUTRISAFE.

Institutional Review Board Statement: The study was conducted according to the guidelines of the Declaration of Helsinki and approved by the ethics committee of the University of Algarve, Faro, Portugal (code CEUAlg Pn°01/2022, approved 21 January 2022).

Informed Consent Statement: Informed consent was obtained from all subjects involved in the study.

Data Availability Statement: Data available on request due to privacy restrictions.

Conflicts of Interest: The authors declare no conflict of interest.

References

1. Simes, D.C.; Viegas, C.S.B.; Araújo, N.; Marreiros, C. Vitamin K as a Diet Supplement with Impact in Human Health: Current Evidence in Age-Related Diseases. *Nutrients* **2020**, *12*, 138. [CrossRef]
2. Simes, D.C.; Viegas, C.S.B.; Araújo, N.; Marreiros, C. Vitamin K as a Powerful Micronutrient in Aging and Age-Related Diseases: Pros and Cons from Clinical Studies. *Int. J. Mol. Sci.* **2019**, *20*, 4150. [CrossRef] [PubMed]
3. Mishima, E.; Ito, J.; Wu, Z.; Nakamura, T.; Wahida, A.; Doll, S.; Tonnus, W.; Nepachalovich, P.; Eggenhofer, E.; Aldrovandi, M.; et al. A non-canonical vitamin K cycle is a potent ferroptosis suppressor. *Nature* **2022**, *608*, 778–783. [CrossRef] [PubMed]
4. Booth, S.L. Vitamin K: Food composition and dietary intakes. *Food Nutr. Res.* **2012**, *56*, 5505. [CrossRef] [PubMed]
5. Shearer, M.J.; Newman, P. Recent trends in the metabolism and cell biology of vitamin K with special reference to vitamin K cycling and MK-4 biosynthesis. *J. Lipid Res.* **2014**, *55*, 345–362. [CrossRef]
6. Thijssen, H.H.; Drittij-Reijnders, M.J. Vitamin K distribution in rat tissues: Dietary phylloquinone is a source of tissue menaquinone-4. *Br. J. Nutr.* **1994**, *72*, 415–425. [CrossRef]
7. Schurgers, L.J.; Vermeer, C. Determination of phylloquinone and menaquinones in food. Effect of food matrix on circulating vitamin K concentrations. *Haemostasis* **2000**, *30*, 298–307.
8. Akbulut, A.C.; Pavlic, J.; Petsophonsakul, P.; Halder, M.; Maresz, K.; Kramann, R.; Schurgers, L. Vitamin K2 Needs an RDI Separate from Vitamin K1. *Nutrients* **2020**, *12*, 1852. [CrossRef]
9. Institute of Medicine (US) Panel on Micronutrients. *Dietary Reference Intakes for Vitamin A, Vitamin K, Arsenic, Boron, Chromium, Copper, Iodine, Iron, Manganese, Molybdenum, Nickel, Silicon, Vanadium, and Zinc*; National Academies Press (US): Washington, DC, USA, 2001.
10. Passarelli, S.; Free, C.M.; Allen, L.H.; Batis, C.; Beal, T.; Biltoft-Jensen, A.P.; Bromage, S.; Cao, L.; Castellanos-Gutiérrez, A.; Christensen, T.; et al. Estimating national and subnational nutrient intake distributions of global diets. *Am. J. Clin. Nutr.* **2022**, *116*, 551–560. [CrossRef]
11. Browner, W.; Newman, T.; Hulley, S. Estimating Sample Size and Power: Applications and Examples. In *Designing Clinical Research: An Epidemiologic Approach*, 4th ed.; Hulley, S., Cummings, S., Browner, W., Grady, D., Newman, T., Eds.; Lippincott Williams & Wilkins: Philadelphia, PA, USA, 2013; pp. 55–83.
12. Bingham, S.A.; Welch, A.A.; McTaggart, A.; Mulligan, A.A.; Runswick, S.A.; Luben, R.; Oakes, S.; Khaw, K.T.; Wareham, N.; Day, N.E. Nutritional methods in the European Prospective Investigation of Cancer in Norfolk. *Public Health Nutr.* **2001**, *4*, 847. [CrossRef]
13. University of Porto; National Health Institute Doutor Ricardo Jorge; University of Lisbon; SilicoLife Lda; Lopes, C.; Torres, D.; Oliveira, A.; Severo, M.; Guiomar, S.; Alarcão, V.; et al. National Food, Nutrition and Physical Activity Survey of the Portuguese general population. *EFSA Support. Publ.* **2017**, *14*, EN-1341. [CrossRef]
14. Bingham, S.A.; Gill, C.; Welch, A.; Cassidy, A.; Runswick, S.A.; Oakes, S.; Lubin, R.; Thurnham, D.I.; Key, T.J.; Roe, L.; et al. Validation of dietary assessment methods in the UK arm of EPIC using weighed records, and 24-hour urinary nitrogen and potassium and serum vitamin C and carotenoids as biomarkers. *Int. J. Epidemiol.* **1997**, *26*, S137–S151. [CrossRef]
15. Presse, N.; Shatenstein, B.; Kergoat, M.J.; Ferland, G. Validation of a Semi-Quantitative Food Frequency Questionnaire Measuring Dietary Vitamin K Intake in Elderly People. *J. Am. Diet Assoc.* **2009**, *109*, 1251–1255. [CrossRef] [PubMed]

16. Dias Mendonça, D.; Zuchinali, P.; Souza, G.C. Development of a food frequency questionnaire to determine vitamin k intake in anticoagulated patients: A pilot study. *Rev. Chil. Nut.* **2018**, *45*, 363–371. [CrossRef]
17. Roe, M.; Pinchen, H.; Church, S.; Finglas, P. McCance and Widdowson's The Composition of Foods Seventh Summary Edition and updated Composition of Foods Integrated Dataset. *Nutr. Bull.* **2015**, *40*, 36–39. [CrossRef]
18. Rees, K.; Takeda, A.; Martin, N.; Ellis, L.; Wijesekara, D.; Vepa, A.; Das, A.; Hartley, L.; Stranges, S. Mediterranean-style diet for the primary and secondary prevention of cardiovascular disease. *Cochrane Database Syst. Rev.* **2019**, *3*, CD009825. [CrossRef]
19. Willett, W. Mediterranean Dietary Pyramid. *Int. J. Environ. Res. Public Health* **2021**, *18*, 4568. [CrossRef]
20. Willett, W. *Nutritional Epidemiology*, 3rd ed.; Oxford University Press: New York, NY, USA, 2013; pp. 70–95.
21. Cade, J.; Thompson, R.; Burley, V.; Warm, D. Development, validation and utilisation of food-frequency questionnaires—A review. *Public Health Nutr.* **2003**, *5*, 567–587. [CrossRef]
22. Nelson, M. The validation of dietary assessment. In *Design Concepts in Nutritional Epidemiology*, 2nd ed.; Barrie, M., Margetts, B.M., Nelson, M., Eds.; Oxford University Press: New York, NY, USA, 1997; pp. 241–272.
23. US Department of Agriculture. FoodData Central. Available online: https://fdc.nal.usda.gov/index.html (accessed on 30 November 2022).
24. Bland, J.M.; Altman, D.G. Statistical methods for assessing agreement between two methods of clinical measurement. *Lancet* **1986**, *1*, 307–310. [CrossRef]
25. Doğan, N.Ö. Bland-Altman analysis: A paradigm to understand correlation and agreement. *Turk. J. Emerg. Med.* **2018**, *18*, 139–141. [CrossRef]
26. Ludbrook, J. Confidence in Altman–Bland plots: A critical review of the method of differences. *Clin. Exp. Pharmacol. Physiol.* **2010**, *37*, 143–149. [CrossRef] [PubMed]
27. Cade, J.E. Measuring diet in the 21st century: Use of new technologies. *Proc. Nutr. Soc.* **2017**, *76*, 276–282. [CrossRef]
28. Shim, J.S.; Oh, K.; Kim, H.C. Dietary assessment methods in epidemiologic studies. *Epidemiol. Health* **2014**, *36*, e2014009. [CrossRef]
29. Schulz, C.A.; Oluwagbemigun, K.; Nöthlings, U. Advances in dietary pattern analysis in nutritional epidemiology. *Eur. J. Nutr.* **2021**, *60*, 4115–4130. [CrossRef] [PubMed]
30. Buitenhuis, H.; Soute, B.; Vermeer, C. Comparison of the vitamins K1, K2 and K3 as cofactors for the hepatic vitamin K-dependent carboxylase. *Biochim. Biophys. Acta* **1990**, *1034*, 170–175. [CrossRef] [PubMed]
31. Hara, K.; Akiyama, Y.; Nakamura, T.; Murota, S.; Morita, I. The inhibitory effect of vitamin K2 (menatetrenone) on bone resorption may be related to its side chain. *Bone* **1995**, *16*, 179–184. [CrossRef]
32. Ambrożewicz, E.; Muszyńska, M.; Tokajuk, G.; Grynkiewicz, G.; Žarković, N.; Skrzydlewska, E. Beneficial Effects of Vitamins K and D3 on Redox Balance of Human Osteoblasts Cultured with Hydroxypatite-Based Biomaterials. *Cells* **2019**, *8*, 325. [CrossRef]
33. Lev, M.; Milford, A. The 3-Ketodihydrosphingosine melaninogenicus: Synthetase of Bacteroides melaninogenicus: Induction by Vitamin K. *Arch. Biochem. Biophys.* **1973**, *157*, 500–508. [CrossRef]
34. Sundaram, K.S.; Lev, M. Regulation of sulfotransferase activity by vitamin k in mouse brain. *Arch. Biochem. Biophys.* **1990**, *277*, 109–113. [CrossRef]
35. Xv, F.; Chen, J.; Duan, L.; Li, S. Research progress on the anticancer effects of vitamin K2. *Oncol. Lett.* **2018**, *15*, 8926–8934. [CrossRef]
36. Thijssen, H.; Drittij-Reijnders, M. Vitamin K status in human tissues: Tissue-specific accumulation of phylloquinone and menaquinone-4. *Br. J. Nutr.* **1996**, *75*, 121–127. [CrossRef]
37. Thijssen, H.H.; Drittij, M.J.; Vermeer, C.; Schoffelen, E. Menaquinone-4 in breast milk is derived from dietary phylloquinone. *Br. J. Nutr.* **2002**, *87*, 219–226. [CrossRef] [PubMed]
38. Booth, S.L.; Sokoll, L.J.; O'Brien, M.E.; Tucker, K.; Dawson-Hughes, B.; Sadowski, J.A. Assessment of dietary phylloquinone intake and vitamin K status in postmenopausal women. *Eur. J. Clin. Nutr.* **1995**, *49*, 832–841.
39. Booth, S.L.; Tucker, K.L.; McKeown, N.M.; Davidson, K.W.; Dallal, G.E.; Sadowski, J.A. Relationships between Dietary Intakes and Fasting Plasma Concentrations of Fat-Soluble Vitamins in Humans. *J. Nutr.* **1997**, *127*, 587–592. [CrossRef] [PubMed]
40. Pritchard, J.M.; Seechurn, T.; Atkinson, S.A. A food frequency questionnaire for the assessment of calcium, vitamin D and vitamin K: A pilot validation study. *Nutrients* **2010**, *2*, 805–819. [CrossRef] [PubMed]
41. Couris, R.R.; Tataronis, G.R.; Booth, S.L.; Dallal, G.E.; Blumberg, J.B.; Dwyer, J.T. Development of a self-assessment instrument to determine daily intake and variability of dietary vitamin K. *J. Am. Coll. Nutr.* **2000**, *19*, 801–807. [CrossRef]
42. Cade, J.E.; Burley, V.J.; Warm, D.L.; Thompson, R.L.; Margetts, B.M. Food-frequency questionnaires: A review of their design, validation and utilisation. *Nutr. Res. Rev.* **2004**, *17*, 5–22. [CrossRef]
43. Cantin, J.; Latour, E.; Ferland-Verry, R.; Morales Salgado, S.; Lambert, J.; Faraj, M.; Nigam, A. Validity and reproducibility of a food frequency questionnaire focused on the Mediterranean diet for the Quebec population. *Nutr. Metab. Cardiovasc. Dis.* **2016**, *26*, 154–161. [CrossRef]
44. Zwakenberg, S.R.; Engelen, A.I.P.; Dalmeijer, G.W.; Booth, S.L.; Vermeer, C.; Drijvers, J.J.M.M.; Ocke, M.C.; Feskens, E.J.M.; van der Schouw, Y.T.; Beulens, J.W.J. Reproducibility and relative validity of a food frequency questionnaire to estimate intake of dietary phylloquinone and menaquinones. *Eur. J. Clin. Nutr.* **2017**, *71*, 1423–1428. [CrossRef]

45. Bu, S.Y.; Choi, M.K.; Jin So, E. Validity and Reliability of a Self-administered Food Frequency Questionnaire to Assess Vitamin K Intake in Korean Adults. *Clin. Nutr. Res.* **2016**, *5*, 153–160.
46. Thane, C.W.; Paul, A.A.; Bates, C.J.; Bolton-Smith, C.; Prentice, A.; Shearer, M.J. Intake and sources of phylloquinone (vitamin K1): Variation with socio-demographic and lifestyle factors in a national sample of British elderly people. *Br. J. Nutr.* **2002**, *87*, 605–613. [CrossRef] [PubMed]

Disclaimer/Publisher's Note: The statements, opinions and data contained in all publications are solely those of the individual author(s) and contributor(s) and not of MDPI and/or the editor(s). MDPI and/or the editor(s) disclaim responsibility for any injury to people or property resulting from any ideas, methods, instructions or products referred to in the content.

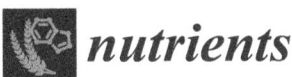

Article

A Bibliometric Analysis of Alternate-Day Fasting from 2000 to 2023

Xiaoxiao Lin, Shuai Wang * and Jinyu Huang *

Affiliated Hangzhou First People's Hospital, Zhejiang University School of Medicine, Hangzhou 310030, China; linxiaoxiao@zcmu.edu.cn
* Correspondence: drwangshuai@zju.edu.cn (S.W.); drhuangjinyu@126.com (J.H.)

Abstract: Alternate-day fasting (ADF) is becoming more popular since it may be a promising diet intervention for human health. Our study aimed to conduct a comprehensive bibliometric analysis to investigate current publication trends and hotspots in the field of ADF. Publications regarding ADF were identified from the Web of Science Core Collection (WOSCC) database. VOSviewer 1.6.16 and Online Analysis Platform were used to analyze current publication trends and hotspots. In total, there were 184 publications from 362 institutions and 39 countries/regions, which were published in 104 journals. The most productive countries/regions, institutions, authors, and journals were the USA, University of Illinois Chicago, Krista A. Varady, and *Nutrients*, respectively. The first high-cited publication was published in *PNAS* and authored by R. Michael Anson, and it was also the first article about ADF. The top five keywords with the highest frequency were as follows: calorie restriction, weight loss, intermittent fasting, obesity, and body weight. In conclusion, this is the first comprehensive bibliometric analysis related to ADF. The main research hotspots and frontiers are ADF for obesity and cardiometabolic risk, and ADF for several different population groups including healthy adults and patients with diabetes, nonalcoholic fatty liver disease (NAFLD), and cancer. The number of studies about ADF is relatively small, and more studies are needed to extend our knowledge about ADF, to improve human health.

Keywords: alternate-day fasting; bibliometric analysis; weight loss; obesity; cardiometabolic risk

Citation: Lin, X.; Wang, S.; Huang, J. A Bibliometric Analysis of Alternate-Day Fasting from 2000 to 2023. *Nutrients* **2023**, *15*, 3724. https://doi.org/10.3390/nu15173724

Academic Editors: António Raposo, Renata Puppin Zandonadi and Raquel Braz Assunção Botelho

Received: 2 August 2023
Revised: 20 August 2023
Accepted: 22 August 2023
Published: 25 August 2023

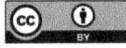

Copyright: © 2023 by the authors. Licensee MDPI, Basel, Switzerland. This article is an open access article distributed under the terms and conditions of the Creative Commons Attribution (CC BY) license (https:// creativecommons.org/licenses/by/ 4.0/).

1. Introduction

Alternate-day fasting (ADF), which is defined as a feast day with usual food, alternated with a fast day with a calorie restriction of about 25% of usual intake (approximately 500 kcal), is a main type of intermittent fasting (IF) [1–6]. ADF is usually used for people with obesity and overweight. A previous systematic review and meta-analysis demonstrated that ADF could effectively lower body fat mass (FM), body weight (BW), total cholesterol (TC), and body mass index (BMI) in individuals with obesity [7]. In addition to obesity, ADF can be used to manage other diseases including non-alcoholic fatty liver disease (NAFLD), diabetes, and asthma. For example, a recent study showed that the combination of exercise with ADF was effective for reducing hepatic steatosis in individuals with NAFLD [8]. In addition, ADF is also beneficial to healthy adults, and Slaven Stekovic et al. found that ADF could reduce low-density lipoprotein, the level of sICAM-1 (an age-associated inflammatory marker), and the metabolic regulator triiodothyronine in healthy and non-obese humans [9]. It seems that ADF could become a beneficial intervention for diverse population groups.

Recently, ADF is becoming more popular since it may be a promising diet intervention for human health. Despite the growing popularity of ADF, there is no bibliometric study summarizing the current publication trends and predicting research hotspots in this field.

Bibliometric study is a comprehensive and timely analysis of countries/regions, institutions, authors, keywords, h-index, and other parameters related to all publication in a specific field. It can provide a detailed overview of a specific area of knowledge and help the researchers know the current publication trends and find hotspots. VOSviewer is a popular software tool used for bibliometric analysis, and the key functions of VOSviewer include the following: (1) network visualization, which allows users to create various types of bibliometric networks, such as co-authorship networks, co-citation networks, and keyword co-occurrence networks; (2) clustering and mapping, which employs advanced algorithms to cluster nodes (authors, articles, or keywords) that are closely related within the network; (3) keyword analysis, which can reveal trends and emerging topics in a particular research area by identifying commonly used terms and their relationships; (4) citation analysis, which helps users explore citation patterns among research articles. This can provide insights into influential articles, research trends, and the evolution of scientific ideas over time. Therefore, our study aimed to conduct a comprehensive bibliometric analysis to determine the frontiers and hotspots in the field of ADF, and then provide a panoramic vision and guidance for future researchers.

2. Materials and Methods

2.1. Search Strategy

In our study, the relevant documents were extracted from Web of Science Core Collection (WoSCC). The database was queried using the following terms: "alternate-day fasting" or "modified alternate day fasting" or "alternate day fasting" or "modified alternate-day fasting" or "alternate day calorie restriction" or "alternate-day calorie restriction" or "modified alternate-day calorie restriction" or "alternate-day modified fasting" from 1 January 2000 to 30 May 2023, with articles and reviews, in the English language.

2.2. Data Collection and Bibliometric Analysis

After the selection, the document in TXT format with "Full Record and Cited References" was downloaded and imported in the VOSviewer 1.6.16 software. We performed a two-step analysis by WoSCC Online Analysis Platform and VOSviewer 1.6.16 software. The information about annual publication number, the top 10 productive countries/regions, institutions, authors, and journals, and the top 20 high-cited publications were exported from WoSCC Online Analysis Platform. VOSviewer 1.6.16 was used to analyze the co-authorship of institutions, countries/regions, authors, citation of journals and references, co-citation of references, and co-occurrence of keywords, and then output relevant figures. In the keyword co-occurrence analysis, we merged the synonyms of "alternate-day fasting" or "modified alternate day fasting" or "alternate day fasting" or "modified alternate-day fasting" or "alternate day calorie restriction" or "alternate-day calorie restriction" or "modified alternate-day calorie restriction" or "alternate-day modified fasting" into the term "alternate-day fasting", "caloric restriction" and "calorie restriction" into the term "caloric restriction", "weight loss" and "weight-loss" into the term "weight loss", "body-composition" and "body composition" into the term "body composition", and "insulin resistance" and "insulin-resistance" into the term "insulin resistance".

3. Results

3.1. Quantity and Trends Analysis of Published Papers

In general, 184 publications including 128 articles and 56 reviews met the inclusion criteria, as shown in Figure 1. The publications, the types of publications, and the subject categories are listed in Figure 2. The top two subjects were nutrition dietetics with 83 publications and endocrinology metabolism with 31 publications. The time periods of publications could be divided into three phases: the first phase included documents published before 2010 (2003–2009), with about 16 documents published on ADF; the second phase included documents published between 2010 and 2018, with no significant increase in the number of publications in the field of ADF; in 2019, the number of publications showed a sharp upward trend, representing the third phase, from 2019 until now.

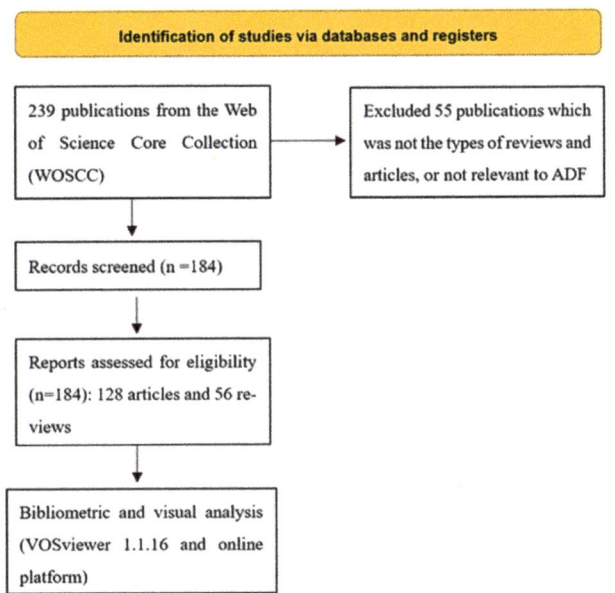

Figure 1. Flowchart of the inclusion and exclusion criteria.

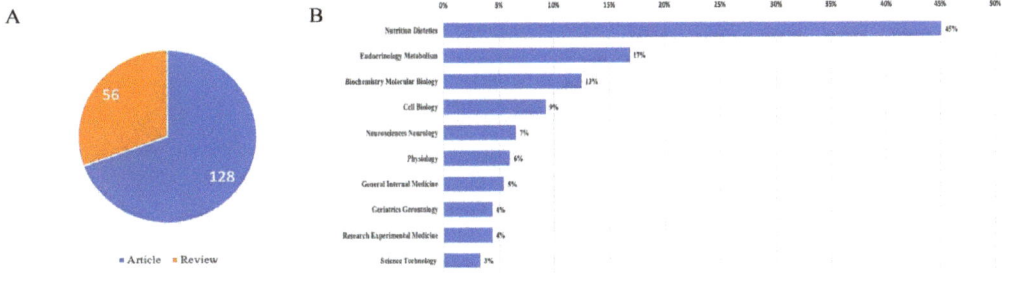

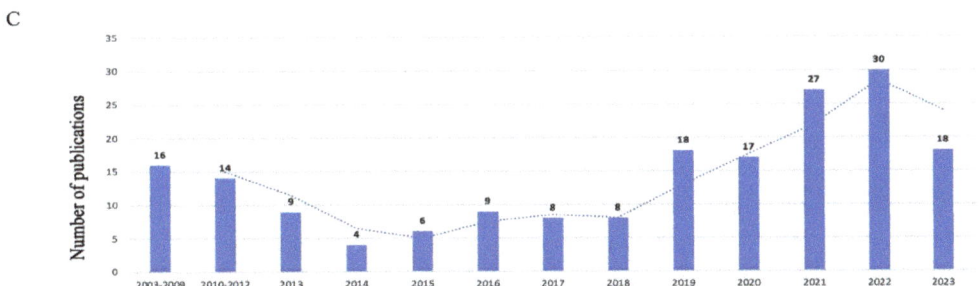

Figure 2. Yearly quantity and literature type of publications on ADF from inception to 30 May 2023. (**A**) Literature type distribution. (**B**) Subject category distribution. (**C**) Annual publication quantitative distribution.

3.2. Analysis of Countries/Regions, Institutions, and Authors

In total, 362 institutions from 39 countries/regions contributed to the field of ADF. The most productive institutions were the University of Illinois Chicago with 37 publications and 2212 citations, the National Institutes of Health (NIH) with 10 publications and 1439 citations, and the University of California System with 9 publications and 490 citations. More than half of total publications were from the USA, accounting for 53.3% (98/184), followed by China with 23 publications, and England with 14 publications. In this field, Krista A. Varady was the most productive author with 43 publications, which is far more than others; she had a high h-index of 25 and a total of 2628 citations. After her, Cynthia M. Kroeger with 17 publications and Monica C. Klempel with 13 publications were the second and third most productive authors. The top 10 most active authors, institutions, and countries/regions in the field of ADF are summarized in Table 1. The network visualization maps of the cooperation relation among authors, organizations, and countries were shown in Figure 3. The top three cooperative authors were Krista A. Varady, Cynthia M Kroeger, and Kelsey Gabel. The top three cooperative institutions were the University of Illinois Chicago, the Medical University of Graz, and the National Institutes of Health (NIH). The top three cooperative countries were the USA, Switzerland, and Germany. The word cloud representing the most frequent authors' keywords is displayed in Figure 4.

Table 1. The top 10 productive authors, institutions and countries based on publications.

Items	Ranking	Country	Publications Number	Citations	C/N	h-Index
Country	1	USA	98	5555	56.7	36
	2	China	23	579	25.2	10
	3	England	14	313	22.4	10
	4	Australia	10	376	37.6	8
	5	Italy	8	226	28.3	7
	6	Brazil	7	52	7.4	4
	7	Canada	7	200	28.6	5
	8	Iran	6	84	14	5
	9	Switzerland	6	301	50.2	4
	10	Austria	5	216	43.2	4
Institution	1	University of Illinois Chicago	37	2212	59.8	23
	2	National Institutes of Health	10	1439	143.9	8
	3	University of California System	9	490	54.4	9
	4	Louisiana State University System	8	1229	153.6	7
	5	Pennington Biomedical Research Center	7	815	116.4	6
	6	Cornell University	5	117	23.4	4
	7	Medical University of Graz	5	216	43.2	4
	8	University of Michigan	5	33	6.6	3
	9	University of Sydney	5	219	43.8	5
	10	Biotechmed Graz	4	216	54	4
Author	1	Krista A. Varady	43	2628	61.1	25
	2	Cynthia M. Kroeger	17	1337	78.6	15
	3	Monica C. Klempel	13	1314	101.1	12
	4	Kelsey Gabel	13	541	41.6	7
	5	John F. Trepanowski	12	1142	95.2	11
	6	Sofia Cienfuegos	12	191	15.9	6
	7	Kristin Hoddy	11	1041	92.2	10
	8	Mark Ezpeleta	10	123	12.3	6
	9	Surabhi Bhutani	9	939	104.3	9
	10	Faiza Kalam	8	115	14.4	6

The average article citation (C/N) = citations/numbers.

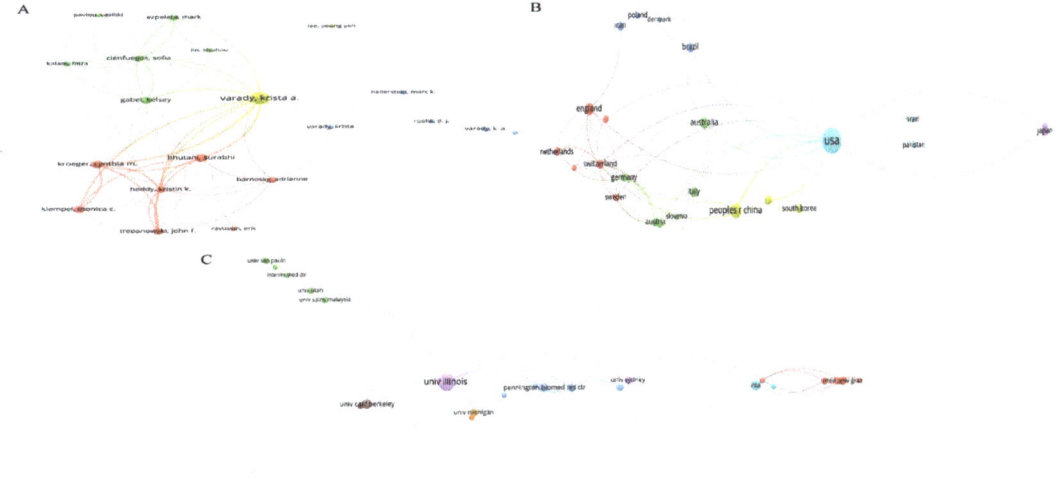

Figure 3. Visualization knowledge maps of authors, institutions, and countries/regions. (**A**) The co-authorship map of authors. (**B**) The co-authorship map of countries/regions. (**C**) The co-authorship map of institutions. Different colors indicate different clusters, and the node size indicates the number of publications. The thickness of the lines represents the link strength of the authors, countries/regions, and institutions.

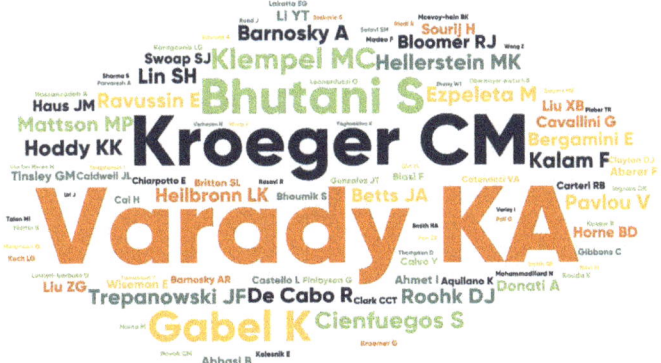

Figure 4. Word cloud of frequent authors' keywords. A word cloud is a visual representation of words, giving greater prominence to words that appear more frequently.

3.3. Analysis of Journals and Highly Cited Publications

Over the last 20 years, 184 documents were published in 104 journals. *Nutrients* was the most productive journal with 18 publications. After it, *American Journal of Clinical Nutrition* and *Obesity* both had six publications. The top 10 productive journals in the field of ADF are shown in Table 2. The characteristics of the top 20 high-cited publications [9–28] are summarized in Table 3, and the most highly cited publication was published in *PNAS* and authored by R. Michael Anson et al., in 2003 [10]. It was also the first article about ADF. In this article, they found that intermittent fasting with ADF had more benefits including increased resistance of neurons to excitotoxic stress in the brain and reduced insulin levels and serum glucose compared with caloric restriction in mice. The second most highly cited publication was published in *Free Radical Biology and Medicine*, authored by James B. Johnson et al., in 2007 [17]. In this article, they found that ADF could decrease the indicators of inflammation, including brain-derived neurotrophic factor and serum tumor necrosis factor-α (TNF-α). The third most highly cited publication was published in *JAMA Internal Medicine* in 2017, authored by Trepanowski et al. [24]. In this article, 69 metabolically healthy obese adults were included. Compared with a daily calorie restriction diet, ADF was not superior in some factors including weight maintenance, weight loss, adherence, and improvement in risk indicators for cardiovascular disease (CVD). The fourth most highly cited publication was published in *American Journal of Clinical Nutrition* in 2007, authored by Dr. Krista A. Varady and Dr. Mark K Hellerstein. In this review, they summarized the human and animal trials in ADF and the prevention of chronic diseases including type 2 diabetes (T2DM) and cardiovascular disease (CVD), since ADF may modulate several risk factors effectively and prevent these chronic diseases to a similar extent to CR. The network visualization maps of citations of journals and references are shown in Figure 5.

Table 2. The top 10 most productive journals.

Ranking	Journal Name	Country	Counts	Citation
1	Nutrients	Switzerland	18	318
2	American Journal of Clinical Nutrition	USA	6	849
3	Obesity	USA	6	528
4	Journal of Nutritional Biochemistry	USA	4	84
5	Mechanisms of Aging and Development	Switzerland	4	123
6	Metabolism Clinical and Experimental	USA	4	217
7	Nutrition Reviews	USA	4	203
8	British Journal of Nutrition	England	3	65
9	Cell Metabolism	USA	3	196
10	Faseb Journal	USA	3	31

Table 3. The top 20 most highly cited references.

Rank	Title	Journal	Total Citations	Year	First Author
1	Intermittent fasting dissociates beneficial effects of dietary restriction on glucose metabolism and neuronal resistance to injury from calorie intake	PNAS	486	2003	R. Michael Anson [10]
2	Alternate-day calorie restriction improves clinical findings and reduces markers of oxidative stress and inflammation in overweight adults with moderate asthma	Free Radical Biology and Medicine	414	2007	James B. Johnson [17]
3	Effect of alternate-day fasting on weight loss, weight maintenance, and cardioprotection among metabolically healthy obese adults: A randomized clinical trial	Jama Internal Medicine	312	2017	John F. Trepanowski [24]
4	Alternate-day fasting and chronic disease prevention: A review of human and animal trials	American Journal of Clinical Nutrition	242	2007	Krista A. Varady [28]
5	Alternate-day fasting in nonobese subjects: Effects on body weight, body composition, and energy metabolism	American Journal of Clinical Nutrition	235	2005	Leonie K. Heilbronn [14]
6	Alternate-day fasting for weight loss in normal weight and overweight subjects: a randomized controlled trial	Nutrition Journal	234	2013	Krista A. Varady [27]

Table 3. Cont.

Rank	Title	Journal	Total Citations	Year	First Author
7	Short-term modified alternate-day fasting: a novel dietary strategy for weight loss and cardioprotection in obese adults	American Journal of Clinical Nutrition	223	2009	Krista A. Varady [26]
8	Alternate-day fasting improves physiological and molecular markers of aging in healthy, non-obese humans	Cell Metabolism	186	2019	Slaven Stekovic [9]
9	Effects of intermittent fasting on body composition and clinical health markers in humans	Nutrition Reviews	170	2015	Grant M. Tinsley [22]
10	Alternate-day fasting and endurance exercise combine to reduce body weight and favorably alter plasma lipids in obese humans	Obesity	170	2013	Surabhi Bhutani [12]
11	A randomized pilot study comparing zero-calorie alternate-day fasting to daily caloric restriction in adults with obesity	Obesity	169	2016	Victoria A. Catenacci [13]
12	Intermittent fasting vs. daily calorie restriction for type 2 diabetes prevention: A review of human findings	Translational Research	164	2014	Adrienne R. Barnosky [11]
13	Intermittent versus daily calorie restriction: Which diet regimen is more effective for weight loss?	Obesity Reviews	153	2011	Krista A. Varady [25]
14	Impact of caloric and dietary restriction regimens on markers of health and longevity in humans and animals: A summary of available findings	Nutrition Journal	138	2011	John F. Trepanowski [23]
15	Effectiveness of intermittent fasting and time-restricted feeding compared to continuous energy restriction for weight loss	Nutrients	134	2019	Corey A. Rynders [20]
16	Health effects of intermittent fasting: Hormesis or harm? A systematic review	American Journal of Clinical Nutrition	122	2015	Benjamin D. Horne [16]
17	Glucose tolerance and skeletal muscle gene expression in response to alternate-day fasting	Obesity Research	122	2005	Leonie K. Heilbronn [14]
18	Do intermittent diets provide physiological benefits over continuous diets for weight loss? A systematic review of clinical trials	Molecular and Cellular Endocrinology	119	2015	Radhika V. Seimon [21]
19	Alternate-day fasting (ADF) with a high-fat diet produces similar weight loss and cardioprotection as ADF with a low-fat diet	Metabolism—Clinical and Experimental	107	2013	Monica C. Klempel [19]
20	Fasting for weight loss: An effective strategy or latest dieting trend?	International Journal of Obesity	96	2015	Alexandra Johnstone [18]

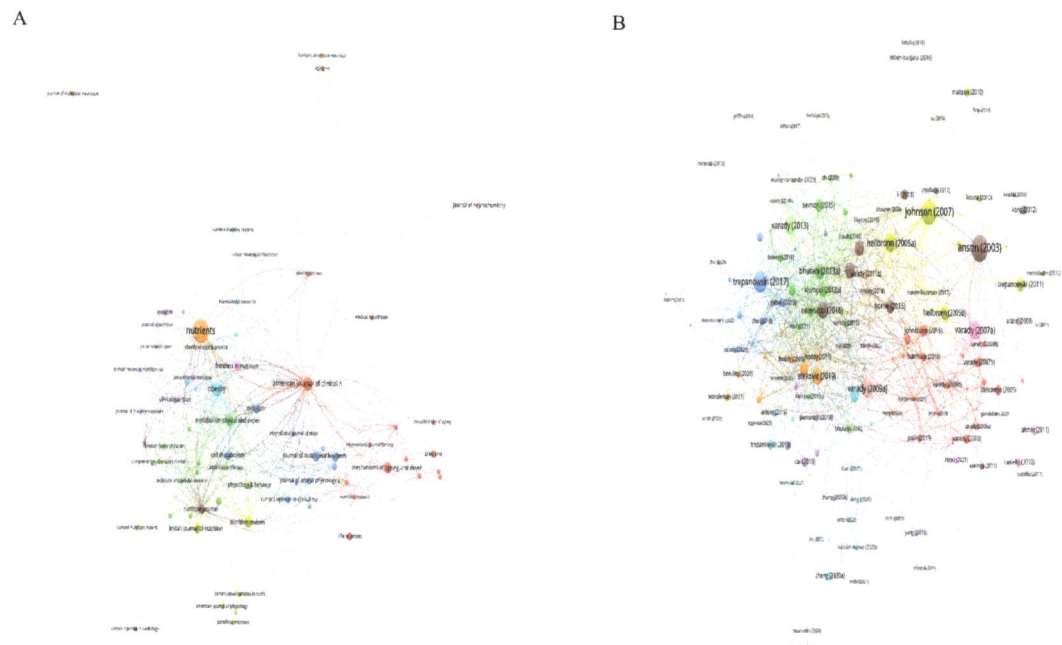

Figure 5. Visualization knowledge maps of journals and references. (**A**) Citation of journals. (**B**) Citation of references. The top three most productive journals were *Nutrients*, *American Journal of Clinical Nutrition*, and *Obesity*. The top three most highly cited publications were "Intermittent fasting dissociates beneficial effects of dietary restriction on glucose metabolism and neuronal resistance to injury from calorie intake" [10], "Alternate-day calorie restriction improves clinical findings and reduces markers of oxidative stress and inflammation in overweight adults with moderate asthma" [17], and "A randomized pilot study comparing zero-calorie alternate-day fasting to daily caloric restriction in adults with obesity" [13].

3.4. Analysis of Document Co-Citation and Clustered Network

Figure 6 shows the co-citation reference in the field of ADF. Co-cited references are defined where one publication is cited by more than one article of the 184 extracted list. The top three co-cited references were Dr. Krista A Varady et al., American journal of clinical nutrition, in 2007 (54 co-citations), Trepanowski et al., *JAMA Internal Medicine*, in 2017 (51 co-citations), and James B. Johnson et al., *Free Radical Biology and Medicine*, in 2007 (50 co-citations), which were described above. The fourth-ranked co-cited reference was published in *Nutrition Journal* with 47 co-citations, authored by Dr. Krista A Varady et al., in 2013. In this randomized controlled trial, they found that ADF was effective for cardioprotection and weight loss in adults with and without overweight. The network visualization map of the co-citation of references is shown in Figure 6.

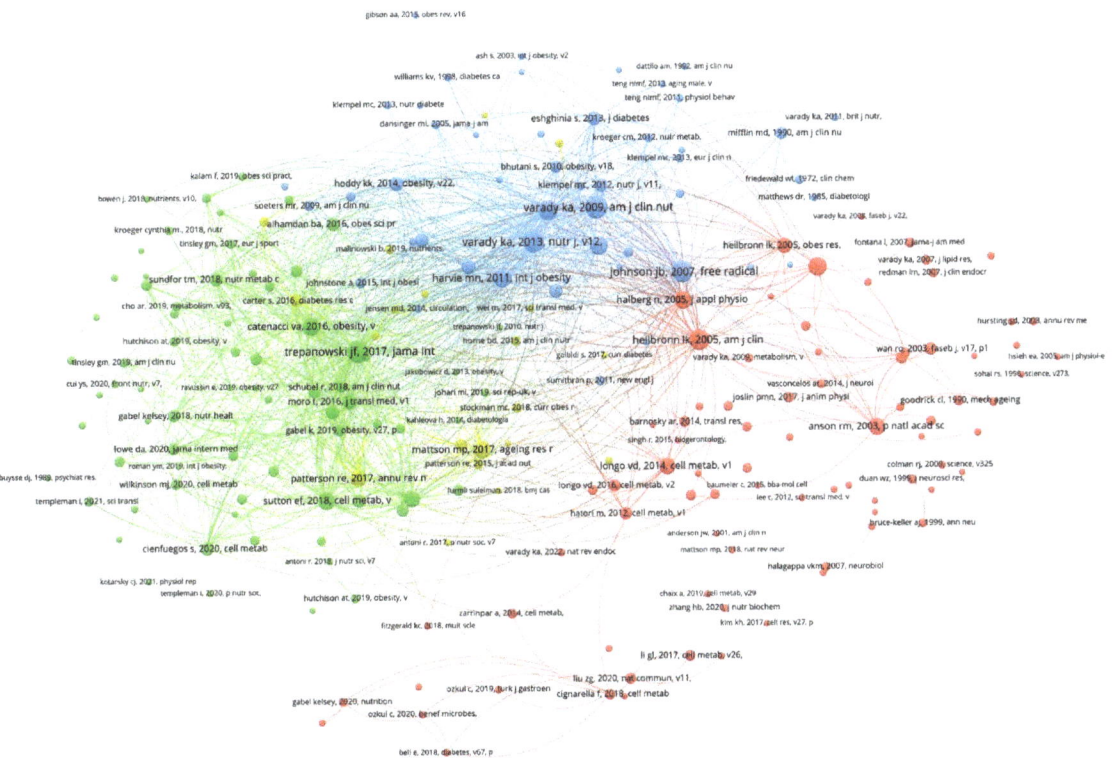

Figure 6. The network visualization map of co-citation of references. The top four co-cited references were "Alternate-day fasting and chronic disease prevention: A review of human and animal trials" [28] (54 co-citations), "Effect of alternate-day fasting on weight loss, weight maintenance, and cardioprotection among metabolically healthy obese adults: A randomized clinical trial" [24] (51 co-citations), "Alternate-day calorie restriction improves clinical findings and reduces markers of oxidative stress and inflammation in overweight adults with moderate asthma" (50 co-citations), and "Alternate-day fasting for weight loss in normal weight and overweight subjects: A randomized controlled trial" [27] (47 co-citations).

3.5. Analysis of Keywords

The co-occurrence of keywords, which could be classified in four clusters, is shown in Figure 7, presenting the frontiers, trends, and hot topics in this field. The green cluster includes alternate-day fasting, weight loss, body weight, and overweight. The red cluster includes caloric restriction, obesity, and metabolism. The blue cluster includes insulin resistance and energy restriction. The yellow cluster includes intermittent fasting, diet, and body composition. The top 10 keywords with the highest frequency aside form alternate-day fasting were calorie restriction (N = 81), weight loss (N = 70), intermittent fasting (N = 62), obesity (N = 62), body weight (N = 41), diet (N = 32), insulin resistance (N = 29), metabolism (N = 28), overweight (N = 23), and body composition (N = 22).

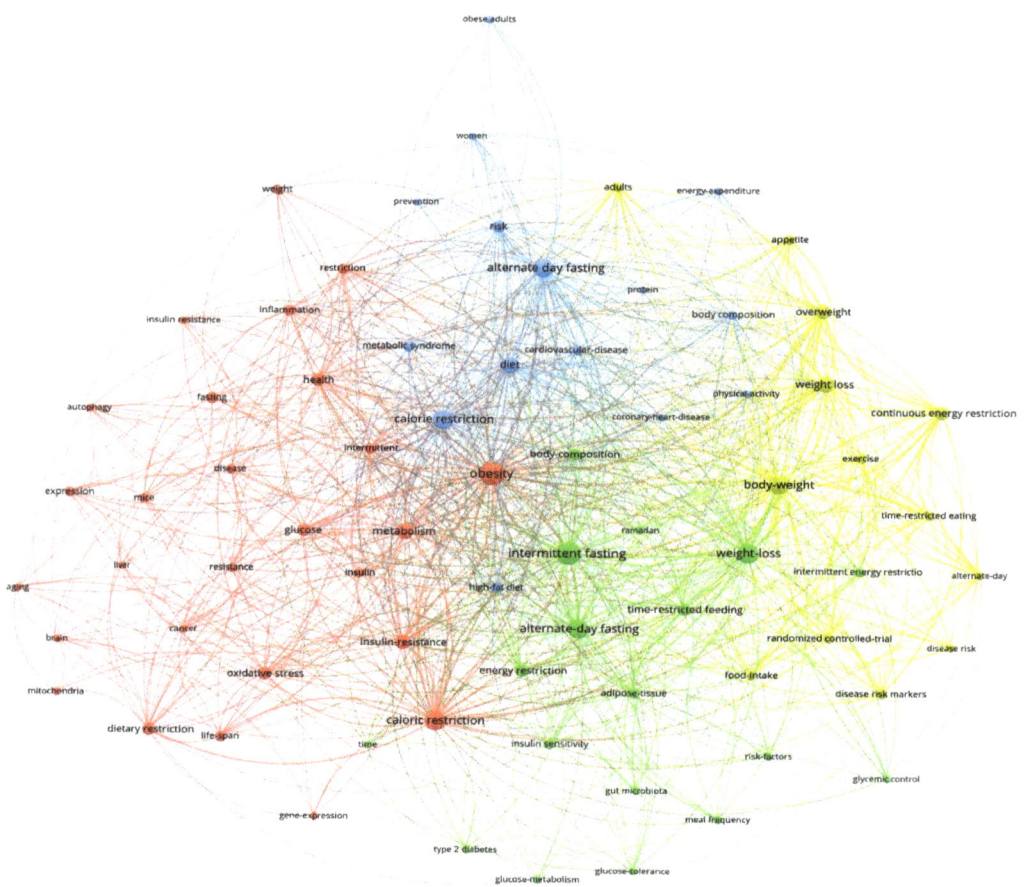

Figure 7. Visualization of keyword co-occurrence analysis. Four clusters are displayed. The top 10 core keywords aside from alternate-day fasting were calorie restriction (N = 81), weight loss (N = 70), intermittent fasting (N = 62), obesity (N = 62), body weight (N = 41), diet (N = 32), insulin resistance (N = 29), metabolism (N = 28), overweight (N = 23), and body composition (N = 22).

4. Discussion

4.1. General Information

To the best of knowledge, this is the first bibliometric analysis related to ADF. ADF is a main type of intermittent fasting, with many benefits for human health, including weight loss and improvements in cardiometabolic parameters and glucose regulation; many previous studies explored the effects of ADF for health conditions including obesity, NAFLD, and diabetes [29,30]. In our analysis, there were 184 publications of 127 articles and 57 reviews from 362 institutions and 39 countries/regions, which were published in 104 journals about ADF. The most productive countries/regions, institutions, authors, and journals were the USA with 98 publications, the University of Illinois Chicago with 37 publications, Krista A. Varady with 43 publications, and Nutrients with 18 publications, respectively. The most highly cited publication was published in PNAS, authored by R. Michael Anson et al., in 2003 [10], and it was also the first article about ADF. The top five keywords with the highest frequency were as follows: calorie restriction, weight loss, intermittent fasting, obesity, and body weight.

4.2. Hotspots and Frontiers

On the basis of current publication trends, important keywords with high frequency, and highly cited publications, the research hotspots in the field of ADF were summarized as follows: (1) **ADF for obesity and cardiometabolic risk.** In the top 20 highly cited references, seven explored the effects of ADF for obesity, and metabolic and cardiometabolic risk [12,13,19,22,24,26,27]. For core keywords, weight loss, body weight, and overweight occurred in the green cluster, while obesity and metabolism were in the red cluster. A meta-analysis demonstrated that ADF could lower body weight, body mass index (BMI), body fat, and total cholesterol in adults with obesity compared with the control in a half year. Daily calorie restriction (CR) is a first-line strategy for adults with obesity to achieve weight loss. However, adherence to CR is difficult to many adults with obesity. Many new strategies have been developed including ADF, time-restricted eating, and a 5:2 diet [2,29,31,32]. ADF is initially used for weight loss. Meanwhile, other benefits, such as improvements in blood pressure, lipid profiles, and insulin sensitivity, have been found in many studies. Many studies have explored the effects of ADF for people with obesity. For example, Varady et al. [27] conducted a study to explore the effects of ADF for coronary artery disease (CAD) risk indicators and body weight in people with obesity, and the results showed that an 8-week ADF intervention could result in a mean weight loss of 5.8% and decrease some several key biomarkers for CAD risk, such as LDL cholesterol, total cholesterol (TC), triacylglycerols, heart rate, and systolic blood pressure (SBP). Hooshiar et al. [33] performed an RCT to investigate the effects of modified alternate-day fasting (MADF) and calorie restriction (CR) on body weight, sleep quality, and daytime sleepiness. They found that ADMF could achieve a greater decrease in weight compared with CR, and MADF might be a beneficial diet for controlling BMI and body weight. (2) **ADF for several different population groups.** In the top 20 highly cited references, seven explored the effects of ADF for non-obese subjects and patients with chronic diseases including diabetes and asthma [9,11,15,17,23,27,28], and insulin resistance occurred in the blue cluster. In addition to obesity, many studies explored the effect of ADF for different populations including healthy, non-obese adults, as well as patients with diabetes and NAFLD. **For healthy, non-obese humans,** ADF is safe, and can increase polyunsaturated free fatty acids (PUFAs), improve the cardiovascular parameters and fat-to-lean ratio, decrease the body weight by 4.5%, and periodically deplete amino acids [9]. **For patients with diabetes,** a randomized controlled trial showed that ADF was effective for glycemic control, while also significantly decreasing BMI, serum triglyceride, body weight, and fat mass [34]. **Two studies investigated the effects of ADF for patients with NAFLD** [8,35]. Johari et al. compared the effects of modified alternate-day calorie restriction (MACR) and normal habitual diet for patients with NAFLD, and they found that ADF was an effective intervention for improving NAFLD-related biomarkers including BMI, weight, and liver transaminases, with a good adherence rate [35]. Recently, a study was conducted to compare the effects of ADF plus exercise to control, exercise alone, and fasting alone on intrahepatic triglyceride (IHTG) content in patients with NAFLD. The results demonstrated that ADF alone was as effective as ADF plus exercise, and they were all better than exercise alone in increasing insulin sensitivity and body weight, fat mass, waist circumference, body weight, and alanine transaminase (ALT) levels [8]. More studies are needed to explore the effects of ADF for diverse populations. It should be noted that sustained ADF may potentiate doxorubicin cardiotoxicity according to a recent study, indicating that the use of ADF should be taken with care in specific populations such as patients receiving doxorubicin treatment [36–38].

There were some limitations in our study. The WoSCC database was used in our study, whereas other databases such as Embase and Pubmed were not used since VOSviewer software cannot analyze and visualize co-citation maps using their data. The overall number of publications in the field of ADF remains relatively small; thus, more studies are urgently needed to extend our knowledge about the effects of ADF for human health, as well as take advantage of this approach to improve human health.

In conclusion, this is the first comprehensive bibliometric analysis related to ADF. The main research hotspots and frontiers were ADF for obesity and cardiometabolic risk, and ADF for diverse populations including healthy adults and patients with diabetes, NAFLD, and cancer. The studies about ADF were limited, and more studies are needed to extend our knowledge about ADF, with the aim of improving human health.

Author Contributions: Methodology, X.L.; Software, X.L.; Validation, X.L.; Formal analysis, X.L.; Resources, J.H.; Data curation, J.H.; Writing—original draft, S.W.; Writing—review & editing, S.W.; Supervision, J.H. All authors have read and agreed to the published version of the manuscript.

Funding: This research was funded by Hangzhou Medical and Health Technology Project (Number Z20210019) and Hangzhou Science and Technology Development Plan (Number 20201203B178).

Institutional Review Board Statement: Not applicable.

Informed Consent Statement: Not applicable.

Data Availability Statement: The data are available from the corresponding authors upon reasonable request.

Conflicts of Interest: The authors declare no conflict of interest.

References

1. Bowen, J.; Brindal, E.; James-Martin, G.; Noakes, M. Randomized Trial of a High Protein, Partial Meal Replacement Program with or without Alternate Day Fasting: Similar Effects on Weight Loss, Retention Status, Nutritional, Metabolic, and Behavioral Outcomes. *Nutrients* **2018**, *10*, 1145. [CrossRef] [PubMed]
2. Patikorn, C.; Roubal, K.; Veettil, S.K.; Chandran, V.; Pham, T.; Lee, Y.Y.; Giovannucci, E.L.; Varady, K.A.; Chaiyakunapruk, N. Intermittent Fasting and Obesity-Related Health Outcomes: An Umbrella Review of Meta-analyses of Randomized Clinical Trials. *JAMA Netw. Open* **2021**, *4*, e2139558. [CrossRef] [PubMed]
3. Templeman, I.; Smith, H.A.; Chowdhury, E.; Chen, Y.-C.; Carroll, H.; Johnson-Bonson, D.; Hengist, A.; Smith, R.; Creighton, J.; Clayton, D.; et al. A randomized controlled trial to isolate the effects of fasting and energy restriction on weight loss and metabolic health in lean adults. *Sci. Transl. Med.* **2021**, *13*, eabd8034. [CrossRef] [PubMed]
4. Trepanowski, J.F.; Kroeger, C.M.; Barnosky, A.; Klempel, M.; Bhutani, S.; Hoddy, K.K.; Rood, J.; Ravussin, E.; Varady, K.A. Effects of alternate-day fasting or daily calorie restriction on body composition, fat distribution, and circulating adipokines: Secondary analysis of a randomized controlled trial. *Clin. Nutr.* **2018**, *37 Pt A*, 1871–1878. [CrossRef]
5. Varady, K.A.; Cienfuegos, S.; Ezpeleta, M.; Gabel, K. Cardiometabolic Benefits of Intermittent Fasting. *Annu. Rev. Nutr.* **2021**, *41*, 333–361. [CrossRef]
6. Zhang, X.; Zou, Q.; Zhao, B.; Zhang, J.; Zhao, W.; Li, Y.; Liu, R.; Liu, X.; Liu, Z. Effects of alternate-day fasting, time-restricted fasting and intermittent energy restriction DSS-induced on colitis and behavioral disorders. *Redox Biol.* **2020**, *32*, 101535. [CrossRef]
7. Park, J.; Seo, Y.G.; Paek, Y.J.; Song, H.J.; Park, K.H.; Noh, H.M. Effect of alternate-day fasting on obesity and cardiometabolic risk: A systematic review and meta-analysis. *Metabolism* **2020**, *111*, 154336. [CrossRef]
8. Ezpeleta, M.; Gabel, K.; Cienfuegos, S.; Kalam, F.; Lin, S.; Pavlou, V.; Song, Z.; Haus, J.M.; Koppe, S.; Alexandria, S.J.; et al. Effect of alternate day fasting combined with aerobic exercise on non-alcoholic fatty liver disease: A randomized controlled trial. *Cell Metab.* **2023**, *35*, 56–70.e3. [CrossRef]
9. Stekovic, S.; Hofer, S.J.; Tripolt, N.; Aon, M.A.; Royer, P.; Pein, L.; Stadler, J.T.; Pendl, T.; Prietl, B.; Url, J.; et al. Alternate Day Fasting Improves Physiological and Molecular Markers of Aging in Healthy, Non-obese Humans. *Cell Metab.* **2019**, *30*, 462–476.e6. [CrossRef]
10. Anson, R.M.; Guo, Z.; de Cabo, R.; Iyun, T.; Rios, M.; Hagepanos, A.; Ingram, D.K.; Lane, M.A.; Mattson, M.P. Intermittent fasting dissociates beneficial effects of dietary restriction on glucose metabolism and neuronal resistance to injury from calorie intake. *Proc. Natl. Acad. Sci. USA* **2003**, *100*, 6216–6220. [CrossRef]
11. Barnosky, A.R.; Hoddy, K.K.; Unterman, T.G.; Varady, K.A. Intermittent fasting vs daily calorie restriction for type 2 diabetes prevention: A review of human findings. *Transl. Res.* **2014**, *164*, 302–311. [CrossRef] [PubMed]
12. Bhutani, S.; Klempel, M.C.; Kroeger, C.M.; Trepanowski, J.F.; Varady, K.A. Alternate Day Fasting and Endurance Exercise Combine to Reduce Body Weight and Favorably Alter Plasma Lipids in Obese Humans. *Obesity* **2013**, *21*, 1370–1379. [CrossRef]
13. Catenacci, V.A.; Pan, Z.X.; Ostendorf, D.; Brannon, S.; Gozansky, W.S.; Mattson, M.P.; Martin, B.; MacLean, P.S.; Melanson, E.L.; Donahoo, W.T. A Randomized Pilot Study Comparing Zero-Calorie Alternate-Day Fasting to Daily Caloric Restriction in Adults with Obesity. *Obesity* **2016**, *24*, 1874–1883. [CrossRef] [PubMed]
14. Heilbronn, L.K.; Civitarese, A.E.; Bogacka, I.; Smith, S.R.; Hulver, M.; Ravussin, E. Glucose tolerance and skeletal muscle gene expression in response to alternate day fasting. *Obes. Res.* **2005**, *13*, 574–581. [CrossRef] [PubMed]

15. Heilbronn, L.K.; Smith, S.R.; Martin, C.K.; Anton, S.D.; Ravussin, E. Alternate-day fasting in nonobese subjects: Effects on body weight, body composition, and energy metabolism. *Am. J. Clin. Nutr.* **2005**, *81*, 69–73. [CrossRef]
16. Horne, B.D.; Muhlestein, J.B.; Anderson, J.L. Health effects of intermittent fasting: Hormesis or harm? A systematic review. *Am. J. Clin. Nutr.* **2015**, *102*, 464–470. [CrossRef]
17. Johnson, J.B.; Summer, W.; Cutler, R.G.; Martin, B.; Hyun, D.H.; Dixit, V.D.; Pearson, M.; Nassar, M.; Telljohann, R.; Maudsley, S.; et al. Alternate day calorie restriction improves clinical findings and reduces markers of oxidative stress and inflammation in overweight adults with moderate asthma. *Free Radic. Biol. Med.* **2007**, *42*, 665–674. [CrossRef]
18. Johnstone, A. Fasting for weight loss: An effective strategy or latest dieting trend? *Int. J. Obes.* **2015**, *39*, 727–733. [CrossRef]
19. Klempel, M.C.; Kroeger, C.M.; Varady, K.A. Alternate day fasting (ADF) with a high-fat diet produces similar weight loss and cardio-protection as ADF with a low-fat diet. *Metab.-Clin. Exp.* **2013**, *62*, 137–143. [CrossRef]
20. Rynders, C.A.; Thomas, E.A.; Zaman, A.; Pan, Z.X.; Catenacci, V.A.; Melanson, E.L. Effectiveness of Intermittent Fasting and Time-Restricted Feeding Compared to Continuous Energy Restriction for Weight Loss. *Nutrients* **2019**, *11*, 2442. [CrossRef]
21. Seimon, R.V.; Roekenes, J.A.; Zibellini, J.; Zhu, B.; Gibson, A.A.; Hills, A.P.; Wood, R.E.; King, N.A.; Byrne, N.M.; Sainsbury, A. Do intermittent diets provide physiological benefits over continuous diets for weight loss? A systematic review of clinical trials. *Mol. Cell. Endocrinol.* **2015**, *418*, 153–172. [CrossRef] [PubMed]
22. Tinsley, G.M.; La Bounty, P.M. Effects of intermittent fasting on body composition and clinical health markers in humans. *Nutr. Rev.* **2015**, *73*, 661–674. [CrossRef] [PubMed]
23. Trepanowski, J.F.; Canale, R.E.; Marshall, K.E.; Kabir, M.M.; Bloomer, R.J. Impact of caloric and dietary restriction regimens on markers of health and longevity in humans and animals: A summary of available findings. *Nutr. J.* **2011**, *10*, 107. [CrossRef] [PubMed]
24. Trepanowski, J.F.; Kroeger, C.M.; Barnosky, A.; Klempel, M.C.; Bhutani, S.; Hoddy, K.K.; Gabel, K.; Freels, S.; Rigdon, J.; Rood, J.; et al. Effect of Alternate-Day Fasting on Weight Loss, Weight Maintenance, and Cardioprotection Among Metabolically Healthy Obese Adults A Randomized Clinical Trial. *JAMA Intern. Med.* **2017**, *177*, 930–938. [CrossRef]
25. Varady, K.A. Intermittent versus daily calorie restriction: Which diet regimen is more effective for weight loss? *Obes. Rev.* **2011**, *12*, E593–E601. [CrossRef]
26. Varady, K.A.; Bhutani, S.; Church, E.C.; Klempel, M.C. Short-term modified alternate-day fasting: A novel dietary strategy for weight loss and cardioprotection in obese adults. *Am. J. Clin. Nutr.* **2009**, *90*, 1138–1143. [CrossRef]
27. Varady, K.A.; Bhutani, S.; Klempel, M.C.; Kroeger, C.M.; Trepanowski, J.F.; Haus, J.M.; Hoddy, K.K.; Calvo, Y. Alternate day fasting for weight loss in normal weight and overweight subjects: A randomized controlled trial. *Nutr. J.* **2013**, *12*, 146. [CrossRef]
28. Varady, K.A.; Hellerstein, M.K. Alternate-day fasting and chronic disease prevention: A review of human and animal trials. *Am. J. Clin. Nutr.* **2007**, *86*, 7–13. [CrossRef]
29. de Cabo, R.; Mattson, M.P. Effects of Intermittent Fasting on Health, Aging, and Disease. *N. Engl. J. Med.* **2019**, *381*, 2541–2551. [CrossRef]
30. Varady, K.A.; Cienfuegos, S.; Ezpeleta, M.; Gabel, K. Clinical application of intermittent fasting for weight loss: Progress and future directions. *Nat. Rev. Endocrinol.* **2022**, *18*, 309–321. [CrossRef]
31. Li, Z.; Heber, D. Intermittent Fasting. *JAMA* **2021**, *326*, 1338. [CrossRef]
32. Marjot, T.; Tomlinson, J.W.; Hodson, L.; Ray, D.W. Timing of energy intake and the therapeutic potential of intermittent fasting and time-restricted eating in NAFLD. *Gut* **2023**, *72*, 1607–1619. [CrossRef]
33. Hooshiar, S.H.; Yazdani, A.; Jafarnejad, S. Alternate-day modified fasting diet improves weight loss, subjective sleep quality and daytime dysfunction in women with obesity or overweight: A randomized, controlled trial. *Front. Nutr.* **2023**, *10*, 1174293. [CrossRef]
34. Umphonsathien, M.; Rattanasian, P.; Lokattachariya, S.; Suansawang, W.; Boonyasuppayakorn, K.; Khovidhunkit, W. Effects of intermittent very-low calorie diet on glycemic control and cardiovascular risk factors in obese patients with type 2 diabetes mellitus: A randomized controlled trial. *J. Diabetes Investig.* **2022**, *13*, 156–166. [CrossRef] [PubMed]
35. Johari, M.I.; Yusoff, K.; Haron, J.; Nadarajan, C.; Ibrahim, K.N.; Wong, M.S.; Hafidz, M.I.A.; Chua, B.E.; Hamid, N.; Arifin, W.N.; et al. A Randomised Controlled Trial on the Effectiveness and Adherence of Modified Alternate-day Calorie Restriction in Improving Activity of Non-Alcoholic Fatty Liver Disease. *Sci. Rep.* **2019**, *9*, 11232. [CrossRef]
36. Meng, Y.; Sun, J.; Zhang, G.; Yu, T.; Piao, H. Unexpected worsening of doxorubicin cardiotoxicity upon intermittent fasting. *Med* **2023**, *4*, 288–289. [CrossRef] [PubMed]
37. Ozcan, M.; Guo, Z.; Valenzuela Ripoll, C.; Diab, A.; Picataggi, A.; Rawnsley, D.; Lotfinaghsh, A.; Bergom, C.; Szymanski, J.; Hwang, D.; et al. Sustained alternate-day fasting potentiates doxorubicin cardiotoxicity. *Cell Metab.* **2023**, *35*, 928–942.e4. [CrossRef] [PubMed]
38. Pan, H.; Yang, S.; Cheng, W.; Cai, Q.; Shubhra, Q.T.H. Alternate-day fasting exacerbates doxorubicin cardiotoxicity in cancer chemotherapy. *Trends Endocrinol. Metab. TEM* **2023**, *34*, 392–394. [CrossRef] [PubMed]

Disclaimer/Publisher's Note: The statements, opinions and data contained in all publications are solely those of the individual author(s) and contributor(s) and not of MDPI and/or the editor(s). MDPI and/or the editor(s) disclaim responsibility for any injury to people or property resulting from any ideas, methods, instructions or products referred to in the content.

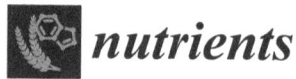

Article

Contribution of Different Food Types to Vitamin A Intake in the Chinese Diet

Xue Li [1,2], Can Guo [1,2], Yu Zhang [1,2], Li Yu [1,2], Fei Ma [1,2], Xuefang Wang [1,2], Liangxiao Zhang [1,2,3,4,*] and Peiwu Li [1,2,3,4,5]

[1] Key Laboratory of Biology and Genetic Improvement of Oil Crops, Ministry of Agriculture and Rural Affairs, Oil Crops Research Institute, Chinese Academy of Agricultural Sciences, Wuhan 430062, China; mafei01@caas.cn (F.M.)
[2] Quality Inspection and Test Center for Oilseed Products, Ministry of Agriculture and Rural Affairs, Oil Crops Research Institute, Chinese Academy of Agricultural Sciences, Wuhan 430062, China
[3] College of Food Science and Engineering, Collaborative Innovation Center for Modern Grain Circulation and Safety, Nanjing University of Finance and Economics, Nanjing 210023, China
[4] Hubei Hongshan Laboratory, Wuhan 430070, China
[5] Xianghu Laboratory, Hangzhou 311231, China
* Correspondence: zhanglx@caas.cn; Tel./Fax: +86-27-86812862

Citation: Li, X.; Guo, C.; Zhang, Y.; Yu, L.; Ma, F.; Wang, X.; Zhang, L.; Li, P. Contribution of Different Food Types to Vitamin A Intake in the Chinese Diet. *Nutrients* 2023, 15, 4028. https://doi.org/10.3390/nu15184028

Academic Editors: António Raposo, Renata Puppin Zandonadi and Raquel Braz Assunção Botelho

Received: 31 July 2023
Revised: 27 August 2023
Accepted: 4 September 2023
Published: 17 September 2023

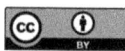

Copyright: © 2023 by the authors. Licensee MDPI, Basel, Switzerland. This article is an open access article distributed under the terms and conditions of the Creative Commons Attribution (CC BY) license (https://creativecommons.org/licenses/by/4.0/).

Abstract: Vitamin A is a fat-soluble micronutrient that is essential for human health. In this study, the daily vitamin A intake of Chinese residents was evaluated by investigating the vitamin A content of various foods. The results show that the dietary intake of vitamin A in common foods was 460.56 ugRAE/day, which is significantly lower than the recommended dietary reference intake of vitamin A (800 ugRAE/day for adult men and 700 ugRAE/day for adult women). Vegetables contributed the most to daily vitamin A dietary intake, accounting for 54.94% of vitamin A intake (253.03 ugRAE/day), followed by eggs, milk, aquatic products, meat, fruit, legumes, coarse cereals, and potatoes. Therefore, an increase in the vitamin A content of vegetables and the fortification of vegetable oils with vitamin A are effective ways to increase vitamin A intake to meet the recommended dietary guidelines in China. The assessment results support the design of fortified foods.

Keywords: vitamin A; vegetables; dietary intake; vegetable oil fortification

1. Introduction

Vitamin A is a compound with the biological activity of retinol. There are two primary groups of substances that provide retinol bioactivity. One is preformed vitamin A (retinol) and the other is provitamin A carotenoids chiefly comprising beta-carotene, alpha-carotene, and cryptoxanthin [1,2]. As an essential fat-soluble micronutrient, vitamin A cannot be synthesized by the human body and needs to be obtained from a regular diet. Vitamin A plays a vital role in ocular function and is involved in preventing xerophthalmia, the maintenance of eye integrity, and cellular division and differentiation [3–5]. Recently, the global prevalence of dry eye disease (DED) has been estimated to be between 5% and 50% [6]. It was concluded from previous investigations that excessive smartphone use in children and adolescents is associated with DED [7–9]. It was concluded in another study that people who use a visual display terminal (VDT) for over 3.71 h per day and occupational VDT users are susceptible to developing DED [10]. Moreover, vitamin A is associated with reproduction, the immune system, and bone and embryonic development [11–13]. Vitamin A deficiency (VAD) has drawn more and more attention from all over the world, and the World Health Organization (WHO) confirmed VAD is one of four major nutritional deficiency diseases. It is common to see chronic VAD and it is hard to detect because it is asymptomatic [14]. Children are commonly found to have VAD, especially preschool-aged children, and boys and girls possess incidences of 0.8% and 0.4%, respectively [15–17].

VAD is the primary cause of childhood xerophthalmia and blindness in developing countries [18] and is associated with poor clinical outcomes in patients with sepsis [19]. In addition, 10–20% of pregnant women in the world lack sufficient vitamin A intake. If lactating women do not intake vitamin A, it will affect the concentration of vitamin A in their infants. As a result, infants with VAD will have wheezing symptoms [20,21]. In addition, the newborns of pregnant women with gestational diabetes have an increased impairment of vitamin A formation [22]. Therefore, increasing vitamin A intake is important to protect the eyes and reduce the incidence of VDA.

Generally, retinol from animal-derived foods and provitamin A carotenoids from plant-derived products are the two primary sources of vitamin A. Retinol can be obtained from eggs, animal liver, fish, and dairy products. The main source of provitamin A carotenoids are yellow and orange fruits as well as dark-green vegetables [23]. β-carotene shows a higher provitamin A activity than β-cryptoxanthin and α-carotene [24]. The dietary intake of vitamin A in Western countries is different from that in developing countries. The typical daily diet in Western countries provides an approximate intake of 20–34% of provitamin A carotenoids, while more than 70% of provitamin A carotenoids were ingested from diets in developing countries [25]. Furthermore, vitamin A-fortified products have appeared on the market, such as fortified wheat flour and milk [26,27]. However, whether the body is deficient in vitamin A and whether more vitamin A should be obtained from the diet and fortified products is not clear. Moreover, acute toxicity can occur if an individual's intake of vitamin A is greater than 3000 ugRAE/day [28,29]. Therefore, it is important to evaluate the vitamin A content in people's daily diets.

A dietary assessment plays an important role in guiding diet intake. It is an investigation of the relationship between diet and health conditions. The US Institute of Medicine recommends estimating the degree of inadequate dietary nutrient intake in a group according to the Estimated Average Requirements (EARs) [30]. The Recommended Dietary Allowance (RDA) is the average daily dietary intake which is adequate to meet the nutritional needs among healthy people. There are many methods used to assess food intake, including food frequency questionnaires (FFQs), 24 h recalls, and weighed and non-weighed food records [31]. Each method has its own advantages and disadvantages. Among these, weighed food records are the gold-standard recommendation, but they are time-consuming and vary depending on the participant [32]. FFQs are commonly used in large dietary epidemiology studies due to their low cost and time efficiency, but they lack specificity [33]. In addition, novel approaches such as image-assisted and image-based methods are applied with the use of mobile devices [34]. In a previous study, the contribution of different foods to the total phytosterol intake of Chinese residents was estimated according to consumption data [35]. In another work, the content of vitamin E in different foods was used to assess vitamin E intake in individuals' daily diet [36]. The simplified dietary assessment (SDA) method was proposed by the International Vitamin A Consultative Group (IVACG) to identify and monitor groups at risk for suboptimal vitamin A intake [37]. The overweight and obese Dominican population was investigated to assess vitamin A and carotenoid intake [38]. However, there is no study that reported on the dietary vitamin A intake in the Chinese diet. Therefore, conducting a dietary assessment of the Chinese population is essential.

In this study, the vitamin A contents in different types of foods and the amount of vitamin A intake in the Chinese daily diet are investigated. In addition, strategies are proposed to increase the vitamin A intake in China.

2. Materials and Methods

2.1. Data Sources

Cereals, vegetable oils, nuts, coarse cereals, potatoes, legumes, vegetables, fruits, meat, eggs, milk, and aquatic products are used to obtain vitamin A according to the Chinese Food Composition Tables released by the National Institute for Nutrition and Health and Chinese Center for Disease Control and Presentation; the production, supply, and distribution (PSD) reports released by the United States Department of Agriculture (USDA) and the Food and Agriculture Organization of the United States (FAOSTAT); the China Population Nutrition and Health Status Monitoring Report; and the China Statistical Yearbook providing the domestic consumption of the main kinds of foods in China. The consumption of major foods in the Chinese diet, including cereals, coarse cereals, potatoes, legumes, vegetables, fruits, nuts, vegetable oils, meat, eggs, milk, and aquatic products, was determined according to the China Population Nutrition and Health Status Monitoring Report and USDA PSD reports. The 16 most frequently consumed kinds of vegetables were selected, and the consumption of each kind of vegetable was obtained from FAOSTAT, while the USDA PSD reports provided the most consumed fruits, which included apples, bananas, pears, grapes, peaches, tangerines, oranges, grapefruits, and cherries. In summary, 45 kinds of foods were used to evaluate vitamin A intake in the Chinese diet.

2.2. Calculation Method

The United States Health and Medicine Division (HMD) defined total vitamin A intake as the sum of 1 µg of retinol, 1/12 µg of dietary β-carotene, and 1/24 µg of dietary α-carotene, expressed as µg of retinol activity equivalents (RAEs). First, the estimated daily vitamin A intake was calculated according to total vitamin A content and the consumption of various foods that are commonly consumed; meanwhile, the contribution of one kind of food to the total vitamin A intake was calculated. Second, the amount of each vegetable required to reach the recommended vitamin A intake if a person were to eat only 1 of the 16 types of vegetables was calculated. Similarly, the amount of each vegetable required if the daily intake of the other 15 vegetables remained unchanged was calculated. In addition, the increase in vitamin A content in each vegetable needed if the daily intake of the other 15 vegetables remained unchanged was calculated.

The data analysis was carried out in Microsoft Excel Version 2021 (Microsoft Corporation, Redmond, WA, USA).

3. Results

3.1. Vitamin A Contents in Various Foods

Vitamin A is a fat-soluble vitamin that is essential for the maintenance of human metabolism and is available from various foods in two forms. One is pre-formed vitamin A (retinol) which is found only in animals, the other is provitamin A carotenoids which is found in plants. Cereals are the staple food for the Chinese population, and are rich in nutrients but contain a low content of provitamin A carotenoids. Vegetable oils and nuts are also widely consumed foods, but also contain low content of provitamin A carotenoids. Therefore, the provitamin A carotenoids content of coarse cereals, potatoes, legumes, vegetables and fruits, the retinol content of meat, eggs, milk, and aquatic products were collected and listed in Table S1. It is evident that vegetables contained the highest content (1088 ugRAE/100 g) of total vitamin A. For example, carrots contained 342 ugRAE/100 g and spinach contained 243 ugRAE/100 g of total vitamin A content, indicating that carrots and spinach are good sources of provitamin vitamin A carotenoids. Meanwhile, eggs have the second highest content of total vitamin A (1045 ugRAE/100 g). All four types of eggs contained high levels of retinol, particularly quail eggs with 337 ugRAE/100 g. In addition, the following retinol contents were detected in aquatic products, milk, and meat. Fruits, beans, potatoes, and coarse cereals had low levels of carotenoids in contrast with other commonly consumed foods.

3.2. Evaluation of the Vitamin A Dietary Intake in the Chinese Diet

The nine food categories including coarse cereals, potatoes, legumes, vegetables, fruits, meat, eggs, milk, and aquatic products were used to calculate the dietary intake of vitamin A. As shown in Figure 1, the dietary intake of vitamin A in these nine kinds of commonly consumed foods was 460.56 ugRAE/day, which was consistent with the vitamin A supply in Asia (431 ugRAE/day) estimated by WHO. However, the recommended dietary reference intakes of vitamin A for adult men and women were 800 ugRAE/day and 700 ugRAE/day in China, respectively [39]. As a result, the actual dietary intake of vitamin A remained inadequate for an adult. The contribution of different foods to vitamin A dietary intake is shown in Figure 1. Vegetables are the first contributor to the dietary intake of vitamin A among the nine food categories, accounting for 54.94% of vitamin A intake (253.03 ugRAE/day), followed by eggs with 18.30% (84.30 ugRAE/day), and the others accounting for less than 10%. The animal foods including milk, aquatic products, and meat contributed 9.80% (45.12 ugRAE/day), 9.45% (43.51 ugRAE/day), and 6.15% (28.32 ugRAE/day), respectively; while fruit, legumes, coarse cereals, and potatoes contributed 0.57% (2.64 ugRAE/day), 0.41% (1.87 ugRAE/day), 0.24% (1.12 ugRAE/day), and 0.14% (0.64 ugRAE/day), respectively.

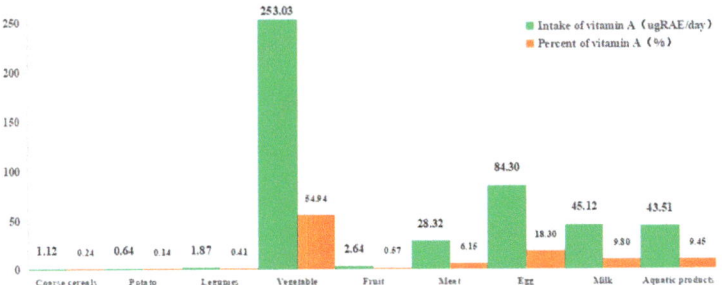

Figure 1. Contribution of different foods to vitamin A dietary intake.

Vegetables were the primary contributor to vitamin A intake, and Table 1 shows the vitamin A content of 16 kinds of vegetables and their contribution to total vitamin A intake. The vitamin A intake of 253.03 ugRAE/day was recorded from vegetables. Carrots and dark green vegetables are rich in provitamin A carotenoids, and the result showed that carrots had the highest contribution to vitamin A intake at 103.49 ugRAE/day and accounted for 28.33% of the 45 kinds of foods. Spinach ranked second at 14.51% (66.83 ugRAE/day). The contributions of Chinese chives, pepper, tomato, asparagus lettuce, lettuce, and pumpkin were 4.78% (22.01 ugRAE/day); 4.13% (19.00 ugRAE/day); 2.62% (12.06 ugRAE/day); 2.57% (11.83 ugRAE/day); 1.96% (9.03 ugRAE/day); and 1.22% (3.08 ugRAE/day), respectively. The total contribution of other vegetables was 1.92% (8.80 ugRAE/day).

Table 1. Contribution of different kinds of vegetables to vitamin A dietary intake.

Vegetables	Vitamin A Content (ugRAE)-100 g	Consumption (%)	Intake of Vitamin A (ugRAE/day)	Percent of Vitamin A (%)
Carrot	342	11.25	103.48	28.33
Kidney bean	18	2.77	1.34	0.29
Cowpea	10	0.25	0.07	0.02
Eggplant	4	11.40	1.23	0.27
Tomato	31	14.46	12.06	2.62
Red pepper	116			
Green pepper	8	5.43	19.00	4.13
Sweet pepper	6			
Cucumber	8	14.32	3.08	0.67
Pumpkin	74	4.53	9.03	1.96
Chinese chives	133	6.15	22.01	4.78
Cabbage	6	8.57	1.38	0.30
Broccoli	13	4.86	1.70	0.37
Spinach	243	10.22	66.83	14.51
Asparagus lettuce	13	5.78	11.83	2.57
Lettuce	63			
Total			253.03	

4. Discussion

The actual average vitamin A daily intake cannot meet the recommended dietary reference intake in the Chinese diet. Nearly 254 million of preschool-aged children were affected by VAD and suffered from night blindness [40]. Meanwhile, the excessive smartphone use potentially increased the DED. The increase in eye diseases requires a greater demand for vitamin A.

Bioavailability was defined as the fraction of an ingested bioactive agent, which reaches the specific site of action in the body. Bioavailability was primarily determined by three factors: bioaccessibility, transformation, and absorption [41]. The main factors limiting the bioavailability of vitamin A were solubility, stability, and dietary composition. Different foods had different bioavailability of vitamin A [42]. However, the recommended dietary reference intake of vitamin A in China for adult men and adult women was 800 ugRAE/day and 700 ugRAE/day, respectively, according to the Chinese dietary reference intakes. The aim of this study was to investigate the amount of vitamin A intake in the Chinese daily diet, rather than the bioavailability of vitamin A. Therefore, effective measures were discussed to increase the vitamin A intake to meet the recommended dietary reference intake of vitamin A.

Firstly, the increase in vegetable consumption is an important measure to obtain the recommended vitamin A dietary intake. Vegetables were rich in vitamins, minerals, and dietary fiber, commonly called the vegetable trio. In addition, the darker vegetables, indicated higher nutritional value [43]. Meanwhile, a survey indicated that vegetables consumption contributes most to dietary happiness over eight days among 14 main food categories [44]. In our study, vegetables had the greatest contributions to vitamin A daily intake among the nine food categories in the Chinese diet, and carrots had the highest content of provitamin A carotenoids and the highest contribution to vitamin A intake among the 16 kinds of vegetables, followed by spinach, Chinese chives, pepper, tomato, asparagus lettuce, lettuce, and pumpkin. Therefore, it was important to improve the amounts of vegetables eaten to increase the vitamin A intake. If one person eats only 1 of the 16 types of vegetables, the amount of each vegetable required is illustrated in Table S2. If the daily intake of the other 15 vegetables remains unchanged, the amount of each vegetable required to be eaten to meet the RDA of vitamin A intake when coarse cereals, potatoes, legumes, fruits, meat, eggs, milk, and aquatic products are consumed normally is illustrated in Table S3. When 1 of the 16 types of vegetables was used to replace all of the vegetables, adult women and men required 144 g and 173 g of carrots, 203 g and 244 g of spinach, and 370 g and 445 g of Chinese chives, respectively. It was recommended to intake 300–500 g of vegetables per day according to the Balanced Diet for Chinese Residents; hence, when eating other vegetables, the intake exceeded the recommended daily allowance for vegetables. If the other 15 vegetables remained unchanged in the diet to meet the RDA of vitamin A intake, adult women and men required 100 g and 130 g of carrots, 126 g and 167 g of spinach, 182 g and 257 g of Chinese chives, and 199 g and 276 g of peppers, respectively. The vitamin A daily intake from other vegetables exceeded the recommended daily intake from vegetables. Generally, carrot intake in Western countries was higher than in China due to differences in dietary habits. Therefore, it is hard to adjust the diet of the Chinese population to increase vegetable intake, especially from carrots and spinach, to meet the guideline of vitamin A intake, which was particularly important for patients with eye diseases, neurological disorders, and skin disorders [40].

It could be concluded that vegetables with a high content of provitamin A carotenoids such as carrot and spinach can meet the recommended intake of vegetables. However, it was hard to eat more than 100 g carrots or more than 120 g spinach per day for all Chinese residents. Therefore, improvement of the vitamin A concentration in vegetables was another strategy to increase the vitamin A intake for the entire Chinese population, and this was also the direction for farmers to pursue. The concentrations required for each vegetable to meet the RDA of vitamin A intake when the other 15 vegetables were included in the diet are listed in Table 2. Dark-green or yellow-green vegetables were good for humans, and most of these vegetables were produced in open fields as commodities with lower production costs and prices as well as high yields per unit area. To obtain vitamin A dietary intake of 700 ugRAE/day and 800 ugRAE/day for adult women and men, respectively, the total vitamin A content of spinach should be increased to 529 ugRAE/100 g and 702 ugRAE/100 g, which is 2.18 and 2.89 times higher than the current level, respectively. Similarly, the total vitamin A content of carrots should be increased to 973 ugRAE/100 g and 1256 ugRAE/100 g, which is 2.85 and 3.67 times of the current content, respectively. It was reported that an Indian farmer developed a carrot variety with β-carotene content of 277 mg/kg, which was the recommended amount that our study obtained based on the results [45]. Therefore, it was critical to increase the provitamin A carotenoids' content of spinach and carrots to meet the daily vitamin A intake. In addition to the common vegetables, vegetables with high provitamin A carotenoids contents were also present in vegetables with low daily consumption. Therefore, we should aim to gradually improve the intake of vegetables with low daily consumption but high provitamin A carotenoids content (e.g., bean curd, amaranth, and kale) and incorporate these into our recipes to increase the intake of vitamin A.

In conclusion, vegetable oil is an ideal matrix to stabilize retinol and delays vitamin A oxidation. Vitamin A can exist in vegetable oil in the form of retinol acetate or retinol palmitate [46]. Therefore, vegetable oil fortification is an important approach to overcome vitamin A deficiency. Rapeseed oil, soybean oil, and peanut oil were the primary types of vegetable oils consumed in China [47], and vitamin A-fortified rapeseed oil and soybean oil were available on the market. These could be used for obtaining the needed vitamin A dietary intake requirements. The recommended intake of vitamin A was 700 ugRAE/day and 800 ugRAE/day for adult women and men, respectively; vegetable oil with 630 ugRAE/100 g and 893 ugRAE/100 g of vitamin A should be implemented into the diets of adult women and men, respectively, when the vegetable oil consumption is 38 g per day. This high value was recommended (893 ugRAE/100 g) as vegetable oil is usually shared by a family. Since lactating women require higher vitamin A intake (1300 ugRAE/day), practical edible oil products with high total vitamin A content for lactating women should be designed. Moreover, the tolerable upper intake level (UL) suggested that the maximum average daily intake may not cause adverse health effects for almost all healthy people. The UL of vitamin A was 3000 ugRAE/day for adults and 700 ugRAE/day for children under 4 years old [38]. Hence, edible oil products with low total vitamin A content for children under 4 years old should be designed. Therefore, the vegetable oil processing industries should design vitamin A-fortified edible oils to meet the recommended daily vitamin A intake.

It has been reported that vitamin A–fortified soybean oil retained 100% of the biological value when the edible oil was heated at 100 °C for 20 min, while it retained 50% of the biological value when the edible oil was used for frying four times at 170 °C [48]. Therefore, vitamin A would not be destroyed during normal cooking. Therefore, consumption of vitamin A-fortified rapeseed oil and soybean oil was a satisfactory way to increase vitamin A intake.

Table 2. The increase in vitamin A content in each vegetable needed if the daily intake of the other 15 vegetables remained unchanged.

Vegetables	Area (ha)	Production (hg/ha)	Population (1000 Person)	per Capita Consumption (g/d)	Vitamin A Concentration Required (ugRAE/100 g)/Women/Men	The Current Concentration (ugRAE/100 g)	Multiple (Women/Men)
Carrot	395,525	459,532	141,260	35.251	973/1256	342	2.85/3.67
Kidney bean	876	113,174	141,260	0.019	1,267,271/1,793,586	18	70,403.94/99,643.67
Cowpea	14,391	10,162	141,260	0.028	855,382/1,214,675	10	85,538.2/121,467.5
Eggplant	804,381	465,690	141,260	72.652	331/469	4	82.75/117.25
Tomato	1,144,821	590,806	141,260	131.181	192/268	31	6.19/8.65
Red pepper						116	
Green pepper	754,718	221,933	141,260	32.486	796/1103	8	6.12/8.48
Sweet pepper						6	
Cucumber	1,292,545	584,874	141,260	146.621	165/234	8	20.63/29.25
Pumpkin	401,581	185,266	141,260	14.430	1722/2415	74	23.27/32.64
Chinese chives	5625	251,302	141,260	0.274	95,419/131,915	133	717.44/991.84
Cabbage	1,002,516	350,046	141,260	68.062	354/501	6	59/83.5
Broccoli	484,031	198,477	141,260	18.633	1294/1831	13	99.54/140.85
Spinach	714,572	417,691	141,260	57.888	529/702	243	2.18/2.89
Asparagus lettuce	607,979	236,321	141,260	27.866	902/1260	13	11.87/16.58
Lettuce						63	

5. Conclusions

In summary, vitamin A is widely found in various consumed foods. However, the daily human intake of vitamin A does not currently meet the recommended dietary intake according to scientific and reasonable calculations as well as the vitamin A intake of 460.56 ugRAE/day of Chinese residents. Among the nine different types of foods, vegetables made the greatest contributions to vitamin A intake, accounting for 54.94% of vitamin A intake (253.03 ugRAE/day). In addition, carrots had the highest provitamin A carotenoids' content, and the contribution of carrots was 28.33% (103.49 ugRAE/day) among the 45 kinds of foods consumed. The current daily intake content is significantly lower than the recommended dietary reference intake of vitamin A (800 ugRAE/day for adult men and 700 ugRAE/day for adult women). Therefore, it is essential to increase vitamin A intake. First, vegetable consumption should be increased to meet the recommended dietary intake. As a result, carrots, spinach, and Chinese chives can meet the recommended daily intake of vegetables. Furthermore, an improvement of the vitamin A concentration in vegetables to meet the recommended dietary intake should be addressed. For example, the concentration in spinach should be increased to 529 ugRAE/100 g and 702 ugRAE/100 g for women and men, respectively. Moreover, increasing the amount of vegetables with low daily consumption but high vitamin A content would be an effective way to increase vitamin A consumption. Additionally, a direct way to increase vitamin A intake is to eat vitamin A-fortified rapeseed oil and soybean oil. Therefore, this study is of great significance to guide the Chinese population to supplement vitamin A intake in a reasonable and scientific manner, thereby meeting the vitamin A dietary intake requirement and reducing the incidence of eye diseases.

Supplementary Materials: The following supporting information can be downloaded at: https://www.mdpi.com/article/10.3390/nu15184028/s1, Table S1: Vitamin A content of main foods; Table S2: The amount of each vegetable needed to be eaten when only eating one of the 16 kinds of vegetables; Table S3: The amount of each vegetable needed to be eaten when the other 15 vegetables' daily intake is kept unchanged.

Author Contributions: Conceptualization, L.Z. and P.L.; methodology, L.Z. and X.L.; software, L.Z.; formal analysis, C.G., Y.Z., L.Y., F.M. and X.W.; data curation, X.L. and Y.Z.; writing—original draft preparation, X.L. and L.Z.; writing—review and editing, L.Z.; supervision, P.L.; funding acquisition, L.Z. and P.L. All authors have read and agreed to the published version of the manuscript.

Funding: This research was funded by the National Key Research and Development Project of China (2021YFD1600101), the Major Project of Hubei Hongshan Laboratory (2022hszd002), the earmarked fund for the China Agriculture Research System (CARS-12 and CARS-13), and the Agricultural Science and Technology Innovation Program of Chinese Academy of Agricultural Sciences (CAAS-ASTIP-2021-OCRI).

Institutional Review Board Statement: Not applicable.

Informed Consent Statement: Not applicable.

Data Availability Statement: The data that support the findings of this study are available on request to the corresponding author.

Conflicts of Interest: The authors declare no conflict of interest.

References

1. Ruhl, R. Non-Pro-Vitamin A and Pro-Vitamin A carotenoids in atopy development. *Int. Arch. Allergy Immunol.* **2013**, *161*, 99–115. [CrossRef] [PubMed]
2. Nebolisa, N.M.; Umeyor, C.E.; Ekpunobi, U.E.; Umeyor, I.C.; Okoye, F.B. Profiling the effects of microwave-assisted and soxhlet extraction techniques on the physicochemical attributes of Moringa oleifera seed oil and proteins. *Oil Crop Sci.* **2023**, *8*, 16–26. [CrossRef]
3. Gonçalves, A.; Estevinho, B.N.; Rocha, F. Microencapsulation of vitamin A: A review. *Trends Food Sci. Technol.* **2016**, *51*, 76–87. [CrossRef]

4. Paiva, A.D.A.; Rondó, P.H.; Vaz-de-Lima, L.R.; Oliveira, C.D.F.; Ueda, M.; Cecilia Gonçalves-Carvalho, C.; Reinaldo, L.G. The impact of vitamin A supplementation on the immune system of vitamin A-deficient children. *Int. J. Vitam. Nutr. Res.* **2010**, *80*, 188–196. [CrossRef]
5. Maheshwari, S.; Kumar, V.; Bhadauria, G.; Mishra, A. Immunomodulatory potential of phytochemicals and other bioactive compounds of fruits: A review. *Food Front.* **2022**, *3*, 221–238. [CrossRef]
6. Al-Marri, K.; Al-Qashoti, M.; Al-Zoqari, H.; Elshaikh, U.; Naqadan, A.; Saeed, R.; Faraj, J.; Shraim, M. The relationship between smartphone use and dry eye disease: A systematic review with a narrative synthesis. *Medicine* **2021**, *100*, 38. [CrossRef]
7. Kim, J.; Hwang, Y.J.; Kang, S.; Kim, M.; Kim, T.S.; Kim, J.; Seo, J.; Ahn, H.; Yoon, S.; Yun, J.P.; et al. Association between Exposure to Smartphones and Ocular Health in Adolescents. *Ophthalmic Epidemiol.* **2016**, *23*, 269–276. [CrossRef]
8. Moon, J.H.; Kim, K.W.; Moon, N.J. Smartphone use is a risk factor for pediatric dry eye disease according to region and age: A case control study. *BMC Ophthalmol.* **2016**, *16*, 188. [CrossRef]
9. Choi, J.H.; Li, Y.; Kim, S.H.; Jin, R.J.; Kim, Y.H.; Cho, W.; You, I.C.; Yoon, K.C. The influences of smartphone use on the status of the tear film and ocular surface. *PLoS ONE* **2018**, *13*, e0206541. [CrossRef] [PubMed]
10. Garg, A.; Bhargav, S.; Arora, T.; Garg, A. Prevalence and Risk Factors of Dry Eye Disease at a Tertiary Care Centre in Haryana, India: A Cross-sectional Study. *J. Clin. Diagn. Res.* **2022**, *16*, NC09–NC129. [CrossRef]
11. Moustakime, Y.; Hazzoumi, Z.; Joutei, K.A. Aromatization of virgin olive oil by seeds of Pimpinella anisum using three different methods: Physico-chemical change and thermal stability of flavored oils. *Grain Oil Sci. Technol.* **2021**, *4*, 108–124. [CrossRef]
12. Maia, S.B.; Souza, A.S.R.; Caminha, M.D.F.C.; Silva, S.L.D.; Cruz, R.D.S.B.L.C.; Santos, C.C.D.; Filho, M.B. Vitamin A and pregnancy: A narrative review. *Nutrients* **2019**, *11*, 681. [CrossRef] [PubMed]
13. Tanumihardjo, S.A. Biological evidence to define a vitamin A deficiency cutoff using total liver vitamin A reserves. *Exp. Biol. Med.* **2021**, *246*, 1045–1053. [CrossRef] [PubMed]
14. Zinder, R.; Cooley, R.; Vlad, L.G.; Molnar, J.A. Vitamin A and Wound Healing. *Nutr. Clin. Pract.* **2019**, *34*, 839–949. [CrossRef] [PubMed]
15. Schaumberg, D.A.; Linehan, M.; Hawley, G.; O'Connor, J.; Dreyfuss, M.; Semba, R.D. Vitamin A deficiency in the South Pacific. *Public Health* **1995**, *109*, 311–317. [CrossRef]
16. Prihastyanti, M.N.U.; Chandra, R.D.; Lukitasari, D.M. How to fulfill carotenoid needs during pregnancy and for the growth and development of infants and children—A review. *efood* **2021**, *2*, 101–112. Available online: https://www.atlantis-press.com/journals/efood (accessed on 9 July 2021). [CrossRef]
17. Arlappa, N.; Balakrishna, N.; Laxmaiah, A.; Nair, K.M.; Brahmam, G.N.V. Prevalence of clinical and sub-clinical vitamin A deficiency among rural preschool children of west Bengal, India. *Indian Pediatr* **2011**, *48*, 47–49. [CrossRef]
18. Ng, F.J.; Mackey, D.A.; O'Sullivan, T.A.; Oddy, W.H.; Seyhan Yazar, S. Is Dietary Vitamin A Associated with Myopia from Adolescence to Young Adulthood? *Trans. Vis. Sci. Technol.* **2020**, *9*, 29. [CrossRef]
19. Zhang, X.P.; Yang, K.Y.; Chen, L.W.; Liao, X.L.; Deng, L.P.; Chen, S.Y.; Ji, Y. Vitamin A deficiency in critically ill children with sepsis. *Crit. Care* **2019**, *23*, 267. [CrossRef]
20. Olang, B.; Naghavi, M.; Bastani, D.; Strandvik, B.; Yngve, A. Optimal vitamin A and suboptimal vitamin D status are common in Iranian infants. *Acta Paediatr.* **2010**, *100*, 439–444. [CrossRef]
21. Luo, Z.X.; Liu, E.M.; Luo, J.; Li, F.R.; Li, S.B.; Zeng, F.Q.; Qu, P.; Fu, Z.; Li, T.Y. Vitamin A deficiency and wheezing. *World J. Pediatr.* **2010**, *6*, 81–84. [CrossRef]
22. Lira, L.Q.D.; Dimenstein, R. Vitamin A and gestational diabetes. *Rev. Assoc. Med. Bras.* **2010**, *56*, 355–359. [CrossRef]
23. Moltedo, A.; Alvarez-Sanchez, C.; Grande, F.; Charrondiere, U.R. The complexity of producing and interpreting dietary vitamin A statistics. *J. Food Compost. Anal.* **2021**, *100*, 103926. [CrossRef]
24. Maurya, V.K.; Shakya, A.; Aggarwal, M.; Gothandam, K.M.; Bohn, T.; Pareek, S. Fate of β-carotene within loaded delivery systems in food: State of knowledge. *Antioxidants* **2021**, *10*, 426. [CrossRef] [PubMed]
25. Loo-Bouwman, C.A.V.; Naber, T.H.J.; Schaafsma, G. A review of vitamin A equivalency of b-carotene in various food matrices for human consumption. *Brit. J. Nutr.* **2014**, *111*, 2153–2166. [CrossRef] [PubMed]
26. Klemm, R.D.W.; West, K.P.; Palmer, A.C., Jr.; Johnson, Q.; Randall, P.; Ranum, P.; Northrop-Clewes, C. Vitamin A fortification of wheat flour: Considerations and current recommendations. *Food Nutr. Bull.* **2010**, *31*, S47–S61. [CrossRef] [PubMed]
27. Yeh, E.B.; Barbano, D.M.; Drake, M. Vitamin fortification of fluid milk. *J. Food Sci.* **2017**, *82*, 856–864. [CrossRef] [PubMed]
28. Allen, L.H.; Haskell, M. Estimating the potential for vitamin A toxicity in women and young children. *J. Nutr.* **2002**, *132*, 2907S–2919S. [CrossRef] [PubMed]
29. Mastroiacovo, P.; Mazzone, T.; Addis, A.; Elephant, E.; Carlier, P.; Vial, T.; Garbis, H.; Robert, E.; Bonati, M.; Ornoy, A.; et al. High vitamin A intake in early pregnancy and major malformations: A multicenter prospective controlled study. *Teratology* **1999**, *59*, 7–11. [CrossRef]
30. US Institute of Medicine. *DRI Dietary Reference Intakes: Applications in Dietary Assessment*; National Academies Press: Washington, DC, USA, 2000. [CrossRef]
31. Fitt, E.; Cole, D.; Ziauddeen, N.; Pell, D.; Stickley, E.; Harvey, A.; Stephen, A.M. DINO (Diet In Nutrients Out) -an integrated dietary assessment system. *Public Health Nutr.* **2014**, *18*, 234–241. [CrossRef]
32. Watkins, S.; Freebor, E.; Mushtaq, S. A validated FFQ to determine dietary intake of vitamin D. *Public Health Nutr.* **2020**, *24*, 4001–4006. [CrossRef] [PubMed]

33. McNutt, S.; Zimmerman, T.P.; Hull, S.G. Development of food composition databases for food frequency questionnaires (FFQ). *J. Food Compos. Anal.* **2008**, *21*, S20–S26. [CrossRef]
34. Boushey, C.J.; Spoden, M.; Zhu, F.M.; Delp, E.J.; Kerr, D.A. New mobile methods for dietary assessment: Review of image-assisted and image-based dietary assessment methods. *Proc. Nutr. Soc.* **2017**, *76*, 283–294. [CrossRef]
35. Yang, R.; Xue, L.; Zhang, L.X.; Wang, X.P.; Qi, X.; Jiang, J.; Yu, L.; Wang, X.P.; Zhang, W.; Zhang, Q.; et al. Phytosterol contents of edible oils and their contributions to estimated phytosterol intake in the Chinese diet. *Foods* **2019**, *8*, 334. [CrossRef] [PubMed]
36. Zhang, Y.; Qi, X.; Wang, X.Y.; Wang, X.F.; Ma, F.; Yu, L.; Mao, J.; Jiang, J.; Zhang, L.X.; Li, P.W. Contribution of tocopherols in commonly consumed foods to estimated tocopherol intake in the Chinese diet. *Front. Nutr.* **2022**, *9*, 829091. [CrossRef] [PubMed]
37. Nimsakul, S.; Collumbien, M.; Likit-Ekaraj, V.; Suwanarach, C.; Tansuhaj, A.; Fuchs, G.J. Simplified dietary assessment to detect vitamin A deficiency. *Nutr. Res.* **1994**, *14*, 325–336. [CrossRef]
38. Durán-Cabral, M.; Fernández-Jalao, I.; Estévez-Santiago, R.; Olmedilla-Alonso, B. Assessment of individual carotenoid and vitamin A dietary intake in overweight and obese Dominican subjects. *Nutr. Hosp.* **2017**, *34*, 407–415. [CrossRef]
39. Chinese Nutrition Society. *Chinese Dietary Reference Intakes, 2013 ed.*; Beijing Science Press: Beijing, China, 2014.
40. Maurya, V.K.; Shakya, A.; Bashir, K.; Kushwaha, S.C.; McClements, D.J. Vitamin A fortification: Recent advances in encapsulation technologies. *Compr. Rev. Food Sci. Food Saf.* **2022**, *21*, 2772–2819. [CrossRef]
41. McClements, D.J. Enhanced delivery of lipophilic bioactives using emulsions: A review of major factors affecting vitamin, nutraceutical, and lipid bioaccessibility. *Food Funct.* **2018**, *9*, 22. [CrossRef]
42. Rana, S.; Arora, S.; Gupta, C.; Bodemala, H.; Kapila, S. Evaluation of in-vivo model for vitamin A bioavailability from vitamin A loaded caseinate complex. *Food Biosc.* **2021**, *42*, 101174. [CrossRef]
43. Minich, D.M. A review of the science of colorful, plant-based food and practical strategies for "eating the rainbow". *J. Nutr. Metab.* **2019**, *2019*, 2125070. [CrossRef] [PubMed]
44. Wahl, D.R.; Villinger, K.; Konig, L.M.; Ziesemer, K.; Schupp, H.T.; Renner, B. Healthy food choices are happy food choices: Evidence from a real life sample using smartphone based assessments. *Sci. Rep.* **2017**, *7*, 17069. [CrossRef] [PubMed]
45. Ministry of Science & Technology. Biofortified Carrot Variety Developed by Farmer Scientist Benefits Local Farmers. 2020. Available online: https://pib.gov.in/PressReleasePage.aspx?PRID=1612159 (accessed on 8 April 2020).
46. Dary, O.; Mora, J.O. Food fortification to reduce vitamin A deficiency: International vitamin A consultative group recommendations. *J. Nutr.* **2002**, *132*, 2927S–2933S. [CrossRef] [PubMed]
47. Yang, R.N.; Zhang, L.X.; Li, P.W.; Yu, L.; Mao, J.; Wang, X.P.; Zhang, Q. A review of chemical composition and nutritional properties of minor vegetable oils in China. *Trends Food Sci. Technol.* **2018**, *74*, 26–32. [CrossRef]
48. Favaro, R.M.D.; Miyasaaka, C.K.; Desai, I.D.; de Oliveira, J.E.D. Evalution of the effect of heat treatment on the biological value of vitamin A fortified soybean oil. *Nutr. Res.* **1992**, *12*, 1357–1363. [CrossRef]

Disclaimer/Publisher's Note: The statements, opinions and data contained in all publications are solely those of the individual author(s) and contributor(s) and not of MDPI and/or the editor(s). MDPI and/or the editor(s) disclaim responsibility for any injury to people or property resulting from any ideas, methods, instructions or products referred to in the content.

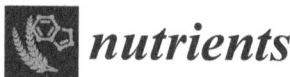

Article

Differences in the Factor Structure of the Eating Attitude Test-26 (EAT-26) among Clinical vs. Non-Clinical Adolescent Israeli Females

Zohar Spivak-Lavi [1,*], Yael Latzer [2,3], Daniel Stein [4,5], Ora Peleg [6] and Orna Tzischinsky [7]

1. Faculty of Social Work, The Max Stern Yezreel Valley College, D.N. Emek Yezreel 1930600, Israel
2. Faculty of Social Welfare and Health Sciences, University of Haifa, Haifa 3498838, Israel; ylatzer@univ.haifa.ac.il
3. Eating Disorders Institution, Psychiatric Division, Rambam Health Care Campus, Haifa 31096, Israel
4. Sackler School of Medicine, Tel Aviv University, Tel Aviv 69978, Israel; prof.daniel.stein@gmail.com
5. Safra Children's Hospital, Sheba Medical Center, Ramat Gan 52621, Israel
6. Education and School Counseling Departments, Max Stern Yezreel Valley College, Yezreel Valley 1930600, Israel
7. Department of Behavioral Sciences, The Max Stern Academic College of Emek Yezreel, Emek Yezreel 1930000, Israel; orna@yvc.ac.il
* Correspondence: zohars@yvc.ac.il

Abstract: In recent years, the diagnostic definitions of eating disorders (EDs) have undergone dramatic changes. The Eating Attitudes Test-26 (EAT-26), which is considered an accepted instrument for community ED studies, has shown in its factorial structure to be inconsistent in different cultures and populations. The aim of the present study was to compare the factor structure of the EAT-26 among clinical and non-clinical populations. The clinical group included 207 female adolescents who were hospitalized with an ED (mean age 16.1). The non-clinical group included 155 female adolescents (mean age 16.1). Both groups completed the EAT-26. A series of factorial invariance models was conducted on the EAT-26. The results indicate that significant differences were found between the two groups regarding the original EAT-26 dimensions: dieting, bulimia and food preoccupation, and oral control. Additionally, the factorial structure of the EAT-26 was found to be significantly different in both groups compared to the original version. In the clinical group, the factorial structure of the EAT-26 consisted of four factors, whereas in the non-clinical sample, five factors were identified. Additionally, a 19-item version of the EAT-26 was found to be considerably more stable and well suited to capture ED symptoms in both groups, and a cutoff point of 22 (not 20) better differentiated clinical samples from non-clinical samples. The proposed shortening of the EAT from 40 to 26 and now to 19 items should be examined in future studies. That said, the shortened scale seems more suited for use among both clinical and non-clinical populations. These results reflect changes that have taken place in ED psychopathology over recent decades.

Keywords: EAT-26; assessment; eating disorders; clinical and non-clinical populations

1. Introduction

1.1. Eating Disorders—Past and Present

Eating disorders (EDs) are severe psychiatric illnesses [1,2], and their rate has steadily increased over the past four decades both in Western and non-Western countries [3,4]. The lifetime prevalence of EDs (according to the DSM 5 (Diagnostic and Statistical Manual of Mental Disorders) diagnostic criteria [5]) is estimated to be about 1–1.5% for anorexia nervosa (AN); 1–2% for bulimia nervosa (BN); and 1–3.5% for binge eating disorder (BED) [6,7]. The prevalence of pathological eating behaviors and a low self-esteem and negative body image among female adolescents and young women, in different studies worldwide, has been estimated to be about 40–70% [8].

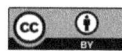

Citation: Spivak-Lavi, Z.; Latzer, Y.; Stein, D.; Peleg, O.; Tzischinsky, O. Differences in the Factor Structure of the Eating Attitude Test (EAT-26) among Clinical vs. Non-Clinical Adolescent Israeli Females. *Nutrients* 2023, *15*, 4168. https://doi.org/10.3390/nu15194168

Academic Editors: Renata Puppin Zandonadi, Raquel Braz Assunção Botelho and António Raposo

Received: 16 August 2023
Revised: 18 September 2023
Accepted: 20 September 2023
Published: 27 September 2023

Copyright: © 2023 by the authors. Licensee MDPI, Basel, Switzerland. This article is an open access article distributed under the terms and conditions of the Creative Commons Attribution (CC BY) license (https://creativecommons.org/licenses/by/4.0/).

Over the past five decades, the clinical picture of EDs, as reflected in the different DSM classifications, has undergone dramatic changes [9]. Bulimia nervosa was added in the early 1980s; BED was added as a provisional diagnosis in the early 1990s; and normal-weight purging disorder, night eating syndrome, and avoidant restrictive feeding and eating disorder (ARFID) for young children were only added around 10 years ago [10].

The changes in the DSM criteria reflect the changes in the prevalence of the different clinical presentations of EDs over the past several decades, and are related, in part, to several important socio-cultural changes. These include the plentitude of food in Westernized countries, increased globalization processes, the exposure of people in non-Westernized countries to societal pressures, and thus, an increase in the risk for EDs [11,12], and changes involved in the distribution and influence of mass media with respect to body image and dieting behaviors, which have increased dramatically in recent decades [13].

In light of these changes, the early detection of individuals who are at a high risk of developing EDs is critical for improvements in prevention, treatment, and prognosis, and the reduction in chronicity [14]. Indeed, over many years, attempts have been made to develop improved assessment tools to better identify these different types of at-risk ED groups [15].

1.2. Self-Reported Screening Tools for Disordered Eating Behaviors

Over the past four decades, a series of assessment tools has been created for the purpose of identifying the presence of at-risk groups for ED symptoms and ED severity. These include the Eating Disorder Inventory (64–91 items depending on the version [16,17]); the Eating Disorder Examination, Screening Version (8 items [18]); the Eating Disorder Examination Questionnaire (36–41 items [19]); the SCOFF Questionnaire (5 items [20]), and the Eating Attitudes Test (EAT; 26–40 items [21–23]).

The EAT questionnaire is commonly used by clinicians and for research purposes in the field of Eds. Its original version, the EAT-40 [22], was developed when AN was characterized mainly by restrictive behaviors [24]. It included seven factors [25]: food preoccupation, a drive for thinness and body-image-related preoccupations, vomiting and laxative abuse, dieting, slow eating, covert eating, and perceived pressure to gain weight. The answers were rated on a 6-point Likert scale, with a cutoff point of 30. A score higher than 30 was considered to identify disturbed eating behavior.

The EAT-40 was found to be valid in patients with AN in a community sample [21]. Nevertheless, it yielded high percentages of false positive scores among potentially high-risk groups—for example, 29% among ballet students and 27% among modeling students [22]. Notwithstanding these limitations, the EAT-40 was considered an effective screening questionnaire for identifying groups at risk of developing EDs [15].

Over the years, the questionnaire was shortened to a 26-item version [21]. The short version includes three scales: dieting, bulimia and food preoccupation, and oral control (i.e., showing self-control overeating, including in conditions when there are environmental pressures and perceived pressures to eat and gain weight). The answers are rated on a 6-point Likert scale, with a cutoff point of 20 or higher showing disturbed eating behavior. Both cutoff points (20 for the EAT-26 and 30 for the EAT-40) have been supported by studies conducted among clinical and non-clinical samples and may assist in identifying people who are at risk of developing an ED [26–30]. The two versions of the EAT have been found to be comparable in the identification of disturbed eating in the general population [15].

The EAT-26 was translated, validated, and adapted into many languages, including Arabic [31], Japanese [32], Italian [33], and Hebrew [34]. In addition, it was examined among diverse ethnic groups, including in Israel [15,25,35], and was declared as the screening instrument of choice for the identification of disordered eating in the general population by the National Eating Disorders Screening Program and by the National Mental Illness Screening Project in 1999 [36].

There are, however, several reasons to suggest that a cutoff point of 20 is no longer a valid cutoff point.

Notwithstanding the generally accepted reliability of the EAT-26 in studies about disordered eating in community populations, concerns have arisen in recent years among clinicians and researchers regarding the use of this instrument. The main suggested reason for this concern stems from recent results of a study conducted by our group in Israel [35], emphasizing that the EAT-26 is used differently, and its results are interpreted differently, in tradition-oriented sub-populations. The results show different factors in different ethnic groups, most of which did not correspond with the original EAT-26 three-factor structure. The analysis yielded two main factors among Israeli Jews, four main factors among Israeli Muslim Arabs, and three main factors among Israeli Christian Arabs, revealing the inconsistencies that were found in its factor structure [37].

Similarly, a few studies in English-speaking countries have reported either three, four, or five factors, with the number of items ranging from 16 to 25 [15]. In non-English-speaking samples, four to six factors were observed, and a new factor was also identified: an awareness of food preoccupation [38]. As for the Hebrew version, it yielded the three original factors, but a fourth factor, an awareness of food preoccupation, was also identified [28].

Another suggested reason is related to the finding that both the EAT-40 and the EAT-26 mainly include items assessing restricting preoccupations and behaviors, with only a few items referring to binging/purging behaviors. This situation likely arose because, at the time of the construction of the two scales, in the late 1970s and early 1980s, respectively, the most studied ED was AN of the restricting type. Following the changes observed over the past decades in the symptoms and psychopathological characteristics of EDs in general and AN in particular, it appears that it is mainly the total score of the EAT-26, rather than its factors, that can be used for the assessment of the severity of ED symptoms in patients with AN, in addition to changes in symptom severity following treatment.

To the best of our knowledge, there have been no studies in which the factor structure of the EAT-26 has been compared between clinical and non-clinical populations.

Hence, several questions have arisen: 1. Does the EAT-26 questionnaire still clearly distinguish between a healthy population and a population with EDs in all its factors? 2. Can the EAT-26 be used today, in 2023, as a screening tool to identify risk groups for the development of EDs in different ethnic populations? 3. Does the cutoff point of 20 allow for a distinction to be made between clinical and non-clinical populations in 2023? 4. Is the factor structure of the EAT-26 similar in clinical and non-clinical populations?

Based on these questions, the main goal of the present study was to examine the factor structure of the EAT-26 questionnaire and the relevant cutoff score in two populations of adolescent girls in Israel: a clinical population and a non-clinical population.

We hypothesized the following:

1. A difference would be found between a clinical population and a non-clinical population in the factor structure of the EAT-26.
2. The clinical group would show a factor structure that is more like the original EAT-26 (three factors) than the non-clinical group would.
3. In accordance with the first hypothesis, a difference would be found between the current EAT-26 cutoff point, reflecting the presence of pathological eating preoccupations and behaviors, and the original cutoff point (20).

2. Materials and Methods

2.1. Participants and Procedure

Two groups were included in the study: a clinical group and a non-clinical group. The clinical group consisted of 207 Jewish Israeli female adolescents who were hospitalized in the Specialized Eating Disorders (EDs) Adolescent Inpatient Department at Safra Children's Hospital, Sheba Medical Center, Tel Hashomer, Israel for the treatment of EDs between the years 2008 and 2020 (masked for review). Of these, 206 participants were under the age of 18, and one participant was 19 years old. She was included in the study because her hospitalization began before she turned 18 and continued until she was 19 years old. It should be noted that, in Israel, the psychiatric care of children is considered to extend up to the age of 21.

The mean age of the patients was 16.1; SD (1.3); and range (12.3–19.0). The most prevalent diagnosis was AN restricting type (n = 94; 45.4%); followed by AN binge/purge type (n = 45; 21.7%); BN (n = 33; 15.95%); and atypical EDs (22; 10.6%). The most prevalent comorbid psychiatric diagnosis was depression (39; 18.8%); followed by ADHD (25; 12.1%); anxiety (10; 4.8%); and obsessive–compulsive disorder OCD (9; 4.3%) (see Table 1).

Table 1. Between-group differences in demographic and clinical parameters.

	Study Group (N = 207)	Control Group (N = 155)	p
Age in years (range)	16.1 ± 1.3 (12.3–19.0)	16.1 ± 1.6 (12–18)	0.99
BMI (range)	17.85 ± 3.46 (10.70–33.60)	21.07 ± 1.61 (14.53–31.64)	<0.001
BMI < 15	35 (16.9)	3 (1.9)	<0.001
BMI > 25	9 (4.4)	31 (19.9)	<0.001
Diagnosis (n/p)			
AN	94 (45.4)		
AN—binge/purge	45 (21.7)	N/A	
BN	33 (15.95)		
Atypical EDs	22 (10.6)		
Co-morbidity (n/p)			
Depression	39 (18.8)		
ADHD	25 (12.1)		
Anxiety	10 (4.8)		
OCD	9 (4.3)		
PTSD	7 (3.4)		
Dysthymia	4 (1.9)		
Social phobia	3 (1.4)		
Panic disorder	3 (1.4)		
Alcohol abuse	2 (1.0)		
Bipolar disorder	2 (1.0)		
Other	8 (3.9)		

BMI—Body Mass Index; ADHD—Attention Deficit/Hyperactivity Disorder; OCD—Obsessive–Compulsive Disorder; PTSD—Post-Traumatic Stress Disorder.

The EAT-26 questionnaires of the clinical sample were filled out during the course of various studies that were conducted in this department, and were all approved by the IRB of the Sheba Medical Center (#2755). The need for informed consent for this specific study was waived due to the study's retrospective nature—namely, a review of electronic medical records. The only other details presented in this study from the medical records were the participants' ages, weights, and heights. The EAT-26 questionnaires were filled out within the first two weeks of hospitalization—that is, when the adolescent was in an acute ED state.

In this department, the diagnosis of an ED is determined by experienced child and adolescent psychiatrists using semi-structured interviews, based on the DSM-IV and DSM-5 criteria. Patients were excluded from study participation if their ED diagnosis was not confirmed unanimously in clinical team meetings of the inpatient department. All patients diagnosed with an ED via the DSM-IV were also re-diagnosed with the same ED when their charts were re-evaluated according to the DSM-5. Comorbid psychiatric diagnoses were similarly determined, using semi-structured interviews, based on the DSM-IV and DSM-5 criteria.

The second group (i.e., the control group) consisted of 156 Jewish Israeli non-clinical female participants of a similar age range to that of the clinical group. One participant was 21 years old, and therefore, was omitted from the sample. Between the years 2011 and 2019, four high schools were recruited for the purpose of the study after receiving ethical approval from the institutional review board (IRB) of the first author's college, the Ministry of Education, the high school principals, the teachers, and the adolescents and their parents. In each high school, one class was sampled from each age group, and those who agreed to participate filled out the questionnaires at school. Informed consent was obtained from the adolescents and their parents. The mean age of the control group ranged from 12 to 18 years. The girls in the clinical group had statistically significantly lower BMIs than their healthy counterparts ($p < 0.001$).

In both study groups, completion of the questionnaires was voluntary, and respondents were told they could stop participating at any point. All participants were assured of anonymity and confidentiality. Controls were excluded if they reported an ED via an open yes/no question. They were also asked to report their weight and height. Only those controls fulfilling these two criteria were included in the study.

2.2. The EAT-26 Instrument

The Eating Attitude Test (EAT-26) [21] is a screening instrument that is commonly used to measure eating attitudes. It comprises 26 items, and scoring is completed on a 6-point scale. The six available response options are "always", "usually", "often", "sometimes", "rarely", or "never". The subscales are dieting, bulimia and food preoccupation, and oral control. Scores range between 0 and 78 points, and higher scores indicate greater pathology. A score of 20 or higher indicates a clinically significant eating pathology level; it is referred to as an EAT-26 "positive score". The EAT-26 has demonstrated high reliability and consistency, and the initial Cronbach's alpha was 0.90 for the total EAT-26 [21]. In the current study, total internal consistency: $\alpha = 0.86$; dieting factor: $\alpha = 80$; bulimia and food preoccupation factor: $\alpha = 67$; and oral control factor: $\alpha = 56$.

2.3. Data Analysis

To estimate whether the Israeli clinical and non-clinical samples manifest EDs in the same way, we conducted a series of factorial invariance models on the EAT-26. In the first model, we tested for *configural invariance* (i.e., pattern invariance), in which one assesses whether similar items measure each construct across groups (i.e., whether EAT-26 dieting, bulimia and food preoccupation, and oral control clusters consist of the same items in clinical and non-clinical samples). In configural invariance models, items are loaded on predefined latent factors, as in Confirmatory Factor Analysis (CFA), such that items' loadings and intercepts are freely estimated for each group (i.e., only the factorial structure is fixed, while the loadings and/or intercepts could be different for each group). Good model fit would support configural invariance. Model fit was estimated via Comparative Fit Index (CFI), Tucker–Lewis Index (TLI), Root Mean Square Error of Approximation (RMSEA), and Standardized Root Mean Square Residual (SRMR). CFI and TLI > 0.90 and RMSEA and SRMR < 0.07 are acceptable. Next, we tested for *metric invariance* (i.e., weak invariance), in which one assesses whether the constructs' factor loadings are similar across groups (i.e., loadings are constrained to be equal across groups); attaining invariance of factor loadings suggests that the constructs have the same meaning to participants across groups. Metric invariance is assessed by comparing the fit of the configural model with that of the metric invariance model; a non-significant chi-squared test would support metric invariance. Of note, metric invariance is not enough to justify the comparison of group means. Next, we tested for *scalar invariance* (i.e., strong invariance), in which one assesses whether items have the same intercepts (i.e., both loadings and intercepts are constrained to be equal across groups). Non-invariance of intercepts may be indicative of potential measurement bias and suggests that there are larger forces such as cultural norms or developmental differences that are influencing the way participants are responding to items across groups. Attainment of scalar invariance justifies comparison of group means. Scalar invariance is assessed by comparing the fit of the metric model with that of the scalar invariance model; a non-significant chi-squared test would support scalar invariance. All models were estimated with the *lavaan* Structural Equation Modeling R package. Missing data were handled with the Full-Information Maximum Likelihood (FIML) method.

Following the assessment of factorial invariance (or lack thereof) between the clinical and non-clinical samples, we employed Exploratory Graph Analysis (EGA; [39]) using *EGAnet* R package—a network psychometrics method that uses undirected network models for the assessment of psychometric properties of questionnaires. Exploratory Graph Analysis was used to verify the number of factors using graphical lasso [40] and the items that are associated with each factor. Network loadings, which are roughly equivalent to factor loadings, are reported using *net.loads()*, with suggested general effect size guidelines for network loadings of 0.15 for small effect sizes, 0.25 for moderate effect sizes, and 0.35 for large effect sizes [41]. The number of factors corroborated other traditional methods—parallel analysis (PA), Velicer's minimum average partial (MAP) test, and the comparison data approach [42]. Next, to examine the stability of the EGAs, we followed the analysis using Bootstrap EGA with 5000 resampling cycles. Finally, we used the novel Unique Variable Analysis (UVA [41]) for detecting redundant items in the EAT-26, and used the *item Stability()* function to detect highly unstable items.

In the final part of the results, we examined the effectiveness of the revised EAT questionnaire in differentiating between clinical and non-clinical samples. To achieve this, we calculated the optimal clinical cutoff point by bootstrapping the optimal cutoff point while maximizing the sensitivity and specificity (i.e., highest Youden's index: sensitivity + specificity—1). We also reported the suggested indexes of the "number needed to diagnose" (NND [43]) (i.e., the number of patients who need to be examined in order to correctly detect one person with the disease of interest in a study population of persons with and without the known disease); "number needed to misdiagnose" (NNM; [1]) (i.e., the number of patients who need to be tested in order for one to be misdiagnosed by the test); and the "likelihood to be diagnosed or misdiagnosed" (LDM [44]), with higher values of LDM (>1) suggesting that a test is more likely to diagnose than misdiagnose.

3. Results

3.1. Assessing Configural Invariance

To assess whether similar items measure the EAT-26 constructs across groups (clinical and non-clinical), we conducted a configural invariance model. The model had a poor fit with the observed data, including $\chi^2_{(227)} = 1041.95$, $p < 0.0001$, *CFI* = 0.77, *TLI* = 0.74, *RMSEA* = 0.13 (90% confidence intervals (CIs) of 0.12 and 0.14), and *SRMR* = 0.10, indicating that the EAT-26 control clusters of dieting, bulimia and food preoccupation, and oral control do not consist of the same items across the groups. We followed the modeling with *modindices()* to examine whether the covariates between the items might improve the model's fit. Eight covariates were identified, yet remodeling the suggested factorial construct with these covariates did not improve the fit, as seen in the following: $\chi^2_{(288)} = 1094.54$, $p < 0.0001$, *CFI* = 0.77, *TLI* = 0.74, *RMSEA* = 0.12 (90% CIs of 0.11 and 0.12), and *SRMR* = 0.10. In other words, the factorial structure of the EAT-26 was found to be significantly different from the original EAT-26 version in Israeli clinical and non-clinical groups (i.e., the configural invariance did not hold). As a result of this finding, we did not further examine the presence of matric or scalar invariances.

3.2. Exploratory Graph Analysis

To assess the factorial structure of the EAT-26 within each group, we conducted an EGA separately for the clinical and non-clinical samples. The EGA network results are presented in Figure 1, and the network loadings are shown in Table 2.

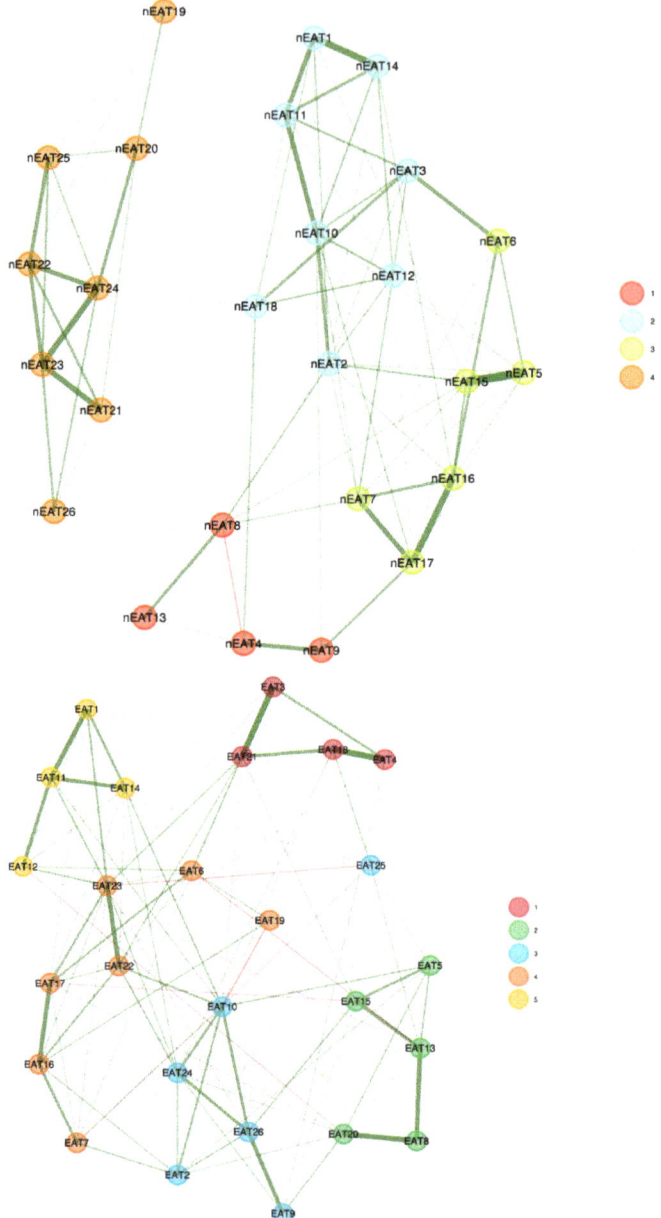

Figure 1. EGA results for clinical (**upper panel**) and non-clinical (**bottom panel**) groups. The factorial structure of the EAT-26 among the clinical group comprised three factors, but with different item configurations than the original EAT-26. The factorial structure among the non-clinical group comprised five factors.

Table 2. (a) Network loadings based on EGA among the clinical group. (b) Network loadings based on EGA among the non-clinical group.

(a)				
	Weight Preoccupation	Binge/Purge Behaviors and Concerns of Others	Dieting and Restricting Symptoms	Eating-Related Concerns
nEAT11	0.35			
nEAT10	0.33			
nEAT1	0.32			
nEAT14	0.30			
nEAT12	0.22			
nEAT3	0.22			
nEAT2	0.18			
nEAT18	0.16			
nEAT8		0.20		
nEAT9		0.18		
nEAT13		0.17		
nEAT4		−0.28		
nEAT16			0.37	
nEAT5			0.31	
nEAT17			0.30	
nEAT15			0.28	
nEAT7			0.26	
nEAT6			0.15	
nEAT23				0.48
nEAT24				0.44
nEAT22				0.40
nEAT21				0.26
nEAT25				0.25
nEAT20				0.22
nEAT26				0.14
nEAT19				0.09

(b)					
	Weight Concerns	Eating-Related Concerns	Food Controls One's Life	One's Own and Others' Control over the Person's Eating	Dieting
EAT11	0.42				
EAT1	0.29				
EAT14	0.26				
EAT12	0.19				
EAT26		0.33			
EAT24		0.25			
EAT10		0.23			
EAT2		0.17			
EAT9		0.16			
EAT25					
EAT18			0.33		
EAT21			0.32		
EAT4			0.30		
EAT3			0.29		
EAT13				0.33	
EAT8				0.32	
EAT20				0.25	
EAT15				0.22	
EAT5				0.20	
EAT16					0.31
EAT17					0.29
EAT23	0.22				0.25
EAT22					0.23
EAT6					0.15
EAT7					--
EAT19					--

Note. General effect size guidelines for network loadings are 0.15 for small, 0.25 for moderate, and 0.35 for large.

3.3. Clinical Sample

The analyses indicated that the factorial structure of the EAT-26 in the clinical group consisted of four factors named "Weight preoccupation", consisting of eight items; "Binge/purge behaviors and concerns of others", consisting of four items; "Dieting and restricting symptoms", consisting of six items; and "Eating-related concerns", consisting of eight items (with item 26, "I enjoy trying new rich foods", and item 19, "I display self-control around food", loading only weakly). A four-factor solution was corroborated by two additional analyses—parallel analysis (eigen values of 7.23, 3.97, 2.04, and 1.45 for the four factors) and Velicer's MAP (squared: 0.016; fourth power: 0.0009). Conversely, the comparison data estimation suggested that five factors must be retained (as compared with one to seven factors).

When estimating the stability of the EGA by bootstrapping with 5000 resampling cycles, the analysis indicated high stability (SE = 0.67), with the CI for the number of factors ranging from 2.69 to 5.31. In addition, the four-factor solution was prevalent in 63.90% of the bootstrap samples, with 23.48% producing a five-factor solution (and 8.64% producing a three-factor solution, and 3.66% producing a six-factor solution). A confirmatory factor analysis (CFA) that was used to corroborate the EGA solution verified the factorial structure as follows: $\chi^2_{(82.99)}$ = 173.96, p < 0.01, CFI = 0.96, TLI = 0.95, $RMSEA$ = 0.073 (90% confidence intervals (CIs) of 0.065 and 0.081), $SRMR$ = 0.08. The CFA is presented in Figure 2a.

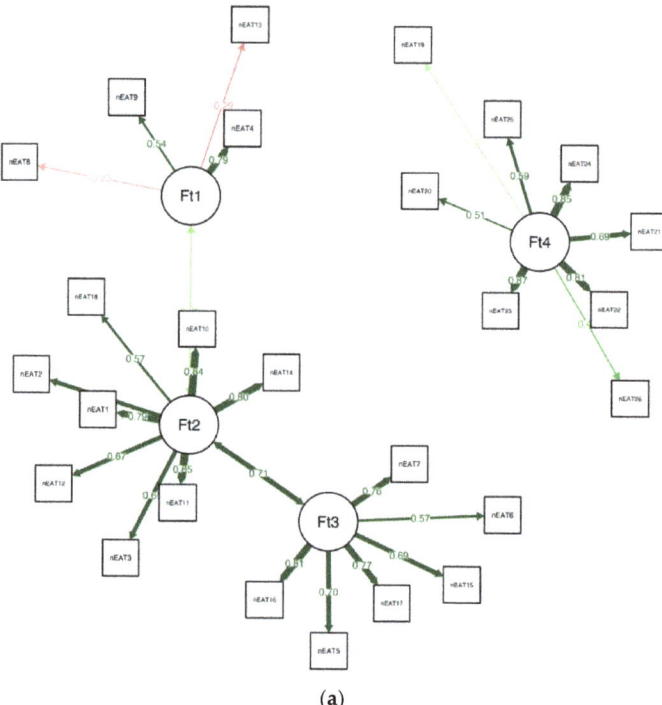

(a)

Figure 2. *Cont.*

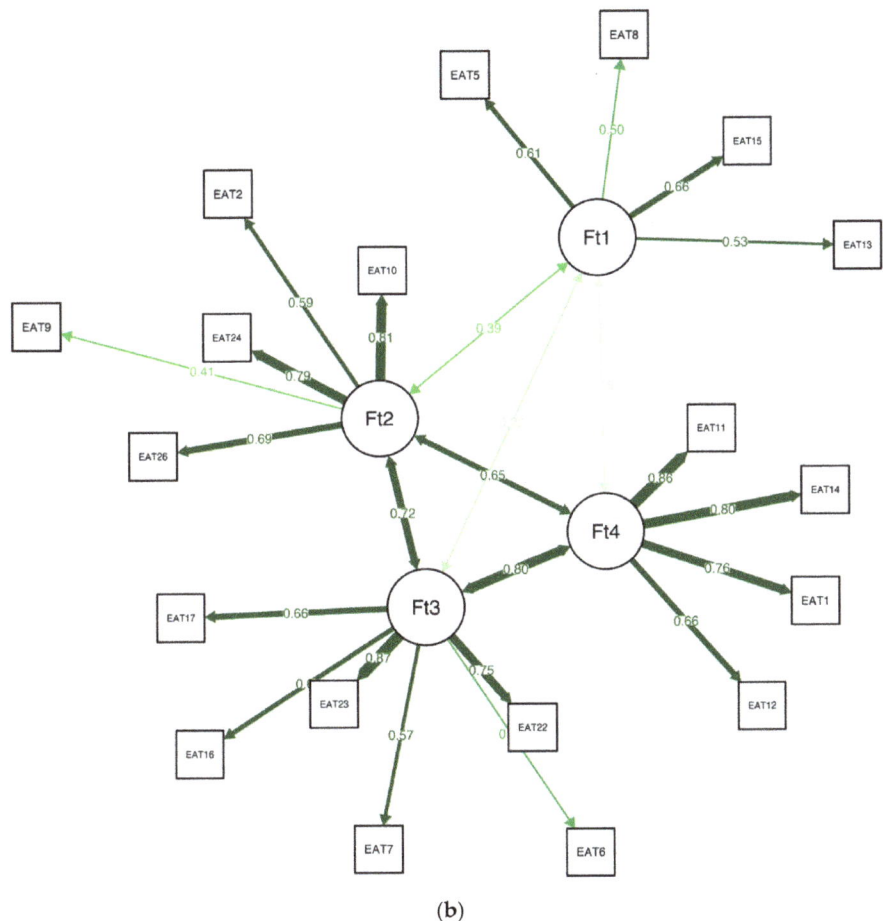

Figure 2. (**a**) The final CFA for clinical samples. (**b**) The final CFA for the suggested 19-item EAT version for non-clinical samples.

3.4. Non-Clinical Sample

The analyses indicated that the factorial structure of the EAT-26 in the non-clinical group consisted of five factors: "Weight concerns", consisting of four items; "Eating-related concerns", consisting of five items; "Food controls one's life", consisting of four items; "One's own and others' control over the person's eating", consisting of five items; and "Dieting", consisting of five items, with item 25 ("have the impulse to vomit after meals"), item 7 ("particularly avoid foods with a high carbohydrate content"), and item 19 ("display self-control around food") not loading significantly on any of the factors. A five-factor solution was corroborated by three additional analyses—parallel analysis, Velicer's MAP (squared: 0.00178), and comparison data (as compared with one to seven factors).

When estimating the stability of the EGA by bootstrapping with 5000 resampling cycles, however, the analysis indicated instability (SE = 0.79), with the CI for the number of factors ranging from 3.44 to 6.56. Although the five-factor solution was the most prevalent (42.94% of the bootstrap samples), a four-factor solution was also frequent, with 40.36% of the sample. This instability might stem from two main processes: redundant items and items with high instability. A unique variable analysis revealed several redundant items, namely, in the presence of item 3 ("find (UVA) myself preoccupied with food"), item 21 ("give too much time and thought to food") is redundant. In the presence of item 4 ("have gone on eating binges where I felt that I may not be able to stop"), item 18 ("feel that food controls my life") is redundant. Finally, in the presence of item 8 ("feel that others would prefer if I ate more"), item 20 ("feel that others pressure me to eat") is redundant.

We omitted the redundant items, conducted an additional EGA with bootstrapping, and used the *itemStability()* function (see Figure 3).

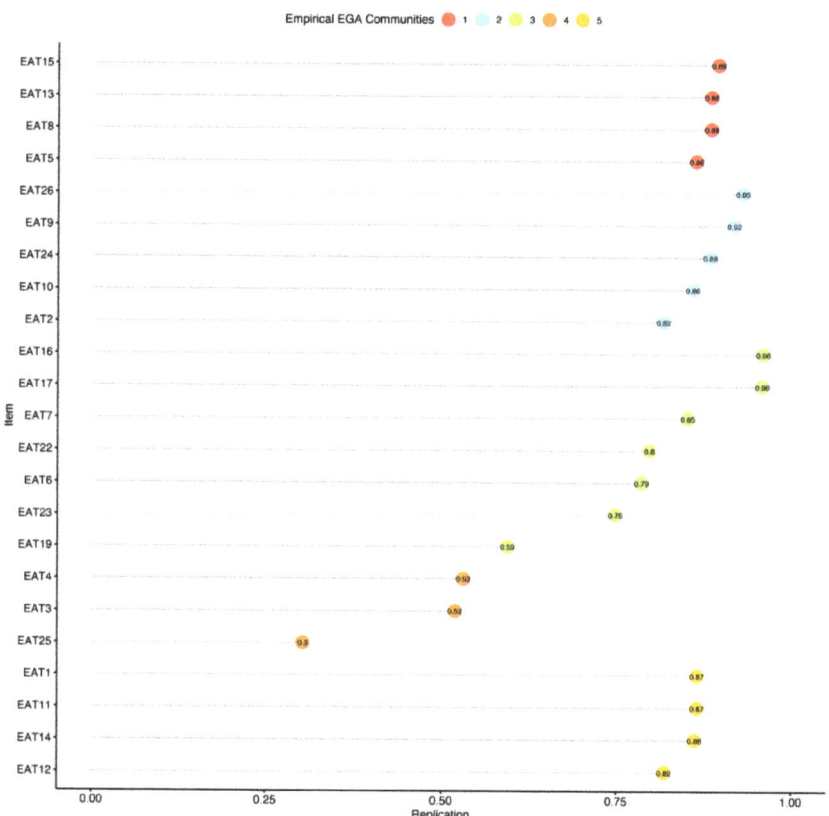

Figure 3. Item stability among the non-clinical sample. Stability below 75% is poor.

The analysis revealed that items 3, 4, 19, and 25 were all unstable. We removed the unstable items and repeated the quality testing (i.e., bootstrapping and testing item stability), and found no additional problems. The final 19-item version of the EAT was found to be considerably more stable than the original 26-item version (SE = 0.55; CI 2.91, 5.09), with 73.40% of the bootstrap samples producing a four-factor solution. A confirmatory factor analysis (CFA) that was used to corroborate the EGA solution verified the factorial structure as follows: $\chi^2_{(42.70)}$ = 82.72, $p < 0.01$, *CFI* = 0.96, *TLI* = 0.95, *RMSEA* = 0.063 (90% confidence intervals (CIs) of 0.052 and 0.072), and *SRMR* = 0.08. The CFA of the suggested EAT-19 questionnaire for the non-clinical samples is presented in Figure 2b, and the network loadings are shown in Table 3.

Table 3. Network loadings based on EGA among the non-clinical group (EAT-19).

	Fat Concerns	Eating-Related Concerns	One's Own and Others' Control over the Person's Eating	Dieting
EAT11	0.42			
EAT1	0.30			
EAT14	0.27			
EAT12	0.19			
EAT26		0.37		
EAT24		0.28		
EAT10		0.27		
EAT9		0.18		
EAT2		0.18		
EAT13			0.40	
EAT15			0.27	
EAT8			0.23	
EAT5			0.19	
EAT17				0.32
EAT23	0.25			0.30
EAT16				0.30
EAT22				0.27
EAT7				0.15
EAT6				0.15

Note. General effect size guidelines for network loadings are 0.15 for small, 0.25 for moderate, and 0.35 for large.

To examine the use of the EAT-19 in the clinical sample as well, we appraised its structure and stability in this population. The EGA produced a four-factor solution (see Figure 4 and Table 4), showing adequate stability when administering a bootstrap EGA ($SE = 0.73$; CI 2.58, 5.42), with 54.02% of the samples reproducing the solution. In addition, 18 out of the 19 items had adequate stability, with item 9 showing only a 51% replication rate. Overall, the EAT-19 seems to be well suited to capture ED symptoms among both non-clinical and clinical samples alike.

Table 4. Network loadings based on EGA among the clinical group (EAT-19).

	Restrictive Weight Concerns	Dieting	Concerns of Others over One's Eating	Eating-Related Concerns
nEAT11	0.36			
nEAT14	0.35			
nEAT1	0.35			
nEAT10	0.34			
nEAT2	0.20			
nEAT12	0.20			
nEAT17		0.37		
nEAT16		0.37		
nEAT5		0.32		
nEAT15		0.28		
nEAT7		0.26		
nEAT6		0.17		
nEAT9		0.07		
nEAT8			0.24	
nEAT13			0.24	
nEAT23				0.54
nEAT24				0.51
nEAT22				0.40
nEAT26				0.19

Note. General effect size guidelines for network loadings are 0.15 for small, 0.25 for moderate, and 0.35 for large.

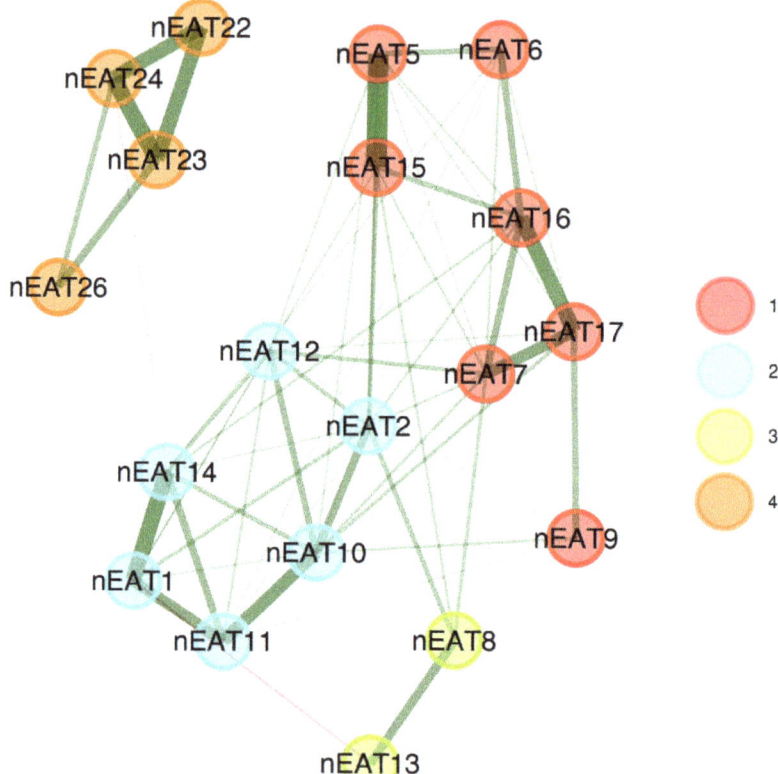

Figure 4. EAT-19 factorial structure among the clinical group.

3.5. Effectiveness of Using the EAT-19 as a Diagnostic Test

Bootstrapping the optimal cutoff point of the suggested EAT-19 revealed that using a cutoff point of 21.68 (i.e., practically rounded to 22) produces a maximum Youden's index of 0.69, with a sensitivity of 83.82% and a specificity of 85.23% (see Figure 5). By using the novel EAT-19 version and the cutoff point of 22, 1.45 patients would need to be examined in order to correctly detect one person with the disease of interest in a study population of persons with and without the known disease (i.e., NND value). In addition, 6.49 patients would need to be tested in order for one person to be misdiagnosed by the test (i.e., NNM value). The overall likelihood to be diagnosed or misdiagnosed is 4.48, which indicates high effectiveness in the diagnosis process.

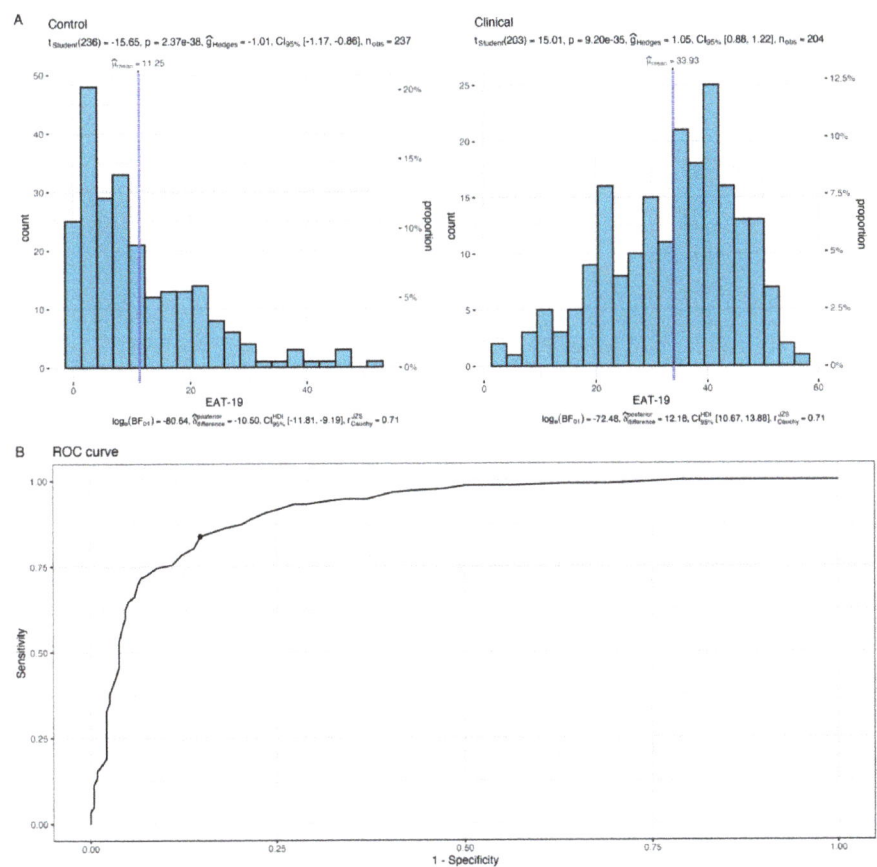

Figure 5. Distribution of EAT-19 scores for the clinical and non-clinical groups (**A**). Vertical blue lines refer to the mean sample score. The test reported in the upper section of panel A examined the difference between the sample mean and the suggested EAT-19 cutoff point (i.e., 22). In (**B**), the ROC curve for the estimation process of the optimal cutoff point is presented, with the black dot indicating the highest Youden's index.

4. Discussion

This study sought to examine whether the EAT-26, which was developed over 40 years ago as a screening tool for identifying individuals who are at a high risk of developing disordered eating and symptoms of EDs, still meets this purpose in 2023. This question is of great relevance given the many changes in the presentation and distribution of ED symptoms that have occurred since the conception of the EAT-26, as well as recent studies casting doubt on the consistency of its three-factor structure in different cultures. Indeed, the present findings indicate that the original EAT-26 three-factor model is not applicable to young Jewish Israeli women, whether from a community (five-factor model) or from a clinical (four-factor solution) sample. Moreover, we found that a 19-item EAT version shows considerably greater stability than the original EAT 26-item version. Overall, we suggest that the adapted 19-item EAT questionnaire might be suitable for identifying individuals who are at risk of developing disordered eating behaviors in clinical and community populations in Israel. The next step is to replicate our findings in non-clinical and clinical populations in other countries around the globe.

Additionally, our findings support the research hypotheses regarding the differences in the factor structure of the EAT-26 between clinical and non-clinical populations (Hypothesis 1), the greater similarity of the clinical group's four-factor solution to the original three-factor EAT-26 model vs. the non-clinical group's five-factor solution (Hypothesis 2), and the difference in the cutoff points for defining pathological eating in both clinical and non-clinical populations in our study (score ≥ 22) vs. the original score of ≥ 20 (Hypothesis 3; [2]). In this respect, it is of note that the differences in the EAT structure in the present study between the clinical and non-clinical samples are in line with the initial research [22] for the EAT-40 [21] and for the EAT-26, showing, for both scales, significant differences between the clinical samples (AN) and the non-clinical samples. Moreover, in the original studies of the questionnaire, significantly higher percentages of participants in the clinical sample vs. the non-clinical sample scored above the cutoff point of 20.

More specifically, the EGA of the EAT-26 in the clinical group yielded four factors: "weight preoccupation", consisting of eight items; "binge/purge behaviors and concerns of others", consisting of four items; "dieting and restricting symptoms", consisting of six items; and "eating-related concerns", consisting of eight items (item 26, "I enjoy trying new rich foods", and item 19, "I display self-control around food", loaded only to a small extent, and were therefore excluded).

The EGA in the non-clinical sample yielded five factors: "weight concerns", consisting of four items; "eating-related concerns", consisting of five items; "food controls one's life", consisting of four items; "one's own and others' control over the person's eating", consisting of five items; and "dieting", consisting of five items (the loadings of item 25, "have the impulse to vomit after meals", item 7, "particularly avoid foods with a high carbohydrate content", and item 19, "display self-control around food" were smaller and therefore excluded).

In recent years, studies in different countries replicated the three-factor structure of the EAT-40 and EAT-26 [45,46]. In a recent study conducted by our group in Israel [35], different factors were observed in different ethnic groups, most of which did not correspond with the original EAT-26 three-factor structure.

The findings of the present study further support this contention in showing differences in the EAT factor structure among clinical populations vs. non-clinical populations.

It should be noted that the previous study, which found that different factors were observed in different ethnic groups in Israel [35], was conducted among adult women, whereas the current study was conducted among teenage girls, and the difference in findings may perhaps be attributed to this age difference. Specifically, it is possible that the questionnaire is experienced differently during adolescence (a period during which there is a high risk for the development of eating disorders) than in adulthood (when there is greater maturity and emotional development).

There are several possible explanations for the differences in the EAT factor structure between the clinical and non-clinical groups. These differences are likely not related to the methodological considerations, as the two groups were of similar age and were studied around the same time period.

One possible explanation for the difference in the EAT-26 between the clinical and non-clinical populations might be the nature of the clinical population. Although there was more than one ED diagnosis among the adolescents in the clinical sample, this group was a more unified group (than the non-clinical group) and was characterized by specific core ED traits. The non-clinical group, for its part, represented other, more diverse non-ED populations, and the female adolescents who made up this group were likely to be more affected by socio-cultural trends (i.e., compared to the female adolescents in the clinical group, who were likely more invested in their illness).

Another possible explanation is that the present results reflect a change in psychopathology in recent decades, whereby many more patients now suffer from the AN binge/purge type rather than the AN restricting type [47] There has also been a significant change in lifestyle habits in recent decades, which is reflected in eating and sports habits, nutrition, and body perception [48]. In addition, there has been a significant change in the media, which broadcasts harmful advertisements related to diets and unreal body image [49]. These advertisements may have harmful effects on the population in general, and on youth in particular, potentially leading to poor body image [50]. These changes may explain various phenomena that have characterized recent years, such as an increased tendency for aesthetic/beauty procedures and surgeries starting at a young age, the use of many harmful techniques for weight regulation, and increases in psychopathology. All of these tendencies may be expressed by both clinical and non-clinical groups [51,52].

4.1. Limitations, Directions for Future Research, and Conclusions

4.1.1. Limitations

The present study had several limitations. First, the sample consisted of female adolescents only (between 12 and 19 years), and EDs may manifest differently in young adults, particularly in BN. Going forward, researchers should examine the effect of age on the current findings regarding the EAT-26 in both groups.

Second, the suggested sample size for the CFA is 200, given that the results can be less stable with smaller sample sizes. Although the sample size was adequate for the clinical group, the non-clinical sample size consisted of 155 participants; as such, the results for the non-clinical sample should be seen as preliminary.

Third, the present study was conducted in Israel, which is a "melting pot" of immigrants and a multicultural country that is both very modern and very traditional and is made up of many different cultures, so the results may not represent other Western countries.

4.1.2. Future Research

At this point, it seems that the EAT-26 questionnaire still allows for a distinction to be made between clinical and non-clinical populations of the same culture with the same cutoff points.

We would suggest that the questionnaire be tested in a clinical population compared to a non-clinical population in future studies. We would also suggest that the proposed cutoff point and the 19-question questionnaire be tested in diverse populations in order to validate the findings of the current study more comprehensively and to test the new cutoff point accordingly.

4.1.3. Clinical Implications

The questionnaire probably remains suitable for the identification of disturbed eating in clinical groups, but less so in non-clinical groups, emphasizing the necessity of adapting the tool to account for changes in the presentation of EDs in recent years.

Given that the psychopathology of EDs seems to have changed in recent decades, we propose revising the questionnaires in order to adapt them to the current situation. In our opinion, the current questionnaire indeed provides a suitable response to the psychopathology of EDs in the 21st century.

The current study's contribution lies in its potential to sharpen clinicians' ability to identify populations in more difficult clinical situations, to aid them in diagnosis, and to help them identify the severity level, so that the therapeutic approach can be better adjusted. Moreover, the abbreviated questionnaire is easier to fill out than the previous one and is also user-friendly.

5. Conclusions

Our findings highlight the differences in the EAT factor structure between our community sample as compared to the original sample, which led to a reduction in the number of scale items from 26 to 19, and led to a change in the cutoff point from 20 to 22.

The EAT, which was developed four decades ago, has thus been reexamined in the current paper and adapted to the requirements of the current era.

The proposed shortening of the EAT from 40 to 26 and now to 19 items must be examined in future studies. However, such a change would render the questionnaire more useful in both clinical and research conditions.

Author Contributions: Writing—original draft, Z.S.-L., Y.L., D.S., O.P. and O.T. All authors have read and agreed to the published version of the manuscript.

Funding: This research received no external funding.

Institutional Review Board Statement: The study was conducted in accordance with the Declaration of Helsinki and approved by the Ethics Committee of Sheba Medical Center, Tel Hashomer, Israel (Protocol No: 2755; date 01/28/16), and Yezreel Valley College Institutional Review Board on 9.12.2019—approval number 3601010170.

Informed Consent Statement: Informed consent was obtained from all subjects involved in the study.

Data Availability Statement: Not applicable.

Conflicts of Interest: The authors declare no conflict of interest.

References

1. Bulik, C.; Yilmaz, Z.; HArdaway, A. Genetics and Epigenetics of Eating Disorders. *Adv. Genom. Genet.* **2015**, *5*, 131–150. [CrossRef] [PubMed]
2. Sharan, P.; Sundar, A.S. Eating Disorders in Women. *Indian J. Psychiatry* **2015**, *57*, 286–295. [CrossRef] [PubMed]
3. Katz, B. Gender and Disordered Eating of Adolescents in Israel. *Isr. J. Psychiatry Relat. Sci.* **2014**, *51*, 137–144. Available online: https://cdn.doctorsonly.co.il/2014/08/10_Gender-and-Disordered.pdf (accessed on 15 September 2023). [PubMed]
4. Latzer, Y.; Spivak-Lavi, Z.; Katz, R. Disordered Eating and Media Exposure among Adolescent Girls: The Role of Parental Involvement and Sense of Empowerment. *Int. J. Adolesc. Youth* **2015**, *20*, 375–391. [CrossRef]
5. American Psychiatric Association. *Diagnostic and Statistical Manual of Mental Disorders (DSM-5®)*; American Psychiatric Publishing: Washington, DC, USA, 2013.
6. Lindvall Dahlgren, C.; Wisting, L.; Rø, Ø. Feeding and Eating Disorders in the DSM-5 Era: A Systematic Review of Prevalence Rates in Non-Clinical Male and Female Samples. *J. Eat. Disord.* **2017**, *5*, 56. [CrossRef] [PubMed]
7. Udo, T.; Grilo, C.M. Prevalence and Correlates of DSM-5–Defined Eating Disorders in a Nationally Representative Sample of US Adults. *Biol. Psychiatry* **2018**, *84*, 345–354. [CrossRef]
8. Slof-Op 't Landt, M.C.T.; van Furth, E.F.; van Beijsterveldt, C.E.M.; Bartels, M.; Willemsen, G.; de Geus, E.J.; Ligthart, L.; Boomsma, D.I. Prevalence of Dieting and Fear of Weight Gain across Ages: A Community Sample from Adolescents to the Elderly. *Int. J. Public. Health* **2017**, *62*, 911–919. [CrossRef]
9. Qian, J.; Wu, Y.; Liu, F.; Zhu, Y.; Jin, H.; Zhang, H.; Wan, Y.; Li, C.; Yu, D. An Update on the Prevalence of Eating Disorders in the General Population: A Systematic Review and Meta-Analysis. *Eat. Weight. Disord.-Stud. Anorex. Bulim. Obes.* **2022**, *27*, 415–428. [CrossRef]
10. Andrea, M. The Evolution of Our Understanding and Treatment of Eating Disorders over the Past 50 Years. *J. Clin. Psychol.* **2019**, *75*, 1380–1391.
11. Keel, P.K.; Klump, K.L. Are Eating Disorders Culture-Bound Syndromes? Implications for Conceptualizing Their Etiology. *Psychol. Bull.* **2003**, *129*, 747–769. [CrossRef]
12. Marks, R.J.; De Foe, A.; Collett, J. The Pursuit of Wellness: Social Media, Body Image and Eating Disorders. *Child. Youth Serv. Rev.* **2020**, *119*, 105659. [CrossRef]
13. Hendrickse, J.; Arpan, L.M.; Clayton, R.B.; Ridgway, J.L. Instagram and College Women's Body Image: Investigating the Roles of Appearance-Related Comparisons and Intrasexual Competition. *Comput. Human. Behav.* **2017**, *74*, 92–100. [CrossRef]
14. Coelho, G.; de Abreu Soares, E.; Innocencio da Silva Gomes, A.; Goncalves Ribeiro, B. Prevention of Eating Disorders in Female Athletes. *Open Access J. Sports Med.* **2014**, *5*, 105–113. [CrossRef] [PubMed]
15. Ocker, L.B.; Lam, E.T.C.; Jensen, B.E.; Zhang, J.J. Psychometric Properties of the Eating Attitudes Test. *Meas. Phys. Educ. Exerc. Sci.* **2007**, *11*, 25–48. [CrossRef]
16. Garner, D.M. *EDI-2 Eating Disorder Inventory-2: Professional Manual*; Psychological Assessment Resources, Inc.: Odessa, FL, USA, 1991.
17. Garner, M.D. *Eating Disorder Inventory-3. Professional Manual*; Psychological Assessment Resources, Inc.: Lutz, FL, USA, 2004.
18. Beglin, S.; Fairburn, C. Evaluation of a New Instrument for the Detection of Eating Disorders in Community Samples. *Psychiatry Res.* **1992**, *4*, 191–201. [CrossRef]
19. Fairburn, C.; Belgin, S. Assessment of Eating Disorders: Interview or Self-report Questionnaire? *Int. J. Eat. Disord.* **1994**, *16*, 363–370. [CrossRef]
20. Farnill, J.; St George', M.; O'brien, A. The SCOFF Questionnaire and Clinical Interview for Eating Disorders in General Practice: Comparative Study. *Br. Med. J.* **2002**, *325*, 755–756. [CrossRef]

21. Garner, D.; Olmsted, M.; Bohr, Y.; Garfinkel, P. The Eating Attitudes Test: Psychometric Features and Clinical Correlates. *Psychol. Med.* **1982**, *12*, 871–878. Available online: https://www.researchgate.net/profile/David_Garner4/publication/313766446_The_Eating_Attitudes_Test_Psychometric_features_and_clinical_correlates/links/5e595921299bf1bdb8443147/The-Eating-Attitudes-Test-Psychometric-features-and-clinical-correlates.pdf (accessed on 19 September 2023). [CrossRef]
22. Garner, D.; Garfinkel, P. Socio-Cultural Factors in the Development of. Anorexia Nervosa. *Psychol. Med.* **1980**, *10*, 647–656. [CrossRef]
23. Garner, D.M.; Garfinkel, P.E. The Eating Attitudes Test: An Index of the Symptoms of Anorexia Nervosa. *Psychol. Med.* **1979**, *9*, 273–279. [CrossRef]
24. Habermas, T. History of Anorexia Nervosa. In *The Wiley Handbook of Eating Disorders*; Levin, M.P., Smolak, L., Eds.; Wiley: New-York, NY, USA, 2015; Volume 1, pp. 1–24. ISBN 9781118573945.
25. Garfinkel, P.E.; Newman, A. The Eating Attitudes Test: Twenty-Five Years Later. *Eat. Weight. Disord.-Stud. Anorex. Bulim. Obes.* **2001**, *6*, 1–21. [CrossRef] [PubMed]
26. Button, E.; Whitehouse, A. Subclinical Anorexia Nervosa. *Psychol. Med.* **1981**, *11*, 509–516. [CrossRef]
27. Gross, J.; Rosen, J.; Leitenberg, H.; Willmuth, M. Validity of the Eating Attitudes Test and the Eating Disorders Inventory in Bulimia Nervosa. *J. Consult. Clin. Psychol.* **1986**, *54*, 875. [CrossRef]
28. Koslowsky, M.; Scheinberg, Z.; Bleich, A.; Mark, M.; Apter, A.; Danon, Y.; Solomon, Z. The Factor Structure and Criterion Validity of the Short Form of the Eating Attitudes Test. *J. Pers. Assess.* **1992**, *58*, 27–35. [CrossRef] [PubMed]
29. Thompson, M.; Schwartz, D. Life Adjustment of Women with Anorexia Nervosa and Anorexic-like Behavior. *Int. J. Eat. Disord.* **1982**, *1*, 47–60. [CrossRef]
30. Túry, F.; Güleç, H.; Kohls, E. Assessment Methods for Eating Disorders and Body Image Disorders. *J. Psychosom. Res.* **2010**, *69*, 601–611. [CrossRef]
31. Nasser, M. The EAT Speaks Many Languages: Review of the Use of the EAT in Eating Disorders Research. *Eat. Weight. Disord. —Stud. Anorex. Bulim. Obes.* **1997**, *2*, 174–181. [CrossRef]
32. Mukai, T.; Crago, M.; Shisslak, C.M. Eating Attitudes and Weight Preoccupation Among Female High School Students in Japan. *J. Child Psychol. Psychiatry* **1994**, *35*, 677–688. [CrossRef]
33. Dotti, A.; Lazzari, R. Validation and Reliability of the Italian EAT-26. *Eat. Weight. Disord.-Stud. Anorex. Bulim. Obes.* **1998**, *3*, 188–194. [CrossRef]
34. Apter, A.; Shah, M.; Iancu, I.; Abramovitc, H.; Weizman, A.; Tyano, S. Cultural Effects on Eating Attitudes in Israeli Subpopulations and Hospitalized Anorectics. *Genet. Soc. Gen. Psychol. Monogr.* **1994**, *120*, 83–99.
35. Spivak-Lavi, Z.; Peleg, O.; Tzischinsky, O.; Stein, D.; Latzer, Y. Differences in the Factor Structure of the Eating Attitude Test-26 (Eat-26) in Different Cultures in Israel: Jews, Muslims, and Christians. *Nutrients* **2021**, *13*, 1899. [CrossRef] [PubMed]
36. NIH National Institute of Mental Health. 1999. Available online: https://www.nih.gov/ (accessed on 15 September 2023).
37. Rogoza, R.; Brytek-Matera, A.; Garner, D.M. Analysis of the EAT-26 in a Non-Clinical Sample. *Arch. Psychiatry Psychother.* **2016**, *2*, 54–58. [CrossRef]
38. Rutt, C.D.; Coleman, K.J. The Evaluation of a Measurement Model for the Body Image Questionnaire and the Eating Attitudes Test in a Hispanic Population. *Hisp. J. Behav. Sci.* **2001**, *23*, 153–170. [CrossRef]
39. Golino, H.; Shi, D.; Christensen, A.P.; Garrido, L.E.; Nieto, M.D.; Sadana, R.; Thiyagarajan, J.A.; Martinez-Molina, A. Investigating the Performance of Exploratory Graph Analysis and Traditional Techniques to Identify the Number of Latent Factors: A Simulation and Tutorial. *Psychol. Methods* **2020**, *25*, 292. [CrossRef] [PubMed]
40. Friedman, J.; Hastie, T.; Tibshirani, R. Sparse Inverse Covariance Estimation with the Graphical Lasso. *Biostatistics* **2008**, *9*, 432–441. [CrossRef]
41. Preprint, P.; Christensen, A.P.; Garrido, L.E.; Golino, H. Unique Variable Analysis: A Novel Approach for Detecting Redundant Variables in Multivariate Data. *PsyArXiv* **2020**, *10*. [CrossRef]
42. Ruscio, J.; Roche, B. Determining the Number of Factors to Retain in an Exploratory Factor Analysis Using Comparison Data of Known Factorial Structure. *Psychol. Assess.* **2012**, *24*, 282–292. [CrossRef]
43. Linn, S.; Grunau, P.D. New Patient-Oriented Summary Measure of Net Total Gain in Certainty for Dichotomous Diagnostic Tests. *Epidemiol. Perspect. Innov.* **2006**, *3*, 11. [CrossRef]
44. Citrome, L.; Ketter, T.A. When Does a Difference Make a Difference? Interpretation of Number Needed to Treat, Number Needed to Harm, and Likelihood to Be Helped or Harmed. *Int. J. Clin. Pract.* **2013**, *67*, 407–411. [CrossRef]
45. Bali, G.; Kokka, I.; Gonidakis, F.; Papakonstantinou, E.; Vlachakis, D.; Chrousos, G.P.; Kanaka-Gantenbein, C.; Bacopoulou, F. Validation of the Eating Habits Questionnaire in Greek Adults. *EMBnet J.* **2023**, *28*, e1029. [CrossRef]
46. McEnery, F.; Fitzgerald, A.; McNicholas, F.; Dooley, B. Fit for Purpose, Psychometric Assessment of the Eating Attitudes Test-26 in an Irish Adolescent Sample. *Eat. Behav.* **2016**, *23*, 52–57. [CrossRef] [PubMed]
47. Serra, R.; Di Nicolantonio, C.; Di Febo, R.; De Crescenzo, F.; Vanderlinden, J.; Vrieze, E.; Bruffaerts, R.; Loriedo, C.; Pasquini, M.; Tarsitani, L. The Transition from Restrictive Anorexia Nervosa to Binging and Purging: A Systematic Review and Meta-Analysis. *Eat. Weight. Disord.* **2022**, *27*, 857–865. [CrossRef] [PubMed]
48. Kiss-Leizer, M.; Tóth-Király, I.; Rigó, A. How the Obsession to Eat Healthy Food Meets with the Willingness to Do Sports: The Motivational Background of Orthorexia Nervosa. *Bulim. Obes.* **2019**, *24*, 465–472. [CrossRef] [PubMed]

49. Aparicio-Martinez, P.; Perea-Moreno, A.-J.; Pilar Martinez-Jimenez, M.; Dolores Redel-Macías, M.; Pagliari, C.; Vaquero-Abellan, M. Social Media, Thin-Ideal, Body Dissatisfaction and Disordered Eating Attitudes: An Exploratory Analysis. *Int. J. Environ. Res. Public Health Artic.* **2019**, *16*, 4177. [CrossRef] [PubMed]
50. Schuck, K.; Munsch, S.; Schneider, S. Body Image Perceptions and Symptoms of Disturbed Eating Behavior among Children and Adolescents in Germany. *Child. Adolesc. Psychiatry Ment. Health* **2018**, *12*, 10. [CrossRef] [PubMed]
51. Chao, A.M.; Wadden, T.A.; Walsh, O.A.; Gruber, K.A.; Alamuddin, N.; Berkowitz, R.I.; Tronieri, J.S. Effects of Liraglutide and Behavioral Weight Loss on Food Cravings, Eating Behaviors, and Eating Disorder Psychopathology. *Obesity* **2019**, *27*, 2005–2010. [CrossRef]
52. Weiss, A.L.; Miller, J.N.; Chermak, R. Adolescent Diet Culture: Where Does It Originate? In *Fad Diets and Adolescents: A Guide for Clinicians, Educators, Coaches and Trainers*; Springer International Publishing: Cham, Switzerland, 2022; pp. 17–24.

Disclaimer/Publisher's Note: The statements, opinions and data contained in all publications are solely those of the individual author(s) and contributor(s) and not of MDPI and/or the editor(s). MDPI and/or the editor(s) disclaim responsibility for any injury to people or property resulting from any ideas, methods, instructions or products referred to in the content.

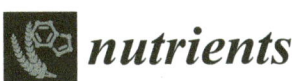

Article

Effects of a Comprehensive Dietary Intervention Program, Promoting Nutrition Literacy, Eating Behavior, Dietary Quality, and Gestational Weight Gain in Chinese Urban Women with Normal Body Mass Index during Pregnancy

Qian Li [1,2], Noppawan Piaseu [1,*], Srisamorn Phumonsakul [1] and Streerut Thadakant [1]

1. Ramathibodi School of Nursing, Faculty of Medicine Ramathibodi Hospital, Mahidol University, 270 Rama 6 Road, Ratchathewi, Bangkok 10400, Thailand; liqian_2021@126.com (Q.L.); srisamorn.phu@mahidol.ac.th (S.P.); streerut.bor@mahidol.edu (S.T.)
2. Ph.D. Candidate in the Doctor of Philosophy Program in Nursing Science (International Program), Faculty of Medicine Ramathibodi Hospital, Faculty of Nursing, Mahidol University, Salaya 73170, Thailand
* Correspondence: noppawan.pia@mahidol.edu

Citation: Li, Q.; Piaseu, N.; Phumonsakul, S.; Thadakant, S. Effects of a Comprehensive Dietary Intervention Program, Promoting Nutrition Literacy, Eating Behavior, Dietary Quality, and Gestational Weight Gain in Chinese Urban Women with Normal Body Mass Index during Pregnancy. *Nutrients* **2024**, *16*, 217. https://doi.org/10.3390/nu16020217

Academic Editors: António Raposo, Renata Puppin Zandonadi and Raquel Braz Assunção Botelho

Received: 4 December 2023
Revised: 2 January 2024
Accepted: 4 January 2024
Published: 10 January 2024

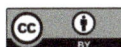

Copyright: © 2024 by the authors. Licensee MDPI, Basel, Switzerland. This article is an open access article distributed under the terms and conditions of the Creative Commons Attribution (CC BY) license (https://creativecommons.org/licenses/by/4.0/).

Abstract: In urban Chinese women with normal body weight during pregnancy, we implemented a comprehensive dietary intervention program aimed at enhancing nutrition literacy, dietary quality, and gestational weight gain. The methods included both online and offline health education on prenatal nutrition, weekly weight monitoring, family back education practices, and real-time dietary guidance. The intervention was delivered to randomly assigned control and intervention group participants from gestational week 12 to week 24. The intervention group ($n = 44$; 100% complete data) showed significant differences (mean (SD)) compared to the control group ($n = 42$; 95.5% complete data) in nutrition literacy (53.39 ± 6.60 vs. 43.55 ± 9.58, $p < 0.001$), restrained eating (31.61 ± 7.28 vs. 28.79 ± 7.96, $p < 0.001$), Diet Quality Distance (29.11 ± 8.52 vs. 40.71 ± 7.39, $p < 0.001$), and weight gain within the first 12 weeks of intervention (4.97 ± 1.33 vs. 5.98 ± 2.78, $p = 0.029$). However, there was no significant difference in the incidence of gestational diabetes (2 (4.5%) vs. 4 (9.5%), $p = 0.629$). Participants in the intervention group reported an overall satisfaction score of 4.70 ± 0.46 for the intervention strategy. These results emphasize the positive role of comprehensive dietary intervention in promoting a healthy diet during pregnancy.

Keywords: pregnancy; health literacy; eating behavior; weight; nutrition; digital; intervention

1. Introduction

Maternal and child health are crucial determinants of a nation's overall health and development. The impact of weight gain during pregnancy on short-term and long-term health outcomes underscores its significance in comprehensive pregnancy health management [1–4]. The findings, based on existing research evidence, suggested that excessive gestational weight gain (GWG) could lead to cesarean section, maternal weight retention, large-for-gestational-age (LGA) infants, gestational hypertension, preeclampsia, and gestational diabetes mellitus (GDM). On the other hand, insufficient GWG was associated with a higher risk of small-for-gestational-age (SGA) infants and preterm birth (PTB).

In a study by Hu that included 1260 Chinese pregnant women, it was found that 60.4% had a normal weight before pregnancy, 19.44% were overweight, and 6.98% were obese based on BMI classification. When comparing their weight gain during pregnancy to the reference values recommended by the American Institute of Medicine (IOM) guidelines in 2009, it was observed that 54.97% had excessive GWG, 34.65% had appropriate GWG, and 10.38% had insufficient GWG [5]. Similar findings were reported in several other surveys conducted on pregnant women in China, indicating that most pregnant women did not meet the weight-gain recommendations outlined by the IOM [6,7]. These statistics highlight the need for attention and intervention to address the issue of inappropriate GWG in China.

GWG, as an indicator of nutritional balance during pregnancy, is closely associated with individual dietary behaviors. While physical activity during pregnancy is acknowledged as a factor influencing GWG, systematic reviews suggest that diet may play a more significant role in determining weight gain during pregnancy [8,9]. Therefore, promoting dietary behaviors during pregnancy becomes crucial for enhancing the health of pregnant women. However, over time, many studies on dietary interventions during pregnancy have yielded mixed results, particularly a significant portion of online dietary intervention studies show no effect [10–14]. This may be related to insufficient key components in the intervention design, which may not have effectively addressed the critical barriers in pregnant women's health dietary practices [15].

Several qualitative studies conducted from the perspective of pregnant women have shed light on the substantial impediments they encounter in their dietary practices [16–41]. These obstacles primarily revolve around deficiencies in the dietary information delivery system, encompassing challenges related to accessing reliable dietary information; cognitive aspects such as understanding, memorization, and the application of dietary information; as well as the skills required to effectively communicate dietary information within the family environment. These findings underscore the pervasive issue of nutritional literacy deficiency among pregnant women [42].

This is in contrast to previous studies that have shown ineffective outcomes, particularly those focusing on online dietary interventions [10–14], which mainly provide static text or video information with limited incorporation of interactive information consultations or regular text responses. However, the acquisition of dietary information does not inherently impart healthy dietary knowledge and skills. Furthermore, it does not imply that pregnant women possess the necessary capacity for healthy self-care. Information acquisition merely marks the beginning of this process [43]. Therefore, researchers should emphasize assessing the proficiency of pregnant women in processing and applying the received information. However, to the best of our knowledge, there is still a lack of research investigating the influence of maternal nutritional literacy on self-care behaviors related to diet during pregnancy.

Digital platforms, with features such as wide accessibility, personalized services, interactivity, real-time updates, and cost-effectiveness, have become ideal tools for implementing comprehensive health education and enhancing health literacy [44]. Nutbeam's health literacy model indicates that health literacy can be effectively improved through tailored information, communication, and education [45].

Therefore, guided by the health literacy model, this study aimed to address the overlooked aspect of maternal health literacy in the provision of general dietary information online. To achieve this goal, an online platform was used to implement a tailored, ongoing, face-to-face health education program. The primary objective was to design a comprehensive, individual-level dietary intervention program that would offer pregnant women easy access to information and help improve their nutritional literacy. By enhancing the dietary behavior of pregnant women in urban China, the study sought to elevate their overall diet quality and nutritional status, ultimately reducing the risk of pregnancy complications.

2. Materials and Methods

2.1. Study Design

This study adopts a two-arm randomized controlled trial design, employing a prospective and pragmatic implementation approach. The variable positioning is based on Orem's self-care theory [46], and the intervention design is grounded in Nutbean's conceptual model of health literacy as an asset [45]. The report follows the CONSORT framework. Approval was obtained from the Human Research Ethics Committee, Faculty of Medicine Ramathibodi Hospital, Mahidol University (MURA2023/590), and the Clinical Research Ethics Committee of the Affiliated Changzhou No. 2. People's Hospital of Nanjing Medical

University ([2023]KY107-01). All methods adhere to relevant guidelines and regulations, such as the Helsinki Declaration. The trial has been registered with the China Clinical Trial Registration Center (ChiCTR2300075082).

2.2. Participants and Recruitment

This study was conducted at an Obstetrics Outpatient Department in Changzhou, China, from August to November 2023. Through systematic sampling based on clinic serial numbers, pregnant women were initially screened by obstetricians, and those in their 6–12 weeks of gestation and primiparous were referred to the eligibility assessment room. Trained midwives conducted a thorough eligibility screening. Inclusion criteria comprised age between 18 and 35, pre-pregnancy BMI between 18.5 kg/m^2 and 24 kg/m^2, primiparous individuals with a single pregnancy, and gestational age less than 12 weeks. Participants needed the ability to use the WeChat application, and households had to include at least one person other than the pregnant woman who served as a cook. Exclusion criteria included various health conditions and behaviors such as diabetes, uncontrolled high blood pressure, thyroid disease, cardiovascular disease, cancer, lung disease, severe gastrointestinal disease, a history of eating disorders or bariatric surgery, serious mental illness, a history of mood and anxiety disorders in the last three months, drug abuse, and a threat of abortion. Participants were withdrawn if they experienced illness or required special dietary needs during the intervention. Eligible pregnant women who provided consent and completed the baseline assessment were randomized into two groups, utilizing the SAS program for full randomization: usual care (n = 44) and Comprehensive Dietary Intervention Program (CDIP) groups (n = 44). The midwives conducting the assessments were unaware of the group assignments. Pregnant women in the control group received standard antenatal care common for Chinese pregnant women, consisting of regular prenatal check-ups and monitoring. Pregnant women in the intervention group received a CDIP intervention alongside routine care based on the standards from the Chinese Dietary Guidelines for Pregnancy and the GWG range recommended by the IOM.

2.3. Sample Size

Based on Deng's randomized controlled trial [47], which reported a GWG of 6.9 ± 3.2 kg in the control group and 4.9 ± 3.1 kg in the intervention group, we determined that each group would require 40 women to achieve 80% power. Assuming a 10% dropout rate between baseline and follow-up, the planned recruitment target is set at 44 women per group.

2.4. Intervention—CDIP

Based on the theoretical foundation of the health literacy model, the CDIP intervention comprised three essential components: tailored information, communication, and education. Behavior change techniques (BCTs) corresponding to these structures were implemented [48], as outlined in Table 1. Following this, specific intervention topics and content were developed in accordance with the established BCTs. The intervention was implemented through a systematic and phased approach.

Phase 1: Offline Intervention

During the face-to-face consultation, participants underwent a 30–40 min session on the day of enrollment at 12 weeks of gestation. This consultation took place in the intervention room, covering topics 1–6. Instruments utilized included a diet booklet (see Figure S1) and food models.

Theme 1: Is your diet healthy? The intervention midwife analyzed baseline survey data with stakeholders, reviewing scores from the nutritional literacy scale to assess participants' literacy levels and knowledge and skill deficiencies. The midwife also examined the intake of ten major nutrients using the diet quality scale, gaining insights into participants' dietary control, food cravings, and home eating environment. The midwife documented individual eating problems and disorders.

Table 1. Comprehensive dietary intervention program structures.

Items	BCTs
Tailored information	• Problem-solving • Instruction on how to perform the behavior • Comparative imagining of future outcomes • Self-monitoring of behavior • Self-monitoring of outcome(s) of behavior • Conserving mental resources
Tailored communication	• Social support • Action planning • Prompts/cues • Feedback on behavior • Feedback on outcome(s) of behavior
Tailored education	• Behavioral practice/rehearsal

Theme 2: What obstacles do you encounter? Participants confirmed the listed barriers, and solutions were discussed. These challenges pertain to difficulties in accessing, comprehending, identifying, and utilizing dietary information, as well as sharing such information with family members. Informing participants of the study schedule addressed these issues. Concerns about consultation time and cost were alleviated by informing participants of the study's free and flexible online intervention. Participants with low self-efficacy were encouraged, and pregnant women lacking motivation were informed of the benefits of following guidelines during pregnancy, with a reward of a free fetal heart rate monitoring project upon completion.

Theme 3: Do you understand this information? Using the self-designed diet education booklet (see Figure S1), participants were introduced to "the Recommended Standards for Weight Gain During Pregnancy for Chinese Women [49]" and "the Chinese Dietary Guidelines During Pregnancy 2022 [50]". They learned how to choose appropriate foods based on preferences, handle food cravings, and self-monitor body weight. Participants were asked to confirm their understanding and provide in-depth clarification if needed.

Theme 4: How is the meal plan implemented? Food models demonstrated daily food calculations based on dietary preferences and Chinese Dietary Guidelines for Pregnancy. This included substituting low-calorie for high-calorie foods, replacing expensive foods with low-cost alternatives, and methods for self-monitoring shared with health providers via WeChat.

Theme 5: Do you believe in yourself? We will help you! Participants were informed that subsequent CDIP interventions would be online, emphasizing convenience and low cost. This included watching pregnancy diet education videos, a family education exercise, weekly weight and meal quality measurement reports, and online discussions. Pregnant women were encouraged to adhere to the schedule, maintaining open communication with investigators.

Theme 6: Enjoy free items! Participants were informed about incentives, such as free fetal heart rate monitoring and continuous online/offline dietary counseling, by following the online intervention plan.

Phase 2: Online Intervention

Delivery was through the WeChat platform, with participants using a communication window for reminders and simultaneous diet education video viewing. The online program included twice-repeated diet education video sessions lasting 35 min (weeks 13 and 20), a 20–30 min return education exercise for family members (week 16), and two 20–30 min in-person meal-planning discussions (weeks 17 and 21). Participants also received a weekly weight-monitoring feedback text message service (SMS).

Theme 7: Did you do it today? During weeks 13 and 20, participants received reminders through WeChat to watch a dietary education video; the content of the dietary education video involves in-depth verbal explanations of the contents found in the dietary education booklet. Focusing on understanding and applying guidelines for pregnant women in China and GWG guidelines, the video explained how to manage energy intake and food cravings.

Theme 8: Pass the knowledge on to your family! At 16 weeks, pregnant women and home cooks met online. Pregnant women explained dietary information to their families based on an educational video. Health providers assessed accuracy, clarifying misconceptions to ensure understanding and utilization.

Theme 9: Let us see your progress! After monitoring food intake at weeks 16 and 20, participants engaged in online meal-planning discussions at weeks 17 and 21. The workshop included summary feedback, analyzing achievement against GWG guidelines, comparing food intake with dietary guidelines, and encouraging participants throughout the process.

Theme 10: What could you do next? The second part of the online discussion focused on individualized meal-plan adjustments based on participants' weight-gain goals. The health provider discussed specific barrier factors and provided solutions. Food frequency measurements at weeks 17 and 21 informed dietary quality adjustments. The health provider advised on changes, maintained the meal plan when aligned with weight-gain goals, and offered encouragement at the consultation's end.

2.5. Compensation

Following the completion of the baseline survey, all enrolled participants received an exquisite photo album and a gift bag (recommended retail value of 80 RMB). Additionally, pregnant women in the CDIP intervention group were provided with complimentary electronic fetal monitoring vouchers (valued at 200 RMB).

2.6. Variables Measures and Measurement Instruments

To achieve the goal of improving dietary behaviors among pregnant women in urban China, a comprehensive assessment of variables based on Orem's self-care theory is planned [46]. Specifically, we are interested in self-care agency, self-care behavior, nutritional status, and relevant pregnancy complications during the process of maternal dietary self-management. Corresponding variables include nutritional literacy, eating behavior, dietary quality, GWG, and the incidence of gestational diabetes.

It is worth noting that this study is an individual-level dietary intervention project, and research suggests that family functioning and physical activity levels may influence maternal dietary behaviors. Therefore, at baseline, this study also measures these two variables to further assess their impact on the outcomes.

The Demographic Questionnaire serves to collect participants' demographic information and comprises two sections—personal characteristics and sociocultural factors—with a total of 8 items. Inquiries encompass age, education level, gestational weeks, pre-pregnancy BMI, family average annual income, ethnic group, religion, cuisine, and family structure.

The Pregnancy Physical Activity Questionnaire in Chinese (PPAQ-C) is employed to assess the baseline physical activity levels of study subjects [51]. In this measurement, participants report their pregnancy activity levels over the past two weeks, covering aspects such as household chores, outdoor activities, occupational tasks, and exercise, totaling 31 items. Through participants' responses to each item, including activity duration and corresponding energy expenditure values, we can calculate the baseline pregnancy activity.

The APGAR questionnaire is utilized to evaluate family functioning, including five aspects: Adaptation, Partnership, Growth, Affection, and Resolve [52]. Each aspect is graded on three levels: "2 points for 'often'", "1 for 'sometimes'", and "0 for 'rarely'". The total score ranges from 0 to 10 points, with higher scores indicating better family functioning.

The Nutrition Literacy Assessment Instrument for Pregnant Women in China (NLAI-P) is employed to measure participants' nutritional literacy [53]. Participants respond to 38 questions across three dimensions: knowledge literacy, behavior literacy, and skill literacy. Scores for each dimension and the total score are calculated based on the scoring criteria provided by the instrument developer, with higher scores indicating higher levels of nutritional literacy during pregnancy.

The Dutch Eating Behavior Questionnaire—Chinese version (DEBQ-C) is used to assess eating behavior [54,55], with participants quickly responding to 33 questions covering three subscales: restrained eating, emotional eating, and external eating. Scores for each subscale and the total score are separately calculated, and higher scores reflect higher levels of eating behavior in the respective dimensions.

The Food Frequency Questionnaire for Pregnant Women (FFQ-P) assesses participants' dietary quality by asking them to recall their dietary habits over the past four weeks [56]. The questionnaire includes 61 food items grouped into ten categories such as meat, fish, vegetables, and fruits. We compare it to the Chinese Diet Balance Index for Pregnancy (DBI-P) to calculate participants' dietary balance index [57]. Details of the DBI scoring are described elsewhere [58,59]. We compute balance coefficients for each food category and the overall dietary quality distance. A score closer to 0 indicates a more balanced diet, while negative distances suggest more severe underconsumption, and positive distances indicate more severe overconsumption.

Assessors in the hospital conducted pre- and post-weight measurements using a standard weight scale. We calculated the weight gain during the twelve-week intervention period (from week 12 to week 24 of pregnancy).

Gestational diabetes mellitus (GDM) diagnosis: GDM diagnosis is based on blood glucose levels obtained from the 75 g Oral Glucose Tolerance Test (OGTT) conducted at 24 weeks of pregnancy, following the diagnostic criteria established by the International Association of Diabetes and Pregnancy Study Group (IADPSG) [60].

2.7. Analysis

Quantitative data analysis was performed using IBM SPSS Statistics v28 (IBM Corp, Armonk, New York, NY, USA). Basic statistics, including the calculation of mean and standard deviation (for normal distribution), median and interquartile range (IQR) (for skewed distribution), as well as frequency and percentage, were conducted. When comparing baseline data, an independent samples t-test was employed if continuous measurement variables met the assumption of normality. Otherwise, the Mann–Whitney U test or Chi-squared test was used to examine differences. For within-group comparisons before and after interventions, a paired samples t-test was applied if the differences in continuous measurement variables met the assumption of normality; otherwise, the Paired Wilcoxon Signed Ranks Test was used. In between-group comparisons after interventions, if continuous variables met the assumptions of normal distribution and homogeneity of variances, the One-way analysis of covariance was used, with baseline data as covariates; otherwise, the Mann–Whitney U test was utilized. For frequency data results with more than 20% cell counts less than the minimum expected count, a Fisher's Chi-squared test was performed. Intergroup comparisons were used to validate research hypotheses, and p-values were obtained using a one-tailed test. In all comparative analyses, $p < 0.05$ was considered statistically significant. Statistical analysis will adhere to the principles of intention-to-treat analysis, and missing data values will be handled using Complete-case analysis [61].

3. Results

3.1. Study Implementation

In this study, the trial was registered with the China Clinical Trial Registration Center under registration number ChiCTR2300075082. This investigation was carried out from August 2023 to November 2023. A total of 2712 individuals were systematically sampled from the Obstetrics Outpatient Department of a tertiary healthcare facility located in Changzhou, China. Among the 88 participants who met the specified inclusion and exclusion criteria and demonstrated a voluntary commitment to participation, they were subjected to a random allocation process, segregating them into two distinct groups, with each cohort comprising 44 individuals.

In the CDIP group, no participants were withdrawn, and compliance and retention were excellent, with no instances of participant attrition. Conversely, the routine care group experienced the attrition of two participants, with one exiting the study due to high-risk pregnancy complications and the other as a result of discontinued communication. Consequently, post-intervention data were acquired from the remaining 42 participants.

Consistent with the principles of intention-to-treat analysis, data from all 88 participants were inclusively considered in the subsequent analysis. A comprehensive recruitment and intervention process is visually depicted in Figure 1 for reference.

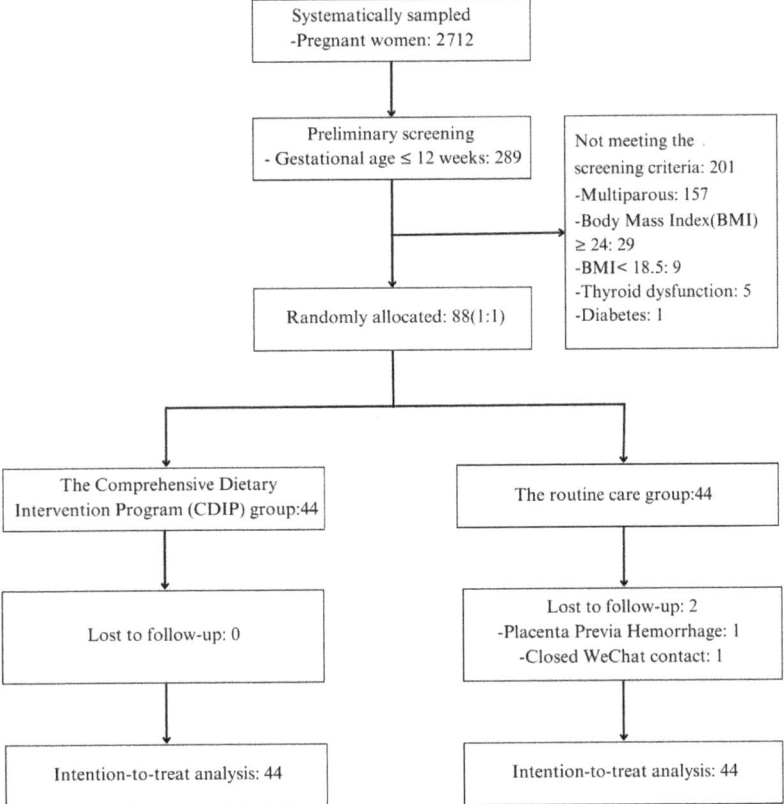

Figure 1. Recruitment and intervention flowchart.

3.2. Comparison of General Characteristics of Study Participants before Intervention

The average age of participants was (26.51 ± 2.96) years, and the two groups showed no statistically significant differences in terms of age, education level, family annual income, and cuisine preference. The average gestational age at baseline was (11.85 ± 0.41) weeks, and the pre-pregnancy Body Mass Index (BMI) was (21.14 ± 1.63) kg/m^2. There were no statistically significant differences between the two groups in terms of gestational age at baseline, pre-pregnancy BMI, family function, and physical activity level indicators. For detailed information on the general characteristics of study participants, please refer to Table 2.

Table 2. General characteristics of study participants at baseline (n = 88).

Variable	Characteristics	CDIP Group	Routine Care Group	Statistics	p-Value
Education Level	Below Associate Degree	9 (20.5%)	15 (35.1%)	2.267 [c]	0.315
	Associate Degree and Bachelor's Degree	30 (68.2%)	26 (59.1%)		
	Bachelor's Degree and Above	5 (11.4%)	3 (6.8%)		
Family Annual Income	<10,000 CNY	5 (11.4%)	12 (27.3%)	5.599 [c]	0.133
	10,000 to 20,000 CNY	27 (61.4%)	20 (45.5%)		
	>20,000 to 40,000 CNY	7 (15.9%)	10 (22.7%)		
	>40,000 CNY	5 (11.4%)	2 (4.5%)		
Cuisine Preference	Hunan Cuisine	4 (9.1%)	4 (9.1%)	0.363 [c]	0.969
	Sichuan Cuisine	5 (11.4%)	6 (13.6%)		
	Anhui Cuisine	7 (15.9%)	8 (18.2%)		
	Jiangsu Cuisine	28 (63.6%)	26 (59.1%)		
Pre-Pregnancy Body Mass Index		20.54 (19.57~22.24)	21.28 (20.23~22.60)	−1.836 [a]	0.066
Family Function		14 (12~15)	14 (11~15)	−0.223 [a]	0.823
Age		26.89 ± 3.47	26.14 ± 2.33	1.190 [b]	0.237
Gestational Age at Baseline		11.89 ± 0.42	11.82 ± 0.40	0.743 [b]	0.459
Physical Activity Level		108.69 ± 29.88	108.74 ± 27.72	−0.009 [b]	0.993

Note: Continuous variables normally distributed are presented as mean ± standard deviation, non-normally distributed continuous variables as median (interquartile range), categorical variables as frequencies (percentages); 'a' indicates Mann–Whitney test; 'b' denotes independent t-test; 'c' signifies Fisher's Chi-squared test.

3.3. Baseline Comparison of Outcome Measures for Participants before Intervention

After conducting statistical analysis on the two groups of study participants, it was found that there were no statistically significant differences between the two groups in terms of baseline prenatal nutritional literacy, eating behavior, dietary quality, and weight gain prior to the pre-test. Specific data can be found in Table 3. The dietary balance coefficients for various nutrient categories showed no statistically significant differences between the two groups. It was also observed that the median coefficients for dietary oil and vegetables were at a balanced zero point during the pre-test. Only the median coefficient for the fruit category was above zero, indicating excess intake, while the other categories were below zero, indicating inadequate intake. Refer to Figure 2 for details.

Table 3. Baseline score comparison of outcome variables for study subjects (N = 88).

Variable	CDIP Group	Routine Care Group	Statistics	p-Value
Total Nutritional Literacy Score	43.28 ± 7.25	43.18 ± 9.24	0.056 [b]	0.955
Knowledge Literacy Dimension	26.77 ± 5.31	26.53 ± 6.57	0.187 [b]	0.852
Behavioral Literacy Dimension	4.36 ± 1.89	4.93 ± 2.22	−1.291 [b]	0.200
Skills Literacy Dimension	13 (10.23~14.48)	13 (10.35~14.05)	−0.367 [a]	0.713
Total Eating Behavior Score	86.09 ± 15.24	85.59 ± 19.12	0.136 [b]	0.892
Restrained Eating Dimension	28.86 ± 6.82	29.20 ± 7.61	−0.221 [b]	0.825
Emotional Eating Dimension	27.20 ± 8.96	26.11 ± 8.82	−0.575 [b]	0.566
External Eating Dimension	30.36 ± 5.64	30.11 ± 7.05	0.184 [b]	0.855
Weight Gain Before Pre-test	0.37 ± 2.37	−0.01 ± 3.18	0.635 [b]	0.527

Table 3. Cont.

Variable	CDIP Group	Routine Care Group	Statistics	p-Value
Total Diet Quality Distance	43.41 ± 7.28	43.68 ± 7.05	−0.179 [b]	0.859
Types of Food	8.50 (8.00~9.00)	8.50 (8.00~10.00)	−0.107 [a]	0.915
Grains and Tubers	−4.00 (−5.00~−1.25)	−4.00 (−5.00~−3.00)	−0.328 [a]	0.743
Meat and Poultry	0 (−1.00~2.00)	−1.00 (−2.00~0)	−1.463 [a]	0.143
Animal Blood or Liver	−6.00 (−6.00~−6.00)	−6.00 (−6.00~−6.00)	−0.575 [a]	0.565
Seafood	−3.00 (−4.00~−1.00)	−4.00 (−4.00~−2.00)	−1.789 [a]	0.074
Eggs	−2.00 (−4.00~0)	−2.00 (−4.00~0)	−1.235 [a]	0.217
Soy and Soy Products	−2.00 (−3.00~−1.00)	−1.00 (−2.00~0)	−1.783 [a]	0.075
Vegetables	0 (−2.00~0)	0 (0~0)	−1.307 [a]	0.191
Seaweed	−2.00 (−2.00~−2.00)	−2.00 (−2.00~−2.00)	−0.633 [a]	0.527
Fruits	5.00 (0~6.00)	5.00 (2.00~6.00)	−1.140 [a]	0.254
Nuts	−3.00 (−3.00~0)	−2.00 (−3.00~0)	−0.600 [a]	0.548
Dairy	−3.00 (−5.00~−1.00)	−4.00 (−5.00~−2.00)	−1.286 [a]	0.198
Water	−3.00 (−5.00~0)	−3.00 (−5.00~−2.00)	−0.702 [a]	0.483
Oil	0 (0~2.00)	0 (0~1.50)	−0.476 [a]	0.634
Salt	2.00 (0~2.00)	2.00 (0~2.00)	−0.217 [a]	0.828

Note: Continuous variables normally distributed are presented as mean ± standard deviation; non-normally distributed continuous variables as median (interquartile range); 'a' indicates Mann–Whitney test; 'b' denotes independent t-test.

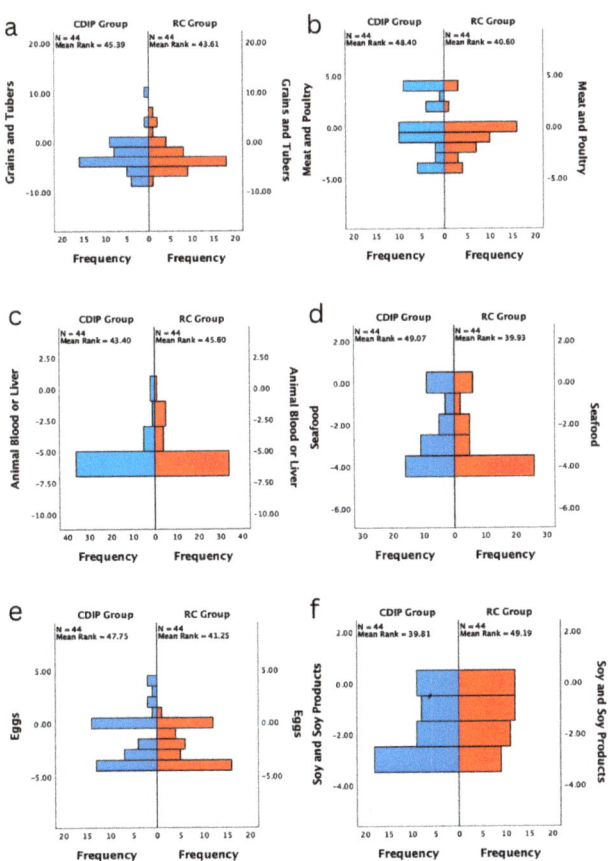

Figure 2. Cont.

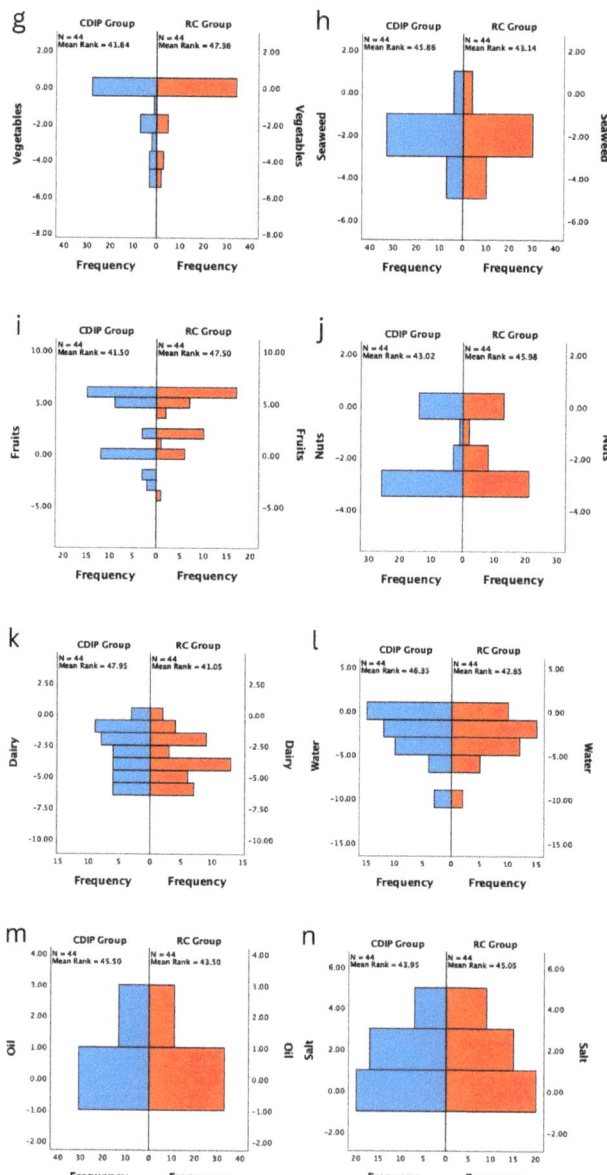

Figure 2. Baseline comparison of balance coefficients for various nutrients in two groups (*n* = 88). Note: (**a**) represents the comparison of frequency distributions in the dietary balance index of grains and tubers between two post-test groups; (**b**) signifies the comparison of frequency distributions in the dietary balance index of meat and poultry between two post-test groups; (**c**) denotes the comparison of frequency distributions in the dietary balance index of animal blood or liver between two post-test groups; (**d**) indicates the comparison of frequency distributions in the dietary balance index of seafood between two post-test groups; (**e**) stands for the comparison of frequency distributions in the dietary balance index of eggs between two post-test groups; (**f**) illustrates the comparison of frequency distributions in the dietary balance index of soy and soy products between two post-test

groups; (**g**) showcases the comparison of frequency distributions in the dietary balance index of vegetables between two post-test groups; (**h**) highlights the comparison of frequency distributions in the dietary balance index of seaweed between two post-test groups; (**i**) focuses on the comparison of frequency distributions in the dietary balance index of fruits between two post-test groups; (**j**) portrays the comparison of frequency distributions in the dietary balance index of nuts between two post-test groups; (**k**) outlines the comparison of frequency distributions in the dietary balance index of dairy between two post-test groups; (**l**) emphasizes the comparison of frequency distributions in the dietary balance index of water between two post-test groups; (**m**) represents the comparison of frequency distributions in the dietary balance index of oil between two post-test groups; (**n**) signifies the comparison of frequency distributions in the dietary balance index of salt between two post-test groups.

3.4. Impact of Intervention on Eating Behavior in Urban Chinese Pregnant Women

Intra-group comparison results show that pregnant women receiving CDIP intervention demonstrated a significant improvement in total eating behavior scores and restrained eating dimension scores compared to baseline ($p < 0.05$). In contrast, pregnant women receiving routine care intervention showed no statistically significant differences in scores compared to baseline. Detailed results are presented in Table 4.

Table 4. Intra-group comparison of eating behavior before and after intervention in two study groups.

Variable	Pre-Test	Post-Test	Statistics	p-Value
CDIP Group				
Total Eating Behavior Score	86.43 ± 14.30	88.36 ± 12.74	−1.781 [b]	0.082
Restrained Eating Dimension	28.86 ± 6.82	31.61 ± 7.28	−4.396 [b]	<0.001
Emotional Eating Dimension	27.20 ± 8.96	26.30 ± 8.75	2.074 [b]	0.044
External Eating Dimension	30.36 ± 5.64	30.45 ± 4.99	−0.146 [b]	0.885
Routine Care Group				
Total Eating Behavior Score	85.52 ± 18.03	84.78 ± 18.49	1.037 [b]	0.306
Restrained Eating Dimension	29.14 ± 7.46	28.59 ± 8.27	1.334 [b]	0.190
Emotional Eating Dimension	26.19 ± 9.02	26.07 ± 8.81	0.280 [b]	0.781
External Eating Dimension	30.19 ± 7.21	30.11 ± 6.46	0.156 [b]	0.877

Note: Continuous variables normally distributed are presented as mean ± standard deviation; "b" indicates paired t-test.

Inter-group comparison results, after adjusting for pre-intervention eating behavior score levels, indicate that following intervention, the total eating behavior score for the CDIP group was significantly higher than the routine care group by an average of 3.87 points (95% CI: 0.336–7.395, $p = 0.032$). Similarly, the restrained eating dimension score for the CDIP group after the intervention was, on average, 3.22 points higher than the routine care group, with a statistically significant difference (95% CI: 1.665–4.768, $p < 0.001$). No statistically significant differences were observed between the two groups in the emotional eating dimension and external eating dimension. The findings of this study suggest that, compared to the control group, CDIP intervention contributes to an improvement in patients' restrained eating behavior. Detailed results can be found in Tables 5 and 6 as well as Figures 3–6.

3.5. Impact of Intervention on Nutrition Literacy in Urban Chinese Pregnant Women

The intra-group comparison results indicate that pregnant women receiving CDIP intervention demonstrated significant improvements in Total Nutritional Literacy Score, Knowledge Literacy Dimension scores, Behavioral Literacy Dimension, and Skills Literacy Dimension compared to baseline ($p < 0.05$). In contrast, pregnant women receiving routine care intervention showed no statistically significant differences in scores compared to baseline. Detailed results are presented in Table 7.

The inter-group comparison results, after adjusting for pre-intervention nutritional literacy levels, reveal that following an intervention, the CDIP group's overall gestational nutritional literacy score was significantly higher than the routine care group, averaging 9.64 points (95% CI: 8.445–10.836, $p < 0.001$). Similarly, the Knowledge Literacy Dimension score for the CDIP group after the intervention was, on average, 5.98 points higher than the routine care group, with a statistically significant difference (95% CI: 5.038–6.921, $p < 0.001$). The Behavioral Literacy Dimension score for the CDIP group after the intervention was, on average, 1.98 points higher than the routine care group, with a statistically significant difference (95% CI: 1.297–2.660, $p < 0.001$). Both groups' Skills Literacy Dimension exhibited a non-normal distribution, with the CDIP group's median surpassing that of the routine care group by 2.05 points after intervention ($p = 0.001$).

Table 5. Inter-group comparison of eating behavior after intervention in two study groups.

Variable	CDIP Group	Routine Care Group	Statistics	p-Value
Total Eating Behavior Score	88.00 ± 13.46	83.93 ± 18.58	2.178 [b]	0.016
Restrained Eating Dimension	31.61 ± 7.28	28.79 ± 7.96	−4.123 [b]	<.001
Emotional Eating Dimension	26.30 ± 8.75	26.07 ± 8.82	−1.196 [b]	0.118
External Eating Dimension	30.45 ± 4.99	30.12 ± 6.46	0.298 [b]	0.383

Note: Continuous variables normally distributed are presented as mean ± standard deviation; 'b' signifies One-way analysis of covariance.

Table 6. Adjusted eating behavior scores after intervention in two study groups.

Eating Behavior Scores	Mean	Standard Error	95% LCI	95% HCI
Total Eating Behavior Score				
CDIP Group	87.900	1.240	85.433	90.366
Routine Care Group	84.034	1.269	81.509	86.558
Restrained Eating Dimension				
CDIP Group	31.803	0.545	30.719	32.887
Routine Care Group	28.587	0.558	27.477	29.697
Emotional Eating Dimension				
CDIP Group	25.836	0.418	25.004	26.668
Routine Care Group	26.553	0.428	25.701	27.405
External Eating Dimension				
CDIP Group	30.392	0.486	29.425	31.359
Routine Care Group	30.185	0.497	29.195	31.174

Note: LCL stands for Lower Confidence Limit, and HCL stands for Upper Confidence Limit.

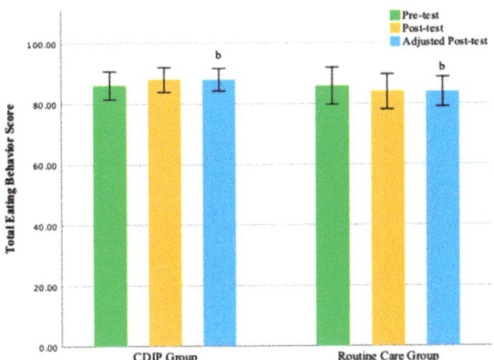

Figure 3. Illustrates the total eating behavior score before and after intervention in two groups. Note: CDIP is the Comprehensive Dietary Intervention Program, 'b' signifies Comparison with the Control Group, $p < 0.05$.

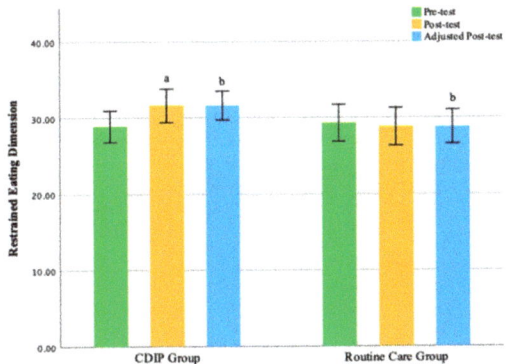

Figure 4. Illustrates the restrained eating dimension before and after intervention in two groups. Note: CDIP is the Comprehensive Dietary Intervention Program, 'a' denotes Intra-group Comparison, $p < 0.05$; 'b' signifies Comparison with the Control Group, $p < 0.05$.

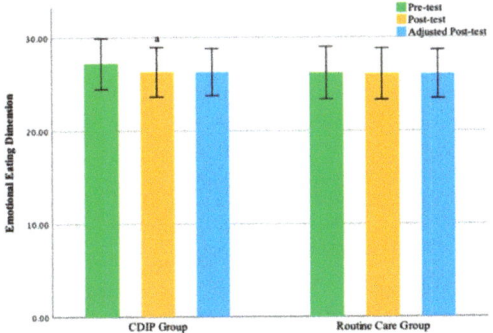

Figure 5. Illustrates the Emotional Eating Dimension Before and After Intervention in Two Groups. Note: CDIP is the Comprehensive Dietary Intervention Program, 'a' denotes Intra-group comparison, $p < 0.05$.

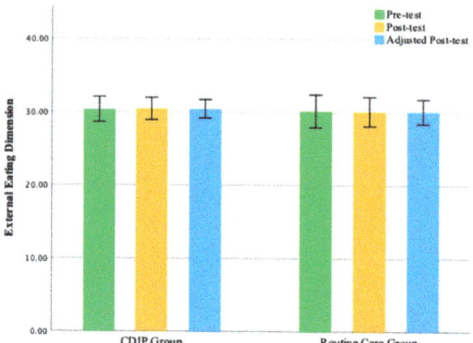

Figure 6. Illustrates the external eating dimension before and after intervention in two groups. Note: CDIP is the Comprehensive Dietary Intervention Program.

Table 7. Intra-group comparison of nutrition literacy before and after intervention in two study groups.

Variable	Pre-Test	Post-Test	Statistics	p-Value
CDIP Group				
Total Nutritional Literacy Score	43.28 ± 7.25	53.39 ± 6.60	−22.293 [b]	<0.001
Knowledge Literacy Dimension	26.77 ± 5.31	33.05 ± 4.70	−17.029 [b]	<0.001
Behavioral Literacy Dimension	4.36 ± 1.89	6.77 ± 2.15	−13.188 [b]	<0.001
Skills Literacy Dimension	13.00 (10.23~14.48)	14.35 (12.75~15.55)	4.660 [a]	<0.001
Routine Care Group				
Total Nutritional Literacy Score	43.07 ± 9.45	43.55 ± 9.58	−1.173 [b]	0.248
Knowledge Literacy Dimension	26.57 ± 6.71	26.89 ± 6.46	−0.935 [b]	0.355
Behavioral Literacy Dimension	4.86 ± 2.25	5.19 ± 2.42	−1.103 [b]	0.277
Skills Literacy Dimension	13.00 (10.30~15.04)	12.30 (10.45~14.10)	−1.350 [a]	0.177

Note: Continuous variables normally distributed are presented as mean ± standard deviation; non-normally distributed continuous variables are presented as median (interquartile range); 'a' indicates Paired Wilcoxon Signed Ranks Test; "b" indicates paired t-test.

The results of this study suggest that, compared to the control group, CDIP intervention contributes to an improvement in nutritional literacy among pregnant women. Detailed results can be found in Tables 8 and 9 and Figures 7–10.

Table 8. Inter-group comparison of nutrition literacy after intervention in two study groups.

Variable	CDIP Group	Routine Care Group	Statistics	p-Value
Total Nutritional Literacy Score	53.39 ± 6.60	43.55 ± 9.58	16.038 [b]	<0.001
Knowledge Literacy Dimension	33.05 ± 4.70	26.89 ± 6.46	12.633 [b]	<0.001
Behavioral Literacy Dimension	6.77 ± 2.15	5.19 ± 2.42	5.774 [b]	<0.001
Skills Literacy Dimension	14.35 (12.75~15.55)	12.30 (10.45~14.10)	−3.234 [a]	0.001

Note: Continuous variables normally distributed are presented as mean ± standard deviation; non-normally distributed continuous variables are presented as median (interquartile range); 'a' indicates Mann–Whitney test; 'b' signifies One-way analysis of covariance.

Table 9. Adjusted nutritional literacy scores after intervention in two study groups.

Variable	Mean	Standard Error	95% LCI	95% HCI
Total Nutritional Literacy Score				
CDIP Group	53.294	0.42	52.459	54.13
Routine Care Group	43.654	0.43	42.798	44.509
Knowledge Literacy Dimension				
CDIP Group	32.961	0.331	32.303	33.619
Routine Care Group	26.981	0.339	26.308	27.655
Behavioral Literacy Dimension				
CDIP Group	6.966	0.239	6.492	7.441
Routine Care Group	4.988	0.244	4.502	5.474

Note: LCL stands for Lower Confidence Limit, and HCL stands for Upper Confidence Limit.

3.6. Impact of Intervention on Diet Quality in Urban Chinese Pregnant Women

The intra-group comparison results indicate that both groups of pregnant women, those receiving CDIP intervention and routine care, demonstrated a significantly shorter Diet Quality Distance compared to baseline ($p < 0.05$). This suggests that the overall dietary balance coefficients for both groups are closer to the balance zero point after the interventions, signifying a significant improvement.

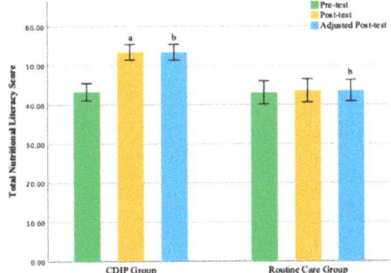

Figure 7. Illustrates the total nutritional literacy score before and after intervention in two groups. Note: CDIP is the Comprehensive Dietary Intervention Program, 'a' denotes Intra-group comparison, $p < 0.05$; 'b' signifies Comparison with the Control Group, $p < 0.05$.

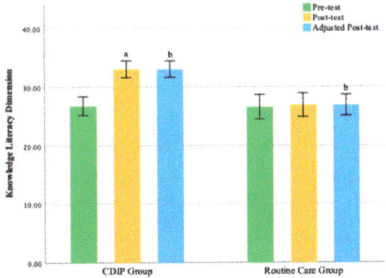

Figure 8. Illustrates the knowledge literacy dimension before and after intervention in two groups. Note: CDIP is the Comprehensive Dietary Intervention Program, 'a' denotes Intra-group comparison, $p < 0.05$; 'b' signifies Comparison with the Control Group, $p < 0.05$.

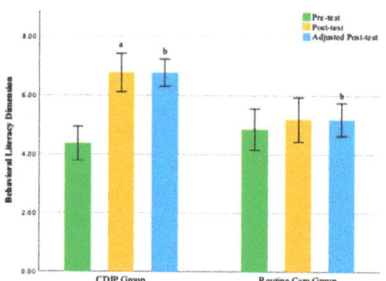

Figure 9. Illustrates the behavioral literacy dimension before and after intervention in two groups. Note: CDIP is the Comprehensive Dietary Intervention Program, 'a' denotes Intra-group comparison, $p < 0.05$; 'b' signifies Comparison with the Control Group, $p < 0.05$.

In the CDIP group, median coefficients for nutrients other than grains and tubers, meat and poultry, and salt are significantly closer to the balance zero point compared to the baseline ($p < 0.05$), and there is an increase in the variety of food types ($p < 0.001$). In the routine care group, significant changes in median coefficients for nutrients other than animal blood or liver, vegetables, oil, and salt were observed compared to baseline ($p < 0.05$). Notably, meat and poultry, as well as eggs, shifted from a negative balance to a positive balance, with a greater distance from the zero point. The post-test median coefficient for fruits was 6, indicating a more positive deviation from the balance zero point compared to the pre-test. Seafood, soy and soy products, seaweed, nuts, dairy, and water showed shorter distances in the negative direction compared to the baseline. Additionally, there is an increase in the variety of food types ($p < 0.001$). Refer to Table 10 for details.

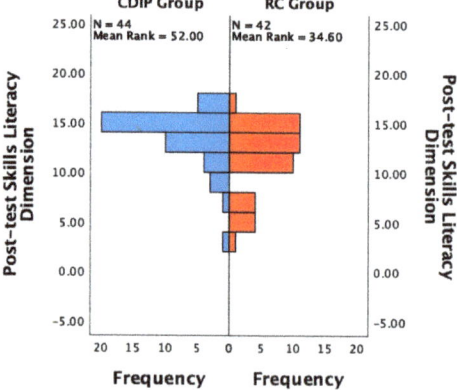

Figure 10. Illustrates the skills literacy dimension after intervention in two groups. Note: CDIP is the Comprehensive Dietary Intervention Program; RC is the routine care.

Table 10. Intra-group comparison of nutrition literacy before and after intervention in CDIP group.

Variable	Pre-Test	Post-Test	Statistics	p-Value
CDIP Group				
Total Diet Quality Distance	43.41 ± 7.28	29.11 ± 8.52	9.403 [b]	<0.001
Types of Food	8.50 (8.00~9.00)	12.00 (11.00~13.00)	−5.330 [a]	<0.001
Grains and Tubers	−4.00 (−5.00~−1.25)	−4.00 (−5.00~−2.00)	−0.662 [a]	0.508
Meat and Poultry	0 (−1.00~2.00)	1.00 (0~1.00)	−1.671 [a]	0.095
Animal Blood or Liver	−6.00 (−6.00~−6.00)	−2.00 (−6.00~0)	−4.373 [a]	<0.001
Seafood	−3.00 (−4.00~−1.00)	−2.00 (−3.00~−2.00)	−2.243 [a]	0.025
Eggs	−2.00 (−4.00~0)	0 (0~0)	−3.835 [a]	<0.001
Soy and Soy Products	−2.00 (−3.00~−1.00)	−1.00 (−2.00~0)	−2.744 [a]	0.006
Vegetables	0 (−2.00~0)	0 (0~0)	−2.994 [a]	0.003
Seaweed	−2.00 (−2.00~−2.00)	0 (−1.50~0)	−4.640 [a]	<0.001
Fruits	5.00 (0~6.00)	0 (0~0)	−4.639 [a]	<0.001
Nuts	−3.00 (−3.00~0)	0 (0~0)	−4.744 [a]	<0.001
Dairy	−3.00 (−5.00~−1.00)	0 (−1.00~0)	−5.035 [a]	<0.001
Water	−3.00 (−5.00~0)	0 (−3.00~0)	−3.950 [a]	<0.001
Oil	0 (0~2.00)	0 (0~0)	−2.449 [a]	0.014
Salt	2.00 (0~2.00)	2.00 (0~2.00)	−1.387 [a]	0.166

Note: Continuous variables normally distributed are presented as mean ± standard deviation; non-normally distributed continuous variables are presented as median (interquartile range); 'a' indicates Paired Wilcoxon Signed Ranks Test"; "b" indicates paired t-test.

The inter-group comparison results, after adjusting for pre-intervention Total Diet Quality Distance levels, indicate that following an intervention, the CDIP group's Total Diet Quality Distance is significantly shorter than the routine care group, averaging 11.49 coefficients less (95% CI: −14.730–8.242, $p < 0.001$). The post-intervention median for the variety of food types in the CDIP group is 3 higher ($p < 0.001$). In the CDIP group, the negative distance for grains and tubers is one coefficient farther compared to the routine care group ($p = 0.042$). The median coefficients for animal blood or liver, seafood, seaweed, fruits, nuts, dairy, and water are closer to the balance zero point compared to the routine care group ($p < 0.05$). There is no statistically significant difference in the post-intervention median coefficients for meat and poultry, eggs, soy and soy products, vegetables, oil, and salt between the two groups ($p > 0.05$).

The results of this study suggest that, compared to the control group, CDIP intervention contributes to the improvement of overall dietary quality in pregnant women. Detailed results can be found in Tables 10–13 and Figures 11 and 12.

Table 11. Intra-group comparison of nutrition literacy before and after intervention in routine care group.

Variable	Pre-Test	Post-Test	Statistics	p-Value
Routine Care Group				
Total Diet Quality Distance	43.71 ± 7.22	40.71 ± 7.39	2.721 [b]	0.010
Types of Food	8.50 (8.00~10.00)	11.00 (9.00~11.70)	−4.526 [a]	<0.001
Grains and Tubers	−4.00 (−5.00~−3.00)	−0.75 (−3.00~0.70)	−2.596 [a]	0.009
Meat and Poultry	−1.00 (−2.00~0)	3.00 (0~4.00)	−4.706 [a]	<0.001
Animal Blood or Liver	−6.00 (−6.00~−6.00)	−6.00 (−6.00~−3.20)	−1.725 [a]	0.084
Seafood	−4.00 (−4.00~−2.00)	0 (−3.00~0)	−2.357 [a]	0.018
Eggs	−2.00 (−4.00~0)	2.00 (0~4.00)	−4.802 [a]	<0.001
Soy and Soy Products	−1.00 (−2.00~0)	0 (−2.00~0)	−2.483 [a]	0.013
Vegetables	0 (0~0)	0 (0~0)	−0.528 [a]	0.598
Seaweed	−2.00 (−2.00~−2.00)	0 (−2.00~0)	−4.491 [a]	<0.001
Fruits	5.00 (2.00~6.00)	6.00 (2.00~6.00)	−3.098 [a]	0.002
Nuts	−2.00 (−3.00~0)	−1.75 (−3.00~0)	−2.701 [a]	0.007
Dairy	−4.00 (−5.00~−2.00)	−1.00 (−1.00~−1.00)	−3.243 [a]	0.001
Water	−3.00 (−5.00~−2.00)	0 (−3.00~0)	−2.114 [a]	0.034
Oil	0 (0~1.50)	2.00 (0~2.00)	−1.414 [a]	0.157
Salt	2.00 (0~2.00)	2.00 (2.00~4.00)	−1.414 [a]	0.157

Note: Continuous variables normally distributed are presented as mean ± standard deviation; non-normally distributed continuous variables are presented as median (interquartile range); 'a' indicates Paired Wilcoxon Signed Ranks Test"; "b" indicates paired t-test.

Table 12. Inter-group comparison of dietary quality after intervention in two study groups.

Variable	CDIP Group	Routine Care Group	Statistics	p-Value
Total Diet Quality Distance	29.11 ± 8.52	40.71 ± 7.39	−7.043 [b]	<0.001
Types of Food	12.00 (11.00~13.00)	9 (9.00~11.00)	−5.305 [a]	<0.001
Grains and Tubers	−4.00 (−5.00~−2.00)	−3.00 (−4.00~−0.75)	2.031 [a]	0.042
Meat and Poultry	1.00 (0~1.00)	0 (−0.25~3.00)	−0.031 [a]	0.975
Animal Blood or Liver	−6.00 (−6.00~−2.00)	−6 (−6.00~−6.00)	−5.030 [a]	<0.001
Seafood	−2.00 (−3.00~−2.00)	−3.00 (−4.00~0)	−2.181 [a]	0.029
Eggs	0 (0~0)	0 (0~2.00)	0.074 [a]	0.941
Soy and Soy Products	−1 (−2.00~0)	−2 (−3.25~0)	−1.708 [a]	0.088
Vegetables	0 (0~0)	0 (−2.00~0)	−0.218 [a]	0.827
Seaweed	0 (−1.50~0)	−2.00 (−2.00~0)	−2.994 [a]	0.003
Fruits	0 (0~0)	2.00 (0~6.00)	3.925 [a]	<0.001
Nuts	0 (0~0)	−3.00 (−3~−1.75)	−6.056 [a]	<0.001
Dairy	0 (−1.00~0)	−1.00 (−4.00~−1.00)	−5.195 [a]	<0.001
Water	0 (−3.00~0)	−3.00 (−5.00~0)	−3.083 [a]	0.002
Oil	0 (0~0)	0 (0~2.00)	−1.407 [a]	0.160
Salt	2.00 (0~2.00)	2.00 (0~2.00)	1.075 [a]	0.282

Note: Continuous variables normally distributed are presented as mean ± standard deviation; non-normally distributed continuous variables are presented as median (interquartile range); 'a' indicates Mann–Whitney test; 'b' signifies One-way analysis of covariance.

Table 13. Adjusted Total Diet Quality Distance after intervention in two study groups.

Total Diet Quality Distance	Mean	Standard Error	95% LCI	95% HCI
CDIP Group	29.169	1.140	26.903	31.436
Routine Care Group	40.656	1.166	38.336	42.976

Note: LCL stands for Lower Confidence Limit, and HCL stands for Upper Confidence Limit.

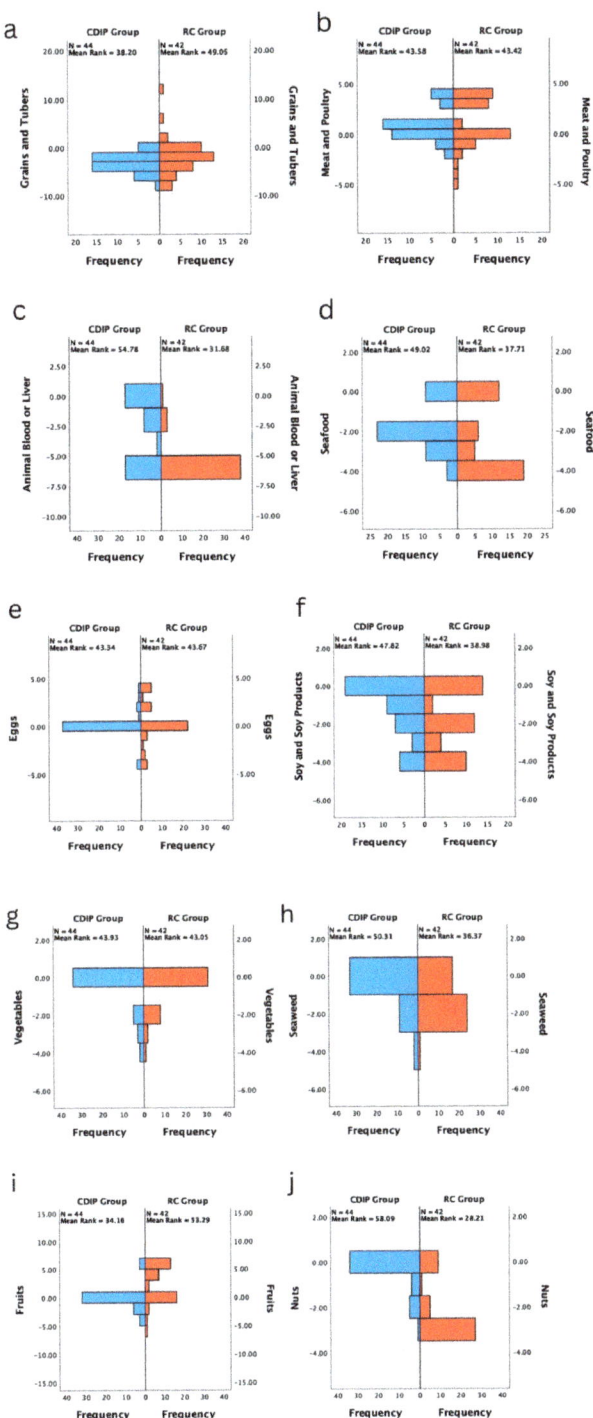

Figure 11. *Cont.*

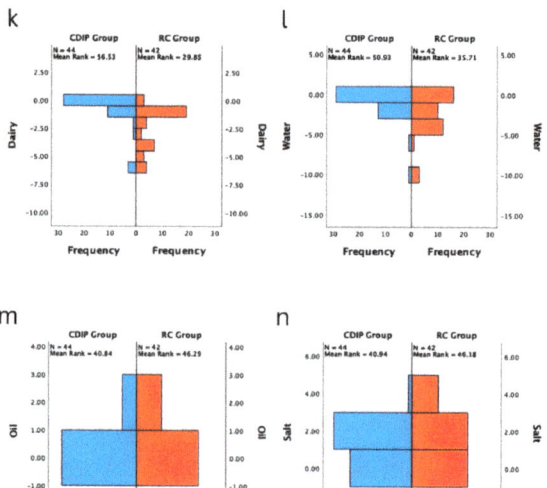

Figure 11. Post-test comparison of balance coefficients for various nutrients in two groups ($n = 86$). Note: (**a**) represents the comparison of frequency distributions in the dietary balance index of grains and tubers between two post-test groups; (**b**) signifies the comparison of frequency distributions in the dietary balance index of meat and poultry between two post-test groups; (**c**) denotes the comparison of frequency distributions in the dietary balance index of animal blood or liver between two post-test groups; (**d**) indicates the comparison of frequency distributions in the dietary balance index of seafood between two post-test groups; (**e**) stands for the comparison of frequency distributions in the dietary balance index of eggs between two post-test groups; (**f**) illustrates the comparison of frequency distributions in the dietary balance index of soy and soy products between two post-test groups; (**g**) showcases the comparison of frequency distributions in the dietary balance index of vegetables between two post-test groups; (**h**) highlights the comparison of frequency distributions in the dietary balance index of seaweed between two post-test groups; (**i**) focuses on the comparison of frequency distributions in the dietary balance index of fruits between two post-test groups; (**j**) portrays the comparison of frequency distributions in the dietary balance index of nuts between two post-test groups; (**k**) outlines the comparison of frequency distributions in the dietary balance index of dairy between two post-test groups; (**l**) emphasizes the comparison of frequency distributions in the dietary balance index of water between two post-test groups; (**m**) represents the comparison of frequency distributions in the dietary balance index of oil between two post-test groups; (**n**) signifies the comparison of frequency distributions in the dietary balance index of salt between two post-test groups.

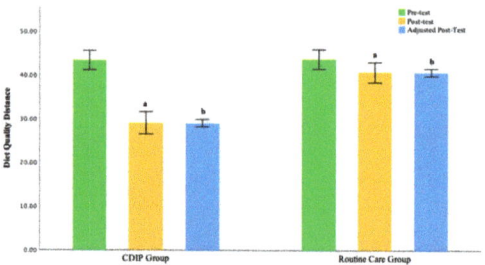

Figure 12. Illustrates the Diet Quality Distance before and after intervention in two groups. Note: CDIP is the Comprehensive Dietary Intervention Program, 'a' denotes Intra-group comparison, $p < 0.05$; 'b' signifies Comparison with the Control Group, $p < 0.05$.

3.7. Impact of Intervention on Weight Gain within 12 Weeks and Gestational Diabetes Status in Urban Chinese Pregnant Women

The inter-group comparison results indicate that, following the intervention, the CDIP group had a significantly lower weight gain within 12 weeks compared to the routine care group, with an average reduction of 1.01 kg (95% CI: −1.911 to −0.105, p = 0.029). According to the recommended standards for weight gain during the mid-pregnancy period of 12 weeks for Chinese pregnant women, which suggests a range of 3.6 to 5.4 kg, 13 individuals (29.5%) in the CDIP group and 22 individuals (52.38%) in the routine care group exceeded this standard. Additionally, two individuals (4.5%) in the CDIP group and nine individuals (37.8%) in the routine care group fell below the standard, and these differences were statistically significant (chi-square = 14.830, p = 0.001). Detailed frequency distributions are shown in Figure 13.

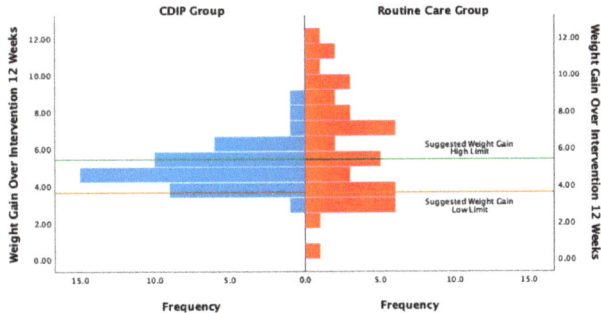

Figure 13. Frequency distribution of weight gain within 12 Weeks in two groups. Note: CDIP is the Comprehensive Dietary Intervention Program.

Regarding the screening and diagnosis of gestational diabetes using the OGTT test at 24 weeks of pregnancy, two individuals in the CDIP group and four individuals in the routine care group were diagnosed. However, this difference was not statistically significant. Refer to Table 14 for more details.

Table 14. Weight gain within 12 weeks and gestational diabetes status in two groups.

Variable	CDIP Group	Routine Care Group	Statistics	p-Value
Weight Gain Over Intervention 12 Weeks	4.97 ± 1.33	5.98 ± 2.78	−2.220 [a]	0.014
Gestational Diabetes Mellitus	2 (4.5%)	4 (9.5%)	0.428 [b]	0.316

Note: Continuous variables normally distributed are presented as mean ± standard deviation; categorical variables are presented as frequencies (percentages); 'a' denotes independent t-test; 'b' signifies Fisher's Chi-squared test.

3.8. Additional Outcome Indicator Description and Analysis

Participants in the CDIP group had 641 online interactions with healthcare providers and collectively sent 1732 interactive WeChat messages over a period of twelve weeks. After watching videos, they provided 76 comments, most of which were positive. One participant expressed concerns about the reliability of the information. During the post-test interviews, healthcare providers asked participants if they encountered any significant difficulties during the engagement process. Four pregnant women mentioned that their busy work schedules left them with insufficient time to participate in midwife interactions.

Pregnant women undergoing CDIP intervention responded to 14 satisfaction-related questions in the post-test. The questionnaire had a 100% response rate. The average satisfaction scores for each question are presented in Table 15. The analysis results indicate that participants expressed high satisfaction with the CDIP intervention.

Table 15. Satisfaction of pregnant women in the Comprehensive Dietary Intervention Program group with the intervention.

Item	Mean ± Std. Deviation
Health Education Theme Setting	4.68 ± 0.47
Health Education Comprehensibility	4.39 ± 0.58
Availability of Health Education Manuals and Video Materials	4.59 ± 0.50
Online and Offline Delivery Methods	4.64 ± 0.49
Program Flexibility	4.55 ± 0.50
Intervention Dosage	4.64 ± 0.49
Communication Methods and Language	4.73 ± 0.50
Interactivity of Health Providers	4.70 ± 0.46
Professionalism of Health Providers	4.68 ± 0.47
Supportive Role of Health Providers	4.68 ± 0.47
Positive Impact on Dietary Behaviors	4.59 ± 0.50
Positive Impact on Weight Control	4.57 ± 0.50
Generalizability	4.55 ± 0.55
Overall Satisfaction	4.70 ± 0.46

3.9. Comparison Analysis of Baseline General Information between Participants Lost to Follow-Up and Those Who Completed the Intervention

During the intervention, two participants were lost to follow-up, leading to incomplete data. Therefore, a comparative analysis was conducted on the baseline general information between those lost to follow-up and those who completed the intervention to determine if there was any bias. The analysis results revealed that there was no statistically significant difference in baseline general information between participants lost to follow-up and those who completed the intervention. The two groups of participants were similar in terms of age, baseline gestational weeks, family annual income, pre-pregnancy Body Mass Index, education level, cuisine preference, family function, and physical activity ($p > 0.05$). Specific results are provided in Table 16.

Table 16. Comparison of baseline general information between lost-to-follow-up and not-lost-to-follow-up study subjects ($n = 88$).

Variable	Characteristics	CDIP Group	Routine Care Group	Statistics	p-Value
Education Level	Below Associate Degree	24 (27.9%)	0 (0)	−1.494 [c]	0.135
	Associate Degree and Bachelor's Degree	54 (62.8%)	2 (100.0%)		
	Bachelor's Degree and Above	8 (9.3%)	0 (0)		
Family Annual Income	<10,000 CNY	17 (19.8%)	0 (0)	2.128 [c]	0.718
	10,000 to 20,000 CNY	46 (53.5%)	1 (50.0%)		
	20,000 to 40,000 CNY	19 (22.1%)	1 (50.0%)		
	>40,000 CNY	4 (4.6%)	0 (0)		
Cuisine Preference	Hunan Cuisine	8 (9.3%)	0 (0)	2.317 [c]	0.626
	Sichuan Cuisine	11 (12.8%)	0 (0)		
	Anhui Cuisine	14 (16.3%)	1 (50%)		
	Jiangsu Cuisine	53 (61.6%)	1 (50%)		
Pre-Pregnancy Body Mass Index		201.00 (19.75~22.58)	21.23 (21.09~)	0.266 [a]	0.790
Family Function		14 (11.75~15)	12 (11~)	−1.014 [a]	0.310

Table 16. *Cont.*

Variable	Characteristics	CDIP Group	Routine Care Group	Statistics	*p*-Value
Age		26.52 ± 2.99	26.00 ± 0	0.246 [b]	0.807
Gestational Age at Baseline		11.85 ± 0.41	12.00 ± 0.40	−0.509 [b]	0.612
Physical Activity Level		108.75 ± 28.98	107.00 ± 4.45	−0.080 [b]	0.936

Note: Continuous variables normally distributed are presented as mean ± standard deviation; non-normally distributed continuous variables are presented as median (interquartile range); categorical variables are presented as frequencies (percentages); 'a' indicates Mann–Whitney test; 'b' denotes independent *t*-test; 'c' signifies Fisher's Chi-squared test.

4. Discussion

The CDIP group exhibited remarkable compliance, indicating the program's effectiveness and participant engagement. This strong adherence enhances the study's internal validity and suggests that the intervention was well-received and valued by participants [62]. The absence of participant attrition in the CDIP group reinforces result reliability, aligning the program closely with participants' expectations and needs [63]. The online intervention's convenience played a pivotal role in maintaining compliance [64]. Its flexibility contributed to sustaining high levels of compliance, reducing participation barriers, and enhancing overall engagement [65]. Online platforms' rich interactivity, enabling real-time interaction with healthcare providers, likely heightened participants' positive experiences and sense of involvement [66,67]. Weekly interactive communication initiated by healthcare providers proved crucial in sustaining active participant engagement, maintaining interest, and facilitating questions and experience sharing [68]. This mode of communication played a key role in the successful implementation of CDIP. Future research can explore the additional functionalities and designs of online platforms to maximize the appeal and effectiveness of health behavior changes. The use of WeChat, the most widely used social platform in China, addresses the digital divide, ensuring broader population benefits [69].

In the baseline comparison of outcome measures, no significant differences were found in prenatal nutritional literacy, eating behavior, dietary quality, and weight gain during the pre-test phase, indicating the homogeneity of the study groups. However, an exploration of baseline dietary quality uncovered predominantly negative values in nutritional category coefficients, consistent with prior research on Chinese pregnant women [70]. This observation may be attributed to the influence of morning sickness, impacting dietary habits and potentially contributing to nutritional deficiencies [71]. Morning sickness, common in early pregnancy, leads to reduced appetite and altered food intake patterns, with pregnant women showing an increased intake of fruits and vegetables, possibly as a response to their comfort-inducing properties during episodes of morning sickness. This finding highlighted the need for tailored dietary guidance, acknowledging the individual variation in nutrient intake levels due to diverse dietary preferences [72]. While there were no significant differences in the median nutrient intake between the groups, the individualized nature of the nutrient intake resulted in a non-normal distribution, underscoring the importance of personalized dietary recommendations. This emphasizes the necessity for comprehensive and flexible dietary intervention programs that consider individual preferences and cultural variations to enhance overall effectiveness [73,74]. As health research evolves, future studies are expected to increasingly focus on personalized health intervention strategies, aligning with individual characteristics to better address diverse needs and expectations.

The CDIP intervention has demonstrated significant effectiveness in enhancing overall dietary behavior, particularly in promoting restrained eating. This success is attributed to a comprehensive approach that includes nutritional education, weekly weight monitoring, and reminders of weight-gain standards. Nutritional education raised the awareness of healthy pregnancy diets [75], influencing a more restrictive attitude towards food intake [76]. Weekly weight monitoring facilitates a real-time understanding of weight changes, promoting proactive restrained eating for better weight control [77]. Reminders of weight-gain standards emphasized healthy weight management goals, guiding pregnant women to consciously choose healthier eating habits [78]. However, the impact on emotional eating was not significant, possibly due to individual differences, physiological changes during pregnancy, and intervention limitations [79–82]. Additionally, the study focused on pregnant women with normal pre-pregnancy BMI, who generally may not have severe emotional eating issues [83]. This may explain why the effect of CDIP intervention on the emotional eating dimension is not significant. Since the study subjects themselves may not have significant emotional eating problems, the observed changes in this specific group may be relatively small. The lack of statistical significance in improving external eating may be attributed to CDIP's focus on the individual level, overlooking environmental and social factors influencing external eating [84]. External eating is shaped by stimuli, social pressure, and emotional factors [85,86], which CDIP may not comprehensively address. Future research should enhance support for social and environmental factors, particularly family and societal influences, and provide comprehensive emotional health support to improve the effectiveness of external eating interventions.

CDIP intervention has demonstrated significant efficacy in improving nutritional literacy among urban Chinese pregnant women, highlighting the scientific and practical value of integrating this intervention with the health literacy framework. In comparison to the baseline, pregnant women receiving CDIP intervention showed notable improvements in overall nutritional literacy scores, knowledge literacy, behavioral literacy, and skills literacy. These findings reveal that the tailored intervention guided by the health literacy framework effectively addresses various aspects of nutritional literacy in pregnant women [87–89]. To further bolster the evidence of the effectiveness of CDIP intervention, inter-group comparisons were conducted across various dimensions of nutritional literacy. Findings revealed that, after adjusting for the baseline level, the Knowledge Literacy Dimension scores for the CDIP group were significantly higher than those for the routine care group, with an average difference of 6.0 points. The significance of this difference lies in the targeted elevation of pregnant women's functional health literacy levels through CDIP intervention. By providing detailed information about prenatal diet, nutritional requirements, and food choices, CDIP encourages participants to develop a deeper understanding of their health goals, thereby enhancing their abilities to acquire information, understand and retain that information, and internalize it into applicable knowledge [90].

This study also reveals that, at the levels of skill literacy and Behavioral Literacy Dimensions, CDIP has achieved satisfactory outcomes through multidimensional intervention strategies. This indicates that CDIP has a significant impact on promoting interactive health literacy and critical health literacy among pregnant women [91]. Firstly, CDIP enhances the ability of pregnant women to disseminate dietary information within their families by training participants to conduct family dietary education themselves rather than having it directly provided by healthcare providers. This unique approach aims to empower pregnant women as leaders in health knowledge, encouraging individual learning and sharing and fostering interaction and communication. This lays the foundation for the development of interactive health literacy, enabling participants to engage in collective learning within the family and enhance health literacy through practical experiences [92]. Secondly, CDIP facilitates effective communication between pregnant women and healthcare providers through regular interactive processes, such as weekly weight-monitoring feedback and interactive dietary counseling. This interactive counseling not only provides opportunities for practical health practices but also guides pregnant women in translating theoretical knowledge into practical health decisions [93]. Through such experiential interactions, pregnant women develop critical health literacy, enabling them to accurately identify strategies that align with their individual circumstances, thereby improving the effectiveness and sustainability of health decision-making. Additionally, CDIP emphasizes interactive health literacy in family dietary education. By encouraging pregnant women to share detailed information about prenatal diet, nutritional requirements, and food choices within their families, this knowledge transfer is not only unidirectional but also involves in-depth interaction with family members, promoting closer communication [94]. This contributes to cultivating pregnant women's understanding and analytical skills regarding different viewpoints, fostering critical thinking about health information, and, ultimately, elevating their critical health literacy [95]. In summary, CDIP, through training, regular interactive processes, and family involvement, establishes a multi-dimensional, interactive health-promotion environment. This environment enhances pregnant women's interactive health literacy, enabling them to participate actively in health decision-making and the learning process. Additionally, it enhances critical health literacy, equipping them with the ability to discern information and make informed decisions.

The CDIP group exhibits a more diverse food intake, particularly in the supplementation of liver and animal blood, algae, and nuts, compared to the routine care group. This may reflect CDIP's emphasis on and attention to less common dietary categories in health education. The routine care group shows relatively poorer performance in these specific dietary categories, possibly due to a lack of awareness of the importance of these nutrient sources or a deficiency in related guidance in traditional prenatal care [70,96,97]. Furthermore, CDIP's intervention shows significant improvement in addressing the inadequate intake of seafood and dairy products. In the southern regions of China, dietary habits often lead pregnant women to insufficiently consume dairy and seafood [70,98,99]. CDIP successfully enhances the intake of these two food categories by emphasizing their nutritional importance. This highlights the positive role of CDIP's intervention in correcting regional dietary habits and providing comprehensive nutritional support to pregnant women. On another note, CDIP emphasizes the standard intake of fruits and alerts participants to the potential adverse effects of excessive fruit consumption. This helps address the common issue of excessive fruit intake among pregnant women in mid-pregnancy [96,100]. By delivering health information on fruit consumption to participants, CDIP effectively promotes a balanced intake of fruits, contributing to preventing overconsumption and slowing the trend of excessive weight gain, thereby maintaining overall maternal health. This nuanced health education approach likely has a positive impact on adjusting dietary patterns and promoting good nutritional habits among pregnant women. However, the lack of a significant effect on salt intake in CDIP intervention results may indicate the relative stability of individual taste preferences [101]. Taste preferences are often influenced by cultural factors, personal preferences, and habits, making it challenging to change pregnant women's preferences for salty flavors through short-term health education alone [102]. This underscores the need for a more comprehensive consideration of the complexity of taste formation in designing interventions. Future research and interventions may require a multidisciplinary approach, incorporating knowledge from psychology, sociology, and other fields, to develop more personalized and practical strategies for reducing salt intake [103].

This study reveals that participants in the routine care group experienced a dual challenge of excessive and insufficient weight gain within the first 12 weeks of mid-pregnancy, aligning with previous research on weight management in Chinese pregnant women [104]. This suggests a prevalent challenge in pregnancy-weight management in China, potentially influenced by specific cultural and lifestyle factors [36]. Furthermore, participants in the control group received general reminders during prenatal check-ups but lacked specific weight-control targets and dietary guidance. In contemporary Chinese society, diverse cultural perspectives on weight may lead to inconsistent responses among pregnant women [36]. Some may ignore the warnings due to a lack of additional information from healthcare providers or a lack of trust, resulting in uncontrolled weight gain [105]. Conversely, women who perceive weight gain as harmful to themselves or their offspring may adopt overly strict dietary measures, impeding normal weight gain [106,107]. In the absence of professional guidance, such restrictive dietary practices, rather than appropriately balancing nutrition and controlling calorie intake, may lead to nutrient deficiencies, posing significant health risks to both the pregnant woman and the fetus [108]. Evidence supporting this inference comes from the CDIP group's intervention results. The CDIP intervention demonstrated a significant positive impact, assisting women in controlling excessive weight gain, with a greater proportion of pregnant women achieving weight gain within the industry-standard range set by the Chinese National Health Commission [109–111]. CDIP, by emphasizing and monitoring weight gain, provided specific and practical weekly weight-gain goals and real-time-adjusted dietary guidance. Weekly comparisons not only delivered real-time weight-management information but also motivated active participation in weight management by stressing the importance of maintaining weight gain within the standard range [112]. This personalized and frequent monitoring approach appeared to positively influence adjustments in pregnant women's weight-gain habits.

This study analyzed the use of OGTT for gestational diabetes screening at 24 weeks. While the CDIP group had two cases, and the routine care group had four, the difference was not statistically significant. Challenges like sample size and study design may have influenced the results [113,114]. Despite the lack of statistical significance, the disparity in diagnosis rates raises practical concerns. This underscores the need for larger studies to understand the impact of dietary interventions on gestational diabetes screening and diagnosis. The findings serve as a starting point for future research and highlight challenges in clinical practice.

When conducting an in-depth analysis of participant satisfaction with the CDIP intervention, a widespread expression of high satisfaction among participants was observed. This reflects the positive evaluation of patients towards the overall intervention. Particularly noteworthy is the significant progress made in health education within the CDIP intervention. Participants gave high scores for the comprehensibility of health education (average score of 4.39 ± 0.58), indicating a high overall level of understanding of the intervention content. They perceived the provided health education materials and information as clear and understandable, contributing to an enhanced ability to make informed decisions regarding their health [45]. However, despite the generally high ratings, there is a recognition of the need to delve deeper into the underlying reasons. Potential causes for lower scores may stem from inadequate explanations of specific topics, the use of professional terminology, or information presentation methods not suitable for certain participants. For instance, the depiction of weight-monitoring charts may be challenging for some to comprehend [115]. During intervention interviews, it was discovered that one pregnant woman expressed concerns about the reliability of information. Although evidence was subsequently provided to substantiate the information's reliability, this situation was surprising. The expressed concern highlights the aspect of patients maintaining a critical mindset in processing health information—an encouraging finding. This critical thinking not only reflects patients' sensitivity to health information but also underscores their proactiveness in the decision-making process [116].

Simultaneously, over the 12 weeks of the intervention, participants exhibited a noticeable trend towards seeking advice on the correctness of their dietary adjustments rather than merely following the recommendations of health providers. This initiative reflects the participants' growth in their ability to make dietary decisions, indicating that they are actively contemplating and adjusting their dietary habits. This insight has important implications for the long-term effectiveness of the intervention and the cultivation of patients' abilities in autonomous health management [117]. Through critical thinking, patients demonstrated unique capabilities in self-health management [118]. They exhibited the ability to judiciously evaluate different dietary information, carefully considering the impact of each decision and avoiding blind conformity [118]. Critical thinking also positions patients as problem solvers, enabling them to analyze the essence of dietary challenges and actively seek practical solutions. Regarding self-monitoring, patients became more attuned to individual dietary behaviors, continuously adjusting and improving dietary plans to better meet personal health needs and goals. This comprehensive development of critical health literacy not only elevated patients' understanding and application of health information but also made them more proactive and rational participants in their dietary management.

In the CDIP intervention, patients gave high ratings (4.70 ± 0.46) to the interactivity with health providers, indicating satisfaction with their interaction with the healthcare team. This positive feedback suggests that patients believe they can effectively engage with healthcare professionals and receive attention in problem-solving and support. However, in a more in-depth analysis, a gap between patient expectations and actual experiences of interactivity was noted. This gap might be related to the expectation that interactions should be initiated by health providers [119], possibly influenced by the reserved social culture in China [120]. Pregnant women may be hesitant to actively burden healthcare professionals but are likely to readily share their experiences once interactions commence. The intervention guidelines of this study are based on the health literacy framework, combining intervention strategies with interactive health literacy viewpoints extensively exploring potential improvements in the interaction between patients and healthcare professionals. Through an understanding of the interactive processes with pregnant women, necessary measures were derived, including actively guiding interactions, encouraging patient participation, clearly expressing openness to communication and questions, and posing questions in a gentler manner to avoid discomfort. Additionally, recommendations were made to provide regular feedback opportunities, encouraging patients to share opinions and feedback, to better understand their expectations and needs and promptly adjust interaction strategies. Implementing these measures can better meet patient expectations for interactivity, simultaneously promoting patients' interactive health literacy, enhancing interaction effectiveness, and increasing patient satisfaction.

It is noteworthy that in the CDIP group, two individuals were diagnosed with gestational diabetes, while in the routine care group, four individuals received the same diagnosis. However, the data indicate that the difference between these two groups did not reach statistical significance. Firstly, a deeper exploration is needed into the reasons why the CDIP group did not demonstrate a superior preventive or diagnostic effect. Although it cannot be simply attributed to the ineffectiveness of the CDIP intervention, challenges such as sample size, study design, and other potential factors in academic research may have influenced the results [113,114]. In this study, the relatively small sample size may be a major contributing factor to the lack of observed significant differences. Secondly, it is crucial to explore whether these statistically non-significant differences hold potential clinical significance in actual clinical practice [121]. Despite the absence of a statistically significant difference, the disparity in the diabetes diagnosis rates between the two groups may raise concerns in practical medical settings. This underscores the distinction between statistical significance and actual clinical relevance, a common challenge in clinical research.

Strengths and Limitations

This study's strengths lie in its comprehensive data analysis, employing a randomized controlled trial design with a 12-week longitudinal approach. The integration of a health literacy framework adds depth to the intervention. However, limitations include a relatively small and region-specific sample size, potential biases in self-reported data, a short intervention duration, and the need for more diverse participant representation. Addressing these limitations and considering potential confounders would strengthen the study's validity and generalizability, providing a more robust foundation for assessing the impact of the CDIP intervention on dietary and health outcomes. The study, being part of a funded program, represents the initial phase of a larger project; future studies may consider comprehensively demonstrating the effectiveness of dietary and behavioral changes in reducing risks in pathological pregnancies.

5. Conclusions

In conclusion, this study investigated the effectiveness of the CDIP for urban Chinese pregnant women. The results indicate positive outcomes in improving nutritional literacy, dietary quality, and restrained eating behaviors. The CDIP demonstrated success in controlling excessive weight gain and promoting a more diverse and balanced food intake. While no significant impact on gestational diabetes screening was observed, the study underscores the need for further research with larger sample sizes to explore clinical significance. Participant feedback highlighted high satisfaction and the development of critical health literacy. Despite limitations, this research contributes valuable insights for future interventions, emphasizing the importance of personalized approaches, interactivity, and long-term follow-ups for sustained impact on maternal and child health.

Supplementary Materials: The following supporting information can be downloaded at: https://www.mdpi.com/article/10.3390/nu16020217/s1, Figure S1—Diet Education Booklet.

Author Contributions: Conceptualization, Q.L., N.P., S.P. and S.T.; methodology, Q.L., N.P., S.P. and S.T.; formal analysis, Q.L.; investigation, Q.L.; data curation, Q.L.; writing—original draft preparation, Q.L.; writing—review and editing, Q.L., N.P., S.P. and S.T.; project administration, Q.L.; funding acquisition, Q.L. All authors have read and agreed to the published version of the manuscript.

Funding: Research grants scholarships to undergraduate students under the Doctor of Philosophy Program in Nursing Science (International Program), Faculty of Medicine Ramathibodi Hospital and Faculty of Nursing, Mahidol University. Student ID: QIAN LI, G6436675.

Institutional Review Board Statement: Approval was obtained from the Human Research Ethics Committee, Faculty of Medicine Ramathibodi Hospital, Mahidol University, Thailand (MURA2023/590, 4 August 2023), and the Clinical Research Ethics Committee of the Affiliated Changzhou No. 2. People's Hospital of Nanjing Medical University, Changzhou, China. ([2023]KY107-01, 20 July 2023).

Informed Consent Statement: Informed consent was obtained from all subjects involved in the study.

Data Availability Statement: The data presented in this study are available upon request from the corresponding author. The data are not publicly available due to privacy issues.

Acknowledgments: We would like to thank all of the Affiliated Changzhou No. 2. People's Hospital of Nanjing Medical University staff who contributed to reviewing the program content and updating and delivering the program. Thanks, also, to the Faculty of Medicine Ramathibodi Hospital, Mahidol University, for their funding support.

Conflicts of Interest: The authors declare no conflicts of interest. The funders had no role in the design of the study; in the collection, analyses, or interpretation of data; in the writing of the manuscript; or in the decision to publish the results.

References

1. Cao, L.J.; Lin, H.Y.; Liang, X.; Chen, Y.J.; Liu, Y.Y.; Zheng, Y.Z.; Wang, X.Y.; Li, W.; Yan, J.; Huang, G.W. Association between Pre-pregnancy Body Mass Index and Offspring Neuropsychological Development from 1 to 24 Months of Age: A Birth Cohort Study in China. *Biomed. Environ. Sci.* **2019**, *32*, 730–738. [PubMed]
2. Eloranta, A.M.; Gunnarsdottir, I.; Thorisdottir, B.; Gunnlaugsson, G.; Birgisdottir, B.E.; Thorsdottir, I.; Einarsdóttir, K. The combined effect of pre-pregnancy body mass index and gestational weight gain on the risk of pre-labour and intrapartum caesarean section-The ICE-MCH study. *PLoS ONE* **2023**, *18*, e0280060. [CrossRef] [PubMed]
3. Ke, J.-F.; Liu, S.; Ge, R.-L.; Ma, L.; Li, M.-F. Associations of maternal pre-pregnancy BMI and gestational weight gain with the risks of adverse pregnancy outcomes in Chinese women with gestational diabetes mellitus. *BMC Pregnancy Childbirth* **2023**, *23*, 414. [CrossRef] [PubMed]
4. Fan, X.; Dai, J.; He, J.; Tian, R.; Xu, J.; Song, J.; Bai, J.; Liu, Y.; Zou, Z.; Chen, X. Optimal gestational weight gain in Chinese pregnant women with gestational diabetes mellitus: A large retrospective cohort study. *J. Obstet. Gynaecol. Res.* **2023**, *49*, 182–193. [CrossRef]
5. Jiajin, H. *Effects of Weight Gain during Pregnancy on Maternal and Child Health Outcomes and Research on Weight Management Methods during Pregnancy*; China Medical University: Taichung, Taiwan, 2019.
6. Tan, J.; Ren, Y.; Qi, Y.; Chen, P.; Tang, L.; He, G.; Li, S.; Sun, X.; Liu, X. The pattern of gestational weight gains among Chinese women: A repeated measure analysis. *Sci. Rep.* **2018**, *8*, 15865. [CrossRef] [PubMed]
7. Zheng, W.; Huang, W.; Zhang, L.; Tian, Z.; Yan, Q.; Wang, T.; Li, G.; Zhang, W. Suggested Gestational Weight Gain for Chinese Women and Comparison with Institute of Medicine Criteria: A Large Population-Based Study. *Obes. Facts* **2021**, *14*, 1–9. [CrossRef] [PubMed]
8. Fair, F.; Soltani, H. A meta-review of systematic reviews of lifestyle interventions for reducing gestational weight gain in women with overweight or obesity. *Obes. Rev.* **2021**, *22*, e13199. [CrossRef]

9. Awoke, M.A.; Skouteris, H.; Makama, M.; Harrison, C.L.; Wycherley, T.P.; Moran, L.J. The Relationship of Diet and Physical Activity with Weight Gain and Weight Gain Prevention in Women of Reproductive Age. *J. Clin. Med.* **2021**, *10*, 2485. [CrossRef]
10. Coughlin, J.W.; Martin, L.M.; Henderson, J.; Dalcin, A.T.; Fountain, J.; Wang, N.Y.; Appel, L.J.; Clark, J.M.; Bennett, W. Feasibility and acceptability of a remotely-delivered behavioural health coaching intervention to limit gestational weight gain. *Obes. Sci. Pract.* **2020**, *6*, 484–493. [CrossRef]
11. Holmes, H.; Palacios, C.; Wu, Y.; Banna, J. Effect of a Short Message Service Intervention on Excessive Gestational Weight Gain in a Low-Income Population: A Randomized Controlled Trial. *Nutrients* **2020**, *12*, 1428. [CrossRef]
12. Li, L.J.; Aris, I.M.; Han, W.M.; Tan, K.H. A Promising Food-Coaching Intervention Program to Achieve Optimal Gestational Weight Gain in Overweight and Obese Pregnant Women: Pilot Randomized Controlled Trial of a Smartphone App. *JMIR Form. Res.* **2019**, *3*, e13013. [CrossRef] [PubMed]
13. Olson, C.M.; Groth, S.W.; Graham, M.L.; Reschke, J.E.; Strawderman, M.S.; Fernandez, I.D. The effectiveness of an online intervention in preventing excessive gestational weight gain: The e-moms roc randomized controlled trial. *BMC Pregnancy Childbirth* **2018**, *18*, 148. [CrossRef]
14. Sandborg, J.; Söderström, E.; Henriksson, P.; Bendtsen, M.; Henström, M.; Leppänen, M.H.; Maddison, R.; Migueles, J.H.; Blomberg, M.; Löf, M. Effectiveness of a Smartphone App to Promote Healthy Weight Gain, Diet, and Physical Activity During Pregnancy (HealthyMoms): Randomized Controlled Trial. *JMIR Mhealth Uhealth* **2021**, *9*, e26091. [CrossRef] [PubMed]
15. Barker, M.; Dombrowski, S.U.; Colbourn, T.; Fall, C.H.; Kriznik, N.M.; Lawrence, W.T.; Norris, S.A.; Ngaiza, G.; Patel, D.; Skordis-Worrall, J. Intervention strategies to improve nutrition and health behaviours before conception. *Lancet* **2018**, *391*, 1853–1864. [CrossRef] [PubMed]
16. Anderson, A.E.; Hure, A.J.; Kay-Lambkin, F.J.; Loxton, D.J. Women's perceptions of information about alcohol use during pregnancy: A qualitative study. *BMC Public Health* **2014**, *14*, 1048. [CrossRef] [PubMed]
17. Anderson, C.K.; Walch, T.J.; Lindberg, S.M.; Smith, A.M.; Lindheim, S.R.; Whigham, L.D. Excess Gestational Weight Gain in Low-Income Overweight and Obese Women: A Qualitative Study. *J. Nutr. Educ. Behav.* **2015**, *47*, 404–411.e1. [CrossRef] [PubMed]
18. Blondin, J.H.; LoGiudice, J.A. Pregnant women's knowledge and awareness of nutrition. *Appl. Nurs. Res.* **2018**, *39*, 167–174. [CrossRef]
19. Bouga, M.; Lean, M.E.J.; Combet, E. Iodine and Pregnancy—A Qualitative Study Focusing on Dietary Guidance and Information. *Nutrients* **2018**, *10*, 408. [CrossRef]
20. Al-Mutawtah, M.; Campbell, E.; Kubis, H.-P.; Erjavec, M. Women's experiences of social support during pregnancy: A qualitative systematic review. *BMC Pregnancy Childbirth* **2023**, *23*, 782. [CrossRef]
21. Daigle Millan, K.; Poccia, S.; Fung, T.T. Information seeking behaviors, attitudes, and beliefs about pregnancy-related nutrition and supplementation: A qualitative study among US women. *Nutr. Health* **2022**, *28*, 563–569. [CrossRef]
22. Duthie, E.A.; Drew, E.M.; Flynn, K.E. Patient-provider communication about gestational weight gain among nulliparous women: A qualitative study of the views of obstetricians and first-time pregnant women. *BMC Pregnancy Childbirth* **2013**, *13*, 231. [CrossRef] [PubMed]
23. Garcia, T.; Duncanson, K.; Shrewsbury, V.A.; Wolfson, J.A. A Qualitative Study of Motivators, Strategies, Barriers, and Learning Needs Related to Healthy Cooking during Pregnancy. *Nutrients* **2021**, *13*, 2395. [CrossRef] [PubMed]
24. Graham, J.E.; Mayan, M.; McCargar, L.J.; Bell, R.C. Making compromises: A qualitative study of sugar consumption behaviors during pregnancy. *J. Nutr. Educ. Behav.* **2013**, *45*, 578–585. [CrossRef] [PubMed]
25. Greene, E.M.; O'Brien, E.C.; Kennelly, M.A.; O'Brien, O.A.; Lindsay, K.L.; McAuliffe, F.M. Acceptability of the Pregnancy, Exercise, and Nutrition Research Study With Smartphone App Support (PEARS) and the Use of Mobile Health in a Mixed Lifestyle Intervention by Pregnant Obese and Overweight Women: Secondary Analysis of a Randomized Controlled Trial. *JMIR Mhealth Uhealth* **2021**, *9*, e17189. [PubMed]
26. Grenier, L.N.; Atkinson, S.A.; Mottola, M.F.; Wahoush, O.; Thabane, L.; Xie, F.; Vickers-Manzin, J.; Moore, C.; Hutton, E.K.; Murray-Davis, B. Be Healthy in Pregnancy: Exploring factors that impact pregnant women's nutrition and exercise behaviours. *Matern. Child. Nutr.* **2021**, *17*, e13068. [CrossRef] [PubMed]
27. Groth, S.W.; Simpson, A.H.; Fernandez, I.D. The Dietary Choices of Women Who Are Low-Income, Pregnant, and African American. *J. Midwifery Womens Health* **2016**, *61*, 606–612. [CrossRef]
28. Hess, C.M.; Maughan, E. Understandings of prenatal nutrition among Argentine women. *Health Care Women Int.* **2012**, *33*, 153–167. [CrossRef] [PubMed]
29. Hromi-Fiedler, A.; Chapman, D.; Segura-Pérez, S.; Damio, G.; Clark, P.; Martinez, J.; Pérez-Escamilla, R. Barriers and Facilitators to Improve Fruit and Vegetable Intake Among WIC-Eligible Pregnant Latinas: An Application of the Health Action Process Approach Framework. *J. Nutr. Educ. Behav.* **2016**, *48*, 468–477.e1. [CrossRef]
30. Lewallen, L.P. Healthy behaviors and sources of health information among low-income pregnant women. *Public Health Nurs.* **2004**, *21*, 200–206. [CrossRef]
31. Loh, A.Z.H.; Oen, K.Q.X.; Koo, I.J.Y.; Ng, Y.W.; Yap, J.C.H. Weight management during pregnancy: A qualitative thematic analysis on knowledge, perceptions and experiences of overweight and obese women in Singapore. *Glob. Health Action* **2018**, *11*, 1499199. [CrossRef]
32. Lucas, C.; Starling, P.; McMahon, A.; Charlton, K. Erring on the side of caution: Pregnant women's perceptions of consuming fish in a risk averse society. *J. Hum. Nutr. Diet.* **2016**, *29*, 418–426. [CrossRef] [PubMed]

33. Lucas, G.; Olander, E.K.; Salmon, D. Healthcare professionals' views on supporting young mothers with eating and moving during and after pregnancy: An interview study using the COM-B framework. *Health Soc. Care Community* **2020**, *28*, 69–80. [CrossRef] [PubMed]
34. McKerracher, L.; Oresnik, S.; Moffat, T.; Murray-Davis, B.; Vickers-Manzin, J.; Zalot, L.; Williams, D.; Sloboda, D.M.; Barker, M.E. Addressing embodied inequities in health: How do we enable improvement in women's diet in pregnancy? *Public Health Nutr.* **2020**, *23*, 2994–3004. [CrossRef]
35. Mehrabi, F.; Ahmaripour, N.; Jalali-Farahani, S.; Amiri, P. Barriers to weight management in pregnant mothers with obesity: A qualitative study on mothers with low socioeconomic background. *BMC Pregnancy Childbirth* **2021**, *21*, 779. [CrossRef] [PubMed]
36. Mo, X.; Cao, J.; Tang, H.; Miyazaki, K.; Takahashi, Y.; Nakayama, T. Inability to control gestational weight gain: An interpretive content analysis of pregnant Chinese women. *BMJ Open* **2020**, *10*, e038585. [CrossRef]
37. Nagourney, E.M.; Goodman, D.; Lam, Y.; Hurley, K.M.; Henderson, J.; Surkan, P.J. Obese women's perceptions of weight gain during pregnancy: A theory-based analysis. *Public Health Nutr.* **2019**, *22*, 2228–2236. [CrossRef]
38. Pullon, S.; Ballantyne, A.; Macdonald, L.; Barthow, C.; Wickens, K.; Crane, J. Daily decision-making about food during pregnancy: A New Zealand study. *Health Promot. Int.* **2019**, *34*, 469–478. [CrossRef] [PubMed]
39. Super, S.; Beulen, Y.H.; Koelen, M.A.; Wagemakers, A. Opportunities for dietitians to promote a healthy dietary intake in pregnant women with a low socio-economic status within antenatal care practices in the Netherlands: A qualitative study. *J. Health Popul. Nutr.* **2021**, *40*, 35. [CrossRef]
40. Thornton, P.L.; Kieffer, E.C.; Salabarría-Peña, Y.; Odoms-Young, A.; Willis, S.K.; Kim, H.; Salinas, M.A. Weight, diet, and physical activity-related beliefs and practices among pregnant and postpartum Latino women: The role of social support. *Matern. Child Health J.* **2006**, *10*, 95–104. [CrossRef]
41. Tovar, A.; Chasan-Taber, L.; Bermudez, O.I.; Hyatt, R.R.; Must, A. Knowledge, attitudes, and beliefs regarding weight gain during pregnancy among Hispanic women. *Matern. Child Health J.* **2010**, *14*, 938–949. [CrossRef]
42. Papežová, K.; Kapounová, Z.; Zelenková, V.; Riad, A. Nutritional Health Knowledge and Literacy among Pregnant Women in the Czech Republic: Analytical Cross-Sectional Study. *Int. J. Environ. Res. Public Health* **2023**, *20*, 3931. [CrossRef]
43. Andrus, M.R.; Roth, M.T. Health literacy: A review. *Pharmacother. J. Hum. Pharmacol. Drug Ther.* **2002**, *22*, 282–302. [CrossRef] [PubMed]
44. Nutbeam, D. The evolving concept of health literacy. *Soc. Sci. Med.* **2008**, *67*, 2072–2078. [CrossRef] [PubMed]
45. Nutbeam, D. Health literacy as a public health goal: A challenge for contemporary health education and communication strategies into the 21st century. *Health Promot. Int.* **2000**, *15*, 259–267. [CrossRef]
46. Hartweg, D.L.; Metcalfe, S.A. Orem's Self-Care Deficit Nursing Theory: Relevance and Need for Refinement. *Nurs. Sci. Q.* **2021**, *35*, 70–76. [CrossRef]
47. Deng, Y.; Hou, Y.; Wu, L.; Liu, Y.; Ma, L.; Yao, A. Effects of diet and exercise interventions to prevent gestational diabetes mellitus in pregnant women with high-risk factors in China: A randomized controlled study. *Clin. Nurs. Res.* **2022**, *31*, 836–847. [CrossRef]
48. Michie, S.; Richardson, M.; Johnston, M.; Abraham, C.; Francis, J.; Hardeman, W.; Eccles, M.P.; Cane, J.; Wood, C.E. The Behavior Change Technique Taxonomy (v1) of 93 Hierarchically Clustered Techniques: Building an International Consensus for the Reporting of Behavior Change Interventions. *Ann. Behav. Med.* **2013**, *46*, 81–95. [CrossRef]
49. Chinese National Health Commission (NHC). Recommended Standards for Gestational Weight Gain in Pregnant Women (WS/T801—2022). *Chin. J. Perinat. Med.* **2022**, *25*, 1.
50. Chinese Nutrition Society (CNS). *Dietary Guidelines for Chinese Residents*; People's Medical Publishing House: Beijing, China, 2022.
51. Chasan-Taber, L.; Schmidt, M.D.; Roberts, D.E.; Hosmer, D.; Markenson, G.; Freedson, P.S. Development and validation of a pregnancy physical activity questionnaire. *Med. Sci. Sports Exerc.* **2004**, *36*, 1750–1760. [CrossRef]
52. Smilkstein, G. The family APGAR: A proposal for a family function test and its use by physicians. *J. Fam. Pract.* **1978**, *6*, 1231–1239.
53. Zhou, Y.; Lyu, Y.; Zhao, R.; Shi, H.; Ye, W.; Wen, Z.; Li, R.; Xu, Y. Development and validation of nutrition literacy assessment instrument for Chinese pregnant women. *Nutrients* **2022**, *14*, 2863. [CrossRef] [PubMed]
54. Wu, S.; Cai, T.; Luo, X. Validation of the Dutch Eating Behavior Questionnaire (DEBQ) in a sample of Chinese adolescents. *Psychol. Health Med.* **2017**, *22*, 282–288. [CrossRef] [PubMed]
55. Van Strien, T.; Frijter, J.E.; Bergers, G.; Defares, P.B. The Dutch Eating Behavior Questionnaire (DEBQ) for Assessment of Restrained, Emotional, and External Eating Behavior. *Int. J. Eat. Disord.* **1986**, *5*, 295–315. [CrossRef]
56. Zhang, H.; Qiu, X.; Zhong, C.; Zhang, K.; Xiao, M.; Yi, N.; Xiong, G.; Wang, J.; Yao, J.; Hao, L.; et al. Reproducibility and relative validity of a semi-quantitative food frequency questionnaire for Chinese pregnant women. *Nutr. J.* **2015**, *14*, 56. [CrossRef]
57. Huang, S.P.L.; Du, Y.; Xu, G.; Zhang, J.; Liu, Y.; Sun, M.; Xiang, Y.; Shao, J.H. Evaluation on dietary quality for pregnant women with gestational diabetes mellitus by adjusted DBI. *Mod. Prev. Med.* **2020**, *47*, 1376–1380.
58. Wang, Y.; Li, R.; Liu, D.; Dai, Z.; Liu, J.; Zhang, J.; Zhou, R.; Zeng, G. Evaluation of the dietary quality by diet balance index for pregnancy among pregnant women. *Wei Sheng Yan Jiu* **2016**, *45*, 211–216. [PubMed]
59. He, Y.; Zhai, F.; Yang, X.; Ge, K. The Chinese Diet Balance Index revised. *Acta Nutr. Sin.* **2009**, *31*, 532–536.
60. Wendland, E.M.; Torloni, M.R.; Falavigna, M.; Trujillo, J.; Dode, M.A.; Campos, M.A.; Duncan, B.B.; Schmidt, M.I. Gestational diabetes and pregnancy outcomes-a systematic review of the World Health Organization (WHO) and the International Association of Diabetes in Pregnancy Study Groups (IADPSG) diagnostic criteria. *BMC Pregnancy Childbirth* **2012**, *12*, 23. [CrossRef]

61. Bell, M.L.; Fiero, M.; Horton, N.J.; Hsu, C.-H. Handling missing data in RCTs; a review of the top medical journals. *BMC Med. Res. Methodol.* **2014**, *14*, 118. [CrossRef]
62. Carroll, C.; Patterson, M.; Wood, S.; Booth, A.; Rick, J.; Balain, S. A conceptual framework for implementation fidelity. *Implement. Sci.* **2007**, *2*, 40. [CrossRef]
63. Andersen, E. Participant retention in randomized, controlled trials: The value of relational engagement. *Int. J. Hum. Caring* **2007**, *11*, 46–51. [CrossRef]
64. Borghouts, J.; Eikey, E.; Mark, G.; De Leon, C.; Schueller, S.M.; Schneider, M.; Stadnick, N.; Zheng, K.; Mukamel, D.; Sorkin, D.H. Barriers to and facilitators of user engagement with digital mental health interventions: Systematic review. *J. Med. Internet Res.* **2021**, *23*, e24387. [CrossRef] [PubMed]
65. Patel, S.; Akhtar, A.; Malins, S.; Wright, N.; Rowley, E.; Young, E.; Sampson, S.; Morriss, R. The acceptability and usability of digital health interventions for adults with depression, anxiety, and somatoform disorders: Qualitative systematic review and meta-synthesis. *J. Med. Internet Res.* **2020**, *22*, e16228. [CrossRef] [PubMed]
66. Barak, A.; Grohol, J.M. Current and Future Trends in Internet-Supported Mental Health Interventions. *J. Technol. Hum. Serv.* **2011**, *29*, 155–196. [CrossRef]
67. Simblett, S.; Greer, B.; Matcham, F.; Curtis, H.; Polhemus, A.; Ferrão, J.; Gamble, P.; Wykes, T. Barriers to and Facilitators of Engagement With Remote Measurement Technology for Managing Health: Systematic Review and Content Analysis of Findings. *J. Med. Internet Res.* **2018**, *20*, e10480. [CrossRef]
68. Crawford, M.J.; Rutter, D.; Manley, C.; Weaver, T.; Bhui, K.; Fulop, N.; Tyrer, P. Systematic review of involving patients in the planning and development of health care. *BMJ* **2002**, *325*, 1263. [CrossRef]
69. Tu, F. WeChat and civil society in China. *Commun. Public* **2016**, *1*, 343–350. [CrossRef]
70. Wang, S.; Liu, H.; Luo, C.; Zhao, R.; Zhou, L.; Huang, S.; Ge, Y.; Cui, N.; Shen, J.; Yang, X.; et al. Association of maternal dietary patterns derived by multiple approaches with gestational diabetes mellitus: A prospective cohort study. *Int. J. Food Sci. Nutr.* **2023**, *74*, 487–500. [CrossRef]
71. Maslin, K.; Dean, C. Nutritional consequences and management of hyperemesis gravidarum: A narrative review. *Nutr. Res. Rev.* **2022**, *35*, 308–318. [CrossRef]
72. Zhu, S.; Zhao, A.; Lan, H.; Li, P.; Mao, S.; Szeto, I.M.-Y.; Jiang, H.; Zhang, Y. Nausea and Vomiting during Early Pregnancy among Chinese Women and Its Association with Nutritional Intakes. *Nutrients* **2023**, *15*, 933. [CrossRef]
73. Diószegi, J.; Llanaj, E.; Ádány, R. Genetic background of taste perception, taste preferences, and its nutritional implications: A systematic review. *Front. Genet.* **2019**, *10*, 1272. [CrossRef] [PubMed]
74. Chen, P.J.; Antonelli, M. Conceptual Models of Food Choice: Influential Factors Related to Foods, Individual Differences, and Society. *Foods* **2020**, *9*, 1898. [CrossRef] [PubMed]
75. Soliman, A.-Z.; Hassan, A.; Fahmy, H.H. Effect of Nutritional Education Intervention on Knowledge, Attitude and Practice of Pregnant Women towards Dietary habits, Physical activity and Optimal Gestational Weight Gain. *Zagazig Univ. Med. J.* **2021**, *27*, 577–588. [CrossRef]
76. Permatasari, T.A.E.; Rizqiya, F.; Kusumaningati, W.; Suryaalamsah, I.I.; Hermiwahyoeni, Z. The effect of nutrition and reproductive health education of pregnant women in Indonesia using quasi experimental study. *BMC Pregnancy Childbirth* **2021**, *21*, 180. [CrossRef] [PubMed]
77. Shieh, C.; Draucker, C.B. Self-monitoring Lifestyle Behavior in Overweight and Obese Pregnant Women: Qualitative Findings. *Clin. Nurse Spec.* **2018**, *32*, 81–89. [CrossRef] [PubMed]
78. Criss, S.; Oken, E.; Guthrie, L.; Hivert, M.-F. A qualitative study of gestational weight gain goal setting. *BMC Pregnancy Childbirth* **2016**, *16*, 1–8. [CrossRef] [PubMed]
79. Bjelica, A.; Cetkovic, N.; Trninic-Pjevic, A.; Mladenovic-Segedi, L. The phenomenon of pregnancy—A psychological view. *Ginekol. Pol.* **2018**, *89*, 102–106. [CrossRef] [PubMed]
80. Racine, S.E.; Keel, P.K.; Burt, S.A.; Sisk, C.L.; Neale, M.; Boker, S.; Klump, K.L. Individual differences in the relationship between ovarian hormones and emotional eating across the menstrual cycle: A role for personality? *Eat. Behav.* **2013**, *14*, 161–166. [CrossRef]
81. Epel, E.; Laraia, B.; Coleman-Phox, K.; Leung, C.; Vieten, C.; Mellin, L.; Kristeller, J.; Thomas, M.; Stotland, N.; Bush, N. Effects of a mindfulness-based intervention on distress, weight gain, and glucose control for pregnant low-income women: A quasi-experimental trial using the ORBIT model. *Int. J. Behav. Med.* **2019**, *26*, 461–473. [CrossRef]
82. Hutchinson, A.; Charters, M.; Prichard, I.; Fletcher, C.; Wilson, C. Understanding maternal dietary choices during pregnancy: The role of social norms and mindful eating. *Appetite* **2017**, *112*, 227–234. [CrossRef]
83. Dakanalis, A.; Mentzelou, M.; Papadopoulou, S.K.; Papandreou, D.; Spanoudaki, M.; Vasios, G.K.; Pavlidou, E.; Mantzorou, M.; Giaginis, C. The association of emotional eating with overweight/obesity, depression, anxiety/stress, and dietary patterns: A review of the current clinical evidence. *Nutrients* **2023**, *15*, 1173. [CrossRef] [PubMed]
84. Robinson, E.; Blissett, J.; Higgs, S. Social influences on eating: Implications for nutritional interventions. *Nutr. Res. Rev.* **2013**, *26*, 166–176. [CrossRef] [PubMed]
85. Stroebele, N.; De Castro, J.M. Effect of ambience on food intake and food choice. *Nutrition* **2004**, *20*, 821–838. [CrossRef] [PubMed]
86. Rodin, J.; Slochower, J. Externality in the nonobese: Effects of environmental responsiveness on weight. *J. Per. Soc. Psychol.* **1976**, *33*, 338. [CrossRef] [PubMed]

87. Timlin, D.; McCormack, J.M.; Kerr, M.; Keaver, L.; Simpson, E.E.A. Are dietary interventions with a behaviour change theoretical framework effective in changing dietary patterns? A systematic review. *BMC Public Health* **2020**, *20*, 1857. [CrossRef] [PubMed]
88. Walters, R.; Leslie, S.J.; Polson, R.; Cusack, T.; Gorely, T. Establishing the efficacy of interventions to improve health literacy and health behaviours: A systematic review. *BMC Public Health* **2020**, *20*, 1040. [CrossRef] [PubMed]
89. Uemura, K.; Yamada, M.; Okamoto, H. Effects of Active Learning on Health Literacy and Behavior in Older Adults: A Randomized Controlled Trial. *J. Am. Geriatr. Soc.* **2018**, *66*, 1721–1729. [CrossRef]
90. Baker, D.W. The meaning and the measure of health literacy. *J. Gen. Intern. Med.* **2006**, *21*, 878–883. [CrossRef]
91. Nutbeam, D. Defining and measuring health literacy: What can we learn from literacy studies? *Int. J. Public Health* **2009**, *54*, 303–305. [CrossRef]
92. Cheng, G.Z.; Chen, A.; Xin, Y.; Ni, Q.Q. Using the teach-back method to improve postpartum maternal-infant health among women with limited maternal health literacy: A randomized controlled study. *BMC Pregnancy Childbirth* **2023**, *23*, 13. [CrossRef]
93. Schillinger, D.; Piette, J.; Grumbach, K.; Wang, F.; Wilson, C.; Daher, C.; Leong-Grotz, K.; Castro, C.; Bindman, A.B. Closing the loop: Physician communication with diabetic patients who have low health literacy. *Arch. Intern. Med.* **2003**, *163*, 83–90. [CrossRef] [PubMed]
94. Gonzalez, C.; Bollinger, B.; Yip, J.; Pina, L.; Roldan, W.; Nieto Ruiz, C. Intergenerational Online Health Information Searching and Brokering: Framing Health Literacy as a Family Asset. *Health Commun.* **2022**, *37*, 438–449. [CrossRef] [PubMed]
95. Austin, E.W.; Pinkleton, B.E.; Radanielina-Hita, M.L.; Ran, W. The role of parents' critical thinking about media in shaping expectancies, efficacy and nutrition behaviors for families. *Health Commun.* **2015**, *30*, 1256–1268. [CrossRef] [PubMed]
96. Yang, J.; Dang, S.; Cheng, Y.; Qiu, H.; Mi, B.; Jiang, Y.; Qu, P.; Zeng, L.; Wang, Q.; Li, Q. Dietary intakes and dietary patterns among pregnant women in Northwest China. *Public Health Nutr.* **2017**, *20*, 282–293. [CrossRef] [PubMed]
97. Ding, Y.; Xu, F.; Zhong, C.; Tong, L.; Li, F.; Li, Q.; Chen, R.; Zhou, X.; Li, X.; Cui, W. Association between chinese dietary guidelines compliance index for pregnant women and risks of pregnancy complications in the tongji maternal and child health cohort. *Nutrients* **2021**, *13*, 829. [CrossRef] [PubMed]
98. Wang, Z.; Shen, J.; Wu, Y.; Cui, X.; Song, Q.; Shi, Z.; Guo, J.; Su, J.; Zang, J. A China Healthy Diet Index-Based Evaluation of Dietary Quality among Pregnant Women in Shanghai across Trimesters and Residential Areas. *J. Nutr. Sci. Vitaminol.* **2021**, *67*, 301–309. [CrossRef] [PubMed]
99. He, J.-R.; Yuan, M.-Y.; Chen, N.-N.; Lu, J.-H.; Hu, C.-Y.; Mai, W.-B.; Zhang, R.-F.; Pan, Y.-H.; Qiu, L.; Wu, Y.-F.; et al. Maternal dietary patterns and gestational diabetes mellitus: A large prospective cohort study in China. *Br. J. Nutr.* **2015**, *113*, 1292–1300. [CrossRef] [PubMed]
100. Huang, W.-Q.; Lu, Y.; Xu, M.; Huang, J.; Su, Y.-X.; Zhang, C.-X. Excessive fruit consumption during the second trimester is associated with increased likelihood of gestational diabetes mellitus: A prospective study. *Sci. Rep.* **2017**, *7*, 43620. [CrossRef]
101. Ma, Z.; He, J.; Sun, S.; Lu, T. Patterns and stability of food preferences among a national representative sample of young, middle-aged, and elderly adults in China: A latent transition analysis. *Food Qual. Prefer.* **2021**, *94*, 104322. [CrossRef]
102. Li, J.-R.; Hsieh, Y.-H.P. Traditional Chinese food technology and cuisine. *Asia Pac. J. Clin. Nutr.* **2004**, *13*, 147–155.
103. Zhang, P.; He, F.J.; Li, Y.; Li, C.; Wu, J.; Ma, J.; Zhang, B.; Wang, H.; Li, Y.; Han, J. Reducing salt intake in China with "action on salt China"(ASC): Protocol for campaigns and randomized controlled trials. *JMIR Res. Protoc.* **2020**, *9*, e15933. [CrossRef] [PubMed]
104. Wang, X.; Zhang, X.; Zhou, M.; Juan, J.; Wang, X. Association of prepregnancy body mass index, rate of gestational weight gain with pregnancy outcomes in Chinese urban women. *Nutr. Metab.* **2019**, *16*, 54. [CrossRef] [PubMed]
105. Vanstone, M.; Kandasamy, S.; Giacomini, M.; DeJean, D.; McDonald, S.D. Pregnant women's perceptions of gestational weight gain: A systematic review and meta-synthesis of qualitative research. *Matern. Child Nutr.* **2017**, *13*, e12374. [CrossRef] [PubMed]
106. Yong, C.; Liu, H.; Yang, Q.; Luo, J.; Ouyang, Y.; Sun, M.; Xi, Y.; Xiang, C.; Lin, Q. The Relationship between Restrained Eating, Body Image, and Dietary Intake among University Students in China: A Cross-Sectional Study. *Nutrients* **2021**, *13*, 990. [CrossRef] [PubMed]
107. Tang, C.; Cooper, M.; Wang, S.; Song, J.; He, J. The relationship between body weight and dietary restraint is explained by body dissatisfaction and body image inflexibility among young adults in China. *Eat. Weight Disord.-Stud. Anorex. Bulim. Obes.* **2021**, *26*, 1863–1870. [CrossRef] [PubMed]
108. Asim, M.; Ahmed, Z.H.; Nichols, A.R.; Rickman, R.; Neiterman, E.; Mahmood, A.; Widen, E.M. What stops us from eating: A qualitative investigation of dietary barriers during pregnancy in Punjab, Pakistan. *Public Health Nutr.* **2022**, *25*, 760–769. [CrossRef] [PubMed]
109. Huang, A.; Xiao, Y.; Hu, H.; Zhao, W.; Yang, Q.; Ma, W.; Wang, L. Gestational Weight Gain Charts by Gestational Age and Body Mass Index for Chinese Women: A Population-Based Follow-up Study. *J. Epidemiol.* **2020**, *30*, 345–353. [CrossRef]
110. Zhang, C.X.; Lai, J.Q.; Liu, K.Y.; Yang, N.H.; Zeng, G.; Mao, L.M.; Li, Z.N.; Teng, Y.; Xia, W.; Dai, N.; et al. Optimal gestational weight gain in Chinese pregnant women by Chinese-specific BMI categories: A multicentre prospective cohort study. *Public Health Nutr.* **2021**, *24*, 3210–3220. [CrossRef]
111. Gong, X.; Wu, T.; Zhang, L.; You, Y.; Wei, H.; Zuo, X.; Zhou, Y.; Xing, X.; Meng, Z.; Lv, Q.; et al. Comparison of the 2009 Institute of Medicine and 2021 Chinese guidelines for gestational weight gain: A retrospective population-based cohort study. *Int. J. Gynaecol. Obstet.* **2023**, *162*, 1033–1041. [CrossRef]
112. Patel, M.L.; Hopkins, C.M.; Brooks, T.L.; Bennett, G.G. Comparing Self-Monitoring Strategies for Weight Loss in a Smartphone App: Randomized Controlled Trial. *JMIR Mhealth Uhealth* **2019**, *7*, e12209. [CrossRef]

113. Lakens, D. Sample size justification. *Collabra Psychol.* **2022**, *8*, 33267. [CrossRef]
114. Ross, P.T.; Bibler Zaidi, N.L. Limited by our limitations. *Perspect. Med. Educ.* **2019**, *8*, 261–264. [CrossRef] [PubMed]
115. de Jersey, S.; Guthrie, T.; Tyler, J.; Ling, W.Y.; Powlesland, H.; Byrne, C.; New, K. A mixed method study evaluating the integration of pregnancy weight gain charts into antenatal care. *Matern. Child. Nutr.* **2019**, *15*, e12750. [CrossRef] [PubMed]
116. Harzheim, L.; Lorke, M.; Woopen, C.; Jünger, S. Health literacy as communicative action—A qualitative study among persons at risk in the context of predictive and preventive medicine. *Int. J. Environ. Res. Public Health* **2020**, *17*, 1718. [CrossRef]
117. Heijmans, M.; Waverijn, G.; Rademakers, J.; van der Vaart, R.; Rijken, M. Functional, communicative and critical health literacy of chronic disease patients and their importance for self-management. *Patient Educ. Couns.* **2015**, *98*, 41–48. [CrossRef]
118. Kasemsap, K. *The Fundamentals of Health Literacy, in Public Health and Welfare: Concepts, Methodologies, Tools, and Applications*; IGI Global: Hershey, PA, USA, 2017; pp. 1–21.
119. Franklin, M.; Lewis, S.; Willis, K.; Bourke-Taylor, H.; Smith, L. Patients' and healthcare professionals' perceptions of self-management support interactions: Systematic review and qualitative synthesis. *Chronic Illn.* **2017**, *14*, 79–103. [CrossRef]
120. Wu, D.Y.; Tseng, W.-S. *Introduction: The Characteristics of Chinese Culture, in Chinese Culture and Mental Health*; Elsevier: Amsterdam, The Netherlands, 1985; pp. 3–13.
121. Staggs, V.S. Pervasive errors in hypothesis testing: Toward better statistical practice in nursing research. *Int. J. Nurs. Stud.* **2019**, *98*, 87–93. [CrossRef]

Disclaimer/Publisher's Note: The statements, opinions and data contained in all publications are solely those of the individual author(s) and contributor(s) and not of MDPI and/or the editor(s). MDPI and/or the editor(s) disclaim responsibility for any injury to people or property resulting from any ideas, methods, instructions or products referred to in the content.

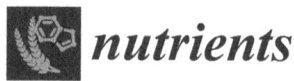

Article

Valorization of *Salicornia patula* Duval-Jouve Young Shoots in Healthy and Sustainable Diets

Irene Sánchez Gavilán [1], Daniela Velázquez Ybarzabal [2], Vicenta de la Fuente [1], Rosa M. Cámara [2], María Cortes Sánchez-Mata [2] and Montaña Cámara [2,*]

[1] Departamento Biología, Facultad de Ciencias, Universidad Autónoma de Madrid, Campus Cantoblanco, 28049 Madrid, Spain; irene.sanchezgavilan@estudiante.uam.es (I.S.G.); vdelafuente@uam.es (V.d.l.F.)

[2] Departamento Nutrición y Ciencia de los Alimentos, Facultad de Farmacia, Universidad Complutense de Madrid, Plaza Ramón y Cajal, s/n, 28040 Madrid, Spain; daniela.velazquezyl@udlap.mx (D.V.Y.); rm.camara@ucm.es (R.M.C.); cortesm@ucm.es (M.C.S.-M.)

* Correspondence: mcamara@ucm.es

Abstract: The revalorization of natural resources in food production is increasing, and the effect of climate change is negatively affecting the production of conventional crops. In recent years, edible halophytes have received more attention due to their ability to tolerate a wide range of salinities. Thus, the use of halophytes that require less water and are strongly adapted to high-salinity soil and coastal areas can provide sustainable agriculture in certain areas. In addition, there is growing interest in the study of the possibilities that these species offer as foods due to their excellent nutritional profile and antioxidant properties. For that reason, the exploitation of plants adapted to these areas is nowadays even more important than in the past to guarantee food security in arid or semiarid salinized territories. The available data about the nutrients and bioactive compounds composition of many non-cultivated edible vegetables traditionally used in the Mediterranean area, such as Salicornia edible young shoots, are still scarce. With the aim of improving the knowledge on their nutritional value, the present study provides new data about the content of some compounds with biological activity, such as fiber and organic acids, in eight samples of young shoots of *S. patula* Duval-Jouve gathered in great mainland and coastal salt marshes in Southwest and Central Spain. Results showed that this vegetable can be considered a healthy food and a very good source of dietary fiber (4.81–6.30 g/100 g fw total fiber). Its organic acid profile showed oxalic, malic, citric and succinic acids. Oxalic acid was the major one, with mean values of 0.151–1.691 g/100 g fw. From the results obtained in this study, *S. patula* shoots could be recommended as an alternative source of fiber for healthy and sustainable diets in the general adult population with no risk of renal disease.

Keywords: halophytes; dietary fiber; organic acids; sustainable diets; healthy diets

Citation: Sánchez Gavilán, I.; Velázquez Ybarzabal, D.; de la Fuente, V.; Cámara, R.M.; Sánchez-Mata, M.C.; Cámara, M. Valorization of *Salicornia patula* Duval-Jouve Young Shoots in Healthy and Sustainable Diets. *Nutrients* **2024**, *16*, 358. https://doi.org/10.3390/nu16030358

Academic Editors: António Raposo, Carol Johnston, Renata Puppin Zandonadi and Raquel Braz Assunção Botelho

Received: 21 December 2023
Revised: 20 January 2024
Accepted: 23 January 2024
Published: 25 January 2024

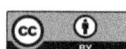

Copyright: © 2024 by the authors. Licensee MDPI, Basel, Switzerland. This article is an open access article distributed under the terms and conditions of the Creative Commons Attribution (CC BY) license (https://creativecommons.org/licenses/by/4.0/).

1. Introduction

A high dietary consumption of vegetables is globally accepted as a key point to reaching a healthy diet. Chronic diseases, such as obesity, cardiovascular disease, metabolic syndrome, and so on, are increasing in Western societies, and some modifiable factors may reduce the risk of these diseases, of which diet is one of the most important [1]. The increase in the presence of plant-based foods in the diet has been proposed to improve the health status of the population. In light of this fact, the recovery of autochthonous species in the diet is a valuable tool to achieve: (i) the diversification of plant-based foods in the diet; (ii) the intake of different nutrients and bioactive compounds from different species, which on the whole may act in a synergistic way; and (iii) the preservation of traditional dietary habits and biodiversity, which contribute to rural development.

These points are within the principles of the Mediterranean Diet, which encourages the use of a wide range of crops for cereals, fruits, and vegetables, not only cultivated products but also wild species, thus sustaining them together with local and traditional knowledge about their use. This dietary pattern has been widely postulated as a healthy model that may reduce the risk of several chronic diseases [2].

The WHO recommends a minimum daily intake of 400 g of vegetables and fruits as a population target. However, the consumption of vegetables and fruits by the Spanish population is below these recommendations, as has been shown in the different nutritional surveys and in the national health surveys [3]. One of the reasons to make this recommendation is the fact that fiber consumption in Western societies is insufficient, and its deficiency is directly linked to certain diseases. Fiber is a key group of compounds that should be present in the diet to provide important health benefits such as the regulation of intestinal transit, satiety, retardation of glucose and fat absorption, lowering cholesterol levels in the plasm and improvement of the gut microbiota. This involves positive effects against constipation, obesity, diabetes, dislipemia and cardiovascular diseases, as well as a reduction in the risk of some colorectal cancers [4,5]. To achieve these benefits, the recommendations for consumption of Total Dietary Fiber in adults, according to the European Food Safety Authority (EFSA), are 25 g/day, including a proportion of 3:1 for insoluble:soluble fiber, based on epidemiological studies that show protection against cardiovascular diseases. Providing the different mechanisms of action of the compounds included in the insoluble and soluble fiber fractions, the intake of both fractions is recommended [5]. The required daily fiber intake can be obtained from foods such as fruits and vegetables, whole grains, legumes, nuts, and others, or by eating foods enriched with fiber as a functional ingredient [6].

It Is well known that many leafy vegetables may have high levels of oxalic acid; this compound, when ingested in high amounts, is excreted in urine, causing hyperoxaluria, which leads to the deposition of calcium oxalate in kidney tissue or crystallization as calcium oxalate kidney calculus (nephrolithiasis). The minimal lethal dose of this organic acid for adults has been established as 5 g per day, which is a very difficult level to reach in a normal and balanced diet. However, people with a sensitivity to this kind of calculus should reduce the amount of oxalic acid in their diet to avoid this problem. Besides this, oxalate forms insoluble complexes with minerals such as Ca and, to a lesser extent, Mg in the gut; the insoluble complexes precipitate and are not absorbed, leading to a lower bioavailability of these minerals and also less absorption of oxalates. Thus, a high intake of these minerals is desirable to impair the negative effects of oxalic acid as both the urinary deposition of absorbed oxalic acid, and the reduction of mineral absorption [7].

The Food and Agriculture Organization of the United Nations (FAO) is concerned about promoting new models of agriculture using locally adapted management practices to provide sustainable agriculture and rural development. FAO highlights soil salinization affecting food security and remarks on "the importance of the selection of salt-tolerant crops and plants, including halophytes, which are able to grow well in such environments" [8].

Severe salinization of agricultural land due to the improper use of irrigation and fertilizers is reducing the area of arable land in the world [9]. Moreover, currently one-sixth of the world population inhabits arid or semiarid regions [10]; in these areas, soil salinization is a key issue with substantial impact on plant productivity, making fresh fruit and vegetable cultivation difficult and representing a serious threat to food security [11]. Harvesting salt-tolerant crops can provide an economic resource in soils with severe salinization. To survive in these saline environments, plants have developed different adaptive mechanisms, including altered growth patterns, osmotic adjustment, and ion homeostasis [12].

Halophytes represent about 1% of the world's flora and are found in salt deserts and saline areas such as beaches, salt marshes, and mangroves. The majority of the crop and forage species used in modern agriculture are salt-sensitive (glycophytes) and can handle only a very limited concentration of salt in their growth media. In fact, halophytes can tolerate a wide range of salinities, even beyond seawater concentration (approx. 500 mM NaCl), and can withstand harsh conditions, such as drought and intense UV radiation [13]. For these reasons, there is a growing economic interest in the study and production of halophytic plants for food uses [14–16], as wild halophyte plants have been traditionally used since ancient times in different areas worldwide, where people living in salinized areas have adapted to the surrounding vegetation.

A health concern regarding the use of halphytes as foods is related to their high Na content. While most vegetables contain a very low Na amount (about 25 mg/100 g or less), many halophytes grow in salinized soils and may accumulate Na up to 1 g/100 g in young shoots and other edible parts [17]. This may be inconvenient, as dietary Na levels should be low to avoid hypertension and reduce cardiovascular risk. For this reason, a maximum intake of sodium of 2 g/day has been recommended by EFSA (2017) [4]. Despite this fact, the use of halophytes to replace common salt in foods such as salads or others may be a good strategy, just as fiber and other nutrients are improved in the diet.

Among halophyte plants, the Chenopodiaceae family is the most, with *Salicornia* species being the most frequently eaten [18,19]. These species grow and have been used as traditional food and in folk medicine in many different regions, particularly in Mediterranean countries such as Spain, Portugal, Italy, and Tunisia [10,11]. In England, France, the USA, and Australia, they were also known as "herbe de Saint Pierre", anglicized in the mid-16th century as samphire, and consumed in situations of extreme need such as famines [20].

In the particular case of *S. patula*, it is well known as an authoctonous species from the Iberin flora, with an essential presence in the habitat of Community Interest No. 1510, "Mediterranean salt steppes", which is mainly present in the autonomous communities of Andalusia, Castilla la Mancha, and Murcia (Spain) in the Natura 2000 European network [21,22]. As with other species of Salicornia, it has been traditionally used as a food in many different regions of the Mediterranean area where it grows. As an example, *S. europaea* L. is often consumed as a salad dressing or as a side dish for fish [19], and it is currently listed as a traditional vegetable in the Apulia region (Italy), where also cultivation attempts of *S. patula* have been made along Lesina lagoon [23,24]. Recently, in Setubal (Portugal), a different halophyte, *S. perennis*, was incorporated as a food ingredient into crackers, like savory snacks, to replace sodium [25]; it has also been powdered, dried, and incorporated into bread to reduce the same amount of sodium [26]. Furthermore, the use of dried *S. ramosissima* as a salt substitute shows great potential as an alternative replacement for sodium-based additives, and their sprouts are steamed and subsequently added to salads or other stews in the Valencian region (Spain) [27], and *S. patula* is also described for food use in Eastern Spain [20].

Thus, looking to safeguard economic and environmental sustainability, the remarkable tolerance of *S. patula* to salinity, drought and high temperatures and its low input needs for cultivation make this plant a resilient crop for the immediate future [28].

In relation to health benefits, some studies have confirmed that *S. patula* is a good source of macronutrients, essential minerals, and some bioactive compounds such as polyphenols, fatty acids, and vitamins [24,29–31]. However, there is a lack of knowledge about the fiber content and some bioactive compounds in the edible parts of this species.

With the aim of improving current diets in a healthy and sustainable way and the valorization of *S. patula* bioactive compounds, the present study is focused on the content of fiber and organic acids in the young shoots of wild *S. patula* samples from different geographical locations in Spain. This knowledge will contribute to revalorizing these wild halophyte species and promoting their crop adaptation for culinary uses, especially in semi-arid regions where the drought seriously threatens the agriculture productivity and compromises food security.

2. Materials and Methods

2.1. Plant Material

Young shoots of wild *S. patula* were collected in their saline natural habitats within the Iberian distribution ranges focused in southwest and central Spain. Eight different geographical locations in Spain, five of them; S1 to S5 are located close to Tinto River area (southwest Spain) and the other three S6 to S8 are located at the center of the Iberian Peninsula, as is shown in Table 1.

Table 1. Description of sites in Spain where *S. patula* Duval-Jouve young shoots were collected.

Sample ID	Site	Grid Reference MGRS
S1	Huelva, La Rábida	29SPB8320
S2	Huelva, Moguer	29SPB7729
S3	Huelva, El Terrón	29SPB4717
S4	Huelva, San Juan del Puerto	29SPB9230
S5	Huelva, Monumento a Colón	29SPB8220
S6	Valladolid Aldeamayor de San Martín	30TUL6196
S7	Madrid, Colmenar de Oreja	31TVK5143
S8	Toledo, Laguna larga de Villacañas	30SYH0928

Plant materials were collected at their optimal status for food consumption: succulent and tender, young shoots. Samples were processed as follows: whole plant was carried to the lab on fridge at 4 °C. Once in the lab, samples were cleaned and young edible shoots were dried in oven at 95 °C and homogenized (dry powder plant material). Then, samples were stored in airtight jars at room temperature and darkness. All analytical determinations were made in triplicate for each sample coming from each collection area.

2.2. Moisture Determination

Moisture was determined by desiccation in an oven at 105 °C for 24 h until a constant weight was reached [32].

2.3. Fiber Determination

The insoluble (IF), soluble (SF), and total dietary fiber (TDF) contents were determined on dried plant material by the enzymatic gravimetric method AOAC 993.19 (FS) and 991.42 (FI) [32,33]. To obtain the insoluble fiber, samples were subject to enzymatic digestion with α-amylase, protease, and amyloglucosidase (Sigma-Aldrich, St. Louis, MO, USA) in order to hydrolyze the protein and starch present in the samples. The liquid obtained was filtrated on Pyrex crucibles with a number 2 filter plate. Insoluble fiber residue was dried in an oven at 100 °C and then weighed. The filtrate was stored in a 500 mL flask with the addition of 400 mL of 96% v/v ethanol and precipitated from one day to the next. Then, it was filtered again through crucibles with the same conditions to obtain the soluble fiber residue. In both residues, the content of protein and ash was determined, and the content corresponding to insoluble and soluble fiber was calculated (with the subtraction of protein and ash).

2.4. Determination of Organic Acids

Individual organic acids were determined by HPLC, based on procedures optimized by [33] and applied to different types of plant samples by [34–36]. Extraction was performed with 0.5 g of dried sample in 25 mL of 4.5% m-phosphoric acid and analyzed using an HPLC-UV methodology.

The HPLC equipment was a liquid chromatographer equipped with an isocratic pump (model PU-II, Micron Analítica, Madrid, Spain), an AS-1555 automatic injector (Jasco, Tokyo, Japan), a Sphereclone ODS (2) 250 × 4.60, 5 mm Phenomenex column (Torrance, CA, USA), a UV detector (Thermo Separation Specta Series UV100, San Jose, CA, USA) working at 215 nm. The mobile phase was 1.8 mmol/L H_2SO_4 (pH 2.6) at 0.4 mL/min flow rate. Data were analyzed using Chromonec XP software (Micronec, Madrid, Spain). Identification was performed comparing retention times with those obtained from commercial pure standards of oxalic, malic, citric, and succinic acids. Quantification was based on the UV signal response, and the resultant peak areas in the chromatograms were plotted against concentrations obtained from standards (Figure 1). Organic acids contents in *S. patula* samples were expressed as mg/100 g of fresh plant material.

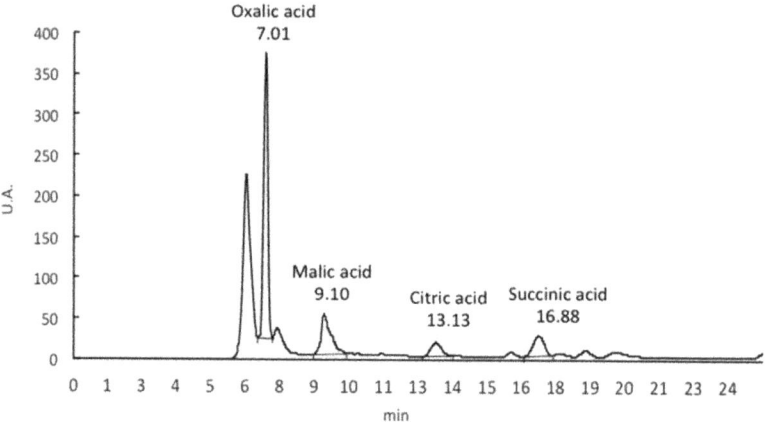

Figure 1. Chromatogram obtained for organic acids in *S. patula* Duval-Jouve edible shoot samples.

2.5. Statistical Analysis

Statistical analysis was performed using Statgraphics 18.0 software. Mean and standard deviations were calculated. The data were transformed logarithmically after verifying normality with the Shapiro–Wilk test ($p > 0.05$). To test the possible differences between three or more groups, they were compared using an ANOVA analysis of variance. Bonferroni corrections between means were calculated only if an F test was significant at $p < 0.05$.

3. Results and Discussion

Table 2 shows the values obtained for the moisture, fiber, and organic acid content (fresh weight, fw) of the fresh *S. patula* shoots belonging to the eight populations analyzed in this study.

Table 2. Total, insoluble, and soluble fiber contents (g/100 g fresh weight) in *S. patula* Duval-Jouve samples, and contribution of each fraction to total dietary fiber content (results presented as mean ± SD).

Sample	Moisture	Insoluble Fiber	Soluble Fiber	Total Fiber
S1	90.121 ± 0.621 [a]	4.417 ± 0.101 [a]	0.841 ± 0.323 [a]	5.269 ± 0.336 [a]
S2	89.876 ± 1.123 [b]	4.800 ± 0.441 [ab]	1.409 ± 0.134 [b]	6.301 ± 0.438 [b]
S3	90.725 ± 0.731 [a]	4.603 ± 0.614 [ab]	1.114 ± 0.190 [b]	5.782 ± 0.811 [a]
S4	91.041 ± 0.775 [ab]	4.612 ± 0.140 [a]	0.488 ± 0.182 [a]	5.104 ± 0.276 [ab]
S5	90.183 ± 1.411 [a]	5.660 ± 0.312 [b]	0.519 ± 0.081 [a]	6.185 ± 0.290 [a]
S6	91.290 ± 1.012 [ab]	5.682 ± 0.129 [a]	0.793 ± 0.073 [a]	6.307 ± 0.273 [ab]
S7	90.763 [a] ± 1.356 [a]	3.996 ± 0.181 [a]	1.034 ± 0.372 [b]	5.038 ± 0.543 [a]
S8	91.111 ± 0.813 [ab]	4.229 ± 0.163 [a]	0.568 ± 0.051 [a]	4.812 ± 0.221 [ab]

In each column, different superscript letters mean statistically significant differences ($p < 0.05$) compared by Shapiro–Wilk test.

S. patula edible shoots had a moisture content with few differences among the analyzed samples between 89.8 and 91.3 g/100 g, which confers them tender and succulent characteristics. The *Salicornia* sample collected in Valladolid, in the center of the Iberian Peninsula, stood out with the highest moisture value (91.3 g/100 g), whereas sample 2 from "Moguer", Huelva, presented the lowest moisture content (89.8 g/100 g) [29,30].

Regarding fiber content, the *S. patula* fresh shoots studied contained between 4.8 g/100 g fw and 6.6 g/100 g fw (53–73 g/100 g dw), with insoluble fiber being the predominant fraction, with an average proportion of 84.79% (Figure 2). Few significant variations can be found in the values reported, with the exception of soluble fiber, where S2, S3, and S7 stood out with higher values than other samples. These variations cannot be attributed exclusively to a single factor, but they may be a product of the natural variability found in biological samples.

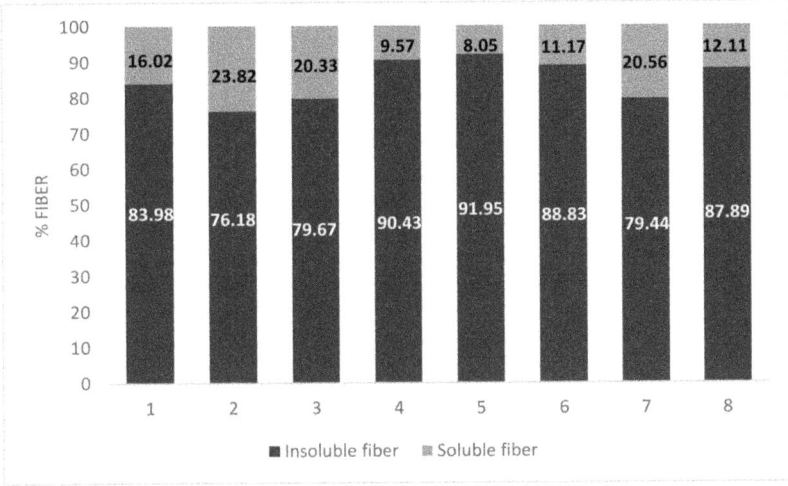

Figure 2. Proportions of insoluble and soluble fiber in *S. patula* Duval-Jouve fresh samples (g/100 g dw).

This is the first report on the fiber content of *S. patula* young shoots. Despite this variability, the comparison with other edible halophyte species shows higher values for *Suaeda fruticosa* Forrsk shoots with 10 and 12 g/100 g fw, similar to *Arthrocnemum macrostachyum* Moric. and *Halocnemum strobilaceum* Pall (M). Bieb., from Tunisia, with 10.1 and 9.1 g/100 g [37].

On the other hand, other halophytes native to Portugal, such as *S. perennis alpini* (Lag) Castroviejo, have been reported to contain 15.3% of total dietary fiber, and *S. ramosissima* J. Woods presented values of 11.2% dw, both of which are being considered as fiber-rich vegetables [11]. *S. patula* young shoots analyzed in this study presented higher values of fiber than both species.

Thus, from the point of view of fiber content, *S. patula* edible parts may be a very good contributor to the diet. The contribution of 4.8–6.6 g of fiber per a portion of 100 g of *S. patula* young shoots is higher than that of other leafy vegetables and could cover up to 19–25% of the recommended intake of total dietary fiber per day, which is a relevant amount. When comparing fiber levels with other vegetables [38], it can be seen that most leafy vegetables present 2–4 g/100 g fiber; *S. patula* provides a higher amount of fiber than most conventional fresh vegetables, being only surpassed by artichokes (about 9 g/100 g). Therefore, the recovery of this vegetable as a food may be a key tool to improve fiber intake in the diet and thus the health status of the population. Regarding the proportions of soluble/insoluble fiber, the analyzed samples present high proportions of insoluble fiber contributing to the effects on intestinal transit and satiety, among others. For those reasons, and according to Regulation (EC) No. 1924/2006 of the European Parliament and of the Council of 20 December 2006 on nutrition and health claims made on food, *S. patula* young shoots could be claimed as "sources of fiber" for providing more than 3 g fiber/100 g fresh plant, and in many cases, as "high amounts of fiber" for providing more than 6 g fiber/100 g [39].

Table 3 shows the organic acid profile and content of the analyzed samples. The identified organic acids were oxalic, malic, citric, and succinic acids. As expected, oxalic acid is predominant, as occurs in other leafy vegetables, with wide variability between 1.73 mg/100 g dw and 18.34 mg/100 g dw, corresponding to 0.151 g/100 g fw and 1.69 g/100 g fw.

Table 3. Organic acids contents (g/100 g fresh weight) in *S. patula* Duval-Jouve samples (results presented as mean ± SD).

Sample	Oxalic Acid	Malic Acid	Citric Acid	Succinic Acid	Oxalic Acid/Ca
S1	0.8224 ± 0.061 [a]	0.016 ± 0.002 [a]	0.072 ± 0.008 [b]	0.033 ± 0.008 [a]	8.132 ± 0.241 [a]
S2	1.060 ± 0.018 [b]	0.015 ± 0.001 [a]	0.020 ± 0.003 [a]	0.012 ± 0.004 [b]	11.381 ± 1.313 [b]
S3	1.691 ± 0.007 [b]	Nd	Nd	Nd	34.006 ± 3.711 [ab]
S4	1.187 ± 0.067 [b]	0.087 ± 0.053 [b]	Nd	0.009 ± 0.003 [a]	11.082 ± 1.192 [a]
S5	1.533 ± 0.045 [b]	0.016 ± 0.011 [a]	Nd	0.077 ± 0.001 [b]	7.581 [a] ± 0.237 [a]
S6	0.151 ± 0.023 [ab]	0.024 ± 0.071 [a]	Nd	Nd	6.689 ± 1.052 [a]
S7	0.758 ± 0.013 [a]	0.019 ± 0.017 [a]	0.004 ± 0.000 [a]	Nd	8.061 ± 1.133 [a]
S8	0.877 ± 0.555 [a]	Nd	0.003 ± 0.000 [a]	Nd	4.763 ± 0.920 [ab]

In each row, different superscript letters mean statistically significant differences ($p < 0.05$) compared by Shapiro–Wilk test. Nd = non detected.

Although it has quite low toxicity (with 5 g as the minimal lethal dose for an adult), this compound may reduce dietary calcium bioaccessibility through the formation of an insoluble complex as well as the formation of calcium oxalate kidney calculus [40]. For those reasons, some authors recommended a molar oxalic acid/Ca ratio not higher than 2.5 in the foods to avoid this effect [41,42].

To calculate the oxalic acid/Ca ratio, the data on the calcium content previously obtained in the analysis of the same Salicornia samples by Inductively Coupled Plasma Mass Spectrometry [29] were used. The ratios obtained are presented in Table 3, showing a ratio higher than 2.5, higher than nutritionally desirable. Samples collected from the "Tinto River", in Southwest Spain (S1 to S5) showed a greater variety and amount of organic acids, with oxalic acid standing out, and the oxalic acid/Ca ratio is higher in these samples than in the material from Central Spain (S6 to S8). The differences in oxalic acid/Ca ratio between young shoots of *S. patula* could be related to the different elemental compositions of the soil. Calcium content is very low in the Tinto River area and higher in soils from central Spain [29].

It can be seen that, although this species should be considered an oxalic-rich vegetable, even samples with the highest amounts of oxalic acid (S3) would not provide more than 1.6 g of this undesirable compound in a standard 100 g portion. Very high amounts of this plant (about 250 g) that are hardly eaten by humans would be necessary to reach toxic doses. Thus, for the general population and with a reasonable consumption (portions lower than 100 g) within the context of a diversified diet, the oxalic acid content of this vegetable would not represent a potential risk for human consumption, according to the results presented. However, given that the content of this compound is high and the low oxalic acid/calcium ratio, young children and people who easily form kidney oxalate calculus should avoid the ingestion of oxalic acid-rich species. Another alternative could be boiling to reduce oxalic acid content by dissolution, as it is done with other vegetables [7,31]. However, highly vulnerable people should avoid this kind of vegetable.

Other minor organic acids present in *S. patula* were malic, citric, and succinic acids but they did not appear in all samples analyzed. Malic acid is present in five of eight analyzed samples, with ranges between 0.157 and 0.979 g/100 g dw. Other authors suggested malic acid accumulation in other *Salicornioideae*, like *S. perennis* from "Mira" (Portugal), under stressful situations, increasing in vegetative stages with high salinity and lower water content [43].

Citric acid was detected only in four of eight samples, with values between 0.201 and 0.719 g/100 g dw. Our results were significantly lower compared to other studies [44], reporting higher content: 8.60 mg/100 g in *Salicornia ramosissima* form "Ría Formosa" (Portugal) and 6.98 mg/100 g dw in *Sarcocornia perennis* (Miller) A. J. Scott and were similar compared with those of *Sarcocornia fructicosa* (L) A. J. Scott and *Salicornia bigelovii* Torr. [15,45]. In some Australian halophytes, *Atriplex nummularia* Lindl, *Suaeda arbusculoides* L.S.Sm, and *Sesuvium portulacastrum* (L) L., higher citric acid values, between 3.33 and 23.9 g/kg dw, have been reported [46].

Succinic acid is present in four of eight, with a content between 0.109 and 0.785 g/100 g dw. Succinic acid in other halophytes like *S. perennis* shows higher content in the vegetative segment than the fruit segment in three different locations of "Ría de Aveiro", with an average of 0.17 and 0.51 µg/mg. Other authors suggested that succinic acts like an osmoprotectant in response to high-salinity environments [47].

Organic acids, either total content or individual profile, can have a significant effect on the sensory, aroma, and flavor of plant-derived foods and, subsequently, consumer acceptance [48]. All these components contribute to reinforcing the interest in this vegetable in the diet. The high presence of sodium, in levels of 1–1.7 g Na/100 g [29], makes it a candidate to be used as a substitute for salt in salads or other different food products, where they are a source of salted flavor at the same time that they provide fiber and other nutrients.

It should be pointed out the importance of a widely diversified intake of many vegetables in the diet, in which all different, either cultivated or wild, autochthonous edible species may be included. In the case of vegetables rich in oxalic acid and/or sodium species such as *S. patula*, boiling is preferable for vulnerable populations (e.g., young children, people who need to control blood pressure), while people at risk of renal disease or infants should avoid these vegetables.

4. Conclusions

In conclusion, the studied young shoots of wild Spanish halophyte, namely *S. patula*, can be considered a healthy food and a very good source of dietary fiber, with the insoluble dietary fiber fraction being the most important one, contributing to improving the nutritional quality of the current diets, even as a common salt substitute providing additional nutrients. The main organic acids present are oxalic, malic, citric, and succinic acids. Oxalic acid was the major one; the contents found would not represent a health problem in an occasional intake of an edible shoot of *S. patula*; however, young children and people who easily form kidney oxalate calculus should avoid the ingestion of oxalic acid-rich species. Boiling could also be advisable to reduce sodium and oxalic acid levels. Thus, *S. patula* could be considered a good alternative to other conventional vegetables for the diversification of sustainable diets with high nutritional potential.

Author Contributions: Conceptualization, V.d.l.F. and M.C.S.-M.; Data curation, M.C.S.-M. and M.C.; Formal analysis, I.S.G. and D.V.Y.; Funding acquisition, V.d.l.F. and M.C.; Investigation, I.S.G. and V.d.l.F.; Methodology, I.S.G., D.V.Y., R.M.C., M.C.S.-M. and M.C.; Project administration, V.d.l.F.; Writing—original draft, I.S.G., R.M.C. and M.C.S.-M.; Writing—review and editing, M.C.S.-M. and M.C. All authors have read and agreed to the published version of the manuscript.

Funding: This research was funded by Ministerio de Ciencia e Innovación, CGL2015-66242-R grant and by UCM-ALIMNOVA Research Group, ref: 951505. Irene Sánchez Gavilán was a recipient of a predoctoral program to "Ministerio de Economía, Industria y Competitividad" (BES 2016-077732).

Institutional Review Board Statement: Not applicable.

Informed Consent Statement: Not applicable.

Data Availability Statement: Data is available only upon request. Tables included in the manuscript show all the data.

Conflicts of Interest: The authors declare no conflict of interest.

References

1. Yokoyama, Y.; Levin, S.M.; Barnard, N.D. Association between plant-based diets and plasma lipids: A systematic review and meta-analysis. *Nutr. Rev.* **2017**, *75*, 683–698. [CrossRef]
2. Guasch-Ferré, M.; Willett, W.C. The Mediterranean diet and health: A comprehensive overview. *J. Intern. Med.* **2021**, *290*, 549–566. [CrossRef] [PubMed]
3. López García, E.; Bretón Lesmes, I.; Díaz Perales, A.; Moreno-Arribas, V.; Portillo Baquedano, M.P.; Rivas Velasco, A.M.; Fresán Salvo, U.; Tejedor Romero, L.; Ortega Porcel, F.B.; Aznar Laín, S.; et al. Informe del Comité Científico de la Agencia Española de Seguridad Alimentaria y Nutrición (AESAN) sobre recomendaciones dietéticas sostenibles y recomendaciones de actividad física para la población española. *Rev. Com. Cient. AESAN* **2022**, *36*, 11–70.

4. European Food Safety Authority (EFSA). Dietary reference values for nutrients: Summary report. *EFSA Support. Publ.* **2017**, *92*, e15121. [CrossRef]
5. Marlett, J.A.; McBurney, M.I.; Slavin, J.L. Position of the American Dietetic Association: Health implications of dietary fiber. *J. Am. Diet. Assoc.* **2002**, *102*, 993–1000. [CrossRef] [PubMed]
6. Cámara, M.; Fernández-Ruiz, V.; Morales, P.; Cortes Sánchez-Mata, M. Fiber compounds and human health. *Curr. Pharm. Des.* **2017**, *23*, 2835–2849. [CrossRef]
7. García-Herrera, P.; Morales, P.; Cámara, M.; Fernández-Ruiz, V.; Tardío, J.; Sánchez-Mata, M.C. Nutritional and phytochemical composition of Mediterranean wild vegetables after culinary treatment. *Foods* **2020**, *9*, 1761. [CrossRef] [PubMed]
8. Benedetti, F.; Caon, L. *Global Soil Laboratory Assessment 2020—Laboratories' Capacities and Needs*; FAO: Rome, Italy, 2021; Available online: https://www.fao.org/3/cb6395en/cb6395en.pdf (accessed on 21 December 2023).
9. Hasnain, M.; Abideen, Z.; Ali, F.; Hasanuzzaman, M.; El-Keblawy, A. Potential of Halophytes as Sustainable Fodder Production by Using Saline Resources: A Review of Current Knowledge and Future Directions. *Plants* **2023**, *12*, 2150. [CrossRef]
10. Khondoker, M.; Mandal, S.; Gurav, R.; Hwang, S. Freshwater Shortage, Salinity Increase, and Global Food Production: A Need for Sustainable Irrigation Water Desalination—A Scoping Review. *Earth* **2023**, *4*, 223–240. [CrossRef]
11. Lopes, M.; Silva, A.S.; Séndon, R.; Barbosa-Pereira, L.; Cavaleiro, C.; Ramos, F. Towards the Sustainable Exploitation of Salt-Tolerant Plants: Nutritional Characterisation, Phenolics Composition, and Potential Contaminants Analysis of Salicornia ramosissima and Sarcocornia perennis alpini. *Molecules* **2023**, *28*, 2726. [CrossRef]
12. Flowers, T.J.; Colmer, T.D. Salinity tolerance in halophytes. *New Phytol.* **2008**, *179*, 945–963. [CrossRef] [PubMed]
13. Vizetto-Duarte, C.; Figueiredo, F.; Rodrigues, M.J.; Polo, C.; Rešek, E.; Custódio, L. Sustainable valorization of halophytes from the mediterranean area: A comprehensive evaluation of their fatty acid profile and implications for human and animal nutrition. *Sustainability* **2019**, *11*, 2197. [CrossRef]
14. Hamed, K.B.; Castagna, A.; Ranieri, A.; Garcia-Caparros, P.; Santin, M.; Hernandez, J.A.; Espin, G.B. Halophyte based Mediterranean agriculture in the contexts of food insecurity and global climate change. *Environ. Exp. Bot.* **2021**, *191*, 104601. [CrossRef]
15. Ventura, Y.; Wuddineh, W.A.; Myrzabayeva, M.; Alikulov, Z.; Khozin-Goldberg, I.; Shpigel, M.; Samocha, T.; Sagi, M. Effect of seawater concentration on the productivity and nutritional value of annual Salicornia and perennial *Sarcocornia halophytes* as leafy vegetable crops. *Sci. Hortic.* **2011**, *128*, 189–196. [CrossRef]
16. Petropoulos, S.A.; Karkanis, A.; Martins, N.; Ferreira, I.C. Halophytic herbs of the Mediterranean basin: An alternative approach to health. *Food Chem. Toxicol.* **2018**, *114*, 155–169. [CrossRef]
17. García-Herrera, P.; Sánchez-Mata, M.D.C. The contribution of wild plants to dietary intakes of micronutrients (II): Mineral Elements. In *Mediterranean Wild Edible Plants: Ethnobotany and Food Composition Tables*; Sánchez-Mata, M., Tardío, J., Eds.; Springer: New York, NY, USA, 2016; pp. 141–171.
18. Cárdenas-Pérez, S.; Piernik, A.; Chanona-Pérez, J.J.; Grigore, M.N.; Perea-Flores, M.J. An overview of the emerging trends of the *Salicornia* L. genus as a sustainable crop. *Environ. Exp. Bot.* **2021**, *191*, 104606. [CrossRef]
19. Loconsole, D.; Cristiano, G.; De Lucia, B. Glassworts: From wild salt marsh species to sustainable edible crops. *Agriculture* **2019**, *9*, 14. [CrossRef]
20. Ríos, S.; Obón, C.; Martínez-Francés, V.; Verde, A.; Ariza, D.; Laguna, E. Halophytes as Food: Gastroethnobotany of Halophytes. In *Handbook of Halophytes: From Molecules to Ecosystems towards Biosaline Agriculture*; Springer: Berlin/Heidelberg, Germany, 2020; pp. 1–36.
21. De la Cruz, M. 1510 Estepas salinas mediterráneas (Limonietalia) (*). In *Bases Ecológicas Preliminares Para la Conservación de los Tipos de Hábitat de Interés Comunitario en España*; Ministerio de Medio Ambiente, y Medio Rural y Marino: Madrid, Spain, 2009; 78p.
22. Rivas Martínez, S.; Herrera, M. Data on *Salicornia* L. (Chenopodiaceae) in Spain. *An. Jard. Bot. Madr.* **1996**, *54*, 149–154.
23. Urbano, M.; Tomaselli, V.; Bisignano, V.; Veronico, G.; Hammer, K.; Laghetti, G. Salicornia patula Duval-Jouve: From gathering of wild plants to some attempts of cultivation in Apulia region (southern Italy). *Genet. Resour. Crop Evol.* **2017**, *64*, 1465–1472. [CrossRef]
24. Accogli, R.; Tomaselli, V.; Direnzo, P.; Perrino, E.V.; Albanese, G.; Urbano, M.; Laghetti, G. Edible halophytes and halo-tolerant species in Apulia region (Southeastern Italy): Biogeography, traditional food use and potential sustainable crops. *Plants* **2023**, *12*, 549. [CrossRef]
25. Clavel-Coibrié, E.; Sales, J.R.; da Silva, A.M.; Barroca, M.J.; Sousa, I.; Raymundo, A. *Sarcocornia perennis*: A salt substitute in savory snacks. *Foods* **2021**, *10*, 3110. [CrossRef]
26. Barroca, M.J.; Flores, C.; Ressurreição, S.; Guiné, R.; Osório, N.; Moreira da Silva, A. Re-Thinking Table Salt Reduction in Bread with Halophyte Plant Solutions. *Appl. Sci.* **2023**, *13*, 5342. [CrossRef]
27. Peris, J.B.; Guillen, A.; Roselló, R.; Laguna, E.; Ferrer-Gallego, P.P.; Gómez-Navarro, J. Les plantes utilitzades en les ensalades campestres valencianes. *Nemus* **2019**, *9*, 46–64.
28. Singh, D.; Buhmann, A.K.; Flowers, T.J.; Seal, C.E.; Papenbrock, J. *Salicornia* as a crop plant in temperate regions: Selection of genetically characterized ecotypes and optimization of their cultivation conditions. *AoB Plants* **2014**, *10*, 6. [CrossRef] [PubMed]
29. Sánchez-Gavilán, I.; Rufo, L.; Rodríguez, N.; de la Fuente, V. On the elemental composition of the Mediterranean euhalophyte *Salicornia patula* Duval-Jouve (Chenopodiaceae) from saline habitats in Spain (Huelva, Toledo and Zamora). *Environ. Sci. Pollut. Res.* **2021**, *28*, 2719–2727. [CrossRef] [PubMed]

30. Sánchez-Gavilán, I.; Ramírez, E.; de la Fuente, V. Bioactive Compounds in *Salicornia patula* Duval-Jouve: A Mediterranean Edible Euhalophyte. *Foods* **2021**, *10*, 410. [CrossRef] [PubMed]
31. Sánchez-Mata, M.C.; Cabrera Loera, R.D.; Morales, P.; Fernández-Ruiz, V.; Cámara, M.; Díez Marqués, C.; Pardo de Santayana, M.; Tardío, J. Wild vegetables of the Mediterranean area as valuable sources of bioactive compounds. *Genet. Resour. Crop Evol.* **2012**, *59*, 431–443. [CrossRef]
32. Horowitz, W.; Latimer, G.W. *Official Methods of Analysis of AOAC International*, 18th ed.; AOAC International: Gaithersburg, MD, USA, 2006.
33. AOAC. *Official Methods of Analysis (Supplement March 1995)*; Ref. 993.19. Vitamins and Other Nutrients; AOAC International: Gaithersburg, MD, USA, 1993.
34. Maieves, H.A.; López-Froilán, R.; Morales, P.; Pérez-Rodríguez, M.L.; Ribani, R.H.; Cámara, M.; Sánchez-Mata, M.C. Antioxidant phytochemicals of *Hovenia dulcis* Thunb. peduncles in different maturity stages. *J. Funct. Foods* **2015**, *18*, 1117–1124. [CrossRef]
35. Arias-Rico, J.; Cruz-Cansino, N.D.S.; Cámara-Hurtado, M.; López-Froilán, R.; Pérez-Rodríguez, M.L.; Sánchez-Mata, M.D.C.; Jaramillo-Morales, O.A.; Barrera-Gálvez, R.; Ramírez-Moreno, E. Study of xoconostle (*Opuntia* spp.) powder as source of dietary fiber and antioxidants. *Foods* **2020**, *9*, 403. [CrossRef]
36. Igual, M.; García-Herrera, P.; Cámara, R.M.; Martínez-Monzó, J.; García-Segovia, P.; Cámara, M. Bioactive compounds in rosehip (*Rosa canina*) powder with encapsulating agents. *Molecules* **2022**, *27*, 4737. [CrossRef]
37. Zaier, M.M.; Ciudad-Mulero, M.; Cámara, M.; Pereira, C.; Ferreira, I.C.; Achour, L.; Kacem, A.; Morales, P. Revalorization of Tunisian wild Amaranthaceae halophytes: Nutritional composition variation at two different phenotypes stages. *J. Food Compos. Anal.* **2020**, *89*, 103463. [CrossRef]
38. BEDCA Database. Available online: https://www.bedca.net/bdpub/ (accessed on 21 December 2023).
39. European Parliament. Regulation (EC) No. 1924/2006 of the European Parliament and of the Council of 20 December 2006 on nutrition and health claims made on foods. *Off. J. Eur. Union* **2006**, *404*, 9.
40. Morales, P.; Ferreira, I.C.; Carvalho, A.M.; Sánchez-Mata, M.C.; Cámara, M.; Fernández-Ruiz, V.; Pardo de Santayana, M.; Tardío, J. Mediterranean non-cultivated vegetables as dietary sources of compounds with antioxidant and biological activity. *LWT-Food Sci. Technol.* **2014**, *55*, 389–396. [CrossRef]
41. Concon, J.M. *Toxicology. Principles and Concepts*; Marcel Dekker: New York, NY, USA, 1988.
42. Derache, R. *Toxicología y Seguridad de los Alimentos*; Omega: Barcelona, Spain, 1990.
43. Magni, N.N.; Veríssimo, A.C.; Silva, H.; Pinto, D.C. Metabolomic Profile of Salicornia perennis Plant's Organs under Diverse in Situ Stress: The Ria de Aveiro Salt Marshes Case. *Metabolites* **2023**, *13*, 280. [CrossRef] [PubMed]
44. Antunes, M.D.; Gago, C.; Guerreiro, A.; Sousa, A.R.; Julião, M.; Miguel, M.G.; Faleiro, M.L.; Panagopoulos, T. Nutritional characterization and storage ability of *Salicornia ramosissima* and *Sarcocornia perennis* for fresh vegetable salads. *Horticulturae* **2021**, *7*, 6. [CrossRef]
45. Lu, D.; Zhang, M.; Wang, S.; Cai, J.; Zhou, X.; Zhu, C. Nutritional characterization and changes in quality of *Salicornia bigelovii* Torr. during storage. *LWT-Food Sci. Technol.* **2010**, *43*, 519–524. [CrossRef]
46. Srivarathan, S.; Phan, A.D.T.; Hong, H.T.; Netzel, G.; Wright, O.R.; Sultanbawa, Y.; Netzel, M.E. Nutritional composition and anti-nutrients of underutilized Australian indigenous edible halophytes—Saltbush, Seablite and Seapurslane. *J. Food Compos. Anal.* **2023**, *115*, 104876. [CrossRef]
47. Kumari, A.; Das, P.; Parida, A.K.; Agarwal, P.K. Proteomics, metabolomics, and ionomics perspectives of salinity tolerance in halophytes. *Front. Plant Sci.* **2015**, *6*, 537. [CrossRef]
48. Jiang, Z.; Huang, Q.; Jia, D.; Zhong, M.; Tao, J.; Liao, G.; Huang, C.; Xu, X. Characterization of Organic Acid Metabolism and Expression of Related Genes During Fruit Development of *Actinidia eriantha* 'Ganmi 6'. *Plants* **2020**, *9*, 332. [CrossRef]

Disclaimer/Publisher's Note: The statements, opinions and data contained in all publications are solely those of the individual author(s) and contributor(s) and not of MDPI and/or the editor(s). MDPI and/or the editor(s) disclaim responsibility for any injury to people or property resulting from any ideas, methods, instructions or products referred to in the content.

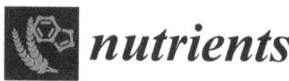

Article

The Role of the Dietitian within Family Therapy for Anorexia Nervosa (FT-AN): A Reflexive Thematic Analysis of Child and Adolescent Eating Disorder Clinician Perspectives

Cliona Brennan [1,2,3,4,*], Julian Baudinet [1,2], Mima Simic [1,2] and Ivan Eisler [1,2]

1 Maudsley Centre for Child and Adolescent Eating Disorders, South London, and Maudsley NHS Foundation Trust, De Crespigny Park, Denmark Hill, London SE5 8AZ, UK; julian.baudinet@kcl.ac.uk (J.B.); mima.simic@slam.nhs.uk (M.S.); ivan.eisler@kcl.ac.uk (I.E.)
2 Institute of Psychiatry, Psychology and Neuroscience, King's College London, De Crespigny Park, London SE5 8AZ, UK
3 Department of Human Nutrition and Dietetics, School of Health Sciences, London Metropolitan University, 166-220 Holloway Road, London N7 8DB, UK
4 Department of Child and Adolescent Psychiatry, Institute of Psychiatry, Psychology and Neuroscience, King's College London, De Crespigny Park, London SE5 8AZ, UK
* Correspondence: cliona.brennan@slam.nhs.uk

Citation: Brennan, C.; Baudinet, J.; Simic, M.; Eisler, I. The Role of the Dietitian within Family Therapy for Anorexia Nervosa (FT-AN): A Reflexive Thematic Analysis of Child and Adolescent Eating Disorder Clinician Perspectives. *Nutrients* **2024**, *16*, 670. https://doi.org/10.3390/nu16050670

Academic Editors: António Raposo, Renata Puppin Zandonadi and Raquel Braz Assunção Botelho

Received: 4 January 2024
Revised: 22 February 2024
Accepted: 23 February 2024
Published: 27 February 2024

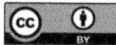

Copyright: © 2024 by the authors. Licensee MDPI, Basel, Switzerland. This article is an open access article distributed under the terms and conditions of the Creative Commons Attribution (CC BY) license (https://creativecommons.org/licenses/by/4.0/).

Abstract: Background: Despite dietitians being important members of the multidisciplinary team delivering family therapy for anorexia nervosa (FT-AN), their specific responsibilities and roles are unclear and their involvement in the treatment can be a contentious issue. Methodology: Clinicians (*n* = 20) experienced in the delivery of FT-AN who were working at a specialist child and adolescent eating disorder service responded to an online survey about their experience of including a dietitian in FT-AN and how they understand the role. Both categorical and open-ended questions were used. Reflexive thematic analysis was used to analyse the qualitative free-text responses of clinician perspectives on the role of the dietitian in FT-AN. Results: All clinicians agreed that dietetics had a role within FT-AN and most frequently sought dietetic involvement in the early phases of FT-AN. Reflexive thematic analysis of responses identified three main themes. These were (1) collaboration is key, (2) confidence as a core consideration and (3) case-by-case approach. These themes evidenced the role of the dietitian within FT-AN and highlighted both the benefits and concerns of this involvement. Conclusions: This study demonstrated that dietitians can take a core role as collaborators within therapy-led teams that facilitate joint working and sharing of expertise. However, dietetic input should be considered on a case-by-case basis, given its potential for creating an over-focus on nutrition and potentially diminishing parental confidence in feeding. When indicated for selected cases, nutritional counselling should be offered in joint sessions with the therapist rather than separately. The findings of the study were limited by the small sample size of participants recruited from a single centre and heterogeneity in the professional background of respondents. Although the integration of dietetics within the multidisciplinary team and the ability of dietitians to individualise patient care can enhance FT-AN treatment, potential benefits and disbenefits should be considered for each case.

Keywords: anorexia nervosa; adolescents; dietetics; family therapy for anorexia nervosa; reflexive thematic analysis

1. Introduction

Anorexia nervosa (AN) is a psychiatric disorder, affecting both physical and mental health. It is the third most common chronic illness among adolescent females and has one of the highest mortality rates amongst all psychiatric conditions [1], ranking second after substance abuse [2]. AN is associated with severe medical, nutritional and psychological consequences and the treatment necessitates input from professionals with specialist skills to manage each of these domains [3–5]. In treatment models for adolescent AN, the family is seen as a valuable resource in supporting the recovery of the young person from the illness [6,7]. As such, interventions employing a family-based approach for treating AN in young people are recommended by the national guidance from Australia and New Zealand [8], the Netherlands [9], Spain [10], the United Kingdom (UK) [11], the United States of America (USA) [12], Denmark [13] and France [14].

Family therapy for anorexia nervosa (FT-AN) is recommended as a first-line treatment for young people with AN by the National Institute for Health and Care Excellence (NICE) [11]. A multidisciplinary team (MDT) approach is described as paramount in both the FT-AN manual [15] and the current UK guidance and standards on specialist child and adolescent eating disorder service structure [16] to ensure that holistic care (including, nutritional, physical monitoring, medication and psychiatric assessment) is offered. Dietitians, alongside other key professions, are described as core members of this MDT [15,16].

Dietitians are skilled in the assessment and management of disordered eating patterns, malnutrition, underweight and nutritional-related deficiencies [17,18]. Restrictive eating, low weight and malnutrition are all salient characteristics of AN [19]. Dietitians are well-placed to support nutritional-related issues arising from the illness. However, eating disorder-associated behaviours and their impact on nutrition are symptoms of the illness, rather than the cause. Dietetic interventions, aimed at managing malnutrition and supporting refeeding, are often recommended as part of the specialist MDT, whereby psychological therapy (such as FT-AN) and medical management are central parts of treatment that are delivered by appropriately qualified and experienced professionals [20,21].

Dietitians are routinely involved in inpatient, residential and day treatments across the life span in AN. However, the role of dietitians across outpatient treatments for children and adolescents with AN is highly variable. Within family approaches to the treatment of AN, there has been some difference in opinion over whether or how a dietitian should be involved. For example, the family-based treatment (FBT) manual does not recommend dietitians as part of the direct treating team; however, dietitians are mentioned as potential members of the consulting team, and in clinical practice, dietitians routinely work in parallel with FBT therapists [22–24]. In FBT, the nutritional guidance on weight restoration delivered by a dietitian is perceived to have the potential to undermine parental confidence in their ability to feed their child and make healthy food choices for them, just as they had done prior to them becoming unwell with AN. In the Maudsley FT-AN manual, however, dietitians extend the nutritional knowledge base of the MDT, providing nutritional psychoeducation in collaboration with therapists and devising standard meal plans that are used to provide guidance in the initial stages of the treatment [15]. In FT-AN, it is suggested that dietitians can also take a more direct advisory role when needed at several stages across treatment. This can include case consultation if weight restoration is not progressing, modifying standard meal plans when there are specific dietary requirements (e.g., coeliac disease) or supporting the young person to move to independent eating. Joint working between the dietitian and therapist is recommended to take place in family sessions to ensure MDT collaboration with the family. Given these conflicting views about how and when to involve dietetics within two very similar treatment models, further research exploring dietetic roles in the outpatient treatment of eating disorders in children and adolescents is needed, in addition to clear guidelines describing the role of the dietitian in FT-AN [18].

Existing research studies mainly concentrate on the role of the dietitian in adult eating disorder treatment and highlight dietitians as essential in the management of malnutrition, whilst also needing to work collaboratively and in accordance with psychological and medical aspects of the treatment [18]. Despite dietitians being skilled in assessing and treating malnutrition, a core characteristic of eating disorders, their involvement in treatment has been raised as a contentious issue [25]. A study by McMaster et al. employed a modified Delphi method to develop consensus guidelines across multiple domains of dietetic involvement within eating disorder treatment for adults. Results identified disagreement between clients and clinicians on essential components of dietetic treatment. Dietetic input was more highly valued by clients than clinicians, and this was raised as a potential barrier to the involvement of dietitians in the treatment, given that access to dietitians is often reliant on referrals being initiated by therapists [25].

Research and guidance on the dietitian's role in adolescent eating disorder treatment are lacking. No empirical studies have been conducted, to date, which assess the effect of nutrition counselling on treatment outcomes in FT-AN or FBT. In the absence of such studies, the ability to advance our understanding of the role of dietitians in treatment remains limited. Though the roles and responsibilities of the dietitian have been conceptualised in FT-AN treatment, further guidance on the role of the dietitian within FT-AN is required to support best practices in this area and ensure consistent evidence-based practice across services delivering this treatment. This study aimed to gather perspectives from experienced clinicians, specialising in the delivery of FT-AN, on the role of the dietitian in FT-AN. The objective of the study was to take an initial step towards gathering evidence that supports further research in this area and will aid the development of consensus guidelines on this role.

2. Materials and Methods

2.1. Sample

All clinicians who were working at the Maudsley Centre for Child and Adolescent Eating Disorders (MCCAED) outpatient service and had experience delivering FT-AN during the data collection period were invited to participate. All clinicians were qualified family therapists, psychiatrists, nurse therapists or clinical psychologists with training and experience in FT-AN. MCCAED provides specialist treatments for all children and adolescents with eating disorders for an area of Southeast London with a population of approximately 2.2 million people. The outpatient service provides specialist family and psychological therapies, psychiatric management, dietetics and physical health reviews. The primary treatment model for anorexia nervosa is FT-AN (see recent publications for service details and outcomes [26,27]).

2.2. Procedure

Approval for this project was granted by South London and Maudsley Child and Adolescent Mental Health Services (CAMHS) service evaluation and audit committee (approval number 330 and date 23 August 2023). Surveys were used to collect data from clinicians via an online platform [28]. Survey questions were informed by MDT consultation about core components of dietetic treatment within FT-AN, barriers to dietetic treatment and outcomes related to dietetic involvement in FT-AN. Surveys were used to allow participants to respond anonymously and remove any potential sources of bias in their responses. Data were collected between June and July 2023. The survey was sent to all clinicians ($n = 35$) with experience in delivering FT-AN and working within the MCCAED team. Surveys recorded the profession of the respondent and were made up of 10 questions allowing quantitative rating and categorical responses. This was followed by 7 open-ended questions, which explored opinions on the role of dietetics in FT-AN, the effects of including a dietitian in FT-AN and potential benefits and challenges that arise when directly or indirectly involving dietetics as part of FT-AN.

2.3. Analysis Plan

Quantitative data from the survey questions are used descriptively rather than to test statistical hypotheses. Qualitative data were separately analysed using reflexive thematic analysis within a critical realist framework, which views meaning and experience as subjective and influenced by social and cultural context. Responses and comments on open-ended questions were initially coded, and initial themes were generated. The themes were reviewed and developed before being defined. Themes were developed through reflexive engagement with the data, with the involvement of two authors who were both working in the service at this time (CB and JB). Themes were cross-checked with survey respondents, and comments or feedback were used to adapt the themes to accurately reflect the views of the team.

2.4. Reflexivity Statement

CB is a cisgender white female working as a dietitian within the FT-AN model in MCCAED, she understands and is aware of the roles and responsibilities that surround being a dietitian in this team and delivering this treatment model. The questions asked within the survey and the themes drawn from responses will inherently contain biases due to their role in the team. The results and conclusions come from their perspective, and their awareness of these biases has been taken into account.

JB is a cisgender white male working as a clinical psychologist within the FT-AN model at MCCAED. He has more than 10 years of experience clinically delivering family-based treatments for adolescent AN, as well as teaching and conducting research in the area. He has provided treatment within both the FBT and FT-AN models and has experience of performing this with and without dietetic input. This experience will inevitably bring bias to the data analysis, although having had the experience of both types of family treatments and performing so with and without a dietitian brings depth to the analysis.

3. Results

3.1. Sample

Twenty clinicians responded to the survey, and these were from a range of professional backgrounds, including nurses ($n = 1$), psychiatrists ($n = 1$), psychologists ($n = 6$) and family therapists ($n = 5$), who represented the MDT. Seven respondents did not disclose their professional background.

3.2. Quantitative Data

Descriptive data for responses to categorical survey questions are displayed in Table 1 for all survey respondents ($n = 20$). All clinicians included in the survey had experience working with a dietitian when delivering FT-AN. Dietetic input was sought for differing proportions of clinicians' caseloads and most frequently for less than 10% ($n = 6$) and up to 25% ($n = 7$) of FT-AN caseloads. All clinicians agreed that dietetics had a role within FT-AN ($n = 20$) and that they most frequently sought involvement in phases 1 and 2 of FT-AN.

Table 1. Quantitative survey response data from participants ($n = 20$).

Survey Question	N	%
What percentage of your caseload have you sought dietetic input for?		
0%	1	5
<10%	6	30
10–25%	7	35
25–50%	2	10
50–75%	1	5
<75%	3	15
Within what phase of FT-AN is dietetic input most valuable?		
No phases	0	0
Phase 1	6	30
Phase 2	6	30
Phase 3	0	0
Phase 4	3	15
All phases	5	25
What phase of treatment would you typically use the standard meal plans?		
Phase 1	15	75
Phase 2	5	30
Phase 3	0	0
Phase 4	0	0

Opinions were divided on the potential for dietetic involvement in FT-AN to be unhelpful, with 45% of clinicians ($n = 9$) stating that there could be unhelpful aspects, whilst 55% ($n = 11$) did not think there were aspects that could be unhelpful. The majority of clinicians agreed that the therapeutic alliance was affected by involving dietetics within FT-AN (65%, $n = 13$). Most clinicians also agreed that there was a greater or differing need for dietetic involvement in atypical cases during FT-AN (65%, $n = 13$).

All clinicians reported that if standardised meal plans were provided, these were used within phases 1 and 2 of FT-AN, with no clinicians reporting their use in phase 3 or 4 (75%, $n = 15$ and 30%, $n = 5$, respectively). All clinicians agreed that there were indirect benefits of having a dietitian as part of the MDT when delivering FT-AN (100%, $n = 20$).

3.3. Qualitative Data

Analysis of free-text responses generated three main themes and eight subthemes that applied to all clinicians (see Table 2). The themes were (1) collaboration is key, (2) confidence as a core consideration and (3) a case-by-case approach. Sub-themes were (1a) working together, (1b) learning from each other and (1c) building trust; (2a) timing matters and (2b) skilling up; (3a) assessing needs, (3b) individualised treatment and (3c) moving on from meal plans. Each one is described further below with relevant illustrative quotations.

Table 2. Themes and subthemes of reflexive thematic analysis.

Themes	Sub-Themes	Codes
Collaboration is key	Working together	1a
	Learning from each other	1b
	Building trust	1c
Confidence as a core consideration	Timing matters	2a
	Skilling up	2b
Case-by-case approach	Assessing needs	3a
	Individualised treatment	3b
	Moving on from meal plans	3c

1. Collaboration is key.

1a. Working together. A core theme that was evident amongst all clinicians related to collaborative working between dietitians and therapists and professionals and families. Responses reinforced fidelity to the FT-AN approach, whereby all MDT members provided specialist input as a cohesive joined-up team. Incorporating dietetics within the treatment rather than as an isolated or separate intervention was important to clinicians. Concerns were raised regarding team splitting and diminished therapeutic alliance when dietetic involvement was offered as a separate intervention.

"I think it is unhelpful if this is done separately and not as part of sessions/treatment. If it is separated it can impact engagement, the therapeutic relationship and learning from each other."

"Most importantly though their role is to be a collaborative partner with the therapist and family against the illness, rather than being a separate voice/perspective."

"Our treatment model is based on delivering treatment within an expert MDT that involves the combined knowledge of all disciplines. Phase one of treatment is based on engaging the family with the MDT approach and creating a secure base for treatment" . . . *"So, all of the above but together with care coordinator/therapist and based on formulation of need to do something different rather than totalistic approaches."*

1b. Learning from each other. Sharing of knowledge and expertise was another core component of dietetic involvement in FT-AN. Clinicians frequently reported that their confidence and knowledge regarding nutritional aspects of treatment were greatly increased by working with a dietitian, which enhanced their ability to deliver FT-AN. The consensus was that this transfer of information and learning from colleagues was bi-directional, whereby therapists and families benefited from dietetic expertise, and similarly, dietitians expanded and improved their practice through learning from therapists and families.

> "I have learned a lot working together with a dietitian over the years and it has contributed to my development and expertise, and I hope this was bidirectional."

> "Working together is essential to safe practice and there is a lot of learning that happens both ways across disciplines."

1c. Building trust. Creating a stable base for FT-AN is essential in the delivery of this treatment. Clinicians felt that collaboration as an MDT, working together and supporting families jointly in psychological and nutritional aspects of treatment were important in building trust and engagement. The consensus from clinicians was that the involvement of a dietitian, as a planned intervention, supported the therapeutic alliance and strengthened families' trust in the treatment.

Bringing in an expert on nutrition in certain cases during FT-AN-aided containment at different phases of treatment, depending on the family's needs. Concerns were raised by clinicians regarding the involvement of a dietitian when a strong therapeutic alliance with the family had not yet been built, or when engagement was already poor. The involvement of dietetics in these scenarios could have a negative impact in terms of undermining the therapist or parents or creating an overreliance on the dietitian in meal planning.

> "I think there are a few ways the dietitian is really helpful" ... "in containing anxiety about families feeling like they are doing the 'right thing', offering support and comfort to the clinician that things are on the right track (more of a distant role) and in providing the same message as the therapist but from a different perspective (e.g., united team front)."

> "I think if families are motivated and on board to see a dietician then it works better. Sometimes it can feel unhelpful when the parents have pre-existing beliefs about a dietician being able to "solve" the young person's eating problems instead of parents needing to take an active role in FT AN."

2. Confidence as a core consideration.

2a. Timing Matters. All clinicians agreed that the timing of dietetic involvement was an important consideration. Parental confidence could be negatively impacted by dietetic intervention too early in treatment, prior to a strong therapeutic alliance being built. Similarly, clinicians voiced concerns regarding dietetic involvement inadvertently undermining parental confidence in meal planning, portioning and feeding if the input was poorly timed.

> "I think if the family is motivated and on board to see a dietician then it works better."

> "Providing expert consultation if the family is really lacking knowledge and confidence in what types of foods to give, in containing anxiety about families feeling like they are doing the 'right thing', offering support and comfort to the clinician that things are on the right track (more of a distant role) and providing the same message as the therapist but from a different perspective (e.g., united team front)."

2b. Skilling up. Survey respondents made multiple references related to the use of dietetic sessions and input to support both clinician and parental confidence in several nutritional aspects of the treatment during FT-AN. There was an overall consensus that dietitians had a central role in sharing expertise on nutritional information, meal planning and intuitive eating with families and in supporting them to feel confident in taking responsibility for these aspects of the treatment. The importance of a collaborative, joint-up approach was reiterated by clinicians. If the approach was split or not collaborative, clinicians felt that the confidence of both clinicians and parents could be negatively impacted.

> "I think it can also affect clinical confidence if not done jointly."

"Helping give confidence and containment to families taking positive risks to have meals not guided by the meal plan which are more in line with "real life"."

3. Case-by-case approach.

3a. Assessment of needs. Dietetic involvement was considered an important and valuable element of treatment within the FT-AN model. However, clinicians felt that an assessment of the needs of the family was crucial before seeking dietetic input. Families requiring dietetic involvement for core purposes such as refeeding management, meal planning, special or complex diets and increasing variety with food were referenced as appropriate uses of dietetic input. In the absence of a clear need, dietetic involvement was seen as unnecessary. Where dietetic involvement was not indicated, clinicians were concerned that the input could lead to an over-focus on nutrition and the potential avoidance of therapeutic work.

"What can also be unhelpful is to take extreme views (i.e., everyone needs to be seen by dietician) as it does not acknowledge the existing processes in place and also other ways that expertise can be shared."

"Sometimes it can feel unhelpful when the parents have pre-existing beliefs about a dietician being able to "solve" the young person's eating problems instead of parents needing to take an active role in FT AN."

"Sometimes the families think that if they 'only got the food right' then the eating disorder would be fixed. Given it is part food part emotion, if we over-focus on the food, I think this can act like an avoidance of the actual issue."

3b. Individualised treatment. Another important role of the dietitian within FT-AN discussed by clinicians was individualising feeding plans, in particular, in adapting meal plans or nutrition advice for bespoke plans and advice. Clinicians felt that this supported a patient-centred approach and helped to ensure that individual needs could be met. Cases with specific dietary needs, complex physical health co-morbidities, atypical presentations or cultural diversity were seen to benefit from direct dietetic input.

"I think it would be very helpful to have more dietetic role in FT-AN especially when working with young people who are not underweight and also binge/purge."

"Would also want dietetic support (in atypical cases) so not promoting any anti-fat messages unintentionally, especially if someone's weight is at higher end."

3c. Moving on from meal plans. Meal plans were discussed by all clinicians, and there was a general consensus that, despite them supporting containment and providing guidance early on in treatment, they could often become unhelpful when families remain "stuck" on them. Clinicians felt that dietitians had a key role in helping families move away from meal plans at various points through FT-AN. During the initial phases, direct or indirect dietetic consultation was used as a tool to educate and guide on refeeding in the absence of a meal plan. In later phases of treatment, the dietitian's role was related to moving off the initially prescribed meal plan and/or incorporating greater dietary variety and flexibility than that provided on standardized meal plans. Again, the theme of building confidence in the nutritional aspects of treatment and working collaboratively to achieve goals was referenced by clinicians.

"When starting to have more independence and eating on their own, going out more, dietetic input would be very helpful. Also, when parents or YP (young people) feel worried to move away from meal plan."

"Planning with the dietitian can make the young person feel safe and confident to take on responsibility for their eating."

"Other times I think older young people need support in understanding the truth about nutrition to help them make better choices, e.g., where social media and googling has provided unhelpful advice."

4. Discussion

Currently, no empirical studies exist that investigate the role of dietitians in family treatments for anorexia nervosa. This study provided initial insights into this topic.

In this study, the exploration of MDT perspectives on the role of the dietitian within FT-AN supported dietetic involvement in some cases. Dietitians were seen by experienced clinicians as a valuable resource, which should be considered and offered when indicated for selected families. Access to dietetic expertise was most valued during the initial phases of the treatment, where nutritional rehabilitation most often takes place, and in atypical cases presenting at healthy weights or for cases with co-morbid complexities. Having said that, direct input from a dietitian was not considered necessary for all and needed to be considered on a case-by-case basis. The involvement of dietetics, where no clinical need was identified, was considered by nearly half of clinicians surveyed to be potentially unhelpful. The findings of this study highlighted several barriers that may discourage therapists from seeking dietetic involvement, including concerns related to diminishing parental confidence in feeding and creating an over-focus on the nutritional aspects of the treatment.

A recent review by Heafala et al. explored the role of dietitians in eating disorder treatment [29], including perspectives of dietitians, MDT members and service users. The themes that were generated from the review were similar to those identified in the current study. The role of dietitians was varied, encompassing roles as collaborators, educators and in supporting individualised patient-centred care [29]. Concerns regarding the impact of dietetic involvement on certain aspects of care that were identified included uncertainty regarding the scope of practice and unclear treatment guidance [29]. McMaster et al. also found that there were a number of barriers to dietetic involvement in eating disorder treatment related to the perception that inexperienced dietitians may discuss weight loss or dieting with patients [30]. The need for clarity on the role of the dietitian, criteria necessitating dietetic involvement and clear guidance on the structure of dietetic involvement within eating disorders has been repeatedly highlighted [29,31,32]. Future directions should include a range of appropriately designed and well-powered empirical studies on this subject to provide much-needed, concrete evidence on the impact that dietitians may have in treatment.

Strengths and Limitations

A strength of this study was in its novel nature, namely that it is the first study that provides an initial important step analysing descriptive, as well as qualitative data on the involvement of dietitians in outpatient FT-AN. Other strengths include its setting, a highly specialised eating disorder centre, where FT-AN was conceptualised, developed and the range of professions included within the sample that spanned multiple disciplines.

The study had a number of limitations. The findings from a convenience sample of self-selecting clinicians from a single centre may not generalise to all clinicians delivering comparable treatments in similar settings. Clinicians who responded may have had more positive views of dietetics, introducing potential biases. However, the use of anonymous surveys aimed to reduce potential biases and support clinicians to answer questions truthfully, including both positive and negative responses. Similarly, although all clinicians surveyed were working primarily as therapists delivering manualised FT-AN, respondents did span a range of professional backgrounds. Experiences and perceptions of the role of the dietitian in FT-AN may have been impacted by professional background. Additionally, this was a single-centre study, meaning that results may not be representative of other eating disorder centres, where experiences and perceptions of the dietitians' role may differ.

5. Conclusions

Although manualised FT-AN clearly describes the dietitian as a core member of the treating team, the roles and responsibilities of dietitians in eating disorders-focused family therapy remain a contentious issue. The findings of this study highlight collaboration as a key component of the dietitian role. To enable the creation of dietetic treatment guidelines that include the MDT perspectives, collaboration with clinicians delivering FT-AN was seen as an important first step. To further advance our understanding of the topic, high-quality research studies are needed. Previously proposed guidance on the dietitians' role in FT-AN originated predominantly from dietitians [33], potentially lacking the diverse perspectives of other professions involved in delivering FT-AN, and the robust research methods required to provide high-quality evidence needed for the development of such guidance. Further research is essential in this area to provide sound evidence on the role of dietitians within family-based treatments for anorexia nervosa.

The overall consensus from clinicians surveyed in our study provided guidance on three important components for dietetic involvement, and further research, in FT-AN. We propose the following treatment implications related to these core components of the role of dietitian within FT-AN.

6. Recommendations for Clinical Practice

1. Dietitians should be recognised as collaborators within therapy-led teams. There should be a focus on joint (family–therapist–dietitian) working that facilitates discussions between therapists and dietitians, working together with parents and families and enhancing the therapeutic alliance through supporting individual patients' goals through collaboration between dietitians, therapists and families.
2. Dietitians should be integrated within the MDT and have direct and indirect involvement in patient care. Dietitians have an important role that involves liaising with dietitians and staff from external teams. Indirect dietetic involvement should include resource creation and professional consultation. Direct involvement should be offered when clinically indicated when co-morbid physical health problems exist, in cases of complex dietary needs, such as allergies, intolerances or sensory sensitivity, and in cases where nutritional requirements are difficult to meet through food alone and supplementation or tube feeding may be required. Dietetic involvement should support increased confidence in the MDT and the sharing of skills and nutritional expertise. Training between dietitians and teams should be bidirectional with knowledge sharing and training occurring from therapist to dietitian and vice versa to support all staff in "singing from the same hymn sheet".
3. Dietitians have a core role in individualising care and ensuring that the diverse needs of families being treated by the service are met. This involves bespoke meal planning when required or providing tailored nutritional recommendations for families with individual needs with co-morbid illnesses, individuals who are highly active or athletic and those who present at higher weights that require additional nutritional advice within FT-AN.

Author Contributions: Conceptualization, C.B., J.B., I.E. and M.S.; methodology, C.B., J.B., I.E. and M.S.; formal analysis, C.B., J.B., I.E. and M.S.; investigation, C.B., J.B., I.E. and M.S.; resources, C.B., J.B., I.E. and M.S.; data curation, C.B., J.B., I.E. and M.S; writing—original draft preparation, C.B., J.B., I.E. and M.S.; writing—review and editing, C.B., J.B., I.E. and M.S.; supervision, J.B., I.E. and M.S.; project administration, C.B., J.B., I.E. and M.S.; funding acquisition, N/A. All authors have read and agreed to the published version of the manuscript.

Funding: This research received no external funding.

Institutional Review Board Statement: The study was conducted according to the guidelines of the Declaration of Helsinki and approved by the Institutional Review Board of South London and Maudsley NHS Hospital on 23/08/2023, approval number 330.

Informed Consent Statement: Informed consent was obtained from all subjects involved in the study.

Data Availability Statement: Data is available on request. Please contact the corresponding author for data requests.

Acknowledgments: We would like to acknowledge all of the participants who took part in the study for their time and support.

Conflicts of Interest: The authors have no conflicts of interest.

References

1. Van Eeden, A.E.; Van Hoeken, D.; Hoek, H.W. Incidence, prevalence and mortality of anorexia nervosa and bulimia nervosa. *Curr. Opin. Psychiatry* **2021**, *34*, 515–524. [CrossRef] [PubMed]
2. Chan, J.K.N.; Correll, C.U.; Wong, C.S.M.; Chu, R.S.T.; Fung, V.S.C.; Wong, G.H.S.; Lei, J.H.C.; Chang, W.C. Life expectancy and years of potential life lost in people with mental disorders: A systematic review and meta-analysis. *eClinicalMedicine* **2023**, *65*, 102294. [CrossRef] [PubMed]
3. Katzman, D.K. Medical complications in adolescents with anorexia nervosa: A review of the literature. *Int. J. Eat. Disord.* **2005**, *37*, S52–S59. [CrossRef] [PubMed]
4. Hudson, L.D.; Chapman, S. Paediatric medical care for children and young people with eating disorders: Achievements and where to next. *Clin. Child Psychol. Psychiatry* **2020**, *25*, 716–720. [CrossRef]
5. Golden, N.H.; Katzman, D.K.; Sawyer, S.M.; Ornstein, R.M.; Rome, E.S.; Garber, A.K.; Kohn, M.; Kreipe, R.E. Update on the medical management of eating disorders in adolescents. *J. Adolesc. Health* **2015**, *56*, 370–375. [CrossRef] [PubMed]
6. Le Grange, D.; Lock, J.; Loeb, K.; Nicholls, D. Academy for eating disorders position paper: The role of the family in eating disorders. *Int. J. Eat. Disord.* **2010**, *43*, 1–5. [CrossRef] [PubMed]
7. Blessitt, E.; Baudinet, J.; Simic, M. Systemic Family Therapy with Children and Adolescents. In *The Handbook of Systemic Family Therapy*; Wampler, K.S., McWey, L.M., Eds.; Wiley-Blackwell: Chichester, UK, 2020; pp. 397–428. ISBN 978-1-119-78839-3.
8. Hay, P.; Chinn, D.; Forbes, D.; Madden, S.; Newton, R.; Sugenor, L.; Touyz, S.; Ward, W. Royal Australian and New Zealand College of Psychiatrists clinical practice guidelines for the treatment of eating disorders. *Aust. N. Z. J. Psychiatry* **2014**, *48*, 977–1008. [CrossRef]
9. Dutch Foundation for Quality Development in Mental Healthcare. *Practice Guideline for the Treatment of Eating Disorders [Zorgstandaard Eetstoornissen]*; Netwerk Kwaliteitsontwikkeling GGz: Utrecht, The Netherlands, 2017.
10. Working Group of the Clinical Practice Guideline for Eating Disorders. Clinical Practice Guideline for Eating Disorders. Quality Plan for the National Health System of the Ministry of Health and Consumer Affairs. Madrid. 2009. Available online: https://portal.guiasalud.es/wp-content/uploads/2019/01/GPC_440_Eat_Disorders_compl_en.pdf (accessed on 20 July 2023).
11. National Insititute of Health and Care Excellence. NICE Guideline (NG69) Eating Disorders: Recognition and Treatment Treatment. 2017. Available online: https://www.nice.org.uk/guidance/ng69 (accessed on 15 June 2023).
12. Yager, J.; Michael Devlin, C.J.; Halmi, K.A.; Herzog, D.B.; Mitchell, J.E., III; Powers, P.; Zerbe, K.J.; McIntyre, J.S.; Anzia, D.J.; Cook, I.A.; et al. Practice Guideline for the Treatment of Patients with Eating Disorders, 3rd ed. 2014. Available online: https://psychiatryonline.org/pb/assets/raw/sitewide/practice_guidelines/guidelines/eatingdisorders.pdf (accessed on 10 July 2023).
13. Danish Health Authority. National Clinical Guideline for the Treatment of Anorexia Nervosa. Quick Guide. 2016. Available online: https://www.sst.dk/da/udgivelser/2016/~/media/36D31B378C164922BCD96573749AA206.ashx (accessed on 22 June 2023).
14. Haute Authorite de Sante. Clinical Practice Guidelines: Anorexia Nervosa Management. 2010. Available online: http://www.has-sante.fr (accessed on 5 May 2023).
15. Simic, M.; Eisler, I. Maudsley Family Therapy for Eating Disorders. In *Encyclopedia of Couple and Family Therapy*, 1st ed.; Lebow, J.L., Chambers, A.L., Breunlin, D.C., Eds.; Springer: Cham, Switzerland, 2018.
16. NHS England. Access and Waiting Time Standard for Children and Young People with an Eating Disorder. July 2015. Available online: https://www.england.nhs.uk/wp-content/uploads/2015/07/cyp-eating-disorders-access-waiting-time-standard-comm-guid.pdf (accessed on 20 May 2023).
17. Judd, P. The role of the dietitian. *Encycl. Hum. Nutr.* **2005**, *70*, 32–38. [CrossRef]
18. Jeffrey, S.; Heruc, G. Balancing nutrition management and the role of dietitians in eating disorder treatment. *J. Eat. Disord.* **2020**, *8*, 8–10. [CrossRef]
19. Rosen, D.S.; Blythe, M.J.; Braverman, P.K.; Breuner, C.C.; Levine, D.A.; Murray, P.J.; O'Brien, R.F.; Seigel, W.M. Clinical report—Identification and management of eating disorders in children and adolescents. *Pediatrics* **2010**, *126*, 1240–1253. [CrossRef]
20. Neale, J.; Hudson, L.D. Anorexia nervosa in adolescents. *Br. J. Hosp. Med.* **2020**, *81*, 1–8. [CrossRef] [PubMed]
21. Royal College of Psychiatrists. CR 233: Medical Emergencies in Eating Disorders (MEED) Guidance on Recognition and Management; 2022, 185p. Available online: https://www.rcpsych.ac.uk/docs/default-source/improving-care/better-mh-policy/college-reports/college-report-cr233-medical-emergencies-in-eating-disorders-(meed)-guidance.pdf?sfvrsn=2d327483_50 (accessed on 3 June 2023).
22. Dalle Grave, R.; Eckhardt, S.; Calugi, S.; Le Grange, D. A conceptual comparison of family-based treatment and enhanced cognitive behavior therapy in the treatment of adolescents with eating disorders. *J. Eat. Disord.* **2019**, *7*, 42. [CrossRef] [PubMed]
23. Lian, B.; Forsberg, S.E.; Fitzpatrick, K.K. Adolescent Anorexia: Guiding Principles and Skills for the Dietetic Support of Family-Based Treatment. *J. Acad. Nutr. Diet.* **2019**, *119*, 17–25. [CrossRef] [PubMed]
24. Lock, J.; Le Grange, D. *Treatment Manual for Anorexia Nervosa—A Family-Based Approach*, 2nd ed.; Guildford Press: New York, NY, USA, 2012.
25. McMaster, C.M.; Wade, T.; Franklin, J.; Hart, S. Development of consensus-based guidelines for outpatient dietetic treatment of eating disorders: A Delphi study. *Int. J. Eat. Disord.* **2020**, *53*, 1480–1495. [CrossRef]

26. Simic, M.; Stewart, C.S.; Konstantellou, A.; Hodsoll, J.; Eisler, I.; Baudinet, J. From efficacy to effectiveness: Child and adolescent eating disorder treatments in the real world (part 1)—Treatment course and outcomes. *J. Eat. Disord.* **2022**, *10*, 27. [CrossRef] [PubMed]
27. Stewart, C.S.; Baudinet, J.; Munuve, A.; Bell, A.; Konstantellou, A.; Eisler, I.; Simic, M. From efficacy to effectiveness: Child and adolescent eating disorder treatments in the real world (Part 2): 7-year follow-up. *J. Eat. Disord.* **2022**, *10*, 14. [CrossRef] [PubMed]
28. Qualtrics. *Qualtrics XM*, April 2021; Qualtrics: Seattle, WA, USA, 2005. Available online: https://www.qualtrics.com (accessed on 5 June 2023).
29. Heafala, A.; Ball, L.; Rayner, J.; Mitchell, L.J. What role do dietitians have in providing nutrition care for eating disorder treatment? An integrative review. *J. Hum. Nutr. Diet.* **2021**, *34*, 724–735. [CrossRef]
30. McMaster, C.M.; Wade, T.; Franklin, J.; Waller, G.; Hart, S. Impact of patient characteristics on clinicians' decisions to involve dietitians in eating disorder treatment. *J. Hum. Nutr. Diet.* **2022**, *35*, 512–522. [CrossRef]
31. Yang, Y.; Conti, J.; McMaster, C.M.; Hay, P. Beyond refeeding: The effect of including a dietitian in eating disorder treatment. A systematic review. *Nutrients* **2021**, *13*, 4490. [CrossRef]
32. McMaster, C.M.; Wade, T.; Basten, C.; Franklin, J.; Ross, J.; Hart, S. Rationale and development of a manualised dietetic intervention for adults undergoing psychological treatment for an eating disorder. *Eat. Weight Disord.* **2020**, *26*, 1467–1481. [CrossRef]
33. O'Connor, G.; Oliver, A.; Corbett, J.; Fuller, S. Developing Clinical Guidelines for Dietitians Treating Young People with Anorexia Nervosa—Family Focused Approach Working Alongside Family Therapists. *Ann. Nutr. Disord. Ther.* **2019**, *6*, 1056.

Disclaimer/Publisher's Note: The statements, opinions and data contained in all publications are solely those of the individual author(s) and contributor(s) and not of MDPI and/or the editor(s). MDPI and/or the editor(s) disclaim responsibility for any injury to people or property resulting from any ideas, methods, instructions or products referred to in the content.

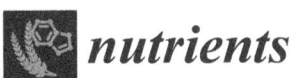

Article

Mediterranean Diet Favors Vitamin K Intake: A Descriptive Study in a Mediterranean Population

Ezequiel Pinto [1,2], Carla Viegas [3,4], Paula Ventura Martins [5], Catarina Marreiros [3], Tânia Nascimento [1,2], Leon Schurgers [6] and Dina Simes [3,4,*]

1. Centro de Estudos e Desenvolvimento em Saúde, Universidade do Algarve, Campus de Gambelas, 8005-139 Faro, Portugal; epinto@ualg.pt (E.P.); tnascimento@ualg.pt (T.N.)
2. Algarve Biomedical Center Research Institute (ABC-RI), Universidade do Algarve, Campus de Gambelas, 8005-139 Faro, Portugal
3. Centre of Marine Sciences (CCMAR), Universidade do Algarve, Campus de Gambelas, 8005-139 Faro, Portugal; caviegas@ualg.pt (C.V.); cimarreiros@ualg.pt (C.M.)
4. GenoGla Diagnostics, Centre of Marine Sciences (CCMAR), Universidade do Algarve, Campus de Gambelas, 8005-139 Faro, Portugal
5. Algarve Cyber-Physical Systems Research Centre (CISCA), Universidade do Algarve, Campus de Gambelas, 8005-139 Faro, Portugal; pventura@ualg.pt
6. Department of Biochemistry, Cardiovascular Research Institute Maastricht, 6200 MD Maastricht, The Netherlands; l.schurgers@maastrichtuniversity.nl
* Correspondence: dsimes@ualg.pt; Tel.: +351-289-800100

Abstract: The Mediterranean diet (MD) is associated with improved longevity and the prevention and management of chronic inflammatory diseases (CIDs). Vitamin K, which is present in MD core components such as leafy green vegetables, is also known as a protective factor for CIDs. Estimates of vitamin K intake in Mediterranean settings are still scarce, and the association between MD and vitamin K intake is yet to be established. This study analyzed vitamin K intake and MD adherence in the Algarve region, in Portugal. We conducted a cross-sectional study in a nonrandom sample of adults using an online questionnaire which included a validated food-frequency questionnaire and a screener for MD adherence. A total of 238 participants were recruited (68% women and 32% men). Adherence to the MD was low (11%). Only 10% of the participants had vitamin K intake below the adequate intake. Adherence to the MD was positively correlated with vitamin K intake (r = 0.463; $p < 0.001$) and age (r = 0.223; $p < 0.001$). Our findings underscore the importance of promoting adherence to the MD for optimal vitamin K intake, and future research should focus on developing effective interventions to promote this dietary pattern, particularly among younger individuals and men.

Keywords: Mediterranean diet; vitamin K; cross-sectional study; dietary intake

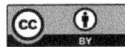

1. Introduction

The Mediterranean diet (MD), recognized as an intangible world heritage by UNESCO, is celebrated for its health-promoting qualities and its respect for the environment [1]. While the MD is traditionally associated with countries bordering the Mediterranean Sea, it has been promoted worldwide as one of the healthiest dietary patterns. The MD primarily emphasizes plant-derived foods, including vegetables, fruit, and legumes, while also encouraging the consumption of unrefined cereals, olive oil, fish (over red meat), and moderate amounts of dairy products and red wine [2]. Due to its high nutritional profile, rich in monounsaturated fatty acids (MUFAs), polyunsaturated fatty acids (PUFAs), different antioxidants, and anti-inflammatory compounds, the MD is now acknowledged for its protective effects against chronic inflammatory diseases (CIDs), commonly referred to as age-associated noncommunicable diseases [3]. Numerous prospective observational studies and trials conducted across diverse populations over several decades have consistently demonstrated that adherence to MD offers benefits in preventing all-cause mortality and managing various CIDs. These include cardiovascular diseases (such as coronary heart disease, stroke, and diabetes), bone diseases (including fragility fractures), cancer, neurodegenerative diseases, cognitive health, depression, and respiratory diseases [4].

Interestingly, vitamin K, abundant in core MD components like green leafy vegetables, also plays a protective role in several CIDs, such as cardiovascular disease, bone-related disorders, cancer, dementia, cognitive impairment, and lung diseases [3,5]. The favorable effects of vitamin K may stem from its function as a cofactor for the gamma-carboxylation of vitamin K-dependent proteins (VKDP), which have diverse physiological roles. Additionally, vitamin K exhibits anti-inflammatory, antioxidant, and transcriptional regulatory properties related to osteoblastic genes, cognitive function, antiferroptosis, and tumor progression inhibition [6–8].

Vitamin K is a liposoluble vitamin that includes phylloquinone (vitamin K1), mostly found in photosynthetic organisms, including green leafy vegetables, herbs, algae, and vegetable oils, and menaquinones (MKn or vitamin K2), which are primarily produced by bacteria and obtained through the consumption of meat, fermented foods, and dairy products [6–9]. Vitamin K1 and K2 sources are mainly dietary [10,11], and vitamin K can be recycled through the vitamin K epoxide reductase cycle (VKOR). However, vitamin K2 can also be produced by human microbiota, and MK-4 can be converted from vitamin K at the tissue level. In fact, vitamin K1 accounts for 90% of the total vitamin K in the diet [12], and vitamin K recommended daily intake (RDI) is based on the median intake of vitamin K1. The adequate intake recommendation (adequate intake—AI) for American adults was set to 120 µg/day for men and 90 µg/day for women [13], and in Europe, 75 µg vitamin K has been recommended as the daily allowance (Commission Directive 2008/100/EC).

Mediterranean populations traditionally follow an eating pattern where vitamin-K-rich foods, such as leafy green vegetables and different types of cheeses, are frequently consumed [14,15]; thus, the association between adherence to this dietary pattern and higher vitamin K intake has been mainly assumed but not established [16,17]. Additionally, estimates of vitamin K populational intake within Mediterranean settings are scarce.

It has been reported that adherence to the MD is decreasing, especially among younger inhabitants of Mediterranean regions [18–21], and recent data for Portugal show that adherence to the MD is low, with prevalences reported at 17% [22] or 8.7% [23]. Given this evidence and recognizing the health benefits of proper vitamin K intake [24–26], the aim of the current study was to analyze populational vitamin K intake and MD adherence in the Algarve region, a Mediterranean setting within Portugal. To the best of our knowledge, this is the first study to describe and analyze the association between MD adherence and vitamin K intake in Portugal.

2. Materials and Methods

2.1. Setting

The Algarve is the southernmost region of Portugal. It spans an area of 4 997 km^2 and was home to 467,495 residents as of 2021 [27]. It is known for its Mediterranean climate and tourism industry, with many residents employed in tourism-related industries, especially during the peak tourist season, which typically occurs in the summer months. The local economy exhibits diversity, with contributions from sectors such as agriculture, fishing, and small-scale industries [28].

Recent demographic data show that the average age of the population stands at 45.3 years, slightly higher than the national average of 44.9 years. The schooling rate, which gauges the percentage of the population aged 3 to 24 attending educational institutions, was 85.9% in 2020, slightly below the national average of 88.4%. Furthermore, educational attainment among the population aged 15 and over in 2021 shows that only 14% hold a higher education degree [28].

2.2. Study Design, Participants, and Data Collection Tools

We conducted a cross-sectional survey in a nonrandom sample of adults using an online, self-fulfillment questionnaire (https://form.jotform.com/222044277445353, accessed on 19 February 2024, NutriK) specifically created for this study, which included questions regarding sociodemographic characteristics, the 14-item Mediterranean Diet Screener, and a previously validated food-frequency questionnaire (FFQ) to assess total vitamin K intake.

The FFQ is composed of 54 food items that contain ≥ 5 µg of vitamin K/100 g of food or, despite having <5 µg of vitamin K/100 g of food, are commonly included in a Mediterranean diet (soft cheese, boiled chickpeas, pumpkin, bell pepper, mackerel, sardines, almonds, walnuts, and coffee) [29]. Data on the vitamin K content of foods were derived from previous research [12], as well as from both McCance and Widdowson's and the United States Department of Agriculture's food composition databases [30,31]. The detailed description of the FFQ and the methods used for its validation are presented elsewhere [32].

Vitamin K intake data provided by the FFQ were presented in µg/day and analyzed considering a 10% threshold around the AI recommendation of 120 µg/day for men and 90 µg/day for women [9]. Thus, an intake of 120 ± 12 µg/day for men and 90 ± 9 µg/day for women was considered as adequate.

The 14-item Mediterranean Diet Adherence Screener (MEDAS) used in this study was the tool created in the "Prevención con Dieta Mediterránea" (PREDIMED) trial [33]. This screener consists of 14 questions related to dietary habits reflecting the key components of the Mediterranean diet, such as the consumption of fruits, vegetables, whole grains, olive oil, nuts, legumes, fish, and moderate alcohol intake, while limiting red meat and processed foods. Each question is scored based on how closely the respondent's diet aligns with the Mediterranean diet pattern. Scores range between 0 and 14 and provide an indication of adherence to the Mediterranean diet, with higher scores indicating better adherence. Scores ≥ 10 indicate good adherence to the MD.

Participation in this study was promoted by publicizing the project through social media using the institutional communication channels and tools of the University of Algarve. Inclusion criteria were (i) age ≥ 18 years; (ii) currently living in the region; and (iii) cognitive ability to fulfill the data collection tools. Exclusion criteria were (i) currently under treatment for serious chronic illness, such as cancer or autoimmune diseases; (ii) diagnosis of a disease that impairs nutrition or food choice, such as Crohn's disease, other malabsorption syndromes, or food allergies.

Sample size calculation, according to methods proposed by Hulley et al. [34] considering a 95% confidence level, a 5% margin of error, and an expected prevalence of adherence to the MD (MEDAS score ≥ 10) of 15%, yielded a minimum sample size of 196 participants. Accounting for a 10% rate for invalid questionnaires, we set the minimum sample size at 216 individuals.

At the end of the data collection phase, 238 valid questionnaires were obtained. Body mass index (BMI) was calculated as the ratio between weight and square of height (kg/m^2).

All respondents gave informed consent for participation, and the study was conducted according to the guidelines of the Declaration of Helsinki and approved by the ethics committee of the University of Algarve, Faro, Portugal (code CEUAlg Pn°01/2022).

2.3. Statistical Analysis

Data were analyzed using IBM SPSS for Windows (version 29.0, 2022, IBM Corporation). Mean, median, standard deviation (SD), and interquartile range (IQR) were computed whenever appropriate, and we used the Kolmogorov–Smirnov test to assess adherence to the normal distribution of quantitative variables (vitamin K intake and age). As the distribution of these variables was non-Gaussian, a nonparametric test (Mann–Whitney) was used for 2-group comparisons. Group comparisons of qualitative variables were assessed with the chi-square test, Fisher's exact test or, when conditions were not met for their use, with the Fisher–Freeman–Halton exact test. We also computed Spearman's correlation coefficient for assessing associations between continuous variables.

Statistical significance for all procedures was set at 0.05.

3. Results

Of the 238 participants, 68% ($n = 161$) were women and 32% were men ($n = 77$). Men had a higher mean BMI than women and a higher prevalence of excess weight or obesity (Table 1).

Table 1. Sociodemographic characteristics, body mass index (BMI), vitamin K intake, and adherence to the Mediterranean diet (MD).

Variable	All ($n = 238$)	Women ($n = 161$)	Men ($n = 77$)	p-Value
Age (years); M ± SD	37.5 ± 1.01	37.2 ± 1.16	38.0 ± 1.99	0.984 *
BMI (kg/m^2); M ± SD	23.8 ± 0.25	23.4 ± 0.31	25.0 ± 0.43	**0.003 ***
Preobese or obese (BMI ≥ 25); %; n	33%; 80	29%; 47	43%; 33	**0.037 ****
Education:				
Less than high school level; %; n	1%; 2	-	3%; 2	
High school; %; n	35%; 82	30%; 49	43%; 33	**0.013 *****
Higher education; %; n	65%; 154	70%; 112	55%; 42	
Vitamin K intake (µg/day); M ± SD	285.2 ± 17.05	317.51 ± 23.65	222.57 ± 18.45	**0.019 ***
Vitamin K adequate intake:				
Below; %; n	10%; 24	4%; 6	22%; 28	
±10%; %; n	5%; 12	6%; 9	4%; 3	**<0.001 ****
Above; %; n	85%; 206	91%; 146	74%; 60	
Adherence to MD; %; n	11%; 26	12%; 20	7%; 6	0.284
MEDAS Score:				
Range (Min–Max)	1- 12	2- 12	1- 12	
M ± SD	6.8 ± 2.18	7.1 ± 2.15	6.3 ± 2.16	
Md; IQR	7; 3	7; 3	6; 4	**0.009 ***

M—mean; SD—standard deviation; Md—Median; IQR—interquartile range; * Mann–Whitney's test; ** chi-square test; *** Fisher–Freeman–Halton's test; statistical significance ($p < 0.05$) is highlighted in **bold**.

Vitamin K intake was higher ($p = 0.019$) in women (Mean = 317.5 ± 23.65 µg/day) than in men (Mean = 222.6 ± 18.45 µg/day). The prevalence of vitamin K intake above AI was also higher ($p < 0.001$) in women (91%; $n = 146$) than in men (74%; $n = 60$).

Adherence to the MD was 11% for all participants: 12% in women and 7% in men. Gender differences in total adherence to MD were statistically not significant ($p = 0.284$), but the MEDAS score was higher in women ($p = 0.009$). This can be explained by gender differences in some specific MD habits: comparatively with women, men report lower use of olive oil for cooking (86% vs. 97%; $p = 0.001$), a higher prevalence of red/processed meat intake at least once a day (74% vs. 58%; $p = 0.001$), a higher prevalence of soda drink intake at least once a day (35% vs. 19%; $p = 0.005$), and a higher prevalence of at least seven glasses of wine a week (14% vs. 5%; $p = 0.013$).

In our population, participants with MD adherence were significantly different from nonadherents in most dietary habits reflecting the key components of the MD, except for the use of olive oil as the main lipid ($p = 0.147$), the infrequent intake of commercial sweets and confectionery ($p = 0.097$), the more frequent poultry intake than red meats ($p = 0.166$), and the frequent use of sofrito sauce ($p = 0.520$) (Table 2).

Table 2. Dietary habits according to adherence to the Mediterranean diet (MD).

Mediterranean Dietary Habits	All (%) (n = 238)	Adherence to MD (%) (n = 26)	Nonadherence to MD (%) (n = 212)	p-Value
Use of olive oil as main culinary lipid	93	100	92	0.147
Olive oil >4 tablespoons	21	50	17	<0.001
Vegetables ≥2 servings/day	52	92	47	<0.001
Fruits ≥3 servings/day	28	58	25	<0.001
Red/processed meats <1/day	37	88	30	<0.001
Butter, cream, margarine <1/day	45	73	41	0.002
Soda drinks <1/day	76	100	73	0.002
Wine glasses ≥7/week	8	23	6	0.003
Legumes ≥3/week	34	77	29	<0.001
Fish/seafood ≥3/week	37	65	33	0.001
Commercial sweets and confectionery ≤2/week	75	88	74	0.097
Tree nuts ≥3/week	27	69	22	<0.001
Poultry more than red meats	69	81	67	0.166
Use of sofrito sauce ≥2/week	80	85	79	0.520

p-value for comparisons between adherent and nonadherent groups computed with the chi-square test; statistical significance ($p < 0.05$) is highlighted in **bold**.

Participants who adhered to the MD had a significantly higher intake of vitamin K (M = 528.5 ± 389.8 µg/day) than nonadherents (M = 257.2 ± 232.1 µg/day) (Table 3).

Table 3. Vitamin K intake according to adherence to the Mediterranean diet (MD).

Vitamin K intake	Adherence to MD (%) (n = 26)	Nonadherence to MD (%) (n = 212)	p-Value
Intake (µg/day); M ± SD	528.5 ± 389.8	257.2 ± 232.1	0.002 *
Adequate intake:			0.096 **
Below; %; n	-	11%; 23	
±10%; %; n	-	5%; 11	
Above; %; n	100%; 26	84%; 178	

M—mean; SD—standard deviation; * Mann–Whitney's test; ** Fisher–Freeman–Halton's test; statistical significance ($p < 0.05$) is highlighted in **bold**.

Additionally, there is a statistically significant positive correlation between vitamin K intake and both the MEDAS score (r = 0.463; $p < 0.001$) and age (r = 0.223; $p < 0.001$). The association between vitamin K intake and MEDAS score is maintained when controlling for age (r = 0.352; $p < 0.001$), both in men (r = 0.455; $p < 0.001$) and in women (r = 0.315; $p < 0.001$), suggesting the significant role of MD habits in vitamin K intake, independent of age and gender.

Vitamin K intake did not correlate with BMI (r = 0.003; $p = 0.958$).

The food items which contributed most to vitamin K intake are presented in Table 4. We did not find any gender differences in specific food items contributing to total vitamin K intake ($p > 0.05$).

Table 4. Foods that contributed the most to total vitamin K intake, presented as mean percentage of total vitamin K intake, in all participants and by gender.

Food	Contribution (%) to Total Vitamin K Intake M ± SD			p-Value *
	All (n = 238)	Women (n = 161)	Men (n = 77)	
Spinach	20 ± 15	22 ± 16	17 ± 12	0.092
Turnip greens, creamed spinach, green vegetable puree	19 ± 14	19 ± 15	19 ± 13	0.896
Broccoli	14 ± 12	13 ± 11	15 ± 13	0.037
Lettuce or mixed green salad	7 ± 8	7 ± 8	7 ± 7	0.217
Cabbage, collard greens, Brussels sprouts	4 ± 5	4 ± 5	3 ± 4	0.754
Stir-fry or stew with vegetables and/or pasta	3 ± 4	3 ± 5	2 ± 2	0.538
Coriander or parsley	3 ± 3	2 ± 3	3 ± 4	0.083
Olive oil	2 ± 5	2 ± 4	3 ± 6	0.323
Watercress and arugula	2 ± 3	2 ± 3	2 ± 3	0.291

M—mean; SD—standard deviation; * Mann–Whitney's test for gender differences.

4. Discussion

In this work, for the first time, we report a correlation between adherence to MD and vitamin K intake in a Portuguese population residing in the Algarve region. Among the participants, 85% exhibited a vitamin K intake of at least 10% above the RI. Specifically, the mean daily vitamin K intake was 317.5 ± 23.65 µg/day for women and 222.6 ± 18.45 µg/day for men.

Globally, estimates of vitamin K intake reveal significant variations across countries and divergent findings among studies. These disparities can be explained by factors such as different methodological approaches for estimations and dietetic patterns [35–40]. A comprehensive assessment of vitamin K intake in Europe, performed by the EFSA Panel on Dietetic Products, Nutrition, and Allergies (NDA), estimated a mean total vitamin K intake ranging between 72 and 196 ug/day in adults aged 18 and above, drawing from data available in Finland, France, Ireland, Italy, Netherlands, Sweden, and the UK [41]. Interestingly, Italy and the Netherlands reported higher mean intake estimates, surpassing 150 µg/day [41]. In the Netherlands, where a high intake of vegetables is part of the dietetic pattern, vitamin K intake was the highest.

Existing studies predominantly focus on vitamin K1 and menaquinones intake, which range between 230–288 ug/day for vitamin K1 and 27–31 ug/day for menaquinones [26,42–44]. Our analysis was limited to total vitamin K due to the scarcity of nutritional composition data and the absence of a validated tool to quantify both vitamin K1 and vitamin K2 intake through self-reported data. Nevertheless, our overall vitamin K estimates align with those observed in the Netherlands. Although vitamin K1 has been demonstrated as the major source of nutritional vitamin K [43], future research should be conducted to distinguish between K1 and K2 dietary sources, physiological functions, and contribution to an MD.

While there are clear overlapping patterns between MD and food items with high vitamin K content, particularly K1 in green vegetables and in olive oil, studies to assess the association between MD and vitamin K intake are, to the best of our knowledge, unknown. One study performed in Italy, comparing vitamin K1 levels between hemodialysis patients and controls, reported a mean of 129.2 ug/day (61.5–380.5) for vitamin K1 in the control group [45]. Although Italy is a Mediterranean country, the authors did not specifically explore the connection between MD adherence and vitamin K1 intake. Additionally, research on the influence of MD on anticoagulation therapy involving vitamin K antagonists has been conducted; however, a direct association between vitamin K intake and adherence to an MD was not established in these studies [16,17]. This relation would potentially add an increment of clinical value to the MD, since vitamin K deficiency has been widely reported to be associated with vascular [46] and renal disease [47].

The question of whether established vitamin K RI is adequate to fulfill vitamin K requirements is still a matter of debate in the scientific community. The RI was based on the maintenance of normal hemostasis, with sufficient vitamin K to maintain proper gamma-carboxylation of blood coagulation factors. However, several extrahepatic VKDP proteins have been shown as incompletely gamma-carboxylated in healthy adults not taking vitamin K supplements [48], with implications in several CIDs [reviewed in [6,7]]. In fact, it was suggested that the Western diet does not contain sufficient vitamin K to fulfill the gamma-carboxylation of extrahepatic tissues, such as the vascular system and bones [48]. Although several interventional clinical trials have established the beneficial effects of vitamin K supplementation in bone and vascular health, others have reported a lack of effects [49–56]. This can be explained by the lack of standardized protocols, the use of different vitamin K vitamers, different follow-up and endpoint measurements, and different approaches to determining vitamin K levels [6,7]. Additional long-term vitamin K interventional studies in healthy subjects and disease cohorts are required to fully understand the optimal vitamin K levels and the impact of vitamin K supplementation on health status.

In our study, we observed a significant association between lower vitamin K intake and poorer adherence to the Mediterranean diet (MD). This finding leads us to hypothesize that promoting the MD could potentially enhance vitamin K intake. However, it should be noted that despite low adherence to the MD, some participants achieved adequate or above-average vitamin K intake, particularly among women. This phenomenon might be partially explained by research indicating that dietary patterns with reduced meat consumption can still facilitate the intake of vitamin-K-rich foods, even if they deviate from the traditional MD [24,46]. Nevertheless, it is crucial to note that these alternative diets may lack the comprehensive health benefits associated with adherence to the MD.

A large body of evidence associates diverse health benefits with higher adherence to the MD, including decreased mortality and prevention of cardiovascular diseases, diabetes, cancer, and neurogenerative diseases [57]. Furthermore, the MD principles align with healthier lifestyles, potentially influencing other healthy choices and, nutritionally, promoting a synergistic interplay, as the MD is not just a collection of isolated nutrients [57–59].

Olive oil, one of the main features of MD, might enhance vitamin K absorption, while fiber provided by adequate amounts of vegetables could slow down digestion, allowing for better utilization [60]. This combined effect could amplify the benefits of individual components, such as vitamin K.

Adherence to the MD for all participants was 11%, lower than the one estimated by the last National Food, Nutrition, and Physical Activity Survey of the Portuguese General Population [61], showing adherences of 18% (95% CI: 17.3–19.1) at the national level and 20% for Algarve. The data for this national survey were collected in 2015–2016, and recent studies suggest that MD adherence has been declining, with estimates that only around 10–15% of adults maintain most dietary habits associated with an MD. The results of the same study, reporting adherence to the MD and its association with country-specific socioeconomic characteristics, suggest that the level of adherence may be influenced by socioeconomic factors and, thus, decreased during the recent economic crisis [20,62].

Our results on MD adherence are also aligned with the literature, suggesting that adherence to the MD is lower in men and in younger individuals [19,63]. In our study, men had a significantly lower ($p = 0.009$) MEDAS score (M = 6.3 ± 2.16) than women (7.1 ± 2.15), but it is important to note that these results could be biased due to the low representativeness of men in our sample. In addition, the positive correlation between MEDAS score and age suggests that older participants have a higher adherence to the MD.

The literature also suggests that the dietary features of the MD that are most commonly being lost seem to be mainly driven by excess meat consumption [64]. Our data support these claims, with low adherence to MD coexisting with a high intake of red/processed meats (63% of participants reported an intake of at least once a day).

We obtained 238 valid replies to our questionnaire, mostly from women (68%). This number of participants surpassed the minimum estimated to achieve a representative sample, according to our calculations, but some sociodemographic characteristics of our participants differ from the available populational data for the Algarve region.

The gender distribution for the participants was 68% for women and 32% for men. Census data for Portugal [65] show that the gender distribution in the Algarve, for adults, is approximately 52% women and 48% men.

Our participants also had a significantly higher rate of higher education than the estimated for the Algarve region: 65% of all participants (70% in women and 55% in men) had concluded some higher education degree, contrasting with the data from the 2021 census showing a rate of 44% for Portugal and just 8% for the Algarve, which is well below the national average. This may have introduced some bias in our results and is in accordance with some research showing that women, especially those with a higher educational level, are generally more likely to participate in health and nutrition studies compared with men [66,67]. It is suggested that women tend to be more interested in health topics, more actively seek health information, and may perceive themselves at higher risk for certain health conditions and thus be more motivated to participate in research related to those conditions [66]. Women may also be subjected to cultural beliefs, traditions, norms, and values that increase their feeling of being helpful and contributing to health knowledge [68,69].

Our participants reported heights and weights that resulted in a 33% combined prevalence for preobesity (BMI between 25–29.9 kg/m^2) and obesity (BMI $\geq$ 30 kg/m^2), significantly higher (p = 0.0037) in men (43%) than in women (29%). These data are below national and regional estimates from the last populational survey [61]. Data available from adults at the national level suggest rates of 36.5% of preobesity and 21.6% for obesity, i.e., around 58% for the combined prevalence of preobesity and obesity. The same survey suggests, in Algarve, rates of 36.3% for preobesity and 19.2% for obesity, resulting in around 56% combined prevalence. The underestimation of weight is a well-documented phenomenon in the scientific literature across various populations and settings, which makes a case for the limited use of self-reported anthropometric measurements in health research [70,71]. However, due to the methodology applied in our study, this was considered the only way to have a general characterization of our participants. We believe that our results are not significantly biased, as it was not an objective of our research to perform a proper assessment of nutritional status.

Despite the limitations of our research related to the cross-sectional design that precludes analyzing causality, the self-reported intake assessment, and the nonrandom nature of our sample, we found a significant association between adherence to MD and vitamin K intake. Additional research, employing larger and more diverse samples, as well as longitudinal designs with biomarkers and dietary records, could enhance the validity of these findings and provide a deeper understanding of the relationship between dietary patterns, vitamin K intake, and health outcomes.

5. Conclusions

Our results indicate that adherence to the MD is low, particularly among younger individuals. Vitamin K intake for most participants is either comparable to or exceeds the recommended adequate intake. Men exhibit both lower adherence to the MD and a higher prevalence of values below the recommended intake.

Our data suggest a positive association between MD adherence and vitamin K intake, indicating that the MD favors intake of vitamin K. Furthermore, our findings underscore the significance of promoting adherence to the MD, especially among individuals with low vitamin K intake.

Future research should prioritize developing effective interventions to promote this dietary pattern, particularly among younger individuals and men, to mitigate the risk of age-related diseases.

Considering the scientific evidence linking improved adherence to MD with health benefits and environmental sustainability, future research and initiatives should raise public awareness about the health and environmental advantages associated with higher MD adherence. Additionally, efforts should focus on enhancing accessibility to the MD for diverse communities worldwide.

Author Contributions: Conceptualization, E.P., C.V. and D.S.; methodology, E.P., P.V.M. and C.M.; software, P.V.M.; formal analysis, E.P. and T.N.; investigation, E.P., C.V. and D.S.; resources, L.S.; writing—original draft preparation, E.P., C.V. and D.S.; writing—review and editing, E.P., C.V., C.M., L.S. and D.S.; project administration, E.P. and D.S.; funding acquisition, E.P., C.V., P.V.M. and D.S. All authors have read and agreed to the published version of the manuscript.

Funding: This research was funded by the Portuguese National Funds from FCT—Foundation for Science and Technology, through transitional provision DL57/2016/CP1361/CT0006, projects EXPL/BTM-TEC/0990/2021, UIDB/04326/2020, UIDP/04326/2020 and LA/P/0101/2020 and AAC n° 41/ALG/2020—Project No. 072583—NUTRISAFE.

Institutional Review Board Statement: This study was conducted according to the guidelines of the Declaration of Helsinki and approved by the ethics committee of the University of Algarve, Faro, Portugal (code CEUAlg Pn°01/2022, approved 21 January 2022).

Informed Consent Statement: Informed consent was obtained from all subjects involved in the study.

Data Availability Statement: The data presented in this study are available on request from the corresponding author due to privacy restrictions.

Conflicts of Interest: Dina Simes and Carla Viegas are cofounders of Genogla Diagnostics. Leon Schurgers receives grants from institutions from Gnosis by Lesaffre, Bayer, and Boehringer Ingelheim, is a consultant for IDS, and is a shareholder of Coagulation Profile. The authors declare that there are no conflicts of interest regarding the publication of this paper.

References

1. Serra-Majem, L.; Medina, F.X. Mediterranean diet: A long journey toward intangible cultural heritage and sustainability. In *The Mediterranean Diet: An Evidence-Based Approach*; Elsevier: Amsterdam, The Netherlands, 2020; pp. 13–24.
2. Castro-Quezada, I.; Román-Viñas, B.; Serra-Majem, L. The Mediterranean Diet and Nutritional Adequacy: A Review. *Nutrients* **2014**, *6*, 231. [CrossRef] [PubMed]
3. Dominguez, L.J.; Di Bella, G.; Veronese, N.; Barbagallo, M. Impact of Mediterranean Diet on Chronic Non-Communicable Diseases and Longevity. *Nutrients* **2021**, *13*, 2028. [CrossRef] [PubMed]
4. Tosti, V.; Bertozzi, B.; Fontana, L. Health Benefits of the Mediterranean Diet: Metabolic and Molecular Mechanisms. *J. Gerontol. A Biol. Sci. Med. Sci.* **2018**, *73*, 318–326. [CrossRef] [PubMed]
5. Martínez-González, M.A.; Gea, A.; Ruiz-Canela, M. The Mediterranean Diet and Cardiovascular Health. *Circ. Res.* **2019**, *124*, 779–798. [CrossRef] [PubMed]
6. Simes, D.C.; Viegas, C.S.B.; Araújo, N.; Marreiros, C. Vitamin K as a Powerful Micronutrient in Aging and Age-Related Diseases: Pros and Cons from Clinical Studies. *Int. J. Mol. Sci.* **2020**, *20*, 4150. [CrossRef] [PubMed]
7. Simes, D.C.; Viegas, C.S.B.; Araújo, N.; Marreiros, C. Vitamin K as a diet supplement with impact in human health: Current evidence in age-related diseases. *Nutrients* **2020**, *12*, 138. [CrossRef] [PubMed]
8. Mishima, E.; Ito, J.; Wu, Z.; Nakamura, T.; Wahida, A.; Doll, S.; Tonnus, W.; Nepachalovich, P.; Eggenhofer, E.; Aldrovandi, M.; et al. A non-canonical vitamin K cycle is a potent ferroptosis suppressor. *Nature* **2022**, *608*, 778–783. [CrossRef]
9. Booth, S.L. Vitamin K: Food composition and dietary intakes. *Food Nutr. Res.* **2012**, *56*, 5505. [CrossRef] [PubMed]
10. Thijssen, H.; Drittij-Reijnders, M. Vitamin K status in human tissues: Tissue-specific accumulation of phylloquinone and menaquinone-4. *Br. J. Nutr.* **1996**, *75*, 121–127. [CrossRef]
11. Shearer, M.; Newman, P. Metabolism and cell biology of vitamin K. *Thromb. Haemost.* **2008**, *100*, 530–547.
12. Schurgers, L.J.; Vermeer, C. Determination of phylloquinone and menaquinones in food. Effect of food matrix on circulating vitamin K concentrations. *Haemostasis* **2000**, *30*, 298–307.
13. Institute of Medicine (US) Panel on Micronutrients. *Dietary Reference Intakes for Vitamin A, Vitamin K, Arsenic, Boron, Chromium, Copper, Iodine, Iron, Manganese, Molybdenum, Nickel, Silicon, Vanadium, and Zinc*; National Academies Press: Washington, DC, USA, 2001.
14. Widmer, R.J.; Flammer, A.J.; Lerman, L.O.; Lerman, A. The Mediterranean diet, its components, and cardiovascular disease. *Am. J. Med.* **2015**, *128*, 229–238. [CrossRef]
15. Guasch-Ferré, M.; Willett, W.C. The Mediterranean diet and health: A comprehensive overview. *J. Intern. Med.* **2021**, *290*, 549–566. [CrossRef] [PubMed]
16. Castro-Barquero, S.; Ribó-Coll, M.; Lassale, C.; Tresserra-Rimbau, A.; Castañer, O.; Pintó, X.; Martínez-González, M.Á.; Sorlí, J.V.; Salas-Salvadó, J.; Lapetra, J.; et al. Mediterranean Diet Decreases the Initiation of Use of Vitamin K Epoxide Reductase Inhibitors and Their Associated Cardiovascular Risk: A Randomized Controlled Trial. *Nutrients* **2020**, *12*, 3895. [CrossRef]

17. Pignatelli, P.; Pastori, D.; Vicario, T.; Bucci, T.; Del Ben, M.; Russo, R.; Tanzilli, A.; Nardoni, M.L.; Bartimoccia, S.; Nocella, C.; et al. Relationship between Mediterranean diet and time in therapeutic range in atrial fibrillation patients taking vitamin K antagonists. *Europace* **2015**, *17*, 1223–1228. [CrossRef]
18. Iaccarino Idelson, P.; Scalfi, L.; Valerio, G. Adherence to the Mediterranean Diet in children and adolescents: A systematic review. *Nutr. Metab. Cardiovasc. Dis.* **2017**, *27*, 283–299. [CrossRef] [PubMed]
19. Archero, F.; Ricotti, R.; Solito, A.; Carrera, D.; Civello, F.; Di Bella, R.; Bellone, S.; Prodam, F. Adherence to the Mediterranean Diet among School Children and Adolescents Living in Northern Italy and Unhealthy Food Behaviors Associated to Overweight. *Nutrients* **2018**, *10*, 1322. [CrossRef] [PubMed]
20. Bonaccio, M.; Donati, M.; Iacoviello, L.; de Gaetano, G. Socioeconomic Determinants of the Adherence to the Mediterranean Diet at a Time of Economic Crisis: The Experience of the MOLI-SANI Study1. *Agric. Agric. Sci. Procedia* **2016**, *8*, 741–747. [CrossRef]
21. Rosi, A.; Paolella, G.; Biasini, B.; Scazzina, F.; Alicante, P.; De Blasio, F.; dello Russo, M.; Rendina, D.; Tabacchi, G.; Cairella, G.; et al. Dietary habits of adolescents living in North America, Europe or Oceania: A review on fruit, vegetable and legume consumption, sodium intake, and adherence to the Mediterranean Diet. *Nutr. Metab. Cardiovasc. Dis.* **2019**, *29*, 544–560. [CrossRef]
22. Andrade, V.; Jorge, R.; García-Conesa, M.T.; Philippou, E.; Massaro, M.; Chervenkov, M.; Ivanova, T.; Maksimova, V.; Smilkov, K.; Ackova, D.G.; et al. Mediterranean Diet Adherence and Subjective Well-Being in a Sample of Portuguese Adults. *Nutrients* **2020**, *12*, 3837. [CrossRef]
23. Mendonça, N.; Gregório, M.J.; Salvador, C.; Henriques, A.R.; Canhão, H.; Rodrigues, A.M. Low Adherence to the Mediterranean Diet Is Associated with Poor Socioeconomic Status and Younger Age: A Cross-Sectional Analysis of the EpiDoC Cohort. *Nutrients* **2022**, *14*, 1239. [CrossRef] [PubMed]
24. Mladěnka, P.; Macáková, K.; Kujovská Krčmová, L.; Javorská, L.; Mrštná, K.; Carazo, A.; Protti, M.; Remião, F.; Nováková, L. Vitamin K—sources, physiological role, kinetics, deficiency, detection, therapeutic use, and toxicity. *Nutr. Rev.* **2022**, *80*, 677–698. [CrossRef] [PubMed]
25. Camacho-Barcia, L.; García-Gavilán, J.; Martínez-González, M.Á.; Fernández-Aranda, F.; Galié, S.; Corella, D.; Cuenca-Royo, A.; Romaguera, D.; Vioque, J.; Alonso-Gómez, Á.M.; et al. Vitamin K dietary intake is associated with cognitive function in an older adult Mediterranean population. *Age Ageing* **2022**, *51*, afab246. [CrossRef] [PubMed]
26. Juanola-Falgarona, M.; Salas-Salvadó, J.; Martínez-González, M.A.; Corella, D.; Estruch, R.; Ros, E.; Fitó, M.; Arós, F.; Gómez-Gracia, E.; Fiol, M.; et al. Dietary intake of vitamin K is inversely associated with mortality risk. *J. Nutr.* **2014**, *144*, 743–750. [CrossRef] [PubMed]
27. Comissao de Coordenação e Desenvolvimento Regional do Algarve (CCDR) Algarve-Censos 2021 (Resultados Preliminares). Available online: https://www.ccdr-alg.pt/site/info/algarve-censos-2021-resultados-preliminares (accessed on 12 February 2024).
28. Comissao de Coordenação e Desenvolvimento Regional do Algarve (CCDR) Região Algarve Em Números. Available online: https://www.ine.pt/ngt_server/attachfileu.jsp?look_parentBoui=550105507&att_display=n&att_download=y (accessed on 11 February 2024).
29. Willett, W. Mediterranean Dietary Pyramid. *Int. J. Environ. Res. Public Health* **2021**, *18*, 4568. [CrossRef] [PubMed]
30. U. S. Department of Agriculture FoodData Central. Available online: https://fdc.nal.usda.gov/ (accessed on 11 February 2024).
31. Roe, M.; Pinchen, H.; Church, S.; Finglas, P. McCance and Widdowson's The Composition of Foods Seventh Summary Edition and updated Composition of Foods Integrated Dataset. *Nutr. Bull.* **2015**, *40*, 36–39. [CrossRef]
32. Pinto, E.; Viegas, C.; Martins, P.V.; Nascimento, T.; Schurgers, L.; Simes, D. New Food Frequency Questionnaire to Estimate Vitamin K Intake in a Mediterranean Population. *Nutrients* **2023**, *15*, 3012. [CrossRef]
33. Martínez-González, M.A.; García-Arellano, A.; Toledo, E.; Salas-Salvadó, J.; Buil-Cosiales, P.; Corella, D.; Covas, M.I.; Schröder, H.; Arós, F.; Gómez-Gracia, E.; et al. A 14-Item Mediterranean Diet Assessment Tool and Obesity Indexes among High-Risk Subjects: The PREDIMED Trial. *PLoS ONE* **2012**, *7*, e43134. [CrossRef] [PubMed]
34. Hulley, S.B.; Cummings, S.R.; Browner, W.S.; Grady, D.G.; Newman, T.B. *Designing Clinical Research*; LWW: Philadelphia, PA, USA, 2013.
35. Duggan, P.; Cashman, K.D.; Flynn, A.; Bolton-Smith, C.; Kiely, M. Phylloquinone (vitamin K1) intakes and food sources in 18-64-year-old Irish adults. *Br. J. Nutr.* **2004**, *92*, 151–158. [CrossRef]
36. Booth, S.L.; Tucker, K.L.; Chen, H.; Hannan, M.T.; Gagnon, D.R.; Cupples, L.A.; Wilson, P.W.F.; Ordovas, J.; Schaefer, E.J.; Dawson-Hughes, B.; et al. Dietary vitamin K intakes are associated with hip fracture but not with bone mineral density in elderly men and women. *Am. J. Clin. Nutr.* **2000**, *71*, 1201–1208. [CrossRef]
37. Booth, S.L.; Pennington, J.A.T.; Sadowski, J.A. Food sources and dietary intakes of vitamin K-1 (phylloquinone) in the American diet: Data from the FDA Total Diet Study. *J. Am. Diet. Assoc.* **1996**, *96*, 149–154. [CrossRef] [PubMed]
38. Presse, N.; Shatenstein, B.; Kergoat, M.J.; Ferland, G. Validation of a semi-quantitative food frequency questionnaire measuring dietary vitamin K intake in elderly people. *J. Am. Diet. Assoc.* **2009**, *109*, 1251–1255. [CrossRef] [PubMed]
39. Nimptsch, K.; Rohrmann, S.; Kaaks, R.; Linseisen, J. Dietary vitamin K intake in relation to cancer incidence and mortality: Results from the Heidelberg cohort of the European Prospective Investigation into Cancer and Nutrition (EPIC-Heidelberg). *Am. J. Clin. Nutr.* **2010**, *91*, 1348–1358. [CrossRef] [PubMed]

40. Thane, C.W.; Paul, A.A.; Bates, C.J.; Prentice, A.; Shearer, M.J. Intake and sources of phylloquinone (vitamin K 1): Variation with socio-demographic and lifestyle factors in a national sample of British elderly people. *Br. J. Nutr.* **2002**, *87*, 605–613. [CrossRef] [PubMed]
41. Turck, D.; Bresson, J.L.; Burlingame, B.; Dean, T.; Fairweather-Tait, S.; Heinonen, M.; Hirsch-Ernst, K.I.; Mangelsdorf, I.; McArdle, H.J.; Naska, A.; et al. Dietary reference values for vitamin K. *EFSA J.* **2017**, *15*, e04780. [PubMed]
42. Geleijnse, J.M.; Vermeer, C.; Grobbee, D.E.; Schurgers, L.J.; Knapen, M.H.J.; Van Der Meer, I.M.; Hofman, A.; Witteman, J.C.M. Dietary Intake of Menaquinone Is Associated with a Reduced Risk of Coronary Heart Disease: The Rotterdam Study. *J. Nutr.* **2004**, *134*, 3100–3105. [CrossRef] [PubMed]
43. Schurgers, L.J.; Geleijnse, J.M.; Grobbee, D.E.; Pols, H.A.P.; Hofman, A.; Witteman, J.C.M.; Vermeer, C. Nutritional Intake of Vitamins K1 (Phylloquinone) and K2 (Menaquinone) in The Netherlands. *J. Nutr. Environ. Med.* **1999**, *9*, 115–122. [CrossRef]
44. Gast, G.C.M.; De Roos, N.M.; Sluijs, I.; Bots, M.L.; Beulens, J.W.J.; Geleijnse, J.M.; Witteman, J.C.; Grobbee, D.E.; Peeters, P.H.M.; Van Der Schouw, Y.T. A high menaquinone intake reduces the incidence of coronary heart disease. *Nutr. Metab. Cardiovasc. Dis.* **2009**, *19*, 504–510. [CrossRef]
45. Fusaro, M.; D'Alessandro, C.; Noale, M.; Tripepi, G.; Plebani, M.; Veronese, N.; Iervasi, G.; Giannini, S.; Rossini, M.; Tarroni, G.; et al. Low vitamin K1 intake in haemodialysis patients. *Clin. Nutr.* **2017**, *36*, 601–607. [CrossRef]
46. Bellinge, J.W.; Dalgaard, F.; Murray, K.; Connolly, E.; Blekkenhorst, L.C.; Bondonno, C.P.; Lewis, J.R.; Sim, M.; Croft, K.D.; Gislason, G.; et al. Vitamin k intake and atherosclerotic cardiovascular disease in the danish diet cancer and health study. *J. Am. Heart Assoc.* **2021**, *10*, e020551. [CrossRef]
47. Dai, L.; Li, L.; Erlandsson, H.; Jaminon, A.M.G.; Qureshi, A.R.; Ripsweden, J.; Brismar, T.B.; Witasp, A.; Heimbürger, O.; Jørgensen, H.S.; et al. Functional Vitamin K insufficiency, vascular calcification and mortality in advanced chronic kidney disease: A cohort study. *PLoS ONE* **2021**, *16*, e0247623. [CrossRef]
48. Theuwissen, E.; Smit, E.; Vermeer, C. The Role of Vitamin K in Soft-Tissue Calcification. *Adv. Nutr.* **2012**, *3*, 166–173. [CrossRef] [PubMed]
49. Gage, B.F.; Birman-Deych, E.; Radford, M.J.; Nilasena, D.S.; Binder, E.F. Risk of osteoporotic fracture in elderly patients taking warfarin: Results from the National Registry of Atrial Fibrillation 2. *Arch. Intern. Med.* **2006**, *166*, 241–246. [CrossRef] [PubMed]
50. Lafforgue, P.; Daver, L.; Monties, J.R.; Chagnaud, C.; de Boissezon, M.C.; Acquaviva, P.C. Bone mineral density in patients given oral vitamin K antagonists. *Rev. Rhum. Engl. Ed.* **1997**, *64*, 249–254. [PubMed]
51. Vlasschaert, C.; Goss, C.J.; Pilkey, N.G.; McKeown, S.; Holden, R.M. Vitamin K Supplementation for the Prevention of Cardiovascular Disease: Where Is the Evidence? A Systematic Review of Controlled Trials. *Nutrients* **2020**, *12*, 2909. [CrossRef]
52. Shea, M.K.; O'Donnell, C.J.; Hoffmann, U.; Dallal, G.E.; Dawson-Hughes, B.; Ordovas, J.M.; Price, P.A.; Williamson, M.K.; Booth, S.L. Vitamin K supplementation and progression of coronary artery calcium in older men and women. *Am. J. Clin. Nutr.* **2009**, *89*, 1799–1807. [CrossRef]
53. Braam, L.A.J.L.M.; Hoeks, A.P.G.; Brouns, F.; Halmuyák, K.; Gerichhausen, M.J.W.; Vermeer, C. Beneficial effects of vitamins D and K on the elastic properties of the vessel wall in postmenopausal women: A follow-up study. *Thromb. Haemost.* **2004**, *91*, 373–380. [CrossRef]
54. Knapen, M.H.J.; Schurgers, L.J.; Vermeer, C. Vitamin K 2 supplementation improves hip bone geometry and bone strength indices in postmenopausal women. *Osteoporos. Int.* **2007**, *18*, 963–972. [CrossRef]
55. Martini, L.A.; Booth, S.L.; Saltzman, E.; Do Rosário Dias De Oliveira Latorre, M.; Wood, R.J. Dietary phylloquinone depletion and repletion in postmenopausal women: Effects on bone and mineral metabolism. *Osteoporos. Int.* **2006**, *17*, 929–935. [CrossRef]
56. Fu, X.; Moreines, J.; Booth, S.L. Vitamin K supplementation does not prevent bone loss in ovariectomized Norway rats. *Nutr. Metab.* **2012**, *9*, 12. [CrossRef]
57. Dinu, M.; Pagliai, G.; Casini, A.; Sofi, F. Mediterranean diet and multiple health outcomes: An umbrella review of meta-analyses of observational studies and randomised trials. *Eur. J. Clin. Nutr.* **2018**, *72*, 30–43. [CrossRef] [PubMed]
58. Grosso, G.; Fresán, U.; Bes-rastrollo, M.; Marventano, S.; Galvano, F. Environmental Impact of Dietary Choices: Role of the Mediterranean and Other Dietary Patterns in an Italian Cohort. *Int. J. Environ. Res. Public Health* **2020**, *17*, 1468. [CrossRef] [PubMed]
59. Grosso, G.; Marventano, S.; Yang, J.; Micek, A.; Pajak, A.; Scalfi, L.; Galvano, F.; Kales, S.N. A comprehensive meta-analysis on evidence of Mediterranean diet and cardiovascular disease: Are individual components equal? *Crit. Rev. Food Sci. Nutr.* **2017**, *57*, 3218–3232. [CrossRef] [PubMed]
60. Román, G.C.; Jackson, R.E.; Gadhia, R.; Román, A.N.; Reis, J. Mediterranean diet: The role of long-chain ω-3 fatty acids in fish; polyphenols in fruits, vegetables, cereals, coffee, tea, cacao and wine; probiotics and vitamins in prevention of stroke, age-related cognitive decline, and Alzheimer disease. *Rev. Neurol.* **2019**, *175*, 724–741. [CrossRef] [PubMed]
61. Lopes, C.; Torres, D.; Oliveira, A.; Severo, M.; Guiomar, S.; Alarcão, V.; Ramos, E.; Rodrigues, S.; Vilela, S.; Oliveira, L.; et al. National Food, Nutrition, and Physical Activity Survey of the Portuguese General Population (2015–2016): Protocol for Design and Development. *JMIR Res. Protoc.* **2018**, *15*, e42. [CrossRef] [PubMed]
62. Damigou, E.; Faka, A.; Kouvari, M.; Anastasiou, C.; Kosti, R.I.; Chalkias, C.; Panagiotakos, D. Adherence to a Mediterranean type of diet in the world: A geographical analysis based on a systematic review of 57 studies with 1,125,560 participants. *Int. J. Food Sci. Nutr.* **2023**, *74*, 799–813. [CrossRef] [PubMed]

63. Obeid, C.A.; Gubbels, J.S.; Jaalouk, D.; Kremers, S.P.J.; Oenema, A. Adherence to the Mediterranean diet among adults in Mediterranean countries: A systematic literature review. *Eur. J. Nutr.* **2022**, *61*, 3327–3344. [CrossRef] [PubMed]
64. Castaldi, S.; Dembska, K.; Antonelli, M.; Petersson, T.; Piccolo, M.G.; Valentini, R. The positive climate impact of the Mediterranean diet and current divergence of Mediterranean countries towards less climate sustainable food consumption patterns. *Sci. Rep.* **2022**, *12*, 8847. [CrossRef] [PubMed]
65. Instituto Nacional de Estatistica Estatísticas Demográficas. Lisboa. 2021. Available online: https://www.ine.pt/xurl/pub/1393 2532 (accessed on 11 February 2024).
66. Clayton, J.A.; Tannenbaum, C. Reporting Sex, Gender, or Both in Clinical Research? *JAMA* **2016**, *316*, 1863–1864. [CrossRef]
67. Leonard, A.; Hutchesson, M.; Patterson, A.; Chalmers, K.; Collins, C. Recruitment and retention of young women into nutrition research studies: Practical considerations. *Trials* **2014**, *15*, 23. [CrossRef]
68. Bartz, D.; Chitnis, T.; Kaiser, U.B.; Rich-Edwards, J.W.; Rexrode, K.M.; Pennell, P.B.; Goldstein, J.M.; O'Neal, M.A.; Leboff, M.; Behn, M.; et al. Clinical Advances in Sex- and Gender-Informed Medicine to Improve the Health of All: A Review. *JAMA Intern. Med.* **2020**, *180*, 574–583. [CrossRef] [PubMed]
69. Das, S.; Mishra, A.J. Dietary practices and gender dynamics: Understanding the role of women. *J. Ethn. Foods* **2021**, *8*, 4. [CrossRef]
70. Robinson, E.; Oldham, M. Weight status misperceptions among UK adults: The use of self-reported vs. measured BMI. *BMC Obes.* **2016**, *3*, 21. [CrossRef] [PubMed]
71. Van Dyke, N.; Drinkwater, E.J.; Rachele, J.N. Improving the accuracy of self-reported height and weight in surveys: An experimental study. *BMC Med. Res. Methodol.* **2022**, *22*, 241. [CrossRef] [PubMed]

Disclaimer/Publisher's Note: The statements, opinions and data contained in all publications are solely those of the individual author(s) and contributor(s) and not of MDPI and/or the editor(s). MDPI and/or the editor(s) disclaim responsibility for any injury to people or property resulting from any ideas, methods, instructions or products referred to in the content.

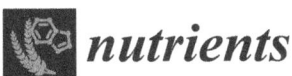

Article

The Role of *PNPLA3*_rs738409 Gene Variant, Lifestyle Factors, and Bioactive Compounds in Nonalcoholic Fatty Liver Disease: A Population-Based and Molecular Approach towards Healthy Nutrition

Meiling Liu [1] and Sunmin Park [2,3,*]

1. Department of Chemical Engineering, Shanxi Institute of Science and Technology, Jincheng 048000, China; liumeiling@sxist.edu.cn
2. Department of Bioconvergence, Hoseo University, Asan 31499, Republic of Korea
3. Department of Food and Nutrition, Institute of Basic Science, Obesity/Diabetes Research Center, Hoseo University, Asan 31499, Republic of Korea
* Correspondence: smpark@hoseo.edu; Tel.: +82-41-540-5345; Fax: +82-41-548-0670

Abstract: This study aimed to investigate the impact of a common non-synonymous gene variant (C>G, rs738409) in patatin-like phospholipase domain-containing 3 (*PNPLA3*), leading to the substitution of isoleucine with methionine at position 148 (*PNPLA3*-I148M), on susceptibility to nonalcoholic fatty liver disease (NAFLD) and explore potential therapeutic nutritional strategies targeting *PNPLA3*. It contributed to understanding sustainable dietary practices for managing NAFLD, recently referred to as metabolic-dysfunction-associated fatty liver. NAFLD had been diagnosed by ultrasound in a metropolitan hospital-based cohort comprising 58,701 middle-aged and older Korean individuals, identifying 2089 NAFLD patients. The interaction between *PNPLA3* and lifestyle factors was investigated. In silico analyses, including virtual screening, molecular docking, and molecular dynamics simulations, were conducted to identify bioactive compounds from foods targeting *PNPLA3*(I148M). Subsequent cellular experiments involved treating oleic acid (OA)-exposed HepG2 cells with selected bioactive compounds, both in the absence and presence of compound C (AMPK inhibitor), targeting *PNPLA3* expression. Carriers of the risk allele *PNPLA3*_rs738409G showed an increased association with NAFLD risk, particularly with adherence to a plant-based diet, avoidance of a Western-style diet, and smoking. Delphinidin 3-caffeoyl-glucoside, pyranocyanin A, delta-viniferin, kaempferol-7-glucoside, and petunidin 3-rutinoside emerged as potential binders to the active site residues of *PNPLA3*, exhibiting a reduction in binding energy. These compounds demonstrated a dose-dependent reduction in intracellular triglyceride and lipid peroxide levels in HepG2 cells, while pretreatment with compound C showed the opposite trend. Kaempferol-7-glucoside and petunidin-3-rutinoside showed potential as inhibitors of *PNPLA3* expression by enhancing AMPK activity, ultimately reducing intrahepatic lipogenesis. In conclusion, there is potential for plant-based diets and specific bioactive compounds to promote sustainable dietary practices to mitigate NAFLD risk, especially in individuals with genetic predispositions.

Keywords: NAFLD; *PNPLA3*; AMPK; *SREBP-1C*; HepG2; compound C

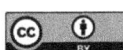

1. Introduction

Nonalcoholic fatty liver disease (NAFLD), a prevalent medical condition characterized by hepatic fat accumulation, liver inflammation, fibrosis, cirrhosis, and the potential to progress to liver cancer [1], has recently been redefined as metabolic-dysfunction-associated fatty liver disease (MAFLD) to reflect its multifactorial nature better and encompass a broader spectrum of liver disorders [2]. While NAFLD and MAFLD share many similarities, including their clinical manifestations and risk factors, they somewhat differ [2]. We have chosen to adhere to the NAFLD definition and terminology. NAFLD affects approximately 15 to 30% of adults globally, highlighting its significant public health impact [3]. While ultrasound scans offer a non-invasive means of detecting liver fat, a liver biopsy remains the gold standard for accurate diagnosis, particularly in cases of mild NAFLD [4]. Despite conducting multiple studies and clinical trials using various treatments, including weight loss drugs, insulin sensitizers, lipid-lowering drugs, and antioxidants such as vitamins C and E, none of them have shown definite efficacy for NAFLD. Recently, the US FDA has approved the drug Rezdiffra (resmetirom) in combination with diet and exercise for the treatment of adult NAFLD/non-cirrhotic nonalcoholic steatohepatitis (NASH) [5]. Certain phytochemicals, including flavonoids, show promise due to their antioxidative properties and ability to improve insulin sensitivity and regulate lipid metabolism, suggesting a potential role in preventing or slowing the progression of NAFLD. Studies have highlighted the ability of some flavonoids to modulate glucose and lipid metabolism, shield the liver, and ameliorate fatty liver. However, the precise mechanisms of action remain incompletely understood [6–9]. Further exploration of medications for NAFLD is warranted.

Understanding the genetic and environmental factors influencing NAFLD development is crucial for effective prevention and treatment with targeted interventions for at-risk individuals. A critical aspect of this interplay between genetic and environmental factors involves AMP-activated protein kinase (AMPK), a pivotal regulator of metabolic pathways that inhibits hepatic lipid synthesis and promotes lipid oxidation, effectively balancing lipid metabolism [10]. Moreover, recent studies have revealed a significant association between the patatin-like phospholipase domain-containing protein-3 (*PNPLA3*)_rs738409C/G polymorphism and NAFLD, highlighting its potential impact on liver fat metabolism [11]. Several studies have shown that *PNPLA3* overexpression induces hepatic steatosis through the carbohydrate response element binding protein (*ChREBP*) and sterol regulatory element binding protein 1c (*SREBP1c*), and its silencing prevents the development of hepatic fat storage and inflammation, thereby effectively preventing the development of NAFLD [12–14]. Furthermore, hepatic lipogenesis is linked to the AMPK pathway, which can modulate *PNPLA3*. However, it remains unclear whether AMPK activation decreases *PNPLA3* expression in the liver and prevents NAFLD and whether the decreased binding energy of bioactive compounds with *PNPLA3* reduces its expression to reduce hepatic lipogenesis.

This study aimed to find a sustainable diet to prevent and mitigate NAFLD in individuals with a genetic predisposition. We explored genetic variants that affect NAFLD risk and their interaction with lifestyle factors, such as nutritional intake, in the middle-aged and elderly individuals of the Korea Genome and Epidemiology Study (KoGES) cohort. Furthermore, we employed a molecular docking system for the *PNPLA3*_rs738409C/G protein to identify bioactive compounds that could potentially interact with the protein. The molecular mechanism of the identified bioactive compounds was further examined in a cell-based experiment using HepG2 cells. By combining epidemiological data, molecular docking, and cell-based experiments, this study contributed to the development of personalized dietary interventions for individuals with a genetic predisposition to NAFLD, ultimately contributing to the prevention and mitigation of the disease.

2. Methods
2.1. Participants

Between 2004 and 2013, 58,701 participants (20,293 males and 38,408 females) voluntarily participated in the hospital-based urban cohort as part of the Korea Genome and Epidemiology Study (KoGES). The sample size was determined using the Gpower calculator, achieving significance at $\alpha = 0.05$, $\beta = 0.99$, with an odds ratio of 1.06 between NAFLD and healthy participants. With over 50,000 participants, this goal was achieved. This study followed the Declaration of Helsinki and was approved by the Institutional Review Boards of the Korea National Institutes of Health (KBP-2019-055) and Hoseo University (1041231-190902-BR-099-01). Every participant completed a written informed consent form.

2.2. Basic Characteristics of the Participants and Biochemical Measurements

Participants were interviewed and queried about their demographics, lifestyle habits, and health status, including their gender, age, education, and income. Household income was divided into three levels ($/month): low income ($2000), middle income ($2000–$4000) and high income ($4000) [15]. The participants were classified into smokers and non-smokers. Those who smoked > 100 cigarettes in the 6 months prior to the participation in the study were considered smokers [16]. Regular physical activity was defined as 150 min per week of moderate physical activity (e.g., mowing, swimming, badminton, or tennis). Anthropometric measurements and biochemical assays of the serum were carried out. Body weight, height, and waist circumference were assessed using established methods [17]. Blood was drawn from the subjects after fasting for more than 12 h. Plasma and serum were separated from the collected blood after centrifugation, and glucose and lipid profiles were assessed in the plasma and serum samples, respectively [18]. Serum total cholesterol, high-density lipoprotein cholesterol (HDL-C), triglycerides, aspartate aminotransferase (AST), and alanine transaminase (ALT) concentrations were measured using an enzyme-linked immunosorbent assay (ELISA) kit (Asan Pharm., Seoul, Republic of Korea).

2.3. Food and Nutrient Intake and Dietary Pattern Using a Semi-Quantitative Food Frequency Questionnaire (SQFFQ)

Dietary habits were assessed using an SQFFQ. Over the previous 12 months, participants reported their typical food intake based on 106 items commonly consumed in the Korean diet. This SQFFQ was validated against four seasons of three-day food records [19,20]. Food intake was determined by multiplying the frequency of consumption for each food by the daily amount, as previously described, and expressed in grams per day. The daily consumption of energy, carbohydrates, fats, proteins, vitamins, and minerals was computed from SQFFQ data using the computer-aided nutritional analysis program CAN-Pro 2.0, developed by the Korean Nutrition Society.

The food items in the SQFFQ were categorized into 30 predetermined food groups, which were utilized in constructing dietary patterns through principal component analysis (PCA). Four distinct dietary patterns were identified by applying eigenvalues greater than 1.5 and employing orthogonal rotation (varimax). The predominant contributing foods in each dietary pattern were assigned factor-loading values of ≥ 0.40. The identified groups were labeled as the Korean balanced diet (KBD), plant-based diet (PBD), Western-style diet (WSD), or rice-based diet (RBD) groups.

2.4. Definition of NAFLD

Since heavy drinking (30 and 20 g of alcohol or higher per day in males and females, respectively) could also induce fatty liver disease, heavy drinkers were excluded. The participants who were diagnosed with NAFLD by a physician with an ultrasound method and had serum AST concentrations ≥ 40 U/L and ALT ≥ 35 U/L were regarded as a risk group ($n = 2089$). The participants with no NAFLD diagnosis and serum AST concentrations < 40 U/L and ALT < 35 U/L were considered normal levels ($n = 48,999$).

2.5. Genotyping and Quality Control

DNA was isolated from the peripheral blood of the participants, and genotyping was conducted using the Affymetrix Genome-Wide Human single-nucleotide polymorphism (SNP) Array 5.0 (Affymetrix, Santa Clara, CA, USA). Genotyping quality and accuracy were determined using the Bayesian robust linear model with the Mahalanobis distance classifier (BRLMM) genotyping algorithm [18]. The exclusion criteria for DNA genotyping were as follows: high genotype deletion detection rate ($\geq 4\%$), low genotyping accuracy (<98%), high heterozygosity (>30%), minor allele frequency (MAF) < 0.01, Hardy–Weinberg equilibrium (HWE) ($p < 0.05$), and having gender bias [18].

2.6. Genetic Variants Affecting NAFLD in Koreans

GWAS analysis explored and identified susceptible genetic variants that increase NAFLD risk. Single-nucleotide polymorphisms (SNPs) influencing NAFLD risk have been identified using PLINK in a Korean population. The age, gender, body mass index (BMI), residential area, physical activity, education, smoking, and energy intake of the participants were used as covariates in the GWAS analysis. The gene names for the SNPs were found by examining the g:Profiler annotation database.

2.7. Screening of Bioactive Compounds in Foods to Have Low Binding Energy with PNPLA3

We first extracted the *PNPLA3* protein sequence in the Fasta format from UniProt (ID: Q9NST1; https://www.uniprot.org/uniprot/Q9NST1, 7 July 2022). Subsequently, we obtained the 5FYA protein using SWISS-MODEL homology modeling. The protein structure was prepared to enhance the protein structure using the Discovery Studio software version 4.5 package. It involved hydrogenating the protein structure, completing missing amino acids, and removing metal ions and water molecules. Additionally, we used the Swiss-PdbViewer to optimize the protein's energy.

We converted 22,589 compounds from food received from Foodb to the protein data bank, partial charge (q), and atom type (t) (pdbqt) format using Open Babel v3.1.0. The Foodb website includes a freely accessible database providing detailed information on the chemical composition of typical unprocessed foods, including micronutrients and macronutrients. The DoGSiteScorer online tool (https://proteins.plus/, 30 July 2022) was employed to predict and elucidate potential binding pockets in the wild and mutated types of *PNPLA3* (I148M) crystals. We examined four molecular dynamics systems using Discover Studio software (Biovia, Discovery Studio Visualizer, software version 20.1.0.19295) to evaluate binding pocket characteristics such as size, surface area, and drug ability score to generate the wild-type *PNPLA3* (WT), mutant *PNPLA3* (MU), *PNPLA3* binding with a small molecule (ligand), and *PNPLA3* mutant binding with a small molecule (ligand-MU). We referred to the CHARMM36 force field parameter table in the Discovery Studio software to define the simulation parameters for the small molecules. The Discovery Studio Visualizer also generated visualizations of the protein–ligand binding structures in both 2D and 3D.

2.8. Molecular Dynamics Simulation (MDS)

MDS is a promising method to examine the conformational changes in the structure of Ile148Met variants relative to the native conformation [21,22]. MDS can detect changes in protein phenotypes, which helps validate the severe implications of disease-associated mutations predicted computationally [23]. MDS of the *PNPLA3*–compound complex was performed using the DS/Standard Dynamics Cascade protocol; the molecule was solvated under periodic boundary conditions, and the CHARMM36 force field was added. The 'Standard Dynamics Cascade' approach was implemented to set the parameters for the MDS of the *PNPLA3* within the solvent system. The default values were used for most parameters, with specific settings: a ramp time of 40 ps, a balancing time of 400 ps, a simulation sampling time of 10,000 ps, and a simulation step size of 2 fs. Various analyses were performed after conducting the simulation for a duration of 10 ns. The root mean square deviation (RMSD), root mean square fluctuation (RMSF), and hydrogen bond values were analyzed to investigate the stability and dynamics of the system.

2.9. Cell Culture

HepG2 cells were cultured in a high-glucose Dulbecco's Modified Eagle Medium (DMEM) and placed in a 37 °C, 5% CO_2 incubator. Oleic acid (OA) was used to simulate in vitro hepatic steatosis. HepG2 cells were exposed to different doses of OA (0, 0.1, 0.3, 0.5, 0.7, 1, 1.5, 2, and 3 mM), the five bioactive compounds (20, 50, 70, 100, 150, and 200 µM), and compound C (AMPK inhibitor). Cell viability was assessed using the 3-(4,5-dimethylthiazol-2-yl)-2,5-diphenyltetrazolium bromide (MTT) assay, which measures cell viability by detecting the conversion of MTT to a purple formazan dye, and the color change was measured at 550 nm. The levels of lipid peroxides in the cells were determined using a thiobarbituric acid reactive substances (TBARS) kit (DoGenBio, Seoul, Republic of Korea).

2.10. Realtime PCR

Total RNA was extracted from the cells using a phenol and guanidine isothiocyanate-based single-phase solution (Trizol reagent, Invitrogen, Rockville, MD, USA). The cDNA synthesis was performed by combining equal amounts of total RNA, superscript III reverse transcriptase, and high-fidelity Taq DNA polymerase. The cDNA was utilized for the polymerase chain reaction (PCR) with the corresponding primers in a real-time PCR machine (BioRad Laboratories, Hercules, CA, USA) to measure the mRNA expression of *PNPLA3* and sterol regulatory element binding protein 1c (*SREBP-1c*) genes. The primers are listed in Supplementary Table S1. The gene expression levels in each sample were quantified using the threshold comparison cycle (CT) method after amplifying the expression by a real-time polymerase chain reaction.

2.11. Statistical Analysis

Statistical analysis was performed using the SPSS software version 21 (IBM Inc., Armonk, NY, USA). All results were presented as mean ± standard deviation. In a population study, the odds ratios (ORs) and 95% confidence intervals (CIs) of NAFLD risk with the biochemical parameters were evaluated using a logistic regression analysis after adjustment for covariates such as age, gender, body mass index (BMI), residential area, physical activity, education, smoking, and energy intake. The interaction between the selected genetic variant for NAFLD risk and lifestyles was evaluated in a two-way analysis of covariance (ANCOVA) while adjusting for the mentioned covariates. Univariate analysis of variance is employed in cellular research to compare the variables associated with metabolic changes among the bioactive compound groups and control group. Multiple groups were analyzed using Tukey's test, with a significance level set at $p < 0.05$.

3. Results

3.1. Basic Characteristics of the Participants

The hospital-based urban cohort consisted of 51,088 participants, out of which 2089 individuals (4%) were diagnosed with NAFLD. Upon adjusting for other factors, women exhibited a 1.3-fold higher incidence of NAFLD than men (Table 1). BMI and waist circumference were significantly associated with NAFLD risk, with 2.6-fold and 1.5-fold higher risks, respectively. Individuals with NAFLD had higher plasma total cholesterol and triglyceride concentrations than those without NAFLD (Table 1). Moreover, the incidence of hypertension and type 2 diabetes in the NAFLD group was 1.3 and 2.3 times higher, respectively, than in the non-NAFLD group. Alcohol consumption and smoking were also more prevalent among the NAFLD group as opposed to the non-NAFLD group. However, there were no significant differences in age, education, income, or dietary nutrient intake between the non-NAFLD and NAFLD groups (Table 1).

Table 1. Participants' socioeconomic level and metabolic characteristics in NAFLD.

	Non-NAFLD (*n* = 48,999)	NAFLD (*n* = 2089)	Adjusted OR (95% CI)
Age (years) [1]	53.77 ± 8.033	54.90 ± 7.886 ***	1.040 (0.945~1.144)
Genders (men: N, %)	14,908 (30.4)	918 (43.9) ***	1.343 (1.176~1.535) ***
BMI (kg/m^2) [2]	23.65 ± 2.775	25.56 ± 3.403 ***	2.581 (2.357~2.827) ***
Waist circumference [3]	79.93 ± 8.35	85.66 ± 9.26 ***	1.479 (1.304~1.678) ***
Plasma total cholesterol (mg/dL) [4]	197 ± 35.22	200 ± 39.97 **	1.259 (1.126~1.408) ***
Plasma triglyceride (mg/dL) [5]	119 ± 76.22	161 ± 126 ***	1.831 (1.635~2.049) ***
Hypertension (N, %) [6]	12,997 (26.5)	849 (40.7) ***	1.317 (1.192~1.456) ***
Type 2 diabetes (N, %) [7]	3641 (7.4)	407 (19.5) ***	2.330 (2.062~2.633) ***

Table 1. Cont.

	Non-NAFLD (n = 48,999)	NAFLD (n = 2089)	Adjusted OR (95% CI)
Education (N, %) [8]			
<High school	14,907 (30.7)	703 (33.9) **	
High school	21,027 (43.3)	837 (40.4)	1.021 (0.910~1.146)
College more	12,616 (26.0)	534 (25.7)	1.002 (0.869~1.155)
Income (N, %) [9]			
<$2000/month	14,379 (31.1)	656 (33.4)	
$2000–4000/month	27,969 (60.5)	1152 (58.7)	0.996 (0.891~1.113)
>$4000/month	3888 (8.4)	154 (7.8)	0.876 (0.694~1.106)
Energy intake (EER %) [10]	98.80 ± 31.66	99.01 ± 32.59	1.093 (0.986~1.211)
CHO (EER %) [11]	71.79 ± 6.93	71.80 ± 7.23	1.029 (0.936~1.131)
Protein (EER %) [12]	13.39 ± 2.56	13.45 ± 2.65	1.033 (0.942~1.133)
Fat (EER %) [13]	13.83 ± 5.38	13.72 ± 5.56	1.077 (0.938~1.237)
Cholesterol intake [14]	169 ± 124	174 ± 138	1.083 (0.951~1.233)
Na intake (mg) [15]	2421 ± 1364	2545 ± 1496 ***	1.001 (0.896~1.118)
Fiber intake(g) [16]	14.61 ± 9.26	15.45 ± 10.51 ***	1.045 (0.936~1.166)
Alcohol (g) [17]	2.09 ± 4.77	3.37 ± 6.35 ***	1.406 (1.116~1.770) **
KBD (%) [18]	15,710 (32.1)	756 (36.2) ***	1.039 (0.938~1.150)
PBD (%) [18]	16,963 (34.6)	638 (30.5) ***	0.948 (0.851~1.056)
WSD (%) [18]	19,151 (39.1)	859 (41.1)	0.940 (0.847~1.043)
RMD (%) [18]	16,276 (33.2)	673 (32.2)	1.014 (0.916~1.121)
Smoking (Number, %)	11,458 (23.5)	717 (34.4) ***	1.167 (1.013~1.345) *

Values represent adjusted means ± standard deviation or the number (N) of participants and percentage. OR, odds ratio; CI, confidence intervals; KBD, Korean balanced diet; PBD, plant-based diet; WSD, Western-style diet; RMD, rice-main diet. The cutoff points of the reference were as follows: [1] 55 years old for age, [2] 25 kg/m^2 BMI, [3] 90 cm for men and 85 cm for women waist circumferences, [4] 230 mg/dL plasma total cholesterol concentrations, [5] 200 mg/dL plasma triglyceride concentrations, [6] 140 mmHg systolic blood pressure (SBP), 90 mmHg diastolic blood pressure (DBP) plus hypertension medication, [7] 126 mL/dL fasting serum glucose plus diabetic drug intake, [8] high school graduation and [9] $2000/month income, [10] <estimated energy requirement (EER), [11] 72 energy percent (En%) for carbohydrate (CHO), [12] 13 En% for protein, [13] 20 En% for fat, [14] 250 mg/day cholesterol intake, [15] 1600 mg for sodium, [16] 20 g for fiber intake, [17] 20 g for alcohol, [18] 75th percentiles of each dietary pattern. Covariates for adjusted means and OR: age, gender, BMI, residence area, physical activity, education, smoking, and energy intake in ANCOVA and logistic regression models, respectively. * Significant differences by NAFLD at $p < 0.05$, ** at $p < 0.01$, *** $p < 0.001$.

3.2. Genetic Variations Associated with NAFLD Risk

GWAS was used to investigate the genetic variations linked to NAFLD risk. The genetic variant found to be significantly associated with NAFLD was *PNPLA3*_rs738409. The adjusted odds ratio (OR) was 1.487, indicating that the risk of NAFLD with the minor allele of the SNP was 1.487 times higher than with the major allele (Table 2). The minor allele of *PNPLA3*_rs738409 was thus the risk allele.

Table 2. Association analysis of *PNPLA3* I148M to influence NAFLD.

CHR	SNP	Position	Mi	Ma	OR	Adjust p Value	MAF	HWE_P	GENE	Function
22	rs738409	44324727	G	C	1.487	1.482×10^{-33}	0.417	0.819	PNPLA3	Missense variant

PNPLA3, patatin-like phospholipase domain-containing protein 3; CHR, chromosome; SNP, single-nucleotide polymorphism; Mi, minor allele; Ma, major allele; OR, odds ratios for NAFLD in the reference of the major allele; adjusted p value, p value for OR adjusted for age, gender, body mass index, residence area, energy intake, physical activity, smoking status, alcohol intake, and education; MAF, minor allele frequency; HWE_P, p-value for Hardy–Weinberg equilibrium.

3.3. Interaction of PNPLA3_rs738409 with Lifestyles

The interaction of *PNPLA3*_rs738409 with smoking significantly affected NAFLD risk. Both major and minor *PNPLA3*_rs738409 alleles were positively associated with NAFLD risk in smokers and non-smokers. However, their association was much higher in former and current smokers (3.12-fold) than in non-smokers (1.89-fold) (Table 3). Among the four dietary patterns (Korean balanced diet, plant-based diet, Western-style diet, and rice-main diet), the plant-based diet (PBD) and Western-style diet (WSD) interacted with *PNPLA3_rs738409*. A PBD was inversely associated with NAFLD risk, but a WSD was positively linked (Table 3). The smoking status also interacted with the NAFLD risk in participants carrying *PNPLA3*_rs738409 minor alleles. However, the interaction between exercise and *PNPLA3*_rs738409 had no significant impact on the risk of NAFLD (Table 3). For participants carrying *PNPLA3*_rs738409 minor alleles, there may also be an increased risk of NAFLD with a low PBD, a high WSD, and smoking.

Table 3. After adjusting the odds ratio of NAFLD risk, rs738409 risk score according to lifestyle pattern.

	Major (n = 17,448)	Hetero (n = 24,821)	Minor (n = 8819)	Gene–Nutrient Interaction p Value
Low energy [1]	1	1.330 (1.167~1.516)	2.342 (2.019~2.716)	0.218
High energy		1.360 (1.109~1.669)	1.941 (1.524~2.473)	
Non-smoke	1	1.310 (1.148~1.495)	1.892 (1.619~2.210)	<0.0001
Former + current smokers		1.386 (1.139~1.686)	3.121 (2.519~3.867)	
Low KBD [2]	1	1.355 (1.181~1.556)	2.206 (1.883~2.584)	0.360
High KBD		1.308 (1.090~1.570)	2.247 (1.823~2.771)	
Low PBD [2]	1	1.367 (1.197~1.562)	2.404 (2.066~2.798)	0.019
High PBD		1.285 (1.056~1.564)	1.896 (1.509~2.383)	
Low WSD [2]	1	1.256 (1.091~1.446)	1.955 (1.660~2.304)	0.017
High WSD		1.475 (1.235~1.760)	2.696 (2.208~3.291)	
Low RMD [2]	1	1.388 (1.214~1.588)	2.299 (1.970~2.682)	0.462
High RMD		1.236 (1.020~1.497)	2.050 (1.644~2.555)	
No exercise [3]	1	1.348 (1.150~1.580)	2.394 (2.000~2.865)	0.072
Exercise		1.329 (1.141~1.549)	2.070 (1.732~2.473)	

Values represent odd ratios and 95% confidence intervals. The cutoff points were as follows: [1] <Estimated energy requirement defined in dietary reference index, [2] <75th percentiles; [3] <moderate exercise for 150 min/day; multiple logistic regression models include the corresponding main effects, interaction terms of SNPs and main effects (energy and nutrient intake), and potential confounders such as age, gender, BMI, residence area, physical activity, education, smoking, and energy intake. Reference was the major.

3.4. Molecular Docking

Molecular docking was performed to gain a deeper understanding of the binding of the bioactive compounds to the *PNPLA3* protein. The docking interactions between the selected bioactive compounds and the wild type (WT) and mutant type (MT) of the *PNPLA3* protein are shown in Table 4, Figures 1 and S1–S4, respectively. The molecular docking analysis showed that the binding energy between the MT of *PNPLA3*_I148M, delphinidin-3-caffeoyl-glucoside, pyranocyanin A, delta-viniferin, kaempferol-7-glucoside, and petunidin-3-rutinoside was lower than the WT of *PNPLA3*_I148M, and they had a higher number of hydrogen bonds between *PNPLA3* and bioactive compounds than others. The more hydrogen bonds the compound has, the stronger and more stable the binding with *PNPLA3* [24]. The binding affinity of *PNPLA3* and the bioactive compounds comprised not only hydrogen bonds but also Van der Waals, alkyl, and carbon–hydrogen bonds. It indicated that the binding affinity between the MT of *PNPLA3*_I148M and the five compounds was higher than with the WT, and the inhibitory effect of the five compounds on the MT of *PNPLA3*_I148M was stronger than that on the WT.

Table 4. The intermolecular binding energy between bioactive compounds and *PNPLA3* active site.

Compound Name	Effective Food	Residues Involved in Hydrogen Bond		Residues Involved in Hydrophobic Interactions		Wild Type	Mutant Type
		Wild-Type	Mutant-Type	Wild-Type	Mutant-Type	Docking Energy, ΔG (kcal mol^{-1})	
Delphinidin 3-caffeoyl-glucoside	grape	His204, Tyr188, Ser152, Cys146, Arg74	Tyr188, Thr200, Ser199, Ser47, Asp166, Arg74	Leu72, Leu51, Pro229, Phe150, Ile148	Phe150, Leu203, Met148, Leu154	−7.6	−9.4

Table 4. *Cont.*

Compound Name	Effective Food	Residues Involved in Hydrogen Bond		Residues Involved in Hydrophobic Interactions		Wild Type	Mutant Type
		Wild-Type	Mutant-Type	Wild-Type	Mutant-Type	Docking Energy, ΔG (kcal mol^{-1})	
Pyranocyanin A	blackcurrant	Arg74, Ser152, Val197, Ser199, Lys198, Pro195, Tyr191	Val197, Lys198, Ser199, Pro195, Asn201, Tyr188, His204, Cys146	His204, Phe150, Pro228, Pro229	Cys15, Met148, Lys198, Tyr188, Phe150, Pro229	−9.1	−10.2
Delta-viniferin	grape	His204, Pro229, Asn201, Pro195	Cys15, Cys146, Arg74, Ser152, Ser199	Pro228, Phe150, Tyr191	Met148, Pro228, Phe150, Pro229	−9	−10
Kaempferol 7-glucoside	flaxseed	Asp166, Ser152, Asn201, Ser199	Cys146, Arg74, Ser152, Tyr191, Pro195, Asn201, His204	Cys15, Tyr188, Ile148, Pro229, Phe150, Pro228	Met148, Phe150, Pro228, Pro229	−8.2	−9.6
Petunidin 3-rutinoside	mulberry	His204, Asn201, Ser199, Lys198	Ser199, Asn201, Tyr191, Arg74, Pro228, Pro22, Ser78, Pro195, Ser152	Phe150, Tyr191, Pro195	Tyr191, Leu154, Met148	−7.9	−9

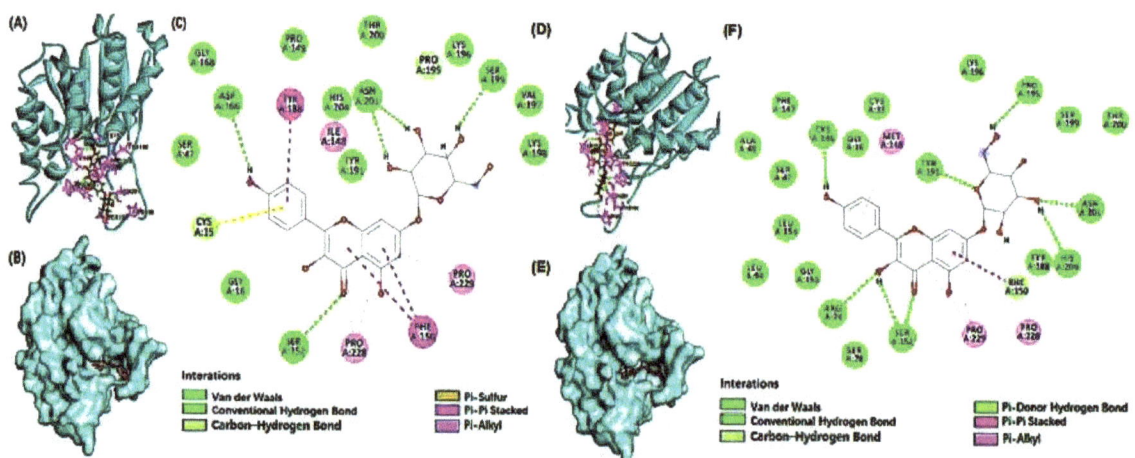

Figure 1. Molecular docking of *PNPLA3* WT (I148) and MT (148M) with kaempferol-7-glucoside. Molecular docking with the bioactive compound and *PNPLA3* wild type (WT, I148) and mutated type (MT; 148M). (**A**,**D**) Diagrammatic representation of the compound (ball and stick model) binding with WT and MT of *PNPLA3*, respectively (**B**,**E**) binding of the compound at the central cavity with WT and MT of *PNPLA3*, respectively, and (**C**,**F**) 2D depiction of *PNPLA3* interacting with the compound and the nature of forces involved in stabilizing complex of –bioactive compound WT and MT of PNPLA3, respectively. *PNPLA3*, phospholipase domain containing 3.

3.5. Molecular Dynamics (MD) Simulation

The RMSD and RMSF were calculated using 100 ns simulations to investigate the stability and dynamics of well-bound ligand–protein complexes with the WT and MT of *PNPLA3*_I148M (Figures 2 and S5–S8). It was observed that the lower the RMSD, the higher the stability of the protein. The RMSD of kaempferol-7-glucose, petunidin-3-rutinoside, delphinidin-3-caffeoyl-glucoside, and delta-viniferin in the WT of *PNPLA3*_I148M was lower than that of the MT, while pyranocyanin A showed the opposite trend (Figures 2 and S5–S8). However, the RMSD ranged between approximately 1.75 and 3.5 nm within 100 s of the wild-type and mutant *PNPLA3*_I148M. The RMSF of the five selected bioactive compounds in the WT and MT *PNPLA3* fluctuated between 0.5 and 3 nm (Figures 2 and S5–S8).

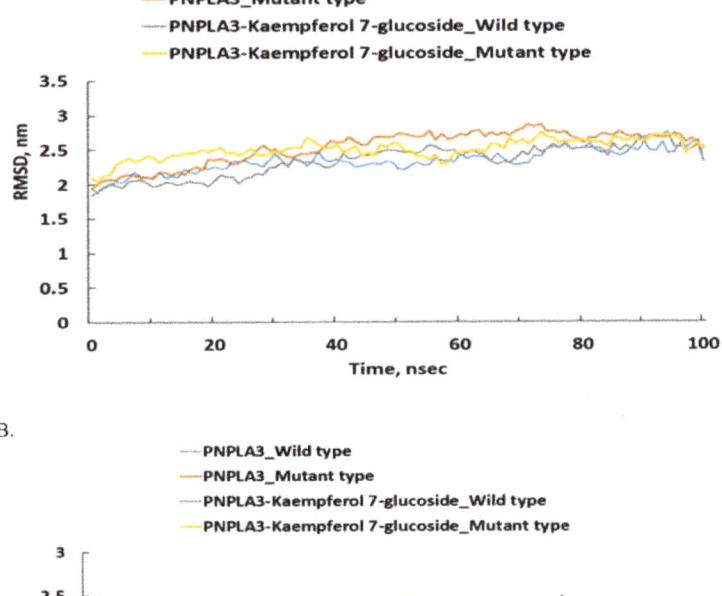

Figure 2. Molecular dynamics (MD) simulation of *PNPLA3* I148 (WT; rs738409) and 148M (MT) and kaempferol-7-glucoside interaction. (**A**) Variation in RMSD (root mean square deviation) of *PNPLA3* alone and *PNPLA3*–compound complex as a function of simulation. (**B**) RMSF (root mean square fluctuation) in *PNPLA3* in the absence and presence of the compound. *PNPLA3*, phospholipase domain containing 3; WT, wild type; MT, mutated type.

3.6. HepG2 Cell Viability

As seen in Figure 3, treatment with OA at concentrations below 2 mM did not affect cell viability after 48 h of incubation. However, when the OA concentration was >2 mM, the viability of the HepG2 cells significantly decreased ($p < 0.05$). Therefore, 2 mM OA was used in the follow-up studies. Oil Red O staining was used to observe the lipid droplet formation with the OA treatment of the HepG2 cells. After treating the HepG2 cells with 2 mM OA for 48 h, many lipid droplets were formed in the cells ($p < 0.01$). Consistent with the Oil Red O staining results, the triglyceride content in the HepG2 cells significantly increased after the 2 mM OA treatment (Figure 3). It suggested that 2 mM of OA could induce lipid accumulation and lipid droplet formation without impacting cell viability in HepG2 cells. At concentrations below 150 μg/mL, delphinidin-3-caffeoyl-glucoside, pyranocyanin A, delta-viniferin, kaempferol-7-glucoside, and petunidin-3-rutinoside did not affect the viability of HepG2 cells (Figure 4).

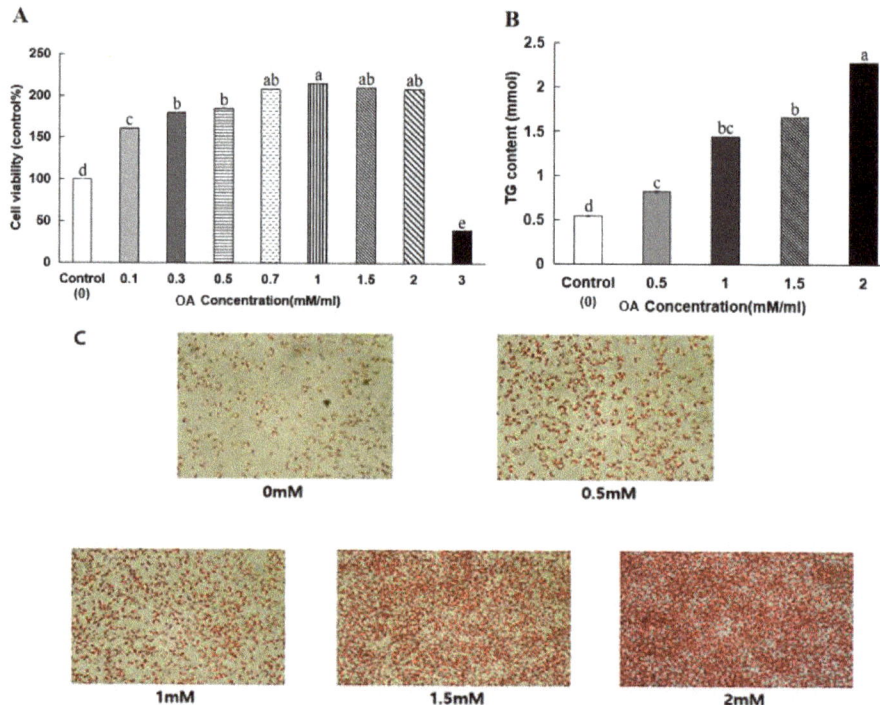

Figure 3. Oleic acid (OA) induces steatosis in HepG2 cells. (**A**) The viability assay of HepG2 cells was treated with different concentrations of oleic acid (OA) for 48 h. (**B**) Measurement of triglyceride content in HepG2 cells after incubation with 2 mM OA for 48 h. (**C**) Oil Red O staining to detect intracellular lipid droplets in HepG2 cells treated with 0, 0.5, 1, 1.5, and 2 mM OA for 48 h. a–e Different letters indicated significant difference between the groups by Tukey test at $p < 0.05$.

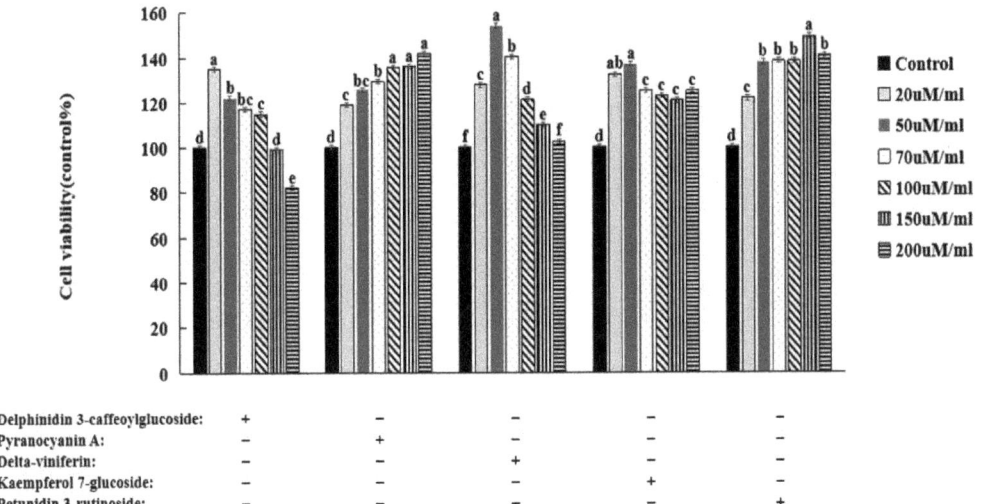

Figure 4. Changes in HepG2 cell viability after treatment with bioactive compounds. a–f Different letters indicated significant difference between the groups by Tukey test at $p < 0.05$.

3.7. Lipid Peroxide Contents in HeG2 Cells

The malondialdehyde contents representing lipid peroxides were measured using the thiobarbituric acid reactive substance (TBARS) quantification method. Compared to no OA, lipid peroxidation significantly increased after the OA treatment, whereas the bioactive compound treatment significantly decreased lipid peroxidation. A high dosage of petunidin 3-rutinoside treatment decreased lipid peroxide contents as much as that seen without OA treatment. The compound C pretreatment suppressed the decrease in lipid peroxide contents due to the treatment with natural compounds. These results indicated that the bioactive compounds potentially exhibited their antioxidant effect through the AMPK pathways in the OA-treated cells (Figure 5A).

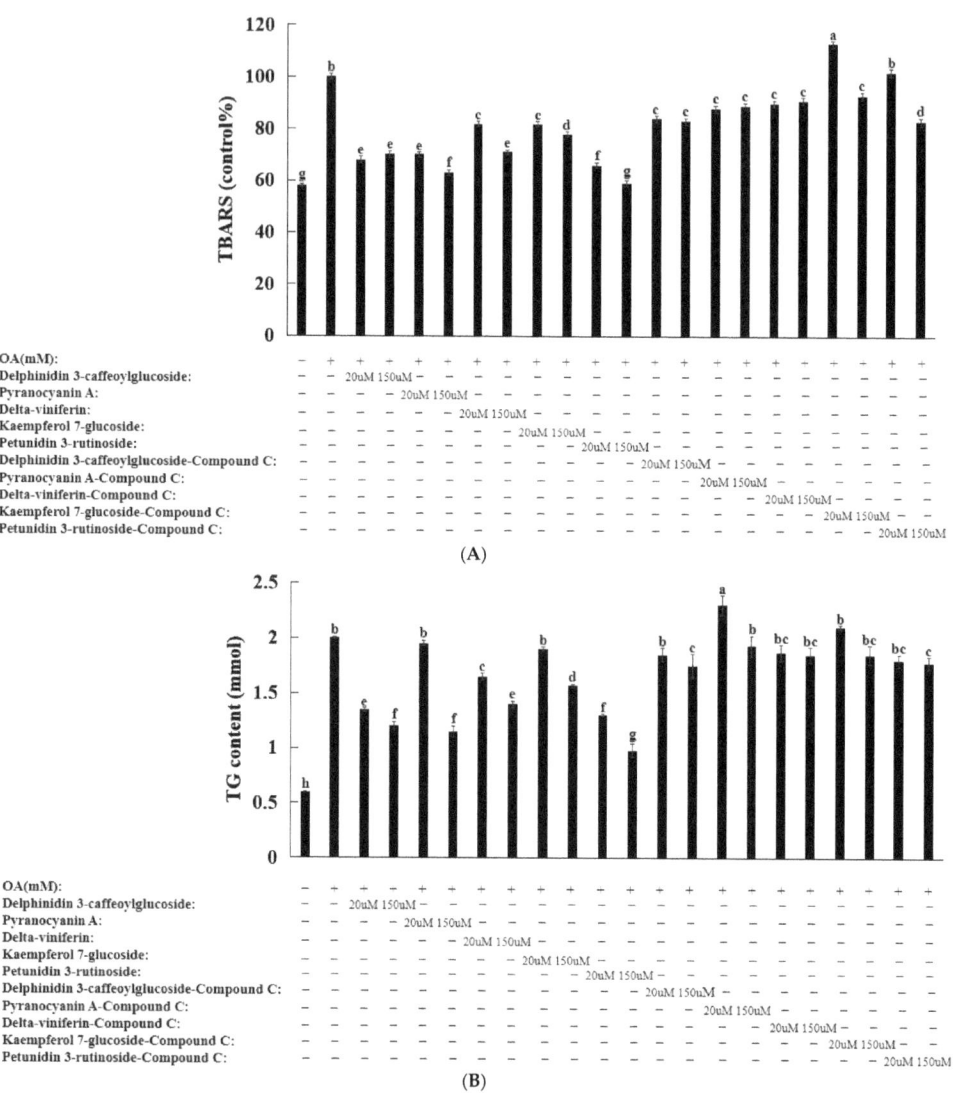

Figure 5. Lipid levels in HepG2 cells after treatment with oleic acid and compounds. (**A**) Lipid peroxide contents. (**B**) Triglyceride contents. a–h Different letters indicated significant difference between the groups by Tukey test at $p < 0.05$.

3.8. Natural Compounds in HepG2 Cells Induced by Oleic Acid

The OA treatment of HepG2 cells induced a morphology similar to hepatic steatosis [25–27]. Treatment with OA alone significantly increased the amounts of intracellular triglycerides. However, the triglyceride contents significantly decreased after treatment with the bioactive compound (Figure 5B). However, pretreatment with compound C blocked its inhibitory effect on cellular triglyceride levels (Figure 5B). The OA treatment increased the mRNA levels of *SREBP-1c* and *PNPLA3*. However, kaempferol 7-glucoside and petunidin 3-rutinoside effectively prevented the increase in mRNA levels (Figure 6). However, pretreatment with compound C inhibited and reversed the bioactive-compound-mediated effects (Figure 6). Collectively, these findings imply that AMPK is involved in adipogenesis gene expression and OA-induced intracellular triglyceride accumulation.

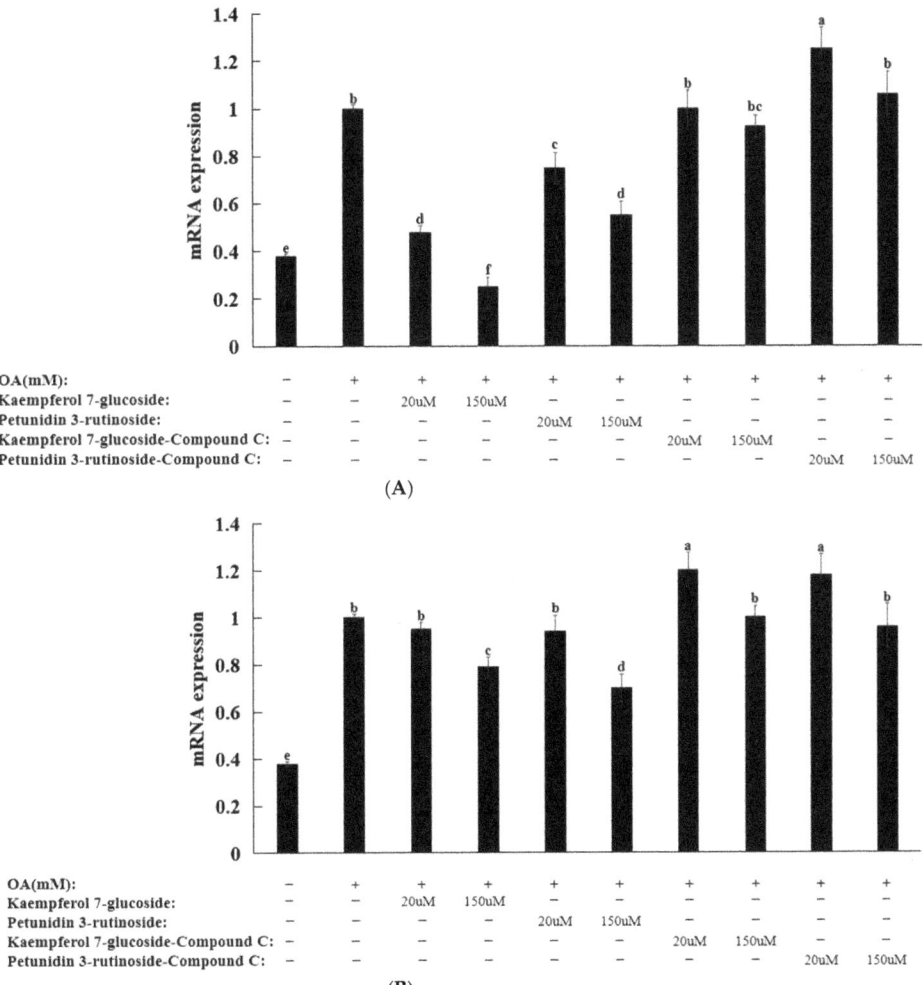

Figure 6. mRNA expression of lipid-metabolism-related genes after pretreatment with compound C and treatment with kaempferol 7-glucoside and petunidin 3-rutinoside. (**A**) *PNPLA3* (**B**) *SREBP-1c PNPLA3*: patatin-like phospholipase domain-containing protein 3; *SREBP-1c*: Sterol regulatory element binding protein. a–f Different letters indicated significant difference between the groups by Tukey test at $p < 0.05$.

4. Discussion

Recent epidemiological projections suggest that the incidence of NAFLD and NASH is likely to increase rapidly in the coming years due to the influence of urbanization [28–30]. This rise is anticipated to impose substantial clinical and economic burdens on the healthcare system in the coming years. Typically, patients with NAFLD and NASH do not exhibit severe symptoms, and their diagnosis usually relies on ultrasound or a liver biopsy [31,32]. Identifying individuals with potential genetic predispositions at an early age is crucial for preventing the development of NAFLD. Across various countries and ethnicities, the *PN-*

*PLA3*_rs738409 polymorphism has been identified as exerting the most significant impact on NAFLD [33,34]. The present study aimed to investigate the impact of the *PNPLA3*_rs738409 polymorphism on NAFLD risk and to explore the interaction between genetic and lifestyle factors on NAFLD risk in participants aged over 45 years. The results may contribute to developing effective strategies for its prevention and management through in silico analysis, cell-based studies, and human studies.

Evidence suggests that the protein expressed by the *PNPLA3* (WT) gene exists in lipid droplet membranes and is responsible for the postprandial remodeling of lipid droplets through its triglyceride hydrolase activity [35,36]. The protein variant *PNPLA3* (I148M) reduces hydrolase activity. It has also been shown to promote the production of profibrotic cytokines (including CCL2 and CCL5), which activate hepatic stellate cells (HSC) and promote inflammation and fibrosis in NAFLD/NASH [37,38]. The present study showed that *PNPLA3* (I148M) elevated NAFLD risk, which might be linked to increased *PNPLA3* gene expression. Therefore, reducing the expression of the *PNPLA3* gene by consuming bioactive compounds may have therapeutic benefits for NAFLD patients with risk alleles [39].

PNPLA3 is a direct target gene of *SREBP-1c*, a key transcription factor that primarily regulates the expression of critical adipose genes of fatty acid synthase (FAS) and acetyl CoA carboxylase 1 (ACC1), and its activity is controlled by AMPK [40,41]. In the present study, *PNPLA3* modulators altered fat accumulation by suppressing AMPK. The increase in liver adipogenesis in NAFLD patients is attributed to *SREBP-1c* activation. As a result, decreasing *SREBP-1* activity is likely to diminish *PNPLA3* expression and ameliorate related steatosis. In this process, AMPK controls *SREBP-1c* to decrease fat deposition. A recent study found that the high expression of human *PNPLA3* (I148M) in the livers of transgenic mice boosted *SREBP-1c* mRNA expression [42]. Furthermore, no evidence has been found to support the regulatory role of *PNPLA3* (I148M) on AMPK, and the mechanism by which *PNPLA3* regulates AMPK needs to be clarified. The present study showed that *SREBP-1c* and *PNPLA3* gene expression increased in OA-treated HepG2 cells, and the AMPK inhibitor further elevated their gene expression. Therefore, it was shown that AMPK controls *PNPLA3* expression through *SREBP-1c*.

The I148M polymorphism of *PNPLA3* (rs738409, C>G) is associated with the occurrence and progression of NAFLD. However, despite significant research in in vitro and in vivo models, the mechanism by which *PNPLA3* (I148M) induces hepatic steatosis is unclear. In vitro investigations have demonstrated that the I148M variant restricts substrate access to the active site of the lipase enzyme, resulting in loss of lipase activity and steatosis [43]. *PNPLA3* (148M) has also been reported to induce hepatic steatosis through the accumulation of *PNPLA3*. Reduction in *PNPLA3* levels by short hairpin RNA (shRNA) knockdown has been shown to reduce liver triglyceride content in mice overexpressing *PNPLA3* (148M) [42]. However, in the livers of mice, neither inactivation nor overexpression of *PNPLA3* resulted in steatosis [42,44]. Therefore, the *PNPLA3* (148M) variant is associated with the accumulation of *PNPLA3*, leading to steatosis. Therapies that lower *PNPLA3* levels can help correct hepatic steatosis in people with the *PNPLA3*(148M) variation [36].

Currently, Rezdiffra (resmetirom) is the first medication approved by the FDA for the treatment of NAFLD. Rezdiffra is a thyroid hormone receptor (THR)-β agonist that acts primarily in the liver. Thyroid hormones, thyroxine, and its active derivative, triiodothyronine, are primary regulators of lipid metabolism, primarily through activation of the THR-β isoform in hepatocytes [45]. Activation of THR-β increases cholesterol metabolism through the expression of the CYP7A1 enzyme and reduces de novo lipogenesis (DNL) through inhibition of *SREBP-1* expression [46]. These activities suggest that Rezdiffra may provide therapeutic benefits in patients with dyslipidemia and increased DNL, which are key features of NAFLD. The accumulation of lipotoxic lipids in the liver is a major driver of the development of NASH and fibrosis. Therefore, drugs that can suppress DNL may represent a promising future approach for NAFLD treatment. The present study showed that *PNPLA3* inhibitors can decrease DNL by potentiating AMPK activity and decreasing *SREBP-1c* expression, further highlighting the potential of targeting lipid metabolism pathways for NAFLD management.

Several plant products and compounds derived from these plants have been proven to benefit liver health. The present study investigated whether bioactive compounds have a protective effect on NAFLD and whether this protective effect comes from regulating energy homeostasis and the AMPK/autophagy signaling pathways linked to *PNPLA3*. We used an AMPK inhibitor (compound C) instead of gene mutation models. The use of inhibitors has several advantages. The inhibitors only need to be added to the culture medium or directly injected into animals and can act on a wide range of cell types. In terms of time, the effect of inhibitors can be achieved relatively quickly, and the dosage and time can be flexibly adjusted. Therefore, inhibitors are relatively simple, flexible, and suitable for many target cell types. We used compound C, an AMPK inhibitor, to validate the effect of AMPK inactivation on the OA-induced activation of HepG2 cells. Compound C inhibits the activation of AMPK. Inactivation of AMPK by compound C resulted in the increased expression of *SREBP-1c* and *PNPLA3*. Our results in HepG2 cells are consistent with the Xu et al. study [47]. These results showed that compound C reversed the flavonoid effects and confirmed the involvement of the flavonoids in the AMPK/autophagy pathway and inhibition of steatosis activated by oleic acid. Increased lipogenesis contributes to hepatic steatosis, and *SREBP-1c* is a transcription factor involved in hepatic lipogenesis. *PNPLA3*, an *SREBP-1c* target gene, is also implicated in lipogenesis. The inhibition of *SREBP-1C* and *PNPLA3* can help reduce hepatic fat accumulation. Treatment with the bioactive compounds, including kaempferol-7-glucoside and petunidin-3-rutinoside, significantly decreased the expression of *SREBP-1c* and *PNPLA3* in oleic acid-treated cells, as well as the malondialdehyde levels, indicating that the bioactive compounds have antioxidant characteristics.

While this study yields valuable insights, several critical limitations merit consideration. First, the study exclusively examined middle-aged and elderly populations, necessitating further investigation into the relationship between *PNPLA3*_rs738409, liver fat content, and metabolic disorders among adolescents and young individuals. Second, the generalizability of our findings across diverse racial groups requires validation. Third, due to the cross-sectional nature of our data derived from a sizable cohort, establishing causal relationships and evaluating the prognostic relevance of *PNPLA3*_rs738409 to NFALD remains infeasible. Prospective studies are essential for addressing these inquiries. Furthermore, despite conducting cell experiments for validation, there needs to be more cell validation for mutated genes and animal experiments that corroborate our findings. Conversely, this study exhibited several notable strengths, including a substantial participant cohort, integration of lifestyle data, a targeted genetic focus, validation through cell-based and in silico methods, clinical relevance, and the potential to contribute to future research. These attributes collectively enhance our comprehension of the intricate interplay between *PNPLA3* rs738409, lifestyle factors, and NAFLD, providing the potential for more efficacious diagnostic and therapeutic approaches for the condition.

5. Conclusions

*PNPLA3*_rs738409 interacted with the PBD, WSD, and smoking status in a large cohort of middle-aged and elderly individuals. For the persons with the *PNPLA3*_rs738409G risk allele, it was better to have a PBD and avoid a WSD and smoking. Notably, specific bioactive compounds, such as delphinidin-3-caffeoyl-glucoside, pyranocyanin A, delta-viniferin, kaempferol-7-glucose, and petunidin-3-rutinoside, exhibited a propensity to lower binding energy with *PNPLA3* I148M in molecular docking analysis. Furthermore, kaempferol-7-glucose and petunidin-3-rutinoside effectively mitigated oleic acid-induced lipid droplet formation and triglyceride levels in HepG2 cells, operating through the AMPK/*SREBP-1C*/*PNPLA3* pathway. Future research should focus on further elucidating the causative relationships between smoking, PBDs, WSDs, and NAFLD, as well as exploring the potential of the identified bioactive compounds as therapeutic agents for individuals with the PNPLA3_rs738409G risk allele.

Supplementary Materials: The following supporting information can be downloaded at: https://www.mdpi.com/article/10.3390/nu16081239/s1. Table S1. List of primers of *PNPLA3* and *SREBP-1c* genes; Figures S1–S4. Molecular docking of *PNPLA3*_rs738409 (I148) and MT (148M) with a bioactive compound; Figures S5–S8. Molecular dynamics (MD) simulation of *PNPLA3*_rs738409 (I148) and MT (148M) and bioactive compound interaction.

Author Contributions: Conceived the study, data collection, data analysis, writing manuscript draft: M.L.: Supervision, critically reviewing and finalizing manuscript: S.P. All authors have read and agreed to the published version of the manuscript.

Funding: This study was supported by a grant from the National Research Foundation of Korea (NRF) funded by the Ministry of Science and ICT (RS-2023-00208567).

Institutional Review Board Statement: The institutional review board (IRB) of the Korea National Institute of Health approved the KoGES (KBP-2015-055, 14 May 2015), and the IRB of Hoseo University accepted the use of the KoGES data to conduct the present study (HR-034-01).

Informed Consent Statement: All participants signed a written informed consent form.

Data Availability Statement: The data was deposited in the Korean biobank (Osong, Republic of Korea) and provided for the research upon request.

Conflicts of Interest: The authors declare no conflict of interest.

References

1. Benedict, M.; Zhang, X. Nonalcoholic fatty liver disease: An expanded review. *World J. Hepatol.* **2017**, *9*, 715. [CrossRef] [PubMed]
2. Gofton, C.; Upendran, Y.; Zheng, M.H.; George, J. MAFLD: How is it different from NAFLD? *Clin. Mol. Hepatol.* **2023**, *29*, S17–S31. [CrossRef] [PubMed]
3. Adams, L.A.; Waters, O.R.; Knuiman, M.W.; Elliott, R.R.; Olynyk, J.K. NAFLD as a risk factor for the development of diabetes and the metabolic syndrome: An eleven-year follow-up study. *Am. Coll. Gastroenterol.* **2009**, *104*, 861–867. [CrossRef] [PubMed]
4. Park, S.; Kang, S. High carbohydrate and noodle/meat-rich dietary patterns interact with the minor haplotype in the 22q13 loci to increase its association with nonalcoholic fatty liver disease risk in Koreans. *Nutr. Res.* **2020**, *82*, 88–98. [CrossRef] [PubMed]
5. Petta, S.; Targher, G.; Romeo, S.; Pajvani, U.B.; Zheng, M.H.; Aghemo, A.; Valenti, L.V.C. The first MASH drug therapy on the horizon: Current perspectives of resmetirom. *Liver Int.* **2024**, *Online ahead of print*. [CrossRef] [PubMed]
6. Peng, C.-H.; Lin, H.-T.; Chung, D.-J.; Huang, C.-N.; Wang, C.-J. Mulberry Leaf Extracts prevent obesity-induced NAFLD with regulating adipocytokines, inflammation and oxidative stress. *J. Food Drug Anal.* **2018**, *26*, 778–787. [CrossRef] [PubMed]
7. Yogalakshmi, B.; Sreeja, S.; Geetha, R.; Radika, M.K.; Anuradha, C.V. Grape seed proanthocyanidin rescues rats from steatosis: A comparative and combination study with metformin. *J. Lipids* **2013**, *2013*, 153897. [CrossRef] [PubMed]
8. Yari, Z.; Rahimlou, M.; Eslamparast, T.; Ebrahimi-Daryani, N.; Poustchi, H.; Hekmatdoost, A. Flaxseed supplementation in nonalcoholic fatty liver disease: A pilot randomized, open labeled, controlled study. *Int. J. Food Sci. Nutr.* **2016**, *67*, 461–469. [CrossRef]
9. Oczkowski, M. Health-promoting effects of bioactive compounds in blackcurrant (*Ribes nigrum* L.) Berries. *Roczniki Państwowego Zakładu Higieny* **2021**, *72*, 229–238. [CrossRef]
10. Day, E.A.; Ford, R.J.; Steinberg, G.R. AMPK as a therapeutic target for treating metabolic diseases. *Trends Endocrinol. Metab.* **2017**, *28*, 545–560. [CrossRef]
11. Kumari, M.; Schoiswohl, G.; Chitraju, C.; Paar, M.; Cornaciu, I.; Rangrez, A.Y.; Wongsiriroj, N.; Nagy, H.M.; Ivanova, P.T.; Scott, S.A. Adiponutrin functions as a nutritionally regulated lysophosphatidic acid acyltransferase. *Cell Metab.* **2012**, *15*, 691–702. [PubMed]
12. Lindén, D.; Ahnmark, A.; Pingitore, P.; Ciociola, E.; Ahlstedt, I.; Andréasson, A.-C.; Sasidharan, K.; Madeyski-Bengtson, K.; Zurek, M.; Mancina, R.M. Pnpla3 silencing with antisense oligonucleotides ameliorates nonalcoholic steatohepatitis and fibrosis in Pnpla3 I148M knock-in mice. *Mol. Metab.* **2019**, *22*, 49–61. [CrossRef] [PubMed]
13. Kumashiro, N.; Yoshimura, T.; Cantley, J.L.; Majumdar, S.K.; Guebre-Egziabher, F.; Kursawe, R.; Vatner, D.F.; Fat, I.; Kahn, M.; Erion, D.M. Role of patatin-like phospholipase domain-containing 3 on lipid-induced hepatic steatosis and insulin resistance in rats. *Hepatology* **2013**, *57*, 1763–1772. [CrossRef] [PubMed]
14. Qiao, A.; Liang, J.; Ke, Y.; Li, C.; Cui, Y.; Shen, L.; Zhang, H.; Cui, A.; Liu, X.; Liu, C. Mouse patatin-like phospholipase domain-containing 3 influences systemic lipid and glucose homeostasis. *Hepatology* **2011**, *54*, 509–521. [CrossRef] [PubMed]

15. Park, S.; Ahn, J.; Lee, B.-K. Self-rated subjective health status is strongly associated with sociodemographic factors, lifestyle, nutrient intakes, and biochemical indices, but not smoking status: KNHANES 2007–2012. *J. Korean Med. Sci.* **2015**, *30*, 1279–1287. [CrossRef] [PubMed]
16. Park, S.; Liu, M.; Kang, S. Alcohol intake interacts with CDKAL1, HHEX, and OAS3 genetic variants, associated with the risk of type 2 diabetes by lowering insulin secretion in Korean adults. *Alcohol. Clin. Exp. Res.* **2018**, *42*, 2326–2336. [CrossRef] [PubMed]
17. Kim, Y.; Han, B.-G.; Group, K. Cohort profile: The Korean genome and epidemiology study (KoGES) consortium. *Int. J. Epidemiol.* **2017**, *46*, e20. [CrossRef] [PubMed]
18. Park, S.; Kang, S. A Western-style diet interacts with genetic variants of the LDL receptor to hyper-LDL cholesterolemia in Korean adults. *Public. Health Nutr.* **2021**, *24*, 2964–2974. [CrossRef] [PubMed]
19. Liu, M.; Jin, H.S.; Park, S. Protein and fat intake interacts with the haplotype of *PTPN11*_rs11066325, *RPH3A*_rs886477, and *OAS3*_rs2072134 to modulate serum HDL concentrations in middle-aged people. *Clin. Nutr.* **2020**, *39*, 942–949. [CrossRef]
20. Doustmohammadian, A.; Amini, M.; Esmaillzadeh, A.; Omidvar, N.; Abtahi, M.; Dadkhah-Piraghaj, M.; Nikooyeh, B.; Neyestani, T.R. Validity and reliability of a dish-based semi-quantitative food frequency questionnaire for assessment of energy and nutrient intake among Iranian adults. *BMC Res. Notes* **2020**, *13*, 95. [CrossRef]
21. Rajendran, V.; Purohit, R.; Sethumadhavan, R. In silico investigation of molecular mechanism of laminopathy caused by a point mutation (R482W) in lamin A/C protein. *Amino Acids* **2012**, *43*, 603–615. [CrossRef]
22. Kumar, A.; Purohit, R. Computational screening and molecular dynamics simulation of disease associated nsSNPs in CENP-E. *Mutat. Res.* **2012**, *738*, 28–37. [CrossRef] [PubMed]
23. Kumar, A.; Rajendran, V.; Sethumadhavan, R.; Purohit, R. Evidence of colorectal cancer-associated mutation in MCAK: A computational report. *Cell Biochem. Biophys.* **2013**, *67*, 837–851. [CrossRef]
24. Khodarahmi, G.; Asadi, P.; Farrokhpour, H.; Hassanzadeh, F.; Dinari, M. Design of novel potential aromatase inhibitors via hybrid pharmacophore approach: Docking improvement using the QM/MM method. *RSC Adv.* **2015**, *5*, 58055–58064. [CrossRef]
25. Araya, J.; Rodrigo, R.; Videla, L.A.; Thielemann, L.; Orellana, M.; Pettinelli, P.; Poniachik, J. Increase in long-chain polyunsaturated fatty acid n−6/n−3 ratio in relation to hepatic steatosis in patients with nonalcoholic fatty liver disease. *Clin. Sci.* **2004**, *106*, 635–643. [CrossRef]
26. Okamoto, Y.; Tanaka, S.; Haga, Y. Enhanced GLUT2 gene expression in an oleic acid-induced in vitro fatty liver model. *Hepatol. Res.* **2002**, *23*, 138–144. [CrossRef] [PubMed]
27. Janorkar, A.V.; King, K.R.; Megeed, Z.; Yarmush, M.L. Development of an in vitro cell culture model of hepatic steatosis using hepatocyte-derived reporter cells. *Biotech. Bioeng.* **2009**, *102*, 1466–1474. [CrossRef]
28. Eslam, M.; George, J. Genetic contributions to NAFLD: Leveraging shared genetics to uncover systems biology. *Nat. Rev. Gastroenterol. Hepatol.* **2020**, *17*, 40–52. [CrossRef]
29. Mantovani, A.; Petracca, G.; Beatrice, G.; Csermely, A.; Tilg, H.; Byrne, C.D.; Targher, G. Nonalcoholic fatty liver disease and increased risk of incident extrahepatic cancers: A meta-analysis of observational cohort studies. *Gut* **2022**, *71*, 778–788. [CrossRef]
30. Estes, C.; Anstee, Q.M.; Arias-Loste, M.T.; Bantel, H.; Bellentani, S.; Caballeria, J.; Colombo, M.; Craxi, A.; Crespo, J.; Day, C.P. Modeling NAFLD disease burden in China, France, Germany, Italy, Japan, Spain, united kingdom, and united states for the period 2016–2030. *J. Hepatol.* **2018**, *69*, 896–904. [CrossRef]
31. Byrne, C.D.; Patel, J.; Scorletti, E.; Targher, G. Tests for diagnosing and monitoring nonalcoholic fatty liver disease in adults. *BMJ* **2018**, *362*, k2734. [CrossRef] [PubMed]
32. Molina-Molina, E.; Krawczyk, M.; Stachowska, E.; Lammert, F.; Portincasa, P. Nonalcoholic fatty liver disease in non-obese individuals: Prevalence, pathogenesis and treatment. *Clin. Res. Hepatol. Gastroenterol.* **2019**, *43*, 638–645. [CrossRef] [PubMed]
33. Chalasani, N.; Guo, X.; Loomba, R.; Goodarzi, M.O.; Haritunians, T.; Kwon, S.; Cui, J.; Taylor, K.D.; Wilson, L.; Cummings, O.W. Genome-wide association study identifies variants associated with histologic features of nonalcoholic fatty liver disease. *Gastroenterology* **2010**, *139*, 1567–1576.e1566. [CrossRef]
34. Sookoian, S.; Pirola, C.J. Meta-analysis of the influence of I148M variant of patatin-like phospholipase domain containing 3 gene (PNPLA3) on the susceptibility and histological severity of nonalcoholic fatty liver disease. *Hepatology* **2011**, *53*, 1883–1894. [CrossRef]
35. Huang, Y.; Cohen, J.C.; Hobbs, H.H. Expression and characterization of a PNPLA3 protein isoform (I148M) associated with nonalcoholic fatty liver disease. *J. Biol. Chem.* **2011**, *286*, 37085–37093. [CrossRef] [PubMed]
36. BasuRay, S.; Wang, Y.; Smagris, E.; Cohen, J.C.; Hobbs, H.H. Accumulation of PNPLA3 on lipid droplets is the basis of associated hepatic steatosis. *Proc. Natl. Acad. Sci. USA* **2019**, *116*, 9521–9526. [CrossRef]
37. Pirazzi, C.; Valenti, L.; Motta, B.M.; Pingitore, P.; Hedfalk, K.; Mancina, R.M.; Burza, M.A.; Indiveri, C.; Ferro, Y.; Montalcini, T. PNPLA3 has retinyl-palmitate lipase activity in human hepatic stellate cells. *Hum. Mol. Genet.* **2014**, *23*, 4077–4085. [CrossRef]
38. Bruschi, F.V.; Claudel, T.; Tardelli, M.; Caligiuri, A.; Stulnig, T.M.; Marra, F.; Trauner, M. The PNPLA3 I148M variant modulates the fibrogenic phenotype of human hepatic stellate cells. *Hepatology* **2017**, *65*, 1875–1890. [CrossRef] [PubMed]
39. Schwartz, B.E.; Rajagopal, V.; Smith, C.; Cohick, E.; Whissell, G.; Gamboa, M.; Pai, R.; Sigova, A.; Grossman, I.; Bumcrot, D. Discovery and targeting of the signaling controls of PNPLA3 to effectively reduce transcription, expression, and function in pre-clinical NAFLD/NASH settings. *Cells* **2020**, *9*, 2247. [CrossRef]
40. Jung, E.-J.; Kwon, S.-W.; Jung, B.-H.; Oh, S.-H.; Lee, B.-H. Role of the AMPK/SREBP-1 pathway in the development of orotic acid-induced fatty liver. *J. Lipid Res.* **2011**, *52*, 1617–1625. [CrossRef]

41. Horton, J.D.; Goldstein, J.L.; Brown, M.S. SREBPs: Activators of the complete program of cholesterol and fatty acid synthesis in the liver. *J. Clin. Investig.* **2002**, *109*, 1125–1131. [CrossRef] [PubMed]
42. Li, J.Z.; Huang, Y.; Karaman, R.; Ivanova, P.T.; Brown, H.A.; Roddy, T.; Castro-Perez, J.; Cohen, J.C.; Hobbs, H.H. Chronic overexpression of PNPLA3 I148M in mouse liver causes hepatic steatosis. *J. Clin. Investig.* **2012**, *122*, 4130–4144. [CrossRef] [PubMed]
43. Pingitore, P.; Pirazzi, C.; Mancina, R.M.; Motta, B.M.; Indiveri, C.; Pujia, A.; Montalcini, T.; Hedfalk, K.; Romeo, S. Recombinant PNPLA3 protein shows triglyceride hydrolase activity and its I148M mutation results in loss of function. *Biochim. Biophys. Acta\Mol. Cell Biol. Lipids* **2014**, *1841*, 574–580. [CrossRef] [PubMed]
44. Basantani, M.K.; Sitnick, M.T.; Cai, L.; Brenner, D.S.; Gardner, N.P.; Li, J.Z.; Schoiswohl, G.; Yang, K.; Kumari, M.; Gross, R.W. Pnpla3/Adiponutrin deficiency in mice does not contribute to fatty liver disease or metabolic syndrome. *J. Lipid Res.* **2011**, *52*, 318–329. [PubMed]
45. Sinha, R.A.; Yen, P.M. Thyroid hormone-mediated autophagy and mitochondrial turnover in NAFLD. *Cell Biosci.* **2016**, *6*, 46. [CrossRef] [PubMed]
46. Lambert, J.E.; Ramos-Roman, M.A.; Browning, J.D.; Parks, E.J. Increased de novo lipogenesis is a distinct characteristic of individuals with nonalcoholic fatty liver disease. *Gastroenterology* **2014**, *146*, 726–735. [CrossRef]
47. Xu, B.; Shen, J.; Li, D.; Ning, B.; Guo, L.; Bing, H.; Chen, J.; Li, Y. Overexpression of microRNA-9 inhibits 3T3-L1 cell adipogenesis by targeting PNPLA3 via activation of AMPK. *Gene* **2020**, *730*, 144260.

Disclaimer/Publisher's Note: The statements, opinions and data contained in all publications are solely those of the individual author(s) and contributor(s) and not of MDPI and/or the editor(s). MDPI and/or the editor(s) disclaim responsibility for any injury to people or property resulting from any ideas, methods, instructions or products referred to in the content.

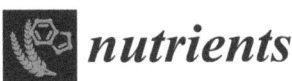

Article

Sociodemographic Trends in Planetary Health Diets among Nutrition Students in Türkiye: Bridging Classroom to Kitchen

Semra Navruz-Varlı [1,†], Hande Mortaş [1,*,†] and Menşure Nur Çelik [2]

1 Department of Nutrition and Dietetics, Faculty of Health Sciences, Gazi University, Ankara 06490, Türkiye; semranavruz@gazi.edu.tr
2 Department of Nutrition and Dietetics, Faculty of Health Sciences, Ondokuz Mayıs University, Samsun 55500, Türkiye; mensurenur.celik@omu.edu.tr
* Correspondence: handeyilmaz@gazi.edu.tr; Tel.: +90-312-216-2639
† These authors contributed equally to this work and share first authorship.

Abstract: This study aimed to investigate the effects of sociodemographic parameters on healthy and sustainable nutrition in nutrition students. This cross-sectional study was conducted with 601 students. Researchers administered questionnaire forms to gather sociodemographic information such as age, gender, geographical region, residence area, accommodation, BMI, and income level. Participants' 24 h dietary records were used to evaluate Healthy Eating Index-2020 (HEI-2020) and Planetary Health Diet Index (PHDI). The mean PHDI scores of the Marmara (53.4 ± 14.9), Aegean (58.2 ± 18.3), Mediterranean (55.3 ± 15.5), and Black Sea (55.5 ± 15.7) regions, which are the coastal regions of Türkiye, were significantly higher than for the Central Anatolia region (46.7 ± 15.1). The PHDI and HEI-2020 score means of students living in metropolitan cities and rural areas were significantly higher than those living in urban areas ($p < 0.05$). Being in the 20–25 years age group increased the probability of being in a lower PHDI group (AOR 1.82; 95% CI 1.07:3.12; $p = 0.028$). While a similar result was found in the 20–25 years age group for HEI-2020, income level and gender did not have a statistically significant effect on these scores. Since students' ages, geographical regions, and residence areas affect PHDI and HEI-2020, it is considered important to take these sociodemographic variables into consideration in guidelines and studies.

Keywords: planetary health diet; sustainable nutrition; diet quality; university students

Citation: Navruz-Varlı, S.; Mortaş, H.; Çelik, M.N. Sociodemographic Trends in Planetary Health Diets among Nutrition Students in Türkiye: Bridging Classroom to Kitchen. *Nutrients* 2024, *16*, 1277. https://doi.org/10.3390/nu16091277

Academic Editors: António Raposo, Renata Puppin Zandonadi and Raquel Braz Assunção Botelho

Received: 3 April 2024
Revised: 22 April 2024
Accepted: 23 April 2024
Published: 25 April 2024

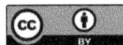

Copyright: © 2024 by the authors. Licensee MDPI, Basel, Switzerland. This article is an open access article distributed under the terms and conditions of the Creative Commons Attribution (CC BY) license (https://creativecommons.org/licenses/by/4.0/).

1. Introduction

It is known that the overweight and obesity situation seen in young adulthood is likely to continue or reach more serious levels in later adulthood [1]. During the university years, which represent a special and important part of young adulthood, social eating habits are shaped, which can significantly affect nutritional status and health in later periods of life. In this regard, it is important to evaluate the diet quality of university students, who are at a stage where the first steps are taken to a new life independent of the family and where basic responsibilities for life such as housing, subsistence, and nutrition are taken individually [2,3]. So, determining the dietary quality of university students, who constitute a significant portion of the young adult group, is important in preventing/controlling health problems that may arise related to nutrition. It is especially important because of their possible role as food preparers in their own future nuclear families and their potential to be role models for the children they will raise [4]. Among university students in Türkiye, the group of students that receive the most intensive nutrition-related education (4 years, theoretical and practical) are the students of departments of nutrition and dietetics [5]. It will be useful in making predictions about the diet quality and sustainable nutrition behavior trends of young people who continue their education in fields other than nutrition. This view is supported by the fact that studies have shown that university students who receive education in the field of health and nutrition are more likely to exhibit positive attitudes and behaviors related to nutrition than those who receive education in science and social fields [6]. In addition, there is a recent study showing that young German medical students who receive long-term nutrition education have better diet quality and more sustainable eating behaviors than the general population [7]. Therefore, determining the nutritional quality and sustainable nutrition behaviors of nutrition students, who were selected as a special subgroup among young adults in our study, is thought to be valuable in terms of evaluating the behavior of this special group, which will raise awareness in this field for the rest of the population.

Effectively implementing sustainable food policies entails addressing various sustainability issues and accommodating a diverse range of food systems, stakeholders, and consumer dietary behaviors [8,9]. Prioritizing the collection of data across these dimensions including sociodemographical issues and ensuring their seamless integration into models are crucial for advancing the sustainable diet agenda. Drawing on country-specific research findings regarding diet quality and sustainability can enhance the accuracy of assessments on the environmental impacts of consumer dietary behaviors in studies focused on sustainability [8,10]. In research conducted for this purpose [10–13], one of the most frequently used tools to evaluate the sustainability dimension of the diet is the Planetary Health Diet Index (PHDI), which is obtained by converting the sustainability and healthy nutrition principles in the EAT-Lancet reference diet into a numerical index [12]. The Planetary Health Diet promotes a high intake of plant-based foods and a low consumption of animal-based foods, following recommended portions for a 2500-kilocalorie daily diet [14].

Considering the statements of the Food and Agriculture Organization [15] that food production must increase in order to meet the needs of the increasing global population [16], it becomes inevitable that updated nutritional guidelines should be created by prioritizing the principle of sustainability. To justify the inclusion of sustainable dietary patterns in these guidelines, the need to compare the PHDI with health-oriented dietary recommendations currently in use has been reported [17]. One of the most commonly used indexes to compare the compliance of individuals' diets with healthy eating recommendations is the Healthy Eating Index (HEI), which was developed to compare compliance with the Dietary Guidelines for Americans [18]. HEI-2020, the latest version of the updated index according to the guide, scores according to threshold values defined according to healthy nutrition recommendations but does not discourage the consumption of animal-sourced foods [17,18]. Additionally, for the HEI, nutritional differences have been demonstrated by gender, income, education, and race/ethnicity [19–21]. However, it is emphasized that the evidence for inequalities in PHDI is insufficient [10,17].

Increasing PHDI scores have been associated with improved diet quality and reductions in obesity and waist circumference [11]. In addition, levels of awareness about diet quality and planetary health tend to be higher in women than in men, in older age groups than young age groups, and in those with higher socioeconomic status than in those with lower socioeconomic status. The region of residence may have a positive or negative effect on diet quality and PHDI scores by restricting access to food or depending on income level [7,17,22].

When evaluating the reflections of differences such as gender, income, education, and ethnicity on the PHDI, there is a need to (1) present country-specific research results and, in doing so, to (2) present the results from the perspective of diet quality in order to add sustainability to existing nutritional recommendations. Therefore, this study aimed to investigate the effects of sociodemographic parameters on healthy and sustainable nutrition in nutrition students who have academic knowledge about sustainable and healthy nutrition approaches. In the study conducted for this purpose, it was hypothesized that sociodemographic variables including gender, age, income level, geographical region, BMI, and accommodation location affect healthy and sustainable nutrition.

2. Materials and Methods

2.1. Participants and Study Design

This cross-sectional study involved 601 adults, comprising 582 females and 19 males, who were enrolled as students in nutrition and dietetics programs at universities in Ankara, the capital city of Türkiye, from September 2023 to December 2023. Non-probabilistic convenience sampling was carried out. This study would require a total of 550 participants with 95% power at the 5% type I error (α) level. Participants were included if they volunteered and were university students studying in the nutrition and dietetics programs, did not follow a specific diet or eating regimen, and did not have any chronic diseases. Exclusions were made for individuals with a daily energy intake below 600 or above 3500 kilocalories according to 24 h dietary records, as well as for pregnant or lactating individuals. Additionally, if any data were missing in the data collection tool questionnaire, that individual was not included in the study.

Ethical approval was obtained from the Ethical Committee of Gazi University (Approval date: 14 July 2023, No: 2023-854). In addition, written informed consent was obtained from the participants in the study. The research was carried out following the Declaration of Helsinki.

2.2. Data Collection Tools

In the study, researchers conducted face-to-face interviews with participants, administering questionnaire forms to gather sociodemographic information such as age, gender, regions where they spent their life until they went to university, residence area, accommodation, and income level. Additionally, participants were asked to complete 24 h dietary record forms for three consecutive days. Height and body weight measurements were self-reported. Body mass index (BMI) was defined as a body weight in kilograms divided by the square of the height in meters (kg/m^2) [23].

Nutritional assessment was conducted based on the data collected from the dietary records. The nutritional content of the dishes consumed was calculated using the Standard Food Recipes book [24]. Subsequently, the data were analyzed using the BeBiS program (version 7.2) to assess total energy and nutrient intake. Participants' nutritional intake was calculated by averaging the data obtained from 24 h dietary record forms for three consecutive days.

The Planetary Health Diet Index (PHDI), devised by Cacau et al. (2021), is based on the dietary guidelines outlined by the EAT-Lancet Commission [12]. This index assesses adherence to these guidelines through a scoring system ranging from 10 to 5 points for each of the 16 diet components, with a total possible score of 0 to 150. Participants' dietary records were used to evaluate these components. Based on their total PHDI score, participants are categorized into tertiles.

The Healthy Eating Index (HEI) was established by the United States Department of Agriculture (USDA) in 1995, aligning with the American Dietary Guidelines [18]. Subsequent updates occurred in 2005, 2010, and 2015, maintaining consistency in components and standards between HEI-2015 and HEI-2020. Despite the name change to emphasize its association with the latest 2020–2025 Dietary Guidelines for Americans, HEI-2020 retains identical criteria and scoring standards to HEI-2015. The HEI-2020 utilized in this study comprises thirteen components, with nine recommended for consumption and four for limited intake. Components recommended for consumption include total fruit, whole fruit, total vegetables, green leafy vegetables and legumes, whole grains, dairy products, protein foods, seafood and plant-based proteins, and fatty acids. Moderation is advised for processed grains, sodium, added sugar, and saturated fats. Higher total scores indicate better nutritional quality across all components [18]. Based on their total HEI-2020 score, participants are categorized into tertiles.

2.3. Statistical Analysis

Continuous variables were expressed as arithmetic mean with standard deviation and categorical variables as percentages. The HEI-2020 total score and PHDI total score were compared according to age groups (<20 years; 20–25 years; >25 years), BMI groups (underweight; normal weight; overweight; obese), gender (female and male), regions of Türkiye (Marmara, Aegean, Mediterranean, Black Sea, Central Anatolia, Eastern Anatolia, Southeast Anatolia), residence areas (metropolis, urban, rural), income level (low, those whose expenses are more than their income; adequate, those whose expenses are equal to their income; high, those whose income exceeds their expenses), and accommodation status (dormitory and home) of the participants. Participants' dietary energy, macronutrient, and micronutrient intakes were shown according to the income levels.

The t-test (in Table 1 for gender and accommodation groups) and one-way ANOVA (in Table 1 for age groups, geographical regions, residence areas, income level groups, and BMI categories; in Table 2 for income level groups) were employed for comparisons in independent groups. Post hoc analysis involved the application of Bonferroni correction for handling multiple pairwise comparisons. Moreover, a series of multivariate ANOVAs (MANOVAs) were conducted with four sociodemographic variables which were found to be significantly different among groups according to Table 1 as independent variables and with the total scores of PHDI and HEI-2020 as dependent variables. The possible effect of age groups (<20 years; 20–25 years; >25 years), geographical regions (Marmara, Aegean, Mediterranean, Black Sea, Central Anatolia, Eastern Anatolia, Southeast Anatolia), residence areas (metropolis, urban, rural), and income level (low; adequate; high) on total scores of the PHDI and the HEI-2020 was analyzed using a multivariate analysis of variance (MANOVA) and the interaction among the factors using the Bonferroni statistic. Furthermore, the effect size was calculated in terms of eta squared (η^2). The results of the MANOVAs are presented in Supplementary Material Tables S1 and S2. The four independent variables included age groups, geographical regions, residence areas, and income level. Of the four sociodemographical variables considered, one to four were entered into the MANOVA at a time, with combinations of sociodemographical variables selected such that cell sizes equaled or exceeded 30 (i.e., sufficient cell size to ensure normalcy of distribution of individual differences). When significant interactions were found, the file was split by both variables and MANOVAs were conducted with the other variable and only the significant findings reported. Parametric statistics were used to confirm the effects obtained via the MANOVAs when Levene's test for homogeneity of variance was significant at the $p > 0.05$ level.

Table 1. Healthy Eating Index-2020 and Planetary Health Diet Index total scores of the students according to the sociodemographic variables.

Variables	Proportion [n (%)]	Total PHDI Score Mean ± SD	95% CI		Total HEI-2020 Score Mean	95% CI	
Total	601 (100)	50.9 ± 15.6	49.7	52.2	47.9 ± 11.7	47.0	48.9
Gender							
Females	582 (96.8)	50.8 ± 15.5	49.6	52.2	47.9 ± 11.6	47.1	48.9
Males	19 (3.2)	52.1 ± 18.1	43.4	60.8	48.0 ± 12.6	41.9	54.1
		t = 0.321 p = 0.748			t = 0.026 p = 0.979		
Age group							
<20 years	215 (35.8)	54.2 ± 15.4 [a]	52.1	56.2	49.9 ± 10.7 [a,b]	48.4	51.3
20–25 years	354 (58.9)	48.8 ± 15.3 [b]	47.2	50.4	46.5 ± 12.0 [b]	45.3	47.8
>25 years	32 (5.3)	53.3 ± 16.1 [a,b]	47.5	59.1	51.4 ± 11.8 [a]	47.1	55.6
		F = 8.635 p < 0.001			F = 7.135 p = 0.001		

Table 1. Cont.

Variables	Proportion [n (%)]	Total PHDI Score Mean ± SD	95% CI		Total HEI-2020 Score Mean	95% CI	
Regions							
Marmara	214 (35.6)	53.4 ± 14.9 [a]	51.4	55.4	49.3 ± 10.4 [a]	47.9	50.7
Aegean	25 (4.2)	58.2 ± 18.3 [a]	50.7	65.7	52.1 ± 12.6 [a,b]	46.9	57.3
Mediterranean	43 (7.2)	55.3 ± 15.5 [a]	50.5	60.0	50.2 ± 13.5 [a,b]	46.1	54.4
Black Sea	33 (5.5)	55.5 ± 15.7 [a]	49.9	61.0	47.6 ± 13.6 [a,b]	42.8	52.1
Central Anatolia	238 (39.5)	46.7 ± 15.1 [b]	44.8	48.6	45.4 ± 11.7 [b]	43.9	46.9
Eastern Anatolia	24 (4.0)	50.0 ± 14.3 [a,b]	43.9	56.1	48.9 ± 10.5 [a,b]	44.1	52.9
Southeast Anatolia	24 (4.0)	50.2 ± 15.5 [a,b]	43.7	56.7	52.8 ± 10.5 [a]	47.8	57.9
		F = 6.096 p < 0.001			F = 3.947 p = 0.001		
Residence area							
Metropolis	265 (44.1)	52.5 ± 15.8 [a]	50.6	54.5	49.7 ± 10.9 [a]	48.4	51.0
Urban	215 (35.8)	47.3 ± 15.2 [b]	45.2	49.3	44.7 ± 11.3 [b]	43.2	46.3
Rural	121 (20.1)	53.9 ± 14.4 [a]	51.4	56.6	49.9 ± 12.5 [a]	47.6	52.2
		F = 9.957 p < 0.001			F = 13.347 p < 0.001		
Income level							
Low	200 (33.3)	53.8 ± 15.6 [a]	51.6	55.9	49.5 ± 10.6 [a]	47.9	50.9
Adequate	328 (54.6)	48.4 ± 15.2 [b]	46.8	50.0	46.9 ± 12.1 [b]	45.6	48.2
High	73 (12.1)	54.5 ± 15.6 [a]	50.9	58.1	48.9 ± 12.1 [a,b]	46.0	51.7
		F = 9.920 p < 0.001			F = 3.285 p = 0.038		
Accommodation							
Dormitory	493 (82.0)	50.6 ± 15.6	49.2	51.9	47.9 ± 11.7	46.9	48.9
Home	108 (18.0)	52.5 ± 15.7	49.5	55.5	48.1 ± 11.7	45.8	50.3
		t = −1.122 p = 0.262			t = −0.103 p = 0.918		
BMI categories							
Underweight	52 (8.7)	56.1 ± 16.6	51.4	60.7	49.2 ± 12.8	45.6	52.7
Normal weight	461 (76.7)	50.2 ± 15.4	48.8	51.6	47.9 ± 11.6	46.9	48.9
Overweight	70 (11.6)	51.5 ± 16.0	47.6	55.3	47.5 ± 11.4	44.8	50.2
Obese	18 (3.0)	53.8 ± 12.5	47.6	60.1	47.9 ± 12.5	41.6	54.1
		F = 2.492 p = 0.059			F = 0.230 p = 0.876		

CI: Confidence interval; BMI: Body mass index; HEI: Healthy Eating Index; PHDI: Planetary Health Index; SD: Standard deviation. [a,b] represent the statistically significant differences among the column groups at $p < 0.05$.

Table 2. Dietary energy, macronutrient, and micronutrient intakes of the students according to income level.

Dietary Intake ($\bar{x} \pm SD$)	Income Level			F	p
	Low	Adequate	High		
Energy (kcal)	1580.1 ± 589.7 [a]	1343.9 ± 501.1 [b]	1370.5 ± 591.7 [b]	12.165	<0.001
Carbohydrates (% of energy)	43.8 ± 9.6	45.9 ± 11.6	43.3 ± 10.7	3.328	0.057
Proteins (% of energy)	15.6 ± 4.6 [a]	14.5 ± 4.6 [b]	16.0 ± 6.3 [a]	5.023	0.007
Fats (% of energy)	40.7 ± 8.9	39.5 ± 10.8	40.8 ± 10.0	0.930	0.395
Cholesterol (mg)	273.7 ± 14.7 [a]	215.2 ± 9.8 [b]	221.9 ± 16.5 [a,b]	6.508	0.002
Saturated fat (g)	24.2 ± 13.3 [a]	19.2 ± 10.1 [b]	20.9 ± 11.7 [a,b]	11.791	<0.001
Fiber (g)	17.5 ± 8.4 [a]	14.3 ± 7.5 [b]	14.7 ± 8.7 [b]	10.068	<0.001
Thiamine (mg)	0.8 ± 0.3 [a]	0.7 ± 0.3 [b]	0.7 ± 0.2 [a,b]	11.407	<0.001
Riboflavin (mg)	1.1 ± 0.5 [a]	0.9 ± 0.6 [b]	1.0 ± 0.4 [a,b]	4.098	0.017

Table 2. Cont.

Dietary Intake ($\bar{x} \pm$ SD)	Low	Income Level Adequate	High	F	p
Niacin (mg)	11.3 ± 6.9 [a]	9.6 ± 7.4 [b]	10.4 ± 6.3 [a,b]	3.589	**0.028**
Folate (mcg)	269.9 ± 12.9 [a]	203.7 ± 11.8 [b]	229.3 ± 13.1 [b]	17.519	**<0.001**
Vitamin A (mcg)	935.3 ± 57.1	829.8 ± 168.4	906.7 ± 96.1	0.137	0.872
Vitamin B_{12} (mcg)	3.7 ± 2.7	3.2 ± 5.2	3.1 ± 2.5	1.087	0.338
Vitamin C (mg)	101.6 ± 78.9 [a]	70.8 ± 61.7 [b]	83.8 ± 59.1 [a,b]	12.960	**<0.001**
Iron (mg)	9.5 ± 5.3 [a]	7.4 ± 3.8 [b]	7.9 ± 4.3 [a,b]	14.708	**<0.001**
Phosphorus (mg)	930.4 ± 353.9 [a]	785.4 ± 353.3 [b]	802.7 ± 307.6 [b]	11.140	**<0.001**
Calcium (mg)	552.7 ± 264.9 [a]	482.1 ± 305.6 [b]	503.7 ± 287.8 [a,b]	3.724	**0.025**
Potassium (mg)	2180.6 ± 902.6 [a]	1696.4 ± 844.8 [b]	1855.688.8 [b]	20	**<0.001**
Zinc (mg)	8.3 ± 3.4 [a]	6.8 ± 3.4 [b]	6.7 ± 3.2 [b]	733	**<0.001**
Magnesium (mg)	239.6 ± 103.9 [a]	185.7 ± 87.1 [b]	203.7 ± 89.2 [b]	20.291	**<0.001**
Copper (mg)	1.2 ± 0.6 [a]	1.0 ± 0.6 [b]	1.0 ± 0.6 [b]	11.799	**<0.001**

SD: Standard deviation. [a,b] represent the statistically significant differences among the column groups at $p < 0.05$. Bold p values indicate statistical significance at the $p < 0.05$ level.

Furthermore, a multivariable logistic regression model (in Tables 3 and 4) was used to identify independent predictors, including dietary energy intake, genders, age groups, income levels, and residence area, of low planetary diet quality defined as T_1. The odds of being in the low planetary diet quality group due to "being female"; "being in <20 years age group"; "having a high income level"; and "living in a metropolis" were examined; and for continuous variables specific intervals were used. The model fit was assessed using appropriate residual and goodness-of-fit statistics. A 5% type I error level was used to infer statistical significance. The IBM Statistical Package for the Social Sciences (SPSS) 28.0.1.0 program was used for statistical analysis, and significance was evaluated at $p < 0.05$.

Table 3. Contrasting low planetary health diet quality to average–high planetary health diet quality in students by the variables.

Variables	Categories of Variables	COR (95% CI)	p Values for COR	AOR (95% CI)	p Values for AOR
Dietary energy		1.01 (1.00–1.01)	**0.007**	1.01 (1.00–1.01)	**0.001**
Genders	Females	1		1	
	Males	0.72 (0.26–2.03)	0.534	0.69 (0.24–2.04)	0.507
Age groups	<20 years	1		1	
	20–25 years	1.75 (1.20–2.55)	**0.003**	1.82 (1.07–3.12)	**0.028**
	>25 years	1.32 (0.59–2.97)	0.498	1.74 (0.72–4.25)	0.221
Income level	Low	0.96 (0.53–1.74)	0.901	1.16 (0.59–2.28)	0.665
	Adequate	1.45 (0.83–2.52)	0.191	1.25 (0.69–2.26)	0.456
	High	1		1	
Residence area	Metropolis	1		1	
	Urban	1.46 (1.00–2.13)	**0.048**	1.17 (0.74–1.87)	0.502
	Rural	0.69 (0.42–1.13)	0.141	0.63 (0.38–1.06)	0.083

AOR: Adjusted odds ratio; CI: Confidence interval; COR: Crude odds ratio; kcal: Kilocalories. Bold p values indicate statistical significance at the $p < 0.05$ level.

Table 4. Contrasting low HEI-2020 tertile to average–high HEI-2020 tertile group in students by the variables.

Variables	Categories of Variables	COR (95% CI)	p Values for COR	AOR (95% CI)	p Values for AOR
Dietary energy		1.01 (1.00–1.01)	0.518	1.00 (1.00–1.00)	0.69
Genders	Females	1		1	
	Males	0.53 (0.17–1.60)	0.258	0.50 (0.16–1.56)	0.233
Age groups	<20 years	1		1	
	20–25 years	2.13 (1.46–3.11)	<0.001	1.45 (0.87–2.43)	0.153
	>25 years	1.07 (0.45–2.53)	0.874	0.88 (0.35–3.22)	0.793
Income level	Low	0.59 (0.33–1.06)	0.076	0.75 (0.39–1.439	0.379
	Adequate	1.23 (0.72–2.09)	0.448	0.92 (0.52–1.62)	0.775
	High	1		1	
Residence area	Metropolis	1		1	
	Urban	2.38 (1.62–3.50)	<0.001	1.83 (1.15–2.91)	**0.011**
	Rural	1.18 (0.73–1.91)	0.501	1.06 (0.63–1.77)	0.840

AOR: Adjusted odds ratio; CI: Confidence interval; COR: Crude odds ratio; kcal: Kilocalories. Bold p values indicate statistical significance at the $p < 0.05$ level.

3. Results

PHDI and HEI-2020 total scores according to individuals' sociodemographic characteristics are shown in Table 1. The mean PHDI and HEI-2020 total scores of the participants were determined as 50.9 ± 15.6 and 47.9 ± 11.7, respectively. There was no statistical difference between the total PHDI and HEI-2020 scores of the participants according to their gender ($p = 0.748$ and $p = 0.979$, respectively). According to age groups, PHDI total score averages of students younger than 20 (54.2 ± 15.4) were significantly higher than for other age groups (48.8 ± 15.3 and 53.3 ± 16.1, respectively, in 20–25 years and >25 years groups; $p < 0.001$). In total HEI-2020 scores, the mean of the >25 years group (51.4 ± 11.8) was found to be statistically higher than that of the 20–25 years group (46.5 ± 12.0; $p = 0.001$) but was not different from the <20 years group (49.9 ± 10.7).

Statistically significant differences were found between Türkiye's total PHDI and HEI-2020 score means according to geographical region. The mean PHDI total scores of the Marmara (53.4 ± 14.9), Aegean (58.2 ± 18.3), Mediterranean (55.3 ± 15.5), and Black Sea (55.5 ± 15.7) regions, which are the coastal regions of Türkiye, were significantly higher than for the Central Anatolia region (46.7 ± 15.1; $p < 0.001$), without any difference among coastal regions. According to geographical region, HEI-2020 total mean scores were shown to be highest in the Southeast Anatolia region (52.8 ± 10.5) and lowest in the Central Anatolia region (45.4 ± 11.7; $p = 0.001$).

The total PHDI and HEI-2020 score means of students living in metropolitan cities and rural areas were significantly higher than those living in urban areas ($p < 0.001$). The mean PHDI scores of individuals in the "adequate" income group (48.4 ± 15.2), whose income was defined as equal to their expenses, were significantly lower than those of individuals in the "high" (54.5 ± 15.6) and "low" (53.8 ± 15.6) income groups ($p < 0.001$). The mean HEI-2020 scores in the "adequate" group (46.9 ± 12.1) were significantly lower than those in individuals in the "low" income group (49.5 ± 10.6; $p = 0.038$) but do not differ from individuals in the "high" income group (48.9 ± 12.1; $p > 0.05$).

There were no statistically significant differences in the students' PHDI and HEI-2020 total mean scores according to their dormitory or home accommodation status ($p = 0.262$ and $p = 0.918$, respectively) and BMI categories ($p = 0.059$ and $p = 0.876$, respectively).

The results of the MANOVAs are presented in Supplementary Material Tables S1 and S2. The four independent variables included age groups, geographical regions, residence areas, and income level. In almost all cases, the results of MANOVAs were confirmed the findings of the ANOVAs. In those cases, the results of the MANOVAs only are reported in Table S2. In cases where significant findings were not found on the tests they were not reported. There are no significant multivariate effects for the variables' combinations in Table S1.

Significant multivariate effects are found for the age groups (F (1, 2) = 0.684, $p < 0.001$, $\eta^2 = 0.003$, CI, 51.106, 59.005), regions (F (1, 5); (2, 5); (3, 5); (4, 5) = 1.265, $p = 0.038$, $\eta^2 = 0.015$, CI, 48.672, 57.012 for 1; 53.099, 66.549 for 2; 50.798, 61.886 for 3; 52.202, 65.242 for 4; 44.768, 53.199 for 5), residence areas (F (1, 2); (2, 3) = 0.696, $p < 0.001$, $\eta^2 = 0.003$, CI, 47.811, 55.824 for 1; 50.402, 58.325 for 2; 52.137, 58.959 for 3), and income levels (F (1, 2); (2, 3) = 1.701, $p = 0.006$, $\eta^2 = 0.007$, CI, 52.721, 61.594 for 1; 49.480, 55.431 for 2; 49.066, 57.389 for 3) in total PHDI scores in Table S2. The large number of samples resulted in smaller effect sizes, i.e., η^2 values. The findings confirmed from Table 1 are shown in Table S2.

Table 2 is presented to reveal whether there are significant differences in energy and nutrient intakes according to participants' income levels. Participants' energy and nutrient intakes according to their income level are shown in Table 2. Mean intakes of energy, protein, cholesterol, saturated fatty acids, fiber, thiamine, niacin, folate, vitamin C, iron, phosphorus, calcium, potassium, zinc, magnesium, and copper were found to be significantly higher in the "low" income group than those in the "adequate" and "high" income groups ($p < 0.05$). There was no statistical difference between income level groups in terms of individuals' mean intake of carbohydrates ($p = 0.057$), fat ($p = 0.395$), vitamin A ($p = 0.872$), and vitamin B_{12} ($p = 0.338$).

In Table 3, when individuals are divided into tertiles according to their PHDI scores (low (T_1)–medium (T_2)–high (T_3)), the risks of being in the lowest tertile category are shown with adjustment (adjusted odds ratio—AOR) and without adjustment (crude odds ratio—COR) according to various sociodemographic characteristics. For categorical variables with an OR higher than one, the odds of being in the T_1 PHDI group were higher than in the reference group. For continuous variables, these odds became higher per specified interval. The probability of being in the T_1 PHDI group increased with increasing dietary energy intake (kcal) (AOR 1.01; 95% CI 1.00:1.01; $p = 0.01$). Being in the 20–25 years age group increased the probability of being in the T_1 PHDI group compared to the reference of the <20 years age group (AOR 1.82; 95% CI 1.07:3.12; $p = 0.028$).

In Table 4, when individuals are divided into tertiles according to their HEI-2020 scores (low (T_1)–medium (T_2)–high (T_3)), the risks of being in the lowest tertile category are shown with adjustment (adjusted odds ratio—AOR) and without adjustment (crude odds ratio—COR) according to various sociodemographic characteristics. For categorical variables with an OR higher than one, the odds of being in the T_1 HEI-2020 group were higher than in the reference group. For continuous variables, these odds became higher per specified interval. Being in the urban residence area group increased the probability of being in the T_1 HEI-2020 group compared to the reference of the metropolis residence area group (AOR 1.83; 95% CI 1.15:2.91; $p = 0.011$).

The percentage distribution of individuals in the T_3 group, which is the highest tertile according to individuals' PHDI score tertiles, in the geographical regions of Türkiye is shown in Figure 1. Geographic regions indicated in darker green indicate higher percentages of participants in the higher PHDI tertile (T_3) in these regions. So, dark green colors visualize higher percentages, and as the green tone becomes lighter, the percentage of individuals in the T_3 tertile decreases. It was found that the individuals with the highest PHDI scores (T_3) were in the Aegean (52%), Black Sea (51.5%), Mediterranean (44.2%), and Marmara (42%) regions of Türkiye, expressed in darker green. These regions were followed by Southeast Anatolia (33.3%), Eastern Anatolia (25%), and Central Anatolia (20.2%).

The percentage distribution of individuals in the T_3 group, which is the highest tertile according to individuals' HEI-2020 score tertiles, in the geographical regions of Türkiye is shown in Figure 2. Geographic regions indicated in darker green indicate higher percentages of participants in the higher HEI-2020 tertile (T_3) in these regions. So, dark green colors visualize higher percentages, and as the green tone becomes lighter, the percentage of individuals in the T_3 tertile decreases. It was found that the individuals with the highest HEI-2020 scores (T_3) were in the Aegean (56%), Eastern Anatolia (45.8%), Southeast Anatolia (41.7%), and Mediterranean (39.5%) regions of Türkiye, expressed in darker green. These regions were followed by Marmara (35.5%), Black Sea (33.3%), and Central Anatolia (27.3%).

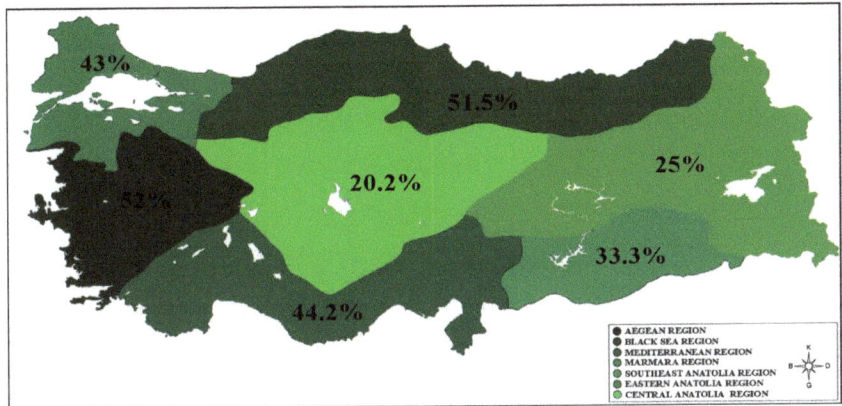

Figure 1. The percentage distribution of individuals in the PHDI T$_3$ group according to Türkiye's geographical regions.

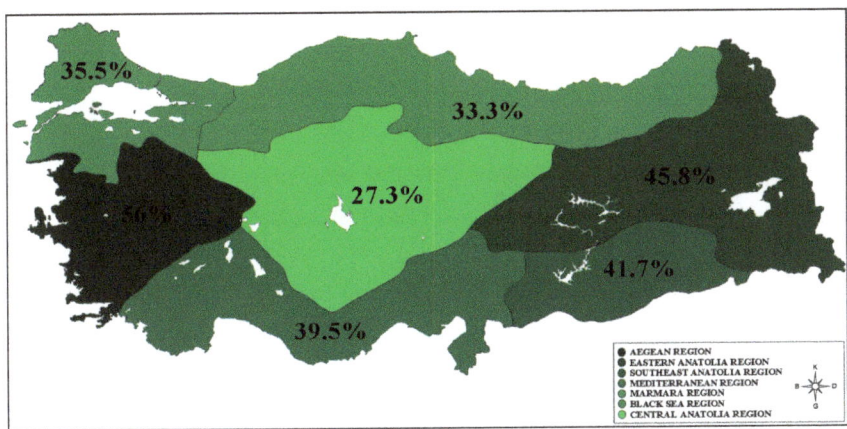

Figure 2. The percentage distribution of individuals in the HEI-2020 T$_3$ group according to Türkiye's geographical regions.

Participants' HEI-2020 and PHDI component scores according to Türkiye's regions are presented in Figure 3. Among the HEI-2020 components, the total vegetable score was highest in the Aegean, Mediterranean, and Black Sea regions, which are the coastal areas of Türkiye. Similarly, seafood and plant protein scores were highest in these regions, while these scores were low in the Central Anatolia and Eastern Anatolia regions. It was seen that the score in the dairy group was highest in the Southeast Anatolia region.

Among the PHDI components, the lowest red meat score was found in the Southeast Anatolia and Eastern Anatolia regions. It was visualized that the fish and seafood scores were lowest in the Central Anatolia and Eastern Anatolia regions and, similarly, the vegetable and whole cereals scores were lowest in these regions.

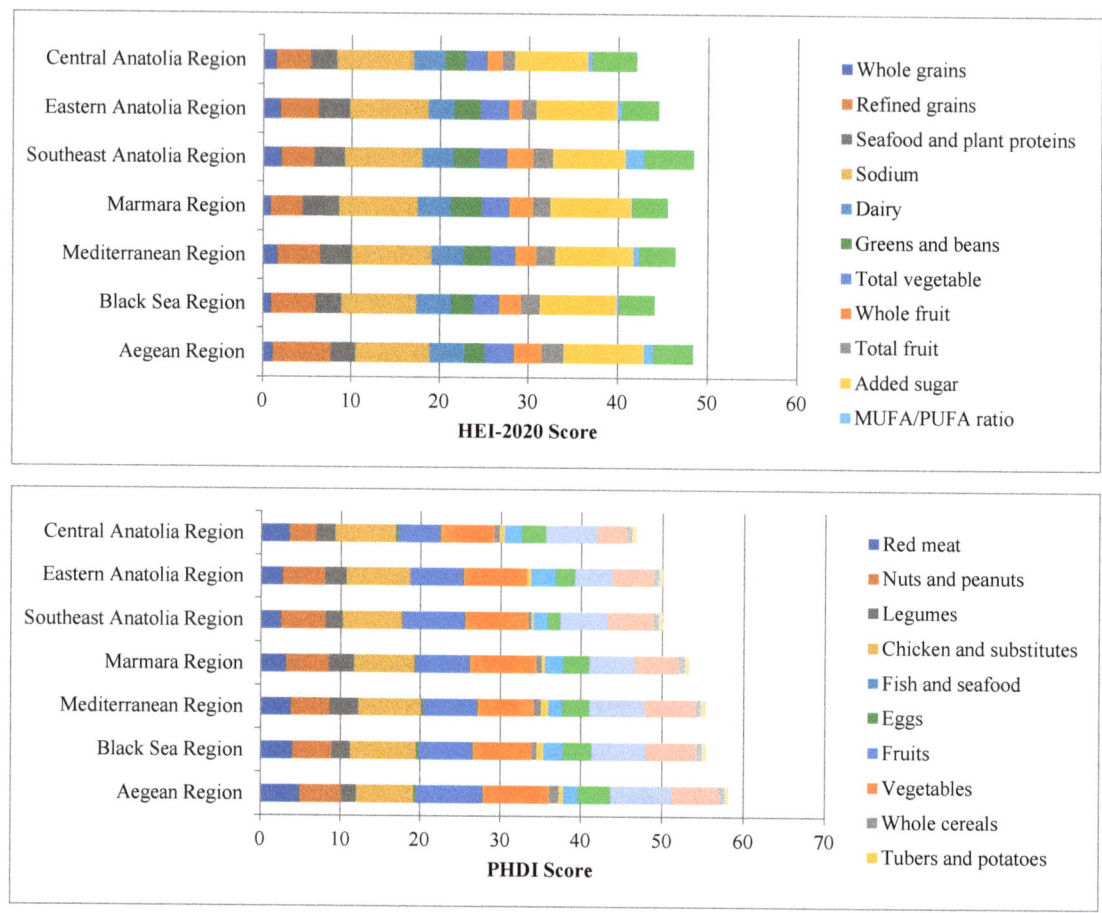

Figure 3. HEI-2020 and PHDI component scores according to Türkiye's regions.

4. Discussion

This study endeavors to explore the impact of sociodemographic factors on the adoption of sustainable and healthy dietary practices among nutrition students well-versed in the principles of sustainable nutrition. To the best of our knowledge, this is the first study to examine PHDI, a nutritional index designed to account for both environmental and health concerns, in Turkish adults in addition to HEI-2020, a nutritional index designed to account only for health concerns, and to assess how well their diets adhered to PHDI. This study found low compliance with EAT-Lancet recommendations and low PHDI scores across all of our geographic regions. It has been shown that age, income level, geographical region, and place of residence are the components that affect the PHDI score. In comparison to other places, high PHDI scores were found in our coastal areas.

Although the PHDI has been tested in the United States population, it is designed for use in a variety of settings. Global diets are neither as healthy nor as sustainable as the EAT-Lancet Commission reference diet. However, it is stated that heterogeneity in how these diets differ from recommendations can be determined by PHDI. Application of the PHDI in diverse global settings could provide a unified framework for directly comparing the health and sustainability of nutrition across countries and monitoring progress over time [25].

PHDI is associated with higher overall nutritional quality and lower greenhouse gas emissions [12,26]. In a study conducted in the Turkish population, it was shown that the average PHDI score was 41.5 when evaluated according to PHDI quartile distributions [10]. In a study conducted in Brazil, PHDI scores were found to be similar (45.9 points) and society's compliance with EAT-Lancet recommendations was evaluated as low [13]. In another study conducted by Cacau et al. in the Brazilian population, the average PHDI score was 60.4, which seems relatively high compared to other countries, but is far from meeting the recommendations [11]. In a recent study, mean PHDI was lower ($p < 0.001$) in men than in women (44.0 and 47.1, respectively) and tended to be lower in younger individuals [17]. On the contrary, in this study, there was no statistical difference between the total PHDI scores of the participants according to their gender, and the average PHDI total score of the participants under the age of 20 was significantly higher than that of the other age groups (Table 1). According to data obtained from all regions of our country, the diet of our population appears to be far from being in line with the evidence presented by EAT-Lancet. It can be said that the average PHDI scores obtained in this study are less than half of the maximum score of 150, and compliance with EAT-Lancet recommendations is low in our country (Table 1). Our results are parallel to previous studies and literature in our country in terms of PHDI score. The fact that PHDI average scores are high, especially in coastal regions (Marmara, Black Sea, Aegean, and Mediterranean) (Table 1, Figures 1 and 2), may be related to the diversity of foods especially food groups such as fish and seafood, vegetables, fruits, dairy, and eggs, which are among the "adequacy" and "optimum" components in the PHDI score, consumed in these regions (Figure 3). In addition, in this study, when the low planetary health diet quality of the participants was compared with the average–high planetary health diet quality according to different variables, being between the ages of 20 and 25, living in a rural area, and increased energy intake were found to be important risk factors for a decrease in the PHDI score (Table 3).

For PHDI to be widely adopted, it must be acceptable to consumers. While there are various factors that influence consumer food choices, such as accessibility, availability, health concerns, and food preferences [27,28], the role of affordability is also considered a key factor that can influence PHDI score [29,30]. While health and sustainability are desirable outcomes of consumer choices, affordability often takes priority, especially for low-income consumers [30–32]. Therefore, it is necessary to understand the cost and affordability of a healthy and sustainable diet such as used in the PHDI for various socioeconomic groups. Two studies conducted in the United Kingdom determined the cost of a healthy, sustainable diet and compared this to the typical diet consumed in that country, finding that there was no increase in cost for following a healthy, sustainable diet [33,34]. On the contrary, in one study conducted in Australia, the typical Australian diet was found to be more costly than a healthy and sustainable diet [35], while in another, the result was found to be the opposite [29]. A PHDI-compliant diet has been shown to be affordable for high-income countries but unaffordable for low-income countries [36]. PHDI and HEI-2020 were found to be higher in those with "low" and "high" income levels and living in "rural" and "metropolitan" areas than those with "sufficient" income levels and living in "urban" areas ($p < 0.05$) (Table 1). When dietary intakes are examined (Table 2), significantly higher saturated fat, cholesterol, phosphorus, and iron intakes in the low-income group show that consumption of animal-based foods is high. However, their high fiber intake suggests that plant sources are included in the diet more than in individuals with other income levels, which positively affects PHDI scores. It is possible that these individuals are individuals living in rural areas. It is thought that this finding was obtained because individuals living in rural areas in our country frequently engage in animal husbandry and the consumption of animal products is common among these individuals. Our findings support our idea that those with high income levels live in metropolises. Although dietary energy intake is low, PHDI and HEI-2020 scores are thought to be high in those living in metropolises due to access to sufficient resources. Individuals with sufficient income levels seem to live in urban areas. Considering city life and daily work pace, it is thought that their dietary intake is not sufficient compared to rural areas, and therefore HEI-2020 and PHDI scores remain low. In addition, although individuals with sufficient and high income levels have similar energy, carbohydrate, fat, and micronutrient intakes, when looking at their diet patterns, it is possible to say that protein intake remains lower at sufficient income levels, and this affects the diet quality of individuals. Considering that the sufficient income group lives in urban areas and the high-income group lives in metropolises, factors such as limited access to resources in urban areas compared to metropolises and the lower income level of those living in urban areas than individuals in metropolitan areas may explain the lower HEI-2020 and PHDI scores in individuals with sufficient income compared to high income levels.

In a study evaluating the obesity consequences of compliance with PHDI, it was observed that individuals with higher compliance with PHDI had lower BMI and waist circumference values [11]. However, another study showed that overweight/obese individuals had higher PHDI scores [13]. One study determined that higher BMI was associated with lower PHDI, with a decrease in BMI associated with an increase in PHDI total scores [10]. Therefore, it is thought that more studies are needed on the effects of obesity on the sustainable environment and the effects of sustainable nutrition on the prevalence of obesity. In this study, no statistically significant difference was found in the PHDI and HEI-2020 total score averages according to BMI categories. Although not statistically significant in the group classified as normal BMI, lower PHDI scores are noteworthy. It is thought that statistical significance may not have been achieved because the majority of the participants in the study (76.7%) were in the normal BMI class (Tables 1 and 2).

Country-specific studies are important due to different cultures, traditions, and access to food in each country, as well as different environmental factors in each country [8]. It is important that this healthy and sustainable diet model is addressed in a way that covers all regions in our country in the context of revealing local differences.

While some studies report that no relationship can be found between dietary energy, protein, and PHDI scores [10,12], the findings of some studies that dietary fiber positively affects nutritional scores are noteworthy [10,37]. Another study also showed that sustainable and healthy eating behaviors and high adherence to PHDI increased with dietary fiber intake [38]. Similarly, in this study, individuals in the "low" income group, whose dietary fiber and folate intake was significantly higher than for other income levels, were found to have higher PHDI scores (Tables 1 and 2).

Low PHDI scores are due to several components. Consumption of moderation components in the United States exceeds targets for added sugars, added fats, saturated fats, trans fats, dairy products, and red and processed meats, reflecting the typical "Western" dietary pattern [25]. This is consistent with other findings regarding animal-derived food consumption in the United States [39]. In addition to overconsumption of moderation ingredients, underconsumption of various adequacy ingredients such as whole grains, fruits, vegetables, legumes, nuts, and seeds has also been reported. Adherence to fruit and vegetable recommendations has been low in the United States [25]. Similar to a cross-sectional study conducted in Brazil [12], adolescents who consumed excessive amounts of animal-derived foods scored lower on the PHDI [12,14]. The scores obtained from the HEI-2020 and PHDI components have an expected distribution in terms of geographical regions in our country. It is expected that seafood and vegetable consumption, and therefore the scores obtained from their consumption, will be high due to agricultural and fishing activities in coastal areas. While the scores obtained from the milk and meat groups were expected to be high in the Eastern and Southeastern Anatolia regions, as they are the regions where the main livestock activities of our country are carried out, the lowest red meat scores were found in the Southeastern Anatolia region. As expected, the scores obtained from milk and its products are highest in the Eastern Anatolia region. Although the Central Anatolia region is described as a "granary", the score obtained from this food group remained low (Figure 3).

The following limitations should be taken into account when evaluating the research findings. It should be kept in mind that this cross-sectional study cannot clearly reveal the cause–effect relationship and can only help us make inferences by providing information about the current situation. The participants' weight and height are based on self-report, which may be misleading. Additionally, supplement use was not taken into account in nutritional intake. However, the goal of EAT-Lancet is to provide a nutritionally adequate diet without the need for nutritional supplements. In this study, we evaluated the situation regarding nutritional intake. Additionally, one of the limitations of the study is that the participants were not distributed evenly in terms of gender. The fact that males are more reluctant than females to participate in research and that the nutrition department students in Türkiye are predominantly female has led to this result. From this perspective, the gender distribution in the study also reflected the distribution of nutrition students in Türkiye. However, the inclusion of only a specific group in the study and the imbalance in gender distribution limit the generalizability of the results to the whole population of Türkiye.

The strengths of the study are as follows: The fact that it evaluated the relationship between diet quality and planetary health across the country suggests that the research sample may reflect Türkiye in terms of sociodemographic variables. In addition, it is important that it is one of the first studies to evaluate individuals' sustainable healthy eating behaviors and the compliance of their diets with PHDI on a regional basis and that it considers PHDI together with HEI-2020, another important dietary index. One of the strengths of the study is that the 24 h recording method, which is thought to be more accurate than the food consumption frequency questionnaire, was used to calculate PHDI. Additionally, although the fact that the study was conducted in the nutrition department as a specific group may seem like a limitation, we think that sustainable and healthy nutrition is low even in a population with basic knowledge about nutrition and that it is valuable to reveal sociodemographic variables.

5. Conclusions

This study seeks to understand how individuals' background influences their choices about eating healthily and sustainably, focusing on nutrition students who are familiar with these concepts. In conclusion, to our knowledge, this study is among the first articles to analyze adherence to the EAT-Lancet universal healthy reference diet by geographical region in a nationally representative sample of adults in Türkiye. Revision of the diet in our country according to EAT-Lancet recommendations will increase nutritional adequacy in terms of some food groups and nutrients. This research shows that participants' PHDI index scores were low. Therefore, adherence to the EAT-Lancet recommendation was determined to be low. No association of BMI with lower PHDI scores was found. However, it was concluded that age, income level, geographical region, and place of residence affect PHDI scores and HEI-2020 scores similarly. Policies are needed to transform food systems and create a more sustainable nutrition pattern. For this reason, in creating sustainable and healthy nutrition behaviors, the importance of developing nutrition guidelines by evaluating the environmental factors affecting them not only across the country but also in geographical and sociodemographic clusters within the same country should not be ignored by policy developers.

It is important for future studies to be conducted on a larger sample that is homogeneously distributed in terms of sociodemographic variables that can represent the country in order to generalize the results. In addition, future studies will be able to reveal the causality between PHDI and sociodemographic variables through longitudinally planned studies. It is thought that this cross-sectional study will be a guide in this direction.

Supplementary Materials: The following supporting information can be downloaded at: https://www.mdpi.com/article/10.3390/nu16091277/s1, Table S1. MANOVA test results including Healthy Eating Index-2020 and Planetary Health Diet Index total scores differences according to the sociodemographic variables interactions. Table S2. MANOVA test results including Healthy Eating Index-2020 and Planetary Health Diet Index total scores differences according to the sociodemographic variables.

Author Contributions: Conceptualization, S.N.-V. and H.M.; data curation, S.N.-V.; formal analysis, H.M.; investigation, S.N.-V. and H.M.; methodology, S.N.-V. and H.M.; project administration, S.N.-V. and M.N.Ç.; resources, H.M. and M.N.Ç.; software, H.M.; supervision, H.M. and S.N.-V.; validation, H.M.; visualization, H.M.; writing, H.M., S.N.-V. and M.N.Ç. All authors have read and agreed to the published version of the manuscript.

Funding: This research received no external funding.

Institutional Review Board Statement: The study was conducted in accordance with the Declaration of Helsinki and approved by the Ethics Committee of Gazi University of Ankara/Turkey (Approval date: 14 July 2023 No: 2023-854).

Informed Consent Statement: Informed consent was obtained from all subjects involved in the study.

Data Availability Statement: The data that support the findings of this study are available from the corresponding author, handeyilmaz@gazi.edu.tr, upon reasonable request due to fact that it is intended to be shared only with researchers working in this field.

Conflicts of Interest: The authors declare no conflicts of interest.

References

1. Brown, J.E. *Nutrition through the Life Cycle*, 8th ed.; Cengage Learning: Boston, MA, USA, 2019.
2. Vadeboncoeur, C.; Foster, C.; Townsend, N. Freshman 15 in England: A longitudinal evaluation of first year university student's weight change. *BMC Obes.* **2016**, *3*, 45. [CrossRef] [PubMed]
3. Mihalopoulos, N.L.; Auinger, P.; Klein, J.D. The Freshman 15: Is it real? *J. Am. Coll. Health* **2010**, *56*, 531–534. [CrossRef] [PubMed]
4. Mortas, H.; Navruz-Varlı, S.; Bilici, S. Adherence to the Planetary Health Diet and its association with diet quality in the young adult population of Türkiye: A large cross-sectional study. *Nutrients* **2024**, *16*, 868. [CrossRef] [PubMed]
5. Yüksek Öğretim Kurumu (YÖK). Mezuniyet Öncesi Beslenme ve Diyetetik Eğitimi Ulusal Çekirdek Eğitim Programı-2016. Available online: https://www.yok.gov.tr/Documents/Kurumsal/egitim_ogretim_dairesi/Ulusal-cekirdek-egitimi-programlari/beslenme_ve_diyetetik.pdf (accessed on 14 April 2024).
6. Navruz Varlı, S.; Bilici, S. Do the sociodemographic factors and body mass index have an impact on food safety knowledge, attitudes and practices? *Tekirdağ Ziraat Fak. Derg.* **2022**, *19*, 496–507. [CrossRef]
7. Helbach, A.; Dumm, M.; Moll, K.; Böttrich, T.; Leineweber, C.G.; Mueller, W.; Matthes, J.; Polidori, M.C. Improvement of dietary habits among German medical students by attending a nationwide online lecture series on nutrition and Planetary Health ("Eat This!"). *Nutrients* **2023**, *15*, 580. [CrossRef] [PubMed]
8. Bertoluci, G.; Masset, G.; Gomy, C.; Mottet, J.; Darmon, N. How to build a standardized country-specific environmental food database for nutritional epidemiology studies. *PLoS ONE* **2016**, *11*, e0150617. [CrossRef] [PubMed]
9. Schröder, H.; Serra-Majem, L.; Subirana, I.; Izquierdo-Pulido, M.; Fitó, M.; Elosua, R. Association of increased monetary cost of dietary intake, diet quality and weight management in Spanish adults. *Br. J. Nutr.* **2016**, *115*, 817–822. [CrossRef]
10. Macit-Çelebi, M.S.; Bozkurt, O.; Kocaadam-Bozkurt, B.; Köksal, E. Evaluation of sustainable and healthy eating behaviors and adherence to the planetary health diet index in Turkish adults: A cross-sectional study. *Front. Nutr.* **2023**, *10*, 1180880. [CrossRef]
11. Cacau, L.T.; Benseñor, I.M.; Goulart, A.C.; Cardoso, L.O.; Lotufo, P.A.; Moreno, L.A.; Marchioni, D.M. Adherence to the planetary health diet index and obesity indicators in the Brazilian longitudinal study of adult health (ELSA-Brasil). *Nutrients* **2021**, *13*, 3691. [CrossRef]
12. Cacau, L.T.; De Carli, E.; de Carvalho, A.M.; Lotufo, P.A.; Moreno, L.A.; Bensenor, I.M.; Marchioni, D.M. Development and validation of an index based on EAT-Lancet recommendations: The Planetary Health Diet Index. *Nutrients* **2021**, *13*, 1698. [CrossRef]
13. Marchioni, D.M.; Cacau, L.T.; De Carli, E.; de Carvalho, A.M.; Rulli, M.C. Low adherence to the EAT-Lancet sustainable reference diet in the Brazilian population: Findings from the national dietary survey 2017–2018. *Nutrients* **2022**, *14*, 1187. [CrossRef] [PubMed]
14. Willett, W.; Rockström, J.; Loken, B.; Springmann, M.; Lang, T.; Vermeulen, S.; Garnett, T.; Tilman, D.; DeClerck, F.; Wood, A.; et al. Food in the Anthropocene: The EAT–Lancet Commission on healthy diets from sustainable food systems. *Lancet* **2019**, *393*, 447–492. [CrossRef]
15. Food and Agriculture Organization of the United Nations. *Dietary Guidelines and Sustainability*; FAO: Rome, Italy, 2019; Available online: http://www.fao.org/nutrition/education/food-dietary-guidelines/background/sustainable-dietaryguidelines/ (accessed on 29 February 2024).
16. United Nations. *Department of Economic and Social Affairs, Population Division*; United Nations: New York, NY, USA, 2019.
17. Frank, S.M.; Jaacks, L.M.; Avery, C.L.; Adair, L.S.; Meyer, K.; Rose, D.; Taillie, L.S. Dietary quality and cardiometabolic indicators in the USA: A comparison of the Planetary Health Diet Index, Healthy Eating Index-2015, and Dietary Approaches to Stop Hypertension. *PLoS ONE* **2024**, *19*, e0296069. [CrossRef] [PubMed]

18. Krebs-Smith, S.M.; Pannucci, T.E.; Subar, A.F.; Kirkpatrick, S.I.; Lerman, J.L.; Tooze, J.A.; Wilson, M.M.; Reedy, J. Update of the healthy eating index: HEI-2015. *J. Acad. Nutr. Diet.* **2018**, *118*, 1591–1602. [CrossRef]
19. Standen, E.C.; Finch, L.E.; Tiongco-Hofschneider, L.; Schopp, E.; Lee, K.M.; Parker, J.E.; Bamishigbin, O.N.; Tomiyama, A.J. Healthy versus unhealthy comfort eating for psychophysiological stress recovery in low-income Black and Latinx adults. *Appetite* **2022**, *176*, 106140. [CrossRef]
20. Liu, J.; Micha, R.; Li, Y.; Mozaffarian, D. Trends in food sources and diet quality among US children and adults, 2003–2018. *JAMA Netw. Open* **2021**, *4*, e215262. [CrossRef]
21. Liu, L.; Xie, T.; Hu, Z.; Liu, J. Association between healthy eating index-2015 and abdominal aortic calcification: A population-based cross-sectional study. *Prev. Med. Rep.* **2023**, *36*, 102421. [CrossRef] [PubMed]
22. Ramón-Arbués, E.; Granada-López, J.M.; Martínez-Abadía, B.; Echániz-Serrano, E.; Antón-Solanas, I.; Jerue, B.A. Factors related to diet quality: A cross-sectional study of 1055 university students. *Nutrients* **2021**, *13*, 3512. [CrossRef]
23. WHO. Fact Sheets. A Healthy Lifestyle-WHO Recommendations. 2010. Available online: https://www.who.int/europe/news-room/fact-sheets/item/a-healthy-lifestyle---who-recommendations (accessed on 6 March 2024).
24. Merdol, T. *Standart Yemek Tarifeleri*, 4th ed.; Hatipoğlu Yayınları: Ankara, Türkiye, 2011.
25. Frank, S.M.; Jaacks, L.M.; Adair, L.S.; Avery, C.L.; Meyer, K.; Rose, D.; Taillie, L.S. Adherence to the Planetary Health Diet Index and correlation with nutrients of public health concern: An analysis of NHANES 2003–2018. *Am. J. Clin. Nutr.* **2024**, *119*, 384–392. [CrossRef]
26. Semba, R.D.; de Pee, S.; Kim, B.; McKenzie, S.; Nachman, K.; Bloem, M.W. Adoption of the 'planetary health diet' has different impacts on countries' greenhouse gas emissions. *Nat. Food* **2020**, *1*, 481–484. [CrossRef]
27. Scott, P. *Global Panel on Agriculture and Food Systems for Nutrition: Food Systems and Diets: Facing the Challenges of the 21st Century*; Springer: London, UK, 2016; p. 132. Available online: http://glopan.org/sites/default/files/ForesightReport.pdf (accessed on 10 March 2024)ISBN 978-0-9956228-0-7.
28. Sautron, V.; Péneau, S.; Camilleri, G.M.; Muller, L.; Ruffieux, B.; Hercberg, S.; Méjean, C. Validity of a questionnaire measuring motives for choosing foods including sustainable concerns. *Appetite* **2015**, *87*, 90–97. [CrossRef]
29. Goulding, T.; Lindberg, R.; Russell, C.G. The affordability of a healthy and sustainable diet: An Australian case study. *Nutr. J.* **2020**, *19*, 109. [CrossRef]
30. Pearson, D.; Friel, S.; Lawrence, M. Building environmentally sustainable food systems on informed citizen choices: Evidence from Australia. *Biol. Agric. Hortic.* **2014**, *30*, 183–197. [CrossRef]
31. Allès, B.; Péneau, S.; Kesse-Guyot, E.; Baudry, J.; Hercberg, S.; Mejean, C. Food choice motives including sustainability during purchasing are associated with a healthy dietary pattern in French adults. *Nutr. J.* **2017**, *16*, 58. [CrossRef] [PubMed]
32. Benedetti, I.; Laureti, T.; Secondi, L. Choosing a healthy and sustainable diet: A three-level approach for understanding the drivers of the Italians' dietary regime over time. *Appetite* **2018**, *123*, 357–366. [CrossRef] [PubMed]
33. Macdiarmid, J.I.; Kyle, J.; Horgan, G.W.; Loe, J.; Fyfe, C.; Johnstone, A.; McNeill, G. Sustainable diets for the future: Can we contribute to reducing greenhouse gas emissions by eating a healthy diet? *Am. J. Clin. Nutr.* **2012**, *96*, 632–639. [CrossRef]
34. Reynolds, C.J.; Horgan, G.W.; Whybrow, S.; Macdiarmid, J.I. Healthy and sustainable diets that meet greenhouse gas emission reduction targets and are affordable for different income groups in the UK. *Public Health Nutr.* **2019**, *22*, 1503–1517. [CrossRef]
35. Barosh, L.; Friel, S.; Engelhardt, K.; Chan, L. The cost of a healthy and sustainable diet–who can afford it? *Aust. N. Z. J. Public Health* **2014**, *38*, 7–12. [CrossRef] [PubMed]
36. Hirvonen, K.; Bai, Y.; Headey, D.; Masters, W.A. Affordability of the EAT–Lancet reference diet: A global analysis. *Lancet Glob. Health* **2020**, *8*, e59–e66. [CrossRef]
37. Cacau, L.T.; Hanley-Cook, G.T.; Huybrechts, I.; De Henauw, S.; Kersting, M.; Gonzalez-Gross, M.; Gottrand, F.; Ferrari, M.; Nova, E.; Castillo, M.J.; et al. Relative validity of the Planetary Health Diet Index by comparison with usual nutrient intakes, plasma food consumption biomarkers, and adherence to the Mediterranean diet among European adolescents: The HELENA study. *Eur. J. Nutr.* **2023**, *62*, 2527–2539. [CrossRef]
38. Alcorta, A.; Porta, A.; Tárrega, A.; Alvarez, M.D.; Vaquero, M.P. Foods for plant-based diets: Challenges and innovations. *Foods* **2021**, *10*, 293. [CrossRef] [PubMed]
39. Zeng, L.; Ruan, M.; Liu, J.; Wilde, P.; Naumova, E.N.; Mozaffarian, D.; Zhang, F.F. Trends in processed meat, unprocessed red meat, poultry, and fish consumption in the United States, 1999–2016. *J. Acad. Nutr. Diet.* **2019**, *119*, 1085–1098. [CrossRef] [PubMed]

Disclaimer/Publisher's Note: The statements, opinions and data contained in all publications are solely those of the individual author(s) and contributor(s) and not of MDPI and/or the editor(s). MDPI and/or the editor(s) disclaim responsibility for any injury to people or property resulting from any ideas, methods, instructions or products referred to in the content.

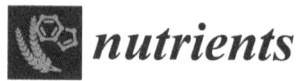

Article

Bariatric Surgery: An Opportunity to Improve Quality of Life and Healthy Habits

Beatriz Vanessa Díaz-González [1,2], Inmaculada Bautista-Castaño [2,3,*], Elisabeth Hernández García [2], Judith Cornejo Torre [2], Juan Ramón Hernández Hernández [2,4] and Lluis Serra-Majem [2,3,4]

1. Triana Primary Health Care Center, Canarian Health Service, 35002 Las Palmas de Gran Canaria, Spain; beatrizvanessa@gmail.com
2. Research Institute of Biomedical and Health Sciences (IUIBS), University of Las Palmas de Gran Canaria, 35016 Las Palmas de Gran Canaria, Spain; elisabethernandez924@gmail.com (E.H.G.); judith.cornejo.dn@gmail.com (J.C.T.); jurahh@yahoo.es (J.R.H.H.); lluis.serra@ulpgc.es (L.S.-M.)
3. Centro de Investigación Biomédica en Red Fisiopatología de la Obesidad y la Nutrición (CIBEROBN), Instituto de Salud Carlos III, 28029 Madrid, Spain
4. Centro Hospitalario Universitario Insular Materno Infantil (CHUIMI), Canarian Health Service, 35016 Las Palmas de Gran Canaria, Spain
* Correspondence: inmaculada.bautista@ulpgc.es

Citation: Díaz-González, B.V.; Bautista-Castaño, I.; Hernández García, E.; Cornejo Torre, J.; Hernández Hernández, J.R.; Serra-Majem, L. Bariatric Surgery: An Opportunity to Improve Quality of Life and Healthy Habits. *Nutrients* 2024, *16*, 1466. https://doi.org/10.3390/nu16101466

Academic Editor: Andras Hajnal

Received: 3 April 2024
Revised: 3 May 2024
Accepted: 8 May 2024
Published: 13 May 2024

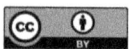

Copyright: © 2024 by the authors. Licensee MDPI, Basel, Switzerland. This article is an open access article distributed under the terms and conditions of the Creative Commons Attribution (CC BY) license (https://creativecommons.org/licenses/by/4.0/).

Abstract: Bariatric surgery therapy (BST) is an effective treatment for obesity; however, little is known about its impacts on health-related quality of life (HRQoL) and related factors. This study aimed to evaluate changes in HRQoL and its relationship with weight loss, depression status, physical activity (PA), and nutritional habits after BST. Data were obtained before and 18 months postprocedure from 56 obese patients who underwent BST. We administered four questionnaires: Short Form-36 health survey for HRQoL, 14-item MedDiet adherence questionnaire, Rapid Assessment of PA (RAPA) questionnaire, and Beck's Depression Inventory-II. Multivariable linear regression analysis was used to identify factors associated with improvement in HRQoL. After the surgery, MedDiet adherence and HRQoL improved significantly, especially in the physical component. No changes in PA were found. Patients without previous depression have better mental quality of life, and patients who lost more than 25% of %TBWL have better results in physical and mental quality of life. In the multivariable analysis, we found that %TBWL and initial PCS (inversely) were related to the improvement in PCS and initial MCS (inversely) with the MCS change. In conclusion, BST is an effective intervention for obesity, resulting in significant weight loss and improvements in HRQoL and nutritional habits.

Keywords: morbid obesity; bariatric surgery; Mediterranean diet; health-related quality of life; physical activity; depression

1. Introduction

Obesity, defined as a body mass index (BMI) ≥ 30 kg/m^2, is a significant public health problem, with its worldwide prevalence growing considerably, tripling between 1975 and 2016 [1]. It is recognized as a disease by the American Medical Association [2], the World Health Organization [1], and the World Obesity Federation [3], and it is a predisposing factor for various pathologies, such as type 2 diabetes mellitus, hypertension, cardiovascular diseases, different cancers, and premature death [4,5].

Severe or morbid obesity, defined as a BMI > 40 (obesity class III), presents a significant therapeutic challenge, as nutritional and pharmacological interventions often prove ineffective in the long term [6].

BST emerges as the most effective treatment option, demonstrating favorable outcomes in terms of weight loss and sustained maintenance [7]. The two most common procedures used currently, the sleeve gastrectomy and gastric bypass, have similar effects on weight loss and diabetes outcomes and similar safety through at least 5-year follow-up. However, emerging evidence suggests that the sleeve procedure is associated with fewer reoperations, and the bypass procedure may lead to more durable weight loss and glycemic control. Different types of bariatric surgery have distinct auxiliary and adverse effects, emphasizing the importance of individualized selection of procedures and risk–benefit conversations for each patient considering bariatric surgery [8,9].

The current data indicate that the perioperative mortality rates of BST range from 0.03% to 0.2%, which has substantially improved since the early 2000s [8,9]. A recent review of 66 health outcomes of bariatric surgery has shown that 56 outcomes were health benefits, including new-onset of diabetes, dyslipidemia, cardiovascular diseases, hypertension, cancers, women's health, and reductions in all-cause mortality and 10 were adverse outcomes, including suicide, fracture, gastroesophageal reflux after sleeve gastrectomy, and neonatal morbidities, but none of the adverse outcomes reached a high level of evidence, warranting the need for further investigation.

In addition to the several pathologies mentioned above, obesity is associated with deterioration in the perceived quality of life, especially its physical component score [10–13]. Mobility problems, reduced self-care, a decreased ability to carry out daily activities, pain, and discomfort are some of the problems suffered by people with obesity. Some characteristics of this pathology prevent patients from making the changes to vital habits that are necessary to promote and maintain a good quality of life, and this is the reason why another widely used outcome measure in obesity treatment is the quality of life and changes thereof [14].

Improvements in health-related quality of life (HRQoL) obtained by weight loss have been reported after BST [15], bariatric endoscopy treatment [16], or conventional treatment of obesity [17]. The impact of bariatric surgery on HRQoL is less well-understood than its clinical effectiveness in terms of weight and comorbidities. Some studies suggest that the physical aspects of HRQoL may improve more than the mental health aspects of HRQoL after bariatric surgery. Due to psychological predispositions, some patients appear to be less likely to benefit from bariatric treatment, whether in terms of HRQOL [10,11].

Moreover obesity is associated with deteriorated quality of life, and there exists a well-known bidirectional relationship between obesity and depression [18,19]. When analyzing various levels of obesity (class I: BMI > 30–<34.9, class II: BMI >35–<39.9, class III: BMI > 40), it seems that the degree of obesity consistently correlates with an increased risk of depression [20,21]. The early identification of such patients and providing them with psychological intervention would likely further improve the outcomes of bariatric treatment.

During the BST follow-up, it is very important to make changes to nutritional and PA habits to improve health and maintain a healthy weight. Regarding nutritional habits, the Mediterranean diet (MedDiet) is suggested as a healthy dietary pattern, consistently demonstrating a positive impact on health and longevity. The MedDiet includes lots of healthy foods like olive oil as the main culinary fat, whole grains, fruits, vegetables, fish, seafood, beans, and nuts, and a low intake of red meat and sweets [22,23].

Several studies have indicated that the MedDiet is not only a preventive measure against cardiovascular and other diseases but could also be highly effective in terms of weight loss, particularly when combined with energy restriction and increased PA [23,24]. Different studies, like the SUN project [25] and the Predimed plus study [26], have shown that in addition to the benefits of cardiovascular risk, higher adherence to the MedDiet pattern is associated with better HRQoL.

Furthermore, PA is recommended as a key component of weight management for preventing weight gain, promoting weight loss, and preventing weight regain after weight loss. PA also yields other positive effects on various health indicators, including overall mortality, cardiovascular disease mortality, incident hypertension, incident type 2 diabetes, incident site-specific cancers, mental health (such as reduced symptoms of anxiety and depression), cognitive health, and sleep [6,7].

Several studies have observed an improvement in quality of life after BST [10–12]; however, there is a lack of studies on factors related to previous depression status, eating habits, or PA that influence changes in quality of life post-BST.

This study aimed to evaluate other factors, different from weight loss, that could influence the improvement of HRQoL post-BST.

2. Material and Methods

2.1. Study Design

We conducted a prospective study involving 56 consecutive patients who underwent BST at Vithas Santa Catalina Hospital in Las Palmas, Spain, between April and July 2015. The BST was offered by the public health service.

Participants were provided with four questionnaires: (a) the SF-36 survey (Spanish version) to measure HRQoL, (b) a 14-item questionnaire assessing adherence to the MedDiet, (c) the Rapid Assessment of Physical Activity (RAPA) questionnaire to measure PA, and (d) Beck's Depression Inventory (BDI) to assess the depression status. The trial was approved by the Institutional Review Board of the CEIC del Hospital Universitario Insular de Gran Canaria (HUIGC).

2.2. Participants

We invited 56 obese patients who were referred for BST after a failed diet and lifestyle intervention to participate in the study. All agreed to take part and answered the questionnaires at baseline and 18 months postprocedure. We delivered the questionnaires during the regular follow-up visit.

The weight, height, and body composition were recorded using the Tanita BC-420MA III, Barcelona, Spain, before the intervention and during the follow-up visits. We reported weight loss outcomes as %total body weight loss (%TBWL).

2.3. Intervention

Regarding the type of procedure, 64.3% (n = 36) underwent restrictive techniques and 35.7% (n = 20) malabsorptive techniques. After the surgery, patients were regularly monitored by both the surgeon and endocrinologist, who provided guidance to enhance physical activity and adhere to a low-calorie Mediterranean diet.

2.4. Questionnaires

At baseline and 18 months after the BST, the patients complete different questionnaires in a face-to-face interview with the research team. All the questionnaires used in the present study had enough reliability and validity and were validated in the European Spanish population (Beck questionnaire for depression [27], RAPA questionnaire for physical activity [28], and SF36 for HRQoL were validated for the Spanish population [29]. The Mediterranean Diet adherence test has also been adequately validated and used in important studies such as the PrediMed study [30].

2.4.1. Short Form Survey-36 (SF-36)

The SF-36 is a well-validated questionnaire for the Spanish population that measures the patients' self-reported opinions on their physical and mental well-being. It has eight domains of HRQoL: general health, physical functioning, role limitations due to physical health, body pain (functional status), energy/vitality, emotional well-being, role limitations due to emotional problems, and social functioning (emotional status). Responses to each question within a domain are combined to generate a score from 0 to 100, where 100 indicates "good health". The domains are calibrated and transformed into the physical component summary (PCS) and mental component summary (MCS), respectively. The SF-36 also includes a global health transition question (HTQ) that asks respondents to rate their general health compared with 12 months ago. We compared the results with the reference Spanish population SF-36 outcomes for the study by Lopez Garcia et al., who prospectively evaluated the HRQoL in 6207 Caucasian noninstitutionalized individuals aged > 18 years from Spain [31].

2.4.2. Fourteen-Item Questionnaires That Assessed Adherence to a MedDiet

The adherence to the MedDiet was assessed using the 14-item MedDiet Adherence Screener (MEDAS), a validated questionnaire, which consisted of 2 questions on dietary habits and 12 questions on food consumption frequency characterizing the MedDiet pattern. Each question was scored 0 or 1. A value of 0 was assigned when the condition was not met. The total score ranged from 0 to 14. The adherence level is determined by adding the values obtained from the 14 items. Three levels are established: (a) a total score ≥ 10 indicates high adherence, (b) a score between 7 and 9 (inclusive) indicates a medium adherence level, and (c) a total sum ≥ 6 suggests low adherence to the MedDiet. To simplify the analysis, the results were recoded into two groups: (a) low adherence < 6 and (b) medium–high adherence ≥ 6 points [30].

2.4.3. Rapid Assessment of Physical Activity (RAPA) Questionnaire

To measure the level of PA, the Rapid Assessment of PA Scale (RAPA) [32] questionnaire was used. This particular test was selected due to its simplicity and ease of performance. RAPA is divided into two categories: RAPA 1, which determines the level of PA: (a) sedentary ('I rarely or never do any physical activities'); (b) little active ('I do some light or moderate PA, but no every week' or 'I do some light PA every week'); (c) moderately active ('I do moderate PA every week, but less than 30 min a day or 5 days a week' or 'I do vigorous physical activities every week, but less than 20 min a day or 3 days a week'); and (d) active ('I do 30 min or more a day of moderate PA, 5 or more days a week' or 'I do 20 min or more a day of vigorous PA, 3 or more days a week'). RAPA 2, which assesses the type of exercise: (a) no muscle strength and flexibility activities; (b) muscle strength activities ('I do activities to increase muscle strength, such as lifting weights or calisthenics, once a week or more'; (c) flexibility activities ('I do activities to improve flexibility, such as stretching or yoga, once a week or more'); or (d) both muscle strength and flexibility activities). For further analysis, participants were divided into two groups according to their RAPA 1 score: "inactive" ("sedentary" + "minimal active") (score 1–3) and "active" ("moderate active" + "active") (score 4–7).

2.4.4. Beck's Depression Inventory-II

The depression level was analyzed with the Beck's Depression Inventory-II (BDI-II) [33]. It is a 21-question (multiple choice) self-report inventory created to provide a quantitative assessment of the severity of depression considering the DSM-IV criteria for diagnosing depressive disorders and includes items measuring cognitive, affective, somatic, and vegetative symptoms of depression. The score scale ranges from 0 to 3 for each question; higher scores indicate more depressive symptoms. Scores of 0–13 are considered to indicate none or minimal depression, 14–19 mild depression, 20–28 moderate depression, and $\geq$29–63 severe depression. For the purpose of the present study, this variable was simplified as none or minimal depression (scores 0–13) and mild–severe depression (scores ≥ 14).

2.5. Outcomes

This study aimed to evaluate changes in HRQoL and its relationship with weight loss, depression status, PA, and nutritional habits after BST.

2.6. Statistical Methods

We expressed continuous variables as mean and measures of dispersion (standard deviation; SD). We reported categorical variables as a percentage. For analysis, we categorized the variables based on (a) gender (male/female), (b) age (≤ 43 or >43 years), (c) initial BMI (<40 or ≥ 40 kg/m^2), (d) procedure type (restrictive or malabsorptive techniques), (e)

PA status (inactive or minimally active/active), (f) MedDiet adherence level (low adherence ≤ 6 and medium–high adherence > 6 points), (g) depression status (none or minimal and mild–severe), and (h) %TBWL (≤25% vs. 25.1–39.9% vs. ≥40%). Bivariate analyses of proportionality of distribution of categorical variables Chi-square test (χ^2). For continuous variables, we used the Kolmogorov–Smirnov test to check that the variables were normally distributed. For comparisons of normally distributed variables, we used the T-Student test or ANOVA. For comparisons of non-normally distributed variables, we used the Mann–Whitney or Kruskal–Wallis tests.

We performed multivariable regression analysis to study the relationship between changes in PSC and MSC scores as dependent variables and age, gender, %TBWL, changes in PA, depression status, and initial summary component values as independent variables.

We performed statistical analysis using IBM SPSS Software 23.0. $p < 0.05$ was considered significant.

3. Results

3.1. Participants Characteristics

The baseline characteristics of the 56 patients are detailed in Table 1. The mean age was 43.8 ± 13.1 years (range 20–69), and most of them were female (n = 41, 73.2%) and with BMI ≥ 40 kg/m² (n = 48, 85.7%).

Table 1. Characteristics of study participants at baseline.

Variables	Patients (n = 56)
Ages years (mean (SD))	43.8 (13.1)
Age groups ≤43 years (n (%)) >43 years (n (%))	29 (51.8%) 27 (48.2%)
Female	41 (73.2%)
Initial weight kg (mean (SD))	128.9 (23.5)
Initial BMI kg/m² (mean (SD))	47.7 (6.4)
Initial BMI group 35–39.9 (n (%)) ≥40 (n (%))	8 (14.3%) 48 (85.7%)

3.2. Weight Loss Outcomes

Regarding the variation in weight parameters, the mean weight loss was 45.2 ± 20.7 kg, the BMI loss was 16.8 ± 7.1 units, and the mean %TBWL was 34.4 ± 13.3. In relation to the surgical technique, a significantly greater weight loss was observed in the malabsorptive compared with restrictive techniques: 54.8 vs. 39.9 kg of weight loss, 19.9 vs. 15.1 units of BMI loss, and 39.6 vs. 31.6% of %TBWL. No significant differences were found by sex with respect to weight loss. By age group, those younger than 43 years lost more weight than those older (50.7 vs. 39.4 kg $p = 0.41$). Finally, in relation to %TBWL, 13 patients (23.2%) lost ≤ 25%, 20 (37.5%) between 25 and 40%, and 21 patients (39.3%) lost ≥ 40%.

3.3. Changes in MedDiet Adherence

After the surgery, the mean score improved significantly from 6.32 (1.9) to 7.62 (1.8) ($p < 0.001$). We did not find any significant relationship between the improvement in MedDiet adherence with gender, surgery procedures, or age group.

Considering the level of adherence, at baseline, 60.4% had low, 35.8% medium, and 3.8% had high levels of adherence to the MedDiet. Postintervention, 32.1% had low, 60.4% medium, and 7.5% high adherence to the MedDiet.

Table 2 shows the changes in the MedDiet group adherence prior to and after the intervention. Most of half the patients with low levels of adherence improve their adherence to a medium–high level ($p = 0.04$).

Table 2. Changes in MedDiet adherence, physical activity, and depression after bariatric surgery.

Variable	Preprocedure	Postprocedure	p
MedDiet adherence group (n (%))			
Low	32 (60.4)	17 (32.1%)	
Medium	19 (35.8)	32 (60.4%)	0.04
High	2 (3.8)	4 (7.5%)	
Physical activity level aerobic			
Inactive	43 (79.6)	24 (44.5)	NS
Active	11 (20.4)	30 (55.5)	
Physical activity level anaerobic			
None	51 (94.4)	45 (84.9)	
Muscle strength	3 (5.6)	6 (11.3)	NS
Flexibility	0	2 (3.8)	
Depression			
Minimal	36 (67.9)	38 (71.7)	NS
Mild–severe	17 (32.1)	15 (28.3)	

3.4. Changes in Physical Activity

Considering the level of PA, for practical purposes, the 54 patients who answered the questionnaire were segregated into two groups: inactive and active. Although the difference was not significant ($p = 0.09$), before the surgery, 79.6% were inactive, and postintervention, only 44.5%. There was also a low improvement in the practice of muscle strength and flexibility exercises.

3.5. Changes in Depression

The Beck questionnaire results showed that pre- and postprocedure depression status was very similar, with less percentage of none or minimal depression status postprocedure (Table 2).

3.6. Changes in HRQoL

The mean baseline PSC score was 51.5 (range 9.5–96.9), and the MSC score was 64.3 (range 1.43–98.6). After the intervention, we found a significant improvement in the PSC score (76.8 vs. 51.5), but we did not find a significant difference in the MSC score. We observed a significant improvement in most of the domains except body pain, social function, emotional role, and mental health domain of the HRQoL. The domains that demonstrated the greatest and most significant improvement were physical function, physical role, vitality, overall health, and health transition (Figure 1 and Table 3).

If we compared the score values of the obese patients with the Spanish population values (Table 3), all of the domains were lower prior to the intervention. Postprocedure, overall health was higher, and physical function and vitality were very similar. The emotional status, except vitality, continues with lower values than the Spanish population's mean values.

When stratified by the baseline characteristics of the PSC and MSC scores, we observed higher PSC initial levels in patients with younger ages (<43 years) and no or minimal depression. The baseline MSC score was better in patients with no or minimal depression. The final MSC score was better in patients with %TBWL 25–40% and in patients with low or minimal depression.

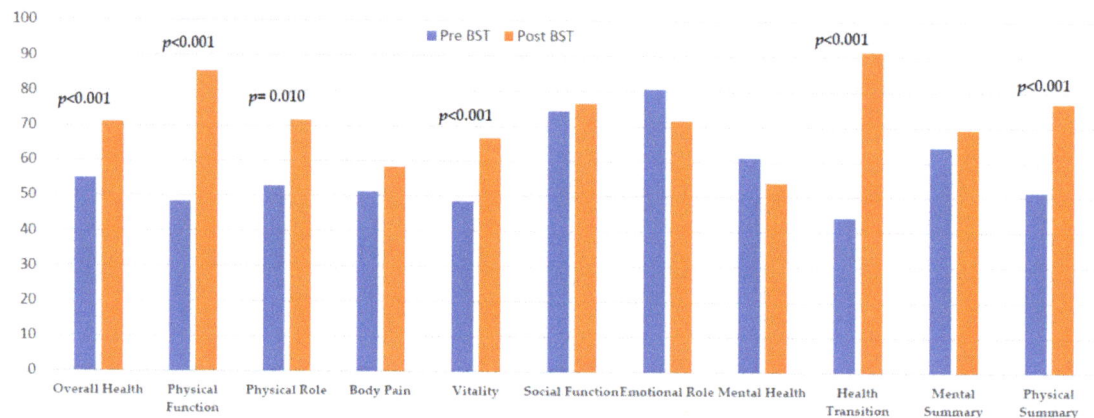

Figure 1. Variation in mean values of SF-36 Health Status components in subjects undergoing bariatric surgery.

Table 3. Variation in mean values of SF-36 Health Status components in a subject undergoing bariatric surgery. Comparison with population values [29].

SF-36 Domains		Spanish Population Mean	Preprocedure Mean	Postprocedure Mean	Mean Difference	p
Functional Status	Overall health	58.3	55.0	71.1	14.2	<0.001
	Physical function	84.7	48.4	85.5	37.3	<0.001
	Physical role	83.2	52.8	71.6	18.6	0.010
	Body pain	79.0	51.2	58.3	7.5	NS
Emotional Status	Vitality	66.9	48.6	66.6	17.3	<0.001
	Social function	90.1	74.5	76.6	0.98	NS
	Emotional role	86.6	80.7	71.7	−7.1	NS
	Mental health	73.3	61.2	54.0	−6.8	0.051
Health transition		---	44.2	91.3	52.4	<0.001
MCS (mental component summary)			64.3	69.3	5.8	NS
PCS (physical component summary)			51.5	76.8	25.1	<0.001

In relation to changes in physical and mental summary scores, we noticed significantly higher PSC score change in those patients who achieved greater %TBWL (>25%). The change in MSC score only results in significance in older patients (≥43 years) and previously inactive patients (Table 4).

We did not find any significative difference in relation to changes in PSC and MSC scores and depression levels, but in the MSC change, the high depression group had better improvement (Table 4).

Table 4. Baseline, final, and variations in physical and mental scores of SF-36 according to selected variables in subjects undergoing bariatric surgery.

	Physical Summary Component (Mean)			Mental Summary Component (Mean)		
	Baseline	Follow-Up	Δ Change	Baseline	Follow-Up	Δ Change
Age						
<43 years	59.6	78.1	18.1	68.9	66	−0.82
≥43 years	42.7	75.6	33.1	59.3	73	13.8
p-value	0.010	NS	NS	NS	NS	0.045

Table 4. Cont.

	Physical Summary Component (Mean)			Mental Summary Component (Mean)		
	Baseline	Follow-Up	Δ Change	Baseline	Follow-Up	Δ Change
Gender						
Male	61.1	79.2	17.4	68	69.3	1.2
Female	48.1	76.1	27.9	63.1	69.4	7.6
p-value	NS	NS	NS	NS	NS	NS
Initial BMI						
<40 kg/m^2	57.4	64.8	7.3	70.1	60.7	−1.3
≥40 kg/m^2	50.5	78.8	28.0	63.6	70.7	6.9
p-value	NS	NS	NS	NS	NS	NS
%TBWL						
≤25	56.1	62.2	6.1	56.6	57.9	1.3
25.1–39.9	53.3	84.0	30.8	68.4	83.0	16.5
≥40	47.4	77.8	30.3	65.2	62.3	−0.7
p-value	NS	0.011	0.020	NS	0.001	NS
Procedure Type						
Restrictive	54.5	78.6	25.8	66.4	72.6	8.4
Malabsortive	49.7	73.8	23.8	60.1	63.4	1.3
p-value	NS	NS	NS	NS	NS	NS
Mediterranean Diet Adherence n (%)						
Low	52.6	77.6	24.2	62.1	69.1	9.0
Medium–High	50.1	75.9	26.4	67.7	69.9	1.1
p-value	NS	NS	NS	NS	NS	NS
Baseline RAPA Aerobic activities n (%)						
Inactive	48.9	77.4	28.1	62.7	71.7	10.2
Active	61.7	75.0	13.1	70.9	60.8	−10.6
p-value	NS	NS	NS	NS	NS	0.019
Depression (Beck)						
None or Minimal	58.9	79.5	20.3	73.7	75.0	1.35
Mild–Severe	36.9	70.3	35.0	45.1	57.0	15.8
p-value	0.001	NS	NS	<0.001	0.041	NS

3.7. Predictive Factors for Improvement in PSC and MSC

In the linear regression analysis, considering the change in the PSC as the dependent variable and the %TBWL, age and sex, initial PSC, and depression status as independent variables, we found that the %TBWL was significantly related to the improvement in the PSC ($p < 0.015$) and the initial PSC was inversely related to this improvement (baseline $p < 0.001$). In the case of the mental summary, considering the change in the MSC as the dependent variable and the %TBWL, age and sex, initial MSC, and depression status as independent variables, we found that the change in this summary was only inversely associated with the initial mental summary ($p < 0.001$) (Table 5).

Table 5. Factors associated with improvement in physical and mental summary components of SF-36 (multivariable linear regression analysis).

Variable	Physical HRQoL (PSC Change)	95% CI	p-Value
	Coefficient β		
%TBWL	0.313	0.126 to 1.151	0.015
Sex	0.043	−10.574 to 15.866	0.689
Age	0.009	−0.565 to 0.602	0.949
Initial PSC score	−0.697	−1.144 to 0.447	0.000

Table 5. *Cont.*

Variable	Physical HRQoL (PSC Change) Coefficient β	95% CI	*p*-Value
Initial Depression	−0.167	−23.397 to 4267	0.170
Variable	Mental HRQoL (MSC change) Coefficient β	95% CI	*p*-value
%TBWL	0.106	−0.359 to 0.751	0.480
Sex	−0.043	−17.804 to 11.985	0.737
Age	0.114	−0.315 to 0.758	0.409
Initial MSC score	−0.677	−1.135 to −0.382	0.000
Initial Depression	−0.191	−29,249 to 8.566	0.246

HRQoL = health-related quality of life; SF-36 = Short Form-36 health survey for HRQoL; PSC = physical component summary; MSC: mental component summary; %TBWL = %total body weight loss.

4. Discussion

The current study demonstrates that following BST, adherence to the MedDiet and HRQoL significantly improved, particularly in the physical component. Additionally, patients without a history of depression and those who achieved a weight loss exceeding 25% of total body weight loss (%TBWL) experienced notably better outcomes in both physical and mental quality of life. However, we did not observe significant changes in PA [34–36].

Regarding HRQoL in the obese population, some authors have found that obesity has negative impacts, particularly affecting physical domains (e.g., physical function, body pain, overall health) and the physical component summary (PCS) of the SF-36 [12,37]. Poor emotional well-being among the obese may be attributed to comorbidity rather than obesity per se [38]. If we compare the initial HRQoL with the general population, our results confirm that the obese population perceives they have a worse quality of life than the non-obese population [31].

BST has consistently demonstrated long-term significant weight loss and a notable improvement in medical comorbidities [39]. Additionally it has been associated with lower rates and fewer symptoms of various mental health conditions, particularly depression, which improved following the intervention [40–42]. However, we did not find improvement in depression levels at 18 months in the present study, which remained similar to the baseline. On the other side, our study aligns with some studies that found higher preoperative depression severity as a predictor of poorer improvement in quality of life change after BST [43,44]. However, different authors have not found clear evidence that preoperative mental health conditions are associated with differential weight loss after surgery [35,45]. In fact, some studies reported that preoperative psychopathology predicted post-operative psychopathology but not weight loss at 2 years [40,46].

Considering the often inversely proportional relationship between weight and self-perceived health [38], weight loss obtained by the BST should improve quality of life. Several authors have suggested a linear correlation between weight changes and HRQoL [47,48]. Studies evaluating HRQoL after BST have demonstrated a favorable change in both physical and mental health at 3 and 6 years and an improvement in PA [49,50]. However, when weight loss is moderate, different authors have not shown improvement in the domains of the SF-36 [51].

Regarding BST, most published trials have found an improvement in HRQoL in physical and mental summary components (SF-36) [51,52]. We found that the best changes in PSC were obtained with better results in weight loss, especially in patients with more than 25% of %total body weight loss (%TBWL). This replicates the findings from Kolotkinn et al., who also found that after a weight loss of 34.2% after gastric bypass surgery, patients experienced significant improvement in HRQoL [53]. Other studies obtained the same results [54].

The mental component summary (MSC), however, did not improve with the intervention, but older and inactive patients prior to the intervention exhibited better positive changes in MSC. Initial MSC was inversely associated with better changes in mental summary postprocedure. Some authors have reported an initial improvement in this sphere and subsequent deterioration at the end of the follow-up period [55]. However, results obtained by Paczkowska et al. have shown that the quality of mental health among patients with morbid obesity significantly depends on gender and the percentage of total weight loss achieved as a result of treatment [56]. Most scientific data have shown that improvement in a patient's mental health is likely attributed to weight loss and resultant gains relating to body image, self-esteem, and self-concept [57].

Our results are similar to those obtained by Brunault et al., with better improvement in physical HRQoL in patients who had higher weight loss and lower preoperative depression severity but are different in the better results in younger patients [44]. We found better results in patients older than 43.

After undergoing BST, patients exhibit enhanced adherence to the MedDiet. However, we did not find a positive association between higher adherence to a MedDiet or better PA habits and better quality of life, as found in other studies [26]. We believe that further studies with longer follow-up times are needed in order to clarify this question.

As for the limitations of the study, we found that the sample size was not very large, and patients with morbid obesity stem from a complex psychological sphere and have lower perceived health across all dimensions of quality of life. While it is true that the results have been assessed at 18 months post-intervention, it is possible that this improvement in the quality of life perceived by the patient is not maintained over time. Therefore, it would be advisable to reevaluate the patients 5 and 10 years after the intervention, considering that there are studies that report an initial improvement that is not sustained over time but is still better than before the intervention [58–60].

On the other hand, the use of SF-36 provides useful information, but it does not contemplate specific problems from obesity, such as body image and social stigma [61], that are better measured by the IWQoL-Lite instrument, developed for use in people with morbid obesity [62], or the OR-WELL-R, a new obesity-related quality-of-life instrument for assessing the "individual experience of overweightness" [63].

Preoperative mental health assessment and management are critical components of comprehensive care in the BST process. Identifying and addressing mental health issues prior to surgery can contribute to more successful outcomes and improved long-term quality of life for patients. It is critical that health care professionals work collaboratively with patients to address these issues and provide comprehensive support.

Health professionals should approach depression cautiously in their obese patients, and in certain instances, addressing this mental health condition might be the first step in managing them.

5. Conclusions

BST is an effective intervention for obesity, resulting in significant weight loss, improvements in HRQoL, and better nutritional habits. Patients without previous depression have better initial and final mental quality of life, and patients with optimal clinical response in weight loss have better results in physical and mental quality of life changes.

It is advisable for all members of the multidisciplinary team responsible for selecting and monitoring patients undergoing bariatric surgery to carefully select the most suitable candidates to benefit from this procedure. Additionally, close monitoring of patients, particularly providing psychological support to those with poorer mental health, is crucial. Well-designed studies with large sample sizes are needed to investigate factors other than weight loss that may be related to improvements in the physical and mental health of patients following bariatric surgery techniques.

Author Contributions: Conceptualization, B.V.D.-G., I.B.-C., J.R.H.H. and L.S.-M.; data curation, B.V.D.-G., E.H.G. and J.C.T.; formal analysis, B.V.D.-G. and I.B.-C.; investigation, B.V.D.-G., I.B.-C., J.R.H.H. and L.S.-M.; methodology, B.V.D.-G., I.B.-C., J.R.H.H. and L.S.-M.; project administration, B.V.D.-G., I.B.-C., J.R.H.H. and L.S.-M.; resources, B.V.D.-G., J.R.H.H. and L.S.-M.; software, B.V.D.-G., E.H.G. and J.C.T.; supervision, B.V.D.-G., I.B.-C. and L.S.-M.; validation, B.V.D.-G., I.B.-C. and L.S.-M.; visualization, B.V.D.-G., I.B.-C. and L.S.-M.; writing—original draft, B.V.D.-G., I.B.-C. and L.S.-M.; writing—review and editing, B.V.D.-G., I.B.-C., E.H.G., J.C.T., J.R.H.H. and L.S.-M. All authors have read and agreed to the published version of the manuscript.

Funding: This research received no external funding.

Institutional Review Board Statement: The study was conducted in accordance with the Declaration of Helsinki, and approved by the Institutional Review Institutional Review Board of the CEIC of the Hospital Universitario Insular de Gran Canaria (HUIGC), CHUMI (Centro Hospitalario Universitario Materno Infantil) code: 2024-093-728. Date: 26 June 2014.

Informed Consent Statement: Informed consent was obtained from all subjects involved in the study.

Data Availability Statement: The data presented in this study are available on request from the corresponding author due to ethical reasons.

Conflicts of Interest: The authors declare no conflicts of interest.

References

1. World Health Organization; Regional Office for Europe. *WHO European Regional Obesity: Report 2022*; World Health Organization: Geneva, Switzerland, 2022.
2. Kyle, T.K.; Dhurandhar, E.J.; Allison, D.B. Regarding Obesity as a Disease: Evolving Policies and Their Implications. *Endocrinol. Metab. Clin. N. Am.* **2016**, *45*, 511–520. [CrossRef]
3. Bray, G.A.; Kim, K.K.; Wilding, J.P.H. Obesity: A chronic relapsing progressive disease process. A position statement of the World Obesity Federation. *Obes. Rev.* **2017**, *18*, 715–723. [CrossRef]
4. Field, A.E.; Coakley, E.H.; Must, A.; Spadano, J.L.; Laird, N.; Dietz, W.H.; Rimm, E.; Colditz, G.A. Impact of Overweight on the Risk of Developing Common Chronic Diseases During a 10-Year Period. *Arch. Intern. Med.* **2001**, *161*, 1581–1586. Available online: http://archinte.jamanetwork.com/ (accessed on 1 February 2024). [CrossRef]
5. Nguyen, N.T.; Magno, C.P.; Lane, K.T.; Hinojosa, M.W.; Lane, J.S. Association of Hypertension, Diabetes, Dyslipidemia, and Metabolic Syndrome with Obesity: Findings from the National Health and Nutrition Examination Survey, 1999 to 2004. *J. Am. Coll. Surg.* **2008**, *207*, 928–934. [CrossRef]
6. Donnelly, J.E.; Blair, S.N.; Jakicic, J.M.; Manore, M.M.; Rankin, J.W.; Smith, B.K. Appropriate Physical Activity Intervention Strategies for Weight Loss and Prevention of Weight Regain for Adults. *Med. Sci. Sports Exerc.* **2009**, *41*, 459–471. [CrossRef]
7. Bull, F.C.; Al-Ansari, S.S.; Biddle, S.; Borodulin, K.; Buman, M.P.; Cardon, G.; Carty, C.; Chaput, J.P.; Chastin, S.; Chou, R.; et al. World Health Organization 2020 guidelines on physical activity and sedentary behaviour. *Br. J. Sports Med.* **2020**, *54*, 1451–1462. [CrossRef]
8. Arterburn, D.E.; Telem, D.A.; Kushner, R.F.; Courcoulas, A.P. Benefits and Risks of Bariatric Surgery in Adults. *JAMA* **2020**, *324*, 879–887. [CrossRef]
9. Kim, M.S.; Kim, J.Y.; Song, Y.S.; Hong, S.; Won, H.; Kim, W.J.; Kwon, Y.; Ha, J.; Fiedorowicz, J.G.; Solmi, M.; et al. Association of bariatric surgery with indicated and unintended outcomes: An umbrella review and meta-analysis for risk–benefit assessment. *Obes. Rev.* **2024**, *25*, e13670. [CrossRef]
10. Coulman, K.D.; Blazeby, J.M. Health-Related Quality of Life in Bariatric and Metabolic Surgery. *Curr. Obes. Rep.* **2020**, *9*, 307–314. [CrossRef]
11. Sierżantowicz, R.; Ładny, J.R.; Lewko, J. Quality of Life after Bariatric Surgery—A Systematic Review. *Int. J. Environ. Res. Public Health* **2022**, *19*, 9078. [CrossRef]
12. Busutil, R.; Espallardo, O.; Torres, A.; Martínez-Galdeano, L.; Zozaya, N.; Hidalgo-Vega, Á. The impact of obesity on health-related quality of life in Spain. *Health Qual. Life Outcomes* **2017**, *15*, 197. [CrossRef]
13. Fontaine, K.R.; Barofsky, I. Obesity and health-related quality of life. *Obes. Rev.* **2001**, *2*, 173–182. [CrossRef]
14. Ballantyne, G.H. Measuring Outcomes following Bariatric Surgery: Weight Loss Parameters, Improvement in Co-morbid Conditions, Change in Quality of Life and Patient Satisfaction. *Obes. Surg.* **2003**, *13*, 954–964. [CrossRef]
15. Sarwer, D.B.; Wadden, T.A.; Moore, R.H.; Eisenberg, M.H.; Raper, S.E.; Williams, N.N. Changes in quality of life and body image after gastric bypass surgery. *Surg. Obes. Relat. Dis.* **2010**, *6*, 608–614. [CrossRef]
16. Lopez-Nava, G.; Asokkumar, R.; Lacruz, T.; Rull, A.; Beltran, L.; Bautista-Castaño, I. The effect of weight loss and exercise on Health-Related Quality of Life (HRQOL) following Endoscopic Bariatric Therapies (EBT) for obesity. *Health Qual. Life Outcomes* **2020**, *18*, 130. [CrossRef]

17. Rogers, M.; Lemstra, M. Improving health-related quality of life through an evidence-based obesity reduction program: The Healthy Weights Initiative. *J. Multidiscip. Healthc.* **2016**, *9*, 103–109. [CrossRef]
18. Luppino, F.S.; de Wit, L.M.; Bouvy, P.F.; Stijnen, T.; Cuijpers, P.; Penninx, B.W.; Zitman, F.G. Overweight, Obesity, and Depression: A systematic review and meta-analysis of longitudinal studies. *Arch. Gen. Psychiatry* **2010**, *67*, 220–229. [CrossRef]
19. Milaneschi, Y.; Simmons, W.K.; van Rossum, E.F.C.; Penninx, B.W. Depression and obesity: Evidence of shared biological mechanisms. *Mol. Psychiatry* **2019**, *24*, 18–33. [CrossRef]
20. Johnston, E.; Johnson, S.; McLeod, P.; Johnston, M. The Relation of Body Mass Index to Depressive Symptoms. *Can. J. Public Health* **2004**, *95*, 179–183. [CrossRef]
21. Preiss, K.; Brennan, L.; Clarke, D. A systematic review of variables associated with the relationship between obesity and depression. *Obes. Rev.* **2013**, *14*, 906–918. [CrossRef]
22. Dussaillant, C.; Echeverría, G.; Urquiaga, I.; Velasco, N.; Rigotti, A. Evidencia actual sobre los beneficios de la dieta mediterránea en salud. *Rev. Méd. Chile* **2016**, *144*, 1044–1052. [CrossRef]
23. Mancini, J.G.; Filion, K.B.; Atallah, R.; Eisenberg, M.J. Systematic Review of the Mediterranean Diet for Long-Term Weight Loss. *Am. J. Med.* **2016**, *129*, 407–415.e4. [CrossRef]
24. Estruch, R.; Ros, E. The role of the Mediterranean diet on weight loss and obesity-related diseases. *Rev. Endocr. Metab. Disord.* **2020**, *21*, 315–327. [CrossRef]
25. Henríquez Sánchez, P.; Ruano, C.; de Irala, J.; Ruiz-Canela, M.; Martínez-González, M.A.; Sánchez-Villegas, A. Adherence to the Mediterranean diet and quality of life in the SUN Project. *Eur. J. Clin. Nutr.* **2012**, *66*, 360–368. [CrossRef]
26. Galilea-Zabalza, I.; Buil-Cosiales, P.; Salas-Salvadó, J.; Toledo, E.; Ortega-Azorín, C.; Díez-Espino, J.; Vazquez-Ruiz, Z.; Zomeño, M.D.; Vioque, J.; Martínez, J.A.; et al. Mediterranean diet and quality of life: Baseline cross-sectional analysis of the PREDIMED-PLUS trial. *PLoS ONE* **2018**, *13*, e0198974. [CrossRef]
27. Sanz, J.; Perdigón, A.L.; Vázquez, C. Adaptación española del Inventario para la Depresión de Beck-II (BDI-II): 2. Propiedades psicométricas en población general. *Clín. Salud* **2003**, *14*, 249–280.
28. Guirao, J.A. Elaboración y Validación de la Versión en Español Europeo de la Escala de Valoración Rápida de Actividad Física (RAPA). Ph.D. Thesis, Universidad de Alicante, Licante, Spain, 2012. Available online: https://dialnet.unirioja.es/servlet/tesis?codigo=64908 (accessed on 30 April 2024).
29. Vilagut, G.; María Valderas, J.; Ferrer, M.; Garin, O.; López-García, E.; Alonso, J. Interpretación de los cuestionarios de salud SF-36 y SF-12 en España: Componentes físico y mental. *Med. Clin.* **2008**, *130*, 726–735. [CrossRef]
30. Schröder, H.; Fitó, M.; Estruch, R.; Martínez-González, M.A.; Corella, D.; Salas-Salvadó, J.; Lamuela-Raventós, R.; Ros, E.; Salaverría, I.; Fiol, M.; et al. A Short Screener Is Valid for Assessing Mediterranean Diet Adherence among Older Spanish Men and Women. *J. Nutr.* **2011**, *141*, 1140–1145. [CrossRef]
31. Lopez-Garcia, E.; Guallar-Castillón, P.; Garcia-Esquinas, E.; Rodríguez-Artalejo, F. Metabolically healthy obesity and health-related quality of life: A prospective cohort study. *Clin. Nutr.* **2017**, *36*, 853–860. [CrossRef]
32. Topolski, T.D.; LoGerfo, J.; Patrick, D.L.; Williams, B.; Walwick, J.; Patrick, M.B. Peer Reviewed: The Rapid Assessment of Physical Activity (RAPA) among older adults. *Prev. Chronic Dis.* **2006**, *3*, A118.
33. Beck, A.T.; Steer, R.A.; Brown, G.K. *Beck Depression Inventory: Second Edition Manual*; The Psychological Corporation: San Antonio, TX, USA, 1996.
34. Friedman, M.A.; Brownell, K.D. Psychological Correlates of Obesity: Moving to the Next Research Generation. *Psychol. Bull.* **1995**, *117*, 3–20. [CrossRef]
35. Livhits, M.; Mercado, C.; Yermilov, I.; Parikh, J.A.; Dutson, E.; Mehran, A.; Ko, C.Y.; Gibbons, M.M. Preoperative predictors of weight loss following bariatric surgery: Systematic review. *Obes. Surg.* **2012**, *22*, 70–89. [CrossRef]
36. Müller, A.; Mitchell, J.E.; Sondag, C.; De Zwaan, M. Psychiatric aspects of bariatric surgery topical collection on eating disorders. *Curr. Psychiatry Rep.* **2013**, *15*, 397. [CrossRef]
37. Barcones-Molero, M.F.; Sánchez-Villegas, A.; Martínez-González, M.A.; Bes-Rastrollo, M.; Martínez-Urbistondo, M.; Santabárbara, J.; Martínez, J.A. Influencia de la obesidad y la ganancia de peso sobre la calidad de vida según el SF-36 en individuos de la cohorte dinámica Seguimiento Universidad de Navarra. *Rev. Clin. Esp.* **2018**, *218*, 408–416. [CrossRef]
38. Doll, H.A.; Petersen, S.E.K.; Stewart-Brown, S.L. Obesity and Physical and Emotional Well-Being: Associations between Body Mass Index, Chronic Illness, and the Physical and Mental Components of the SF-36 Questionnaire. *Obes. Res.* **2000**, *8*, 160–170. [CrossRef]
39. Sjöström, L. Review of the key results from the Swedish Obese Subjects (SOS) trial—A prospective controlled intervention study of bariatric surgery. *J. Intern. Med.* **2013**, *273*, 219–234. [CrossRef]
40. Hayden, M.J.; Murphy, K.D.; Brown, W.A.; O'Brien, P.E. Axis I Disorders in Adjustable Gastric Band Patients: The Relationship Between Psychopathology and Weight Loss. *Obes. Surg.* **2014**, *24*, 1469–1475. [CrossRef]
41. Hayden, M.J.; Dixon, J.B.; Dixon, M.E.; Shea, T.L.; O'Brien, P.E. Characterization of the Improvement in Depressive Symptoms Following Bariatric Surgery. *Obes. Surg.* **2011**, *21*, 328–335. [CrossRef]
42. Booth, H.; Khan, O.; Prevost, A.T.; Reddy, M.; Charlton, J.; Gulliford, M.C. Impact of bariatric surgery on clinical depression. Interrupted time series study with matched controls. *J. Affect. Disord.* **2015**, *174*, 644–649. [CrossRef]
43. Andersen, J.R.; Aasprang, A.; Bergsholm, P.; Sletteskog, N.; Våge, V.; Natvig, G.K. Predictors for health-related quality of life in patients accepted for bariatric surgery. *Surg. Obes. Relat. Dis.* **2009**, *5*, 329–333. [CrossRef]

44. Brunault, P.; Frammery, J.; Couet, C.; Delbachian, I.; Bourbao-Tournois, C.; Objois, M.; Cosson, P.; Réveillère, C.; Ballon, N. Predictors of changes in physical, psychosocial, sexual quality of life, and comfort with food after obesity surgery: A 12-month follow-up study. *Qual. Life Res.* **2015**, *24*, 493–501. [CrossRef]
45. Dawes, A.J.; Maggard-Gibbons, M.; Maher, A.R.; Booth, M.J.; Miake-Lye, I.; Beroes, J.M.; Shekelle, P.G. Mental Health Conditions Among Patients Seeking and Undergoing Bariatric Surgery. *JAMA* **2016**, *315*, 150–163. [CrossRef]
46. Lier, H.Ø.; Biringer, E.; Stubhaug, B.; Tangen, T. Prevalence of psychiatric disorders before and 1 year after bariatric surgery: The role of shame in maintenance of psychiatric disorders in patients undergoing bariatric surgery. *Nord. J. Psychiatry* **2013**, *67*, 89–96. [CrossRef]
47. Kolotkin, R.L.; Andersen, J.R. A systematic review of reviews: Exploring the relationship between obesity, weight loss and health-related quality of life. *Clin. Obes.* **2017**, *7*, 273–289. [CrossRef]
48. Kroes, M.; Osei-Assibey, G.; Baker-Searle, R.; Huang, J. Impact of weight change on quality of life in adults with overweight/obesity in the United States: A systematic review. *Curr. Med. Res. Opin.* **2016**, *32*, 485–508. [CrossRef]
49. Strain, G.W.; Kolotkin, R.L.; Dakin, G.F.; Gagner, M.; Inabnet, W.B.; Christos, P.; Saif, T.; Crosby, R.; Pomp, A. The effects of weight loss after bariatric surgery on health-related quality of life and depression. *Nutr. Diabetes* **2014**, *4*, e132. [CrossRef]
50. Tettero, O.M.; Aronson, T.; Wolf, R.J.; Nuijten, M.A.H.; Hopman, M.T.E.; Janssen, I.M.C. Increase in Physical Activity After Bariatric Surgery Demonstrates Improvement in Weight Loss and Cardiorespiratory Fitness. *Obes. Surg.* **2018**, *28*, 3950–3957. [CrossRef]
51. van Gemert, W.A.M.; van der Palen, J.; Monninkhof, E.M.; Rozeboom, A.; Peters, R.; Wittink, H.; Schuit, A.J.; Peeters, P.H. Quality of Life after Diet or Exercise-Induced Weight Loss in Overweight to Obese Postmenopausal Women: The SHAPE-2 Randomised Controlled Trial. *PLoS ONE* **2015**, *10*, e0127520. [CrossRef]
52. Biter, L.U.; van Buuren, M.M.A.; Mannaerts, G.H.H.; Apers, J.A.; Dunkelgrün, M.; Vijgen, G.H.E.J. Quality of Life 1 Year After Laparoscopic Sleeve Gastrectomy Versus Laparoscopic Roux-en-Y Gastric Bypass: A Randomized Controlled Trial Focusing on Gastroesophageal Reflux Disease. *Obes. Surg.* **2017**, *27*, 2557–2565. [CrossRef]
53. Kolotkin, R.L.; Crosby, R.D.; Gress, R.E.; Hunt, S.C.; Adams, T.D. Two-year changes in health-related quality of life in gastric bypass patients compared with severely obese controls. *Surg. Obes. Relat. Dis.* **2009**, *5*, 250–256. [CrossRef]
54. Albarrán-Sánchez, A.; Ramírez-Rentería, C.; Ferreira-Hermosillo, A.; Rodríguez-Pérez, V.; Espinosa-Cárdenas, E.; Molina-Ayala, M.; Boscó-Gárate, I.; Mendoza-Zubieta, V. Quality of life evaluation in Mexican patients with severe obesity before and after bariatric surgery. *Gac. Med. Mex.* **2023**, *157*, 64–69. [CrossRef]
55. Canetti, L.; Bachar, E.; Bonne, O. Deterioration of mental health in bariatric surgery after 10 years despite successful weight loss. *Eur. J. Clin. Nutr.* **2016**, *70*, 17–22. [CrossRef]
56. Paczkowska, A.; Hoffmann, K.; Raakow, J.; Pross, M.; Berghaus, R.; Michalak, M.; Bryl, W.; Marzec, K.; Kopciuch, D.; Zaprutko, T.; et al. Impact of bariatric surgery on depression, anxiety and stress symptoms among patients with morbid obesity: International multicentre study in Poland and Germany. *BJPsych Open* **2022**, *8*, e32. [CrossRef]
57. O'Brien, P.E. Bariatric surgery: Mechanisms, indications and outcomes. *J. Gastroenterol. Hepatol.* **2010**, *25*, 1358–1365. [CrossRef]
58. Andersen, J.R.; Aasprang, A.; Karlsen, T.I.; Karin Natvig, G.; Våge, V.; Kolotkin, R.L. Health-related quality of life after bariatric surgery: A systematic review of prospective long-term studies. *Surg. Obes. Relat. Dis.* **2015**, *11*, 466–473. [CrossRef]
59. Hachem, A.; Brennan, L. Quality of Life Outcomes of Bariatric Surgery: A Systematic Review. *Obes. Surg.* **2016**, *26*, 395–409. [CrossRef]
60. Rausa, E.; Kelly, M.E.; Galfrascoli, E.; Aiolfi, A.; Cavalcoli, F.; Turati, L.; Bonavina, L.; Sgroi, G. Quality of Life and Gastrointestinal Symptoms Following Laparoscopic Roux-en-Y Gastric Bypass and Laparoscopic Sleeve Gastrectomy: A Systematic Review. *Obes. Surg.* **2019**, *29*, 1397–1402. [CrossRef]
61. Duval, K.; Marceau, P.; Pérusse, L.; Lacasse, Y. An overview of obesity-specific quality of life questionnaires. *Obes. Rev.* **2006**, *7*, 347–360. [CrossRef]
62. Forhan, M.; Vrkljan, B.; MacDermid, J. A systematic review of the quality of psychometric evidence supporting the use of an obesity-specific quality of life measure for use with persons who have class III obesity: Diagnostic in Obesity and Complications. *Obes. Rev.* **2010**, *11*, 222–228. [CrossRef]
63. Camolas, J.; Ferreira, A.; Mannucci, E.; Mascarenhas, M.; Carvalho, M.; Moreira, P.; do Carmo, I.; Santos, O. Assessing quality of life in severe obesity: Development psychometric properties of the ORWELL-R. *Eat. Weight. Disord. Stud. Anorex. Bulim. Obes.* **2016**, *21*, 277–288. [CrossRef]

Disclaimer/Publisher's Note: The statements, opinions and data contained in all publications are solely those of the individual author(s) and contributor(s) and not of MDPI and/or the editor(s). MDPI and/or the editor(s) disclaim responsibility for any injury to people or property resulting from any ideas, methods, instructions or products referred to in the content.

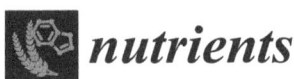

Article

Shift Work, Shifted Diets: An Observational Follow-Up Study on Diet Quality and Sustainability among Healthcare Workers on Night Shifts

Semra Navruz-Varlı and Hande Mortaş *

Department of Nutrition and Dietetics, Faculty of Health Sciences, Gazi University, 06490 Ankara, Türkiye; semranavruz@gazi.edu.tr
* Correspondence: handeyilmaz@gazi.edu.tr; Tel.: +90-312-216-2639

Abstract: This study aimed to investigate the change in diet quality in addition to dietary adherence to the planetary health diet during night shifts in healthcare workers. This observational follow-up study involved 450 healthcare workers working night shifts (327 females, 123 males). A survey form requesting sociodemographic information (gender, age, marital status), job title, sleeping duration during the night shift, 24 h dietary records for pre-night-shift, during night shift, and post-night-shift, and anthropometric measurements (body weight and height) was applied. The scores of the Planetary Health Diet Index (PHDI) and the Healthy Eating Index 2020 (HEI-2020) were calculated according to the dietary records. The total HEI-2020 and PHDI scores decreased significantly ($p < 0.05$) during the night shift (44.0 ± 8.8 and 48.3 ± 13.2, respectively) compared to pre-night-shift (46.1 ± 9.2 and 51.9 ± 13.4, respectively) and increased post-night-shift (44.7 ± 9.9 and 50.6 ± 14.9, respectively), with no statistically significant difference between pre- and post-night-shift. There was a significant main effect of night shift working on total PHDI ($F(896, 2) = 8.208$, $p < 0.001$, $\eta_p^2 = 0.018$) and HEI-2020 scores ($F(894, 2) = 6.277$, $p = 0.002$, $\eta_p^2 = 0.014$). Despite healthcare workers' knowledge of health factors, night shifts lead to poor dietary choices. To improve diet quality and sustainability, it is crucial to enhance access to healthy food options in their work environment.

Keywords: healthcare workers; sustainable nutrition; diet quality; night shift

Citation: Navruz-Varlı, S.; Mortaş, H. Shift Work, Shifted Diets: An Observational Follow-Up Study on Diet Quality and Sustainability among Healthcare Workers on Night Shifts. *Nutrients* **2024**, *16*, 2404. https://doi.org/10.3390/nu16152404

Academic Editors: António Raposo, Renata Puppin Zandonadi and Raquel Braz Assunção Botelho

Received: 29 June 2024
Revised: 20 July 2024
Accepted: 23 July 2024
Published: 24 July 2024

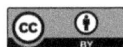

Copyright: © 2024 by the authors. Licensee MDPI, Basel, Switzerland. This article is an open access article distributed under the terms and conditions of the Creative Commons Attribution (CC BY) license (https://creativecommons.org/licenses/by/4.0/).

1. Introduction

Healthcare workers make up one-third of shift workers, while nurses represent the largest group [1]. Shift work schedules are required for individuals to access healthcare services 24 h a day. Almost a quarter of healthcare workers regularly work night shifts [2]. The well-being of healthcare professionals directly affects the health of the patients who need their care. Although practices related to the safety and health of patients come to the fore in healthcare institutions, the safety and health of healthcare professionals should also be supported at the same rate. A natural connection has been reported between the healthcare professional workforce and basic self-care activities (e.g., physical activity, diet quality). In healthcare workers who experience high levels of stress and fatigue, sleep quantity/quality, diet quality, and physical activity cannot reach the desired levels, and this may threaten health [3,4].

Although health professionals have advanced health knowledge, they have difficulty in implementing health-promoting behaviors recommended at the national/international level. The main reasons for this are long working hours and shift work (especially night shift work). These harmful working conditions increase the risk of physiological and psychological disorders. Shift work mainly changes the diet undesirably [5]. When working the night shift, food intake differs from day to night. Night shift workers have a higher meal frequency and lower diet quality than day shift workers [6,7]. As a first step to ensuring the implementation of targeted wellness strategies, it is critical to determine changes in nutrition as well as sleep and physical activity assessments under extended hours and night shift working conditions. The average diet quality of nurses working night shifts is low. Nurses working the night shift need resources to support diet quality to reduce the adverse effects caused by working conditions [8]. Additionally, fatty and salty foods were found to be negatively associated with diet quality in female nurses working night shifts [2]. Attention is drawn to the importance of intervention studies on meal timing and diet quality of healthcare workers working shifts [9].

Global changes in nutrition are associated with intensive production methods that contribute to environmental degradation (greenhouse gas emissions, land use change, land degradation, water pollution, etc.) while causing an increase in non-communicable chronic diseases. The Planetary Health Diet Index (PHDI) was developed to measure compliance with dietary evidence established by the EAT-Lancet Commission. It has been reported that nutritional adequacy in terms of vitamins, fiber, and minerals will be increased by changing diets according to EAT-Lancet recommendations. The need for policy action to support healthier and more-sustainable diets worldwide has been highlighted [10]. It is thought that evaluating the compliance of healthcare professionals, who are pioneers in protecting and improving public health, with the planetary health diet and revealing the current situation will contribute to filling the gap in the literature.

To our knowledge, no study has been found that evaluates the differences in healthcare workers' diet quality and planetary health diet compliance by following up throughout the periods of pre-night-shift, during, and post-night-shift. Therefore, this study aimed to investigate the change in diet quality and dietary adherence to the planetary health diet during night shifts in healthcare workers.

2. Materials and Methods

2.1. Participants and Study Design

This study was conducted as a prospective observational follow-up study with the voluntary participation of 450 nurses, doctors, emergency medical technicians, and ambulance care technicians working in private, university, and state hospitals and private health institutions in Ankara, the capital of Turkey. The study was conducted between June 2023 and January 2024. Criteria for inclusion of healthcare professionals in the study were: being between the ages of 20 and 40 years, not having a disease that affects food consumption (situations that limit the consumption of various foods, such as lactose intolerance and celiac), not being a vegetarian or vegan, not being on a weight loss diet, not having any food allergies, not being pregnant or breastfeeding, and working shifts for at least a year. Individuals (n = 22) who started working the day shift instead of the night shift, who did not provide 24 h dietary records, or who lost communication during the study period were excluded from the study.

Healthcare workers' shift working patterns were 24 h a day, from 08:00 a.m. to 08:00 a.m. the next day. The data obtained in this period were evaluated as "during night shift" in this article. The working schedule of healthcare professionals was 24 h work/24–48 h off. In the article, the day before the 24 h working day was expressed as the "pre-night-shift" (off day). The day after a 24 h working day was defined as the "post-night-shift" (off day). The healthcare workers were followed up for three days: pre-night-shift, during night shift, and post-night-shift.

Ethical approval was obtained from the Ethical Committee of Gazi University (Date: 16 April 2024, No: 2023-851-07). In addition, written informed consent was obtained from the participants in the study. This research was carried out following the Declaration of Helsinki.

2.2. Data Collection Tools

In this study, a survey form requesting sociodemographic information (gender, age, marital status), job title, sleeping duration during the night shift, and 24 h dietary records pre-night-shift, during night shift and post-night-shift was applied by the researchers via a face-to-face interview method. The participants' body weight and height were measured using a BC 532 Innerscan scale (Tanita Corporation, Tokyo, Japan) and stadiometer, respectively. Body mass index (BMI) was calculated as body weight in kilograms divided by the square of the height in meters (kg/m^2) and categorized [11].

The researchers conducted a nutritional assessment by collecting 24 h dietary records from all participants for three days including "pre-", "during" and "post-night-shift". Participants were instructed to log everything they consumed, including foods, beverages, sauces, and condiments. In addition, the mealtimes were recorded, and information was obtained about which meal they consumed that food in. The healthcare workers prepared and brought in the meals they consumed during the night shift from home or obtained them from places such as canteens and cafeterias at work. Individuals self-declared the ingredients of the meals they prepared while keeping 24 h dietary records. However, the ingredients that went into the ready-made meals they purchased from places such as canteens and cafeterias were obtained through the Standard Food Recipes book [12]. The collected data were then analyzed for total energy and nutrient intake using the BeBiS program, version 7.2.

2.3. Instruments to Evaluate Diet Quality and Sustainability

The United States Department of Agriculture (USDA) developed the Healthy Eating Index (HEI) in 1995 based on the American Dietary Guidelines [13]. This index was updated in 2005, 2010, and 2015. The components and standards of the HEI-2015 remained unchanged in the HEI-2020. The HEI-2020 retains the same 13 components and scoring standards as the HEI-2015, despite being renamed to reflect its alignment with the 2020–2025 Dietary Guidelines for Americans.

The HEI-2020, utilized in this study, includes 13 components: nine that should be consumed in adequate amounts and four that should be consumed in moderation. The nine desired components are total fruit, whole fruit, total vegetables, green leafy vegetables and fresh legumes, whole grains, dairy products, protein foods, seafood and plant-based proteins, and fatty acids. The four components to be limited are refined grains, sodium, added sugars, and saturated fats. Each component in the index is scored between 0 and 5 or 0 and 10, with low scores indicating poor nutrition and high scores indicating good nutrition [14].

The Planetary Health Diet Index (PHDI) was created by Cacau et al. (2021) based on the dietary recommendations from the EAT-Lancet Commission [15]. The index scores range from 10 to 5 points per component, with a total possible score of 0–150. Sixteen diet components are assessed using food records. The components and their maximum points are: red meat (10 points), nuts and peanuts (10 points), legumes (10 points), chicken and its substitutes (10 points), fish and seafood (10 points), eggs (10 points), fruit (10 points), vegetables (10 points), the ratio of dark green leafy vegetables to other vegetables (5 points), the ratio of red vegetables to other vegetables (5 points), whole grains (10 points), milk and its products (10 points), unsaturated fats (10 points), animal fats (10 points), and added sugars (10 points).

2.4. Physical Activity Assessment

Healthcare workers' physical activity adequacies were evaluated using the Brief Physical Activity Assessment Tool developed by Marshall et al. (2005) [16]. The assessment includes two questions: one about the frequency and duration of vigorous-intensity physical activity, and the other about the frequency and duration of moderate-intensity activities (including walking) performed in a typical week. A scoring algorithm combines the responses to these questions to determine if individuals are classified as "adequately active".

2.5. Statistical Analysis

Continuous variables were presented as the arithmetic mean with standard deviation, while categorical variables were shown as percentages. The HEI-2020 and PHDI total scores were categorized according to descriptive characteristics, including gender, age group, BMI group, marital status, job title, sleeping status during the night shift, and physical activity adequacy, and the changes between pre-, during and post-night-shift were compared using repeated-measures ANOVA (Table 1). If there was a significant difference in the repeated-measures ANOVA test, Tukey's post-hoc test was used for pairwise comparisons of the parameters. Changes in the HEI-2020 and PHDI total scores and subcomponent scores between pre-, during, and post-night-shift were compared using repeated-measures ANOVA (Table 2). Tukey's post-hoc test was used for pairwise comparisons of the parameters. The effects of individuals' night shift changes (pre-, during, and post-) and, the interactions of the night shift changes with gender, age groups, BMI groups, marital status, branch of work, sleeping status during the night shift, and physical activity on the total PHDI and HEI-2020 scores were analyzed using two-way between-subjects ANOVA (Table 3). The results were interpreted with 95% confidence. Statistical analysis was conducted using IBM SPSS Statistics version 28.0.1.0, with significance determined at $p < 0.05$.

Table 1. Descriptive characteristics of the health workers.

Variables	Percentages n (%)	Total PHDI Score (Mean ± SD)			Total HEI-2020 Score (Mean ± SD)		
		Pre-Night-Shift	During Night Shift	Post-Night-Shift	Pre-Night-Shift	During Night Shift	Post-Night-Shift
Gender							
Female	327 (72.7)	51.9 ± 13.4 [a]	48.2 ± 13.8 [b]	50.8 ± 14.9 [a]	46.6 ± 9.4 [a]	43.8 ± 8.8 [b]	44.6 ± 10.2 [b]
		$F = 10{,}730.176; p < 0.001; \eta^2 = 0.971$			$F = 8034.557; p < 0.001; \eta^2 = 0.985$		
Male	123 (27.3)	51.9 ± 13.3 [a]	48.8 ± 11.7 [b]	50.8 ± 14.9 [a,b]	44.7 ± 8.4	44.6 ± 8.6	45.0 ± 8.9
		$F = 5049.914; p < 0.001; \eta^2 = 0.976$			$F = 18{,}506.432; p = 0.170; \eta^2 = 0.014$		
Age group (years)							
20–25	122 (27.1)	49.3 ± 14.1 [a]	45.5 ± 12.9 [b]	46.2 ± 14.5 [a,b]	45.6 ± 9.6 [a]	43.4 ± 8.4 [b]	42.7 ± 9.9 [b]
		$F = 3830.169; p < 0.001; \eta^2 = 0.969$			$F = 6830.632; p < 0.001; \eta^2 = 0.983$		
26–30	188 (41.8)	52.5 ± 13.2 [a]	49.7 ± 13.1 [b]	51.7 ± 14.9 [a,b]	45.9 ± 9.1 [a,b]	44.4 ± 8.6 [b]	46.1 ± 9.9 [a]
		$F = 6845.947; p < 0.001; \eta^2 = 0.973$			$F = 10{,}859.282; p < 0.001; \eta^2 = 0.983$		
31–40	140 (31.1)	53.4 ± 12.8 [a]	48.9 ± 13.5 [b]	52.9 ± 14.5 [a]	46.7 ± 8.8 [a]	44.1 ± 9.4 [b]	44.7 ± 9.6 [b]
		$F = 5937.575; p < 0.001; \eta^2 = 0.977$			$F = 9026.722; p < 0.001; \eta^2 = 0.985$		
BMI (kg/m²)							
Normal weight	288 (64.0)	51.5 ± 13.3 [a]	48.4 ± 13.3 [b]	51.2 ± 15.4 [a]	46.3 ± 9.5 [a]	44.5 ± 8.5 [b]	45.2 ± 9.9 [a]
		$F = 4.642; p = 0.010; \eta^2 = 0.016$			$F = 3.407; p = 0.034; \eta^2 = 0.012$		
Overweight	135 (30.0)	51.7 ± 13.2 [a]	47.8 ± 13.5 [b]	49.4 ± 13.9 [b]	45.1 ± 8.4 [a]	43.4 ± 9.2 [b]	43.7 ± 9.8 [b]
		$F = 3.057; p = 0.049; \eta^2 = 0.022$			$F = 1.549; p = 0.011; \eta^2 = 0.011$		
Obese	27 (6.0)	56.8 ± 13.7	50.5 ± 11.6	50.4 ± 13.7	48.8 ± 8.8	43.8 ± 9.3	45.5 ± 10.1
		$F = 2.631; p = 0.082; \eta^2 = 0.092$			$F = 2.147; p = 0.127; \eta^2 = 0.076$		
Marital status							
Married	200 (44.4)	53.1 ± 12.8 [a]	49.4 ± 12.9 [b]	51.7 ± 14.6 [a,b]	46.7 ± 8.6 [a]	44.6 ± 9.2 [b]	45.6 ± 9.7 [a,b]
		$F = 8042.590; p < 0.001; \eta^2 = 0.976$			$F = 13{,}786.891; p < 0.001; \eta^2 = 0.986$		
Single	250 (55.6)	50.9 ± 13.8 [a]	47.5 ± 13.5 [b]	49.7 ± 15.1 [b]	45.6 ± 9.6 [a]	43.6 ± 8.4 [b]	44.1 ± 9.9 [a,b]
		$F = 7959.767; p < 0.001; \eta^2 = 0.970$			$F = 13{,}266.537; p < 0.001; \eta^2 = 0.982$		
Job title							
Nurse	267 (59.3)	50.2 ± 13.5 [a]	46.6 ± 12.9 [b]	49.1 ± 15.6 [b]	46.5 ± 9.0 [a]	44.7 ± 8.6 [b]	44.6 ± 10.3 [b]
		$F = 8425.803; p < 0.001; \eta^2 = 0.969$			$F = 14{,}954.402; p < 0.001; \eta^2 = 0.983$		
Doctor	36 (8.0)	50.5 ± 13.2 [a]	46.3 ± 12.9 [b]	52.6 ± 14 [a]	45.6 ± 9.6 [a]	44.9 ± 7.7 [b]	48.9 ± 9.6 [a]
		$F = 1694.439; p < 0.001; \eta^2 = 0.980$			$F = 2088.182; p < 0.001; \eta^2 = 0.984$		
Emergency medical technician	100 (22.2)	54.5 ± 12.8 [a]	49.7 ± 12.4 [b]	51.6 ± 12.4 [a,b]	45.4 ± 9.4 [a]	42.1 ± 8.4 [b]	44.1 ± 9.4 [a,b]
		$F = 4620.098; p < 0.001; \eta^2 = 0.979$			$F = 7232.001; p < 0.001; \eta^2 = 0.987$		
Ambulance care technician	47 (10.4)	57.0 ± 12.1	56.5 ± 14.2	55.6 ± 14.7	45.7 ± 9.2	43.6 ± 10.5	43.9 ± 7.9
		$F = 2685.913; p = 0.881; \eta^2 = 0.003$			$F = 2789.670; p = 0.489; \eta^2 = 0.015$		
Sleeping during night shift							
Not sleeping	118 (26.2)	47.1 ± 11.9 [a]	43.9 ± 13.4 [b]	46.3 ± 13.3 [a,b]	44.9 ± 8.6 [a]	42.8 ± 7.6 [b]	43.4 ± 9.3 [a,b]
		$F = 4145.019; p < 0.001; \eta^2 = 0.973$			$F = 8357.545; p < 0.001; \eta^2 = 0.986$		
0–2 h sleep	332 (73.8)	53.6 ± 13.4 [a]	49.9 ± 13.4 [b]	52.1 ± 15.1 [a]	46.5 ± 9.3 [a]	44.5 ± 9.1 [b]	45.2 ± 10.1 [a,b]
		$F = 13{,}167.330; p < 0.001; \eta^2 = 0.975$			$F = 18{,}804.628; p < 0.001; \eta^2 = 0.983$		
Physical activity status							
Inadequate	170 (37.8)	48.9 ± 13.1 [a]	45.8 ± 12.5 [b]	48.1 ± 15.3 [a,b]	46.7 ± 8.8	45.7 ± 8.4	45.1 ± 9.9
		$F = 10{,}383.005; p < 0.001; \eta^2 = 0.974$			$F = 9883.626; p = 0.189; \eta^2 = 0.010$		
Adequate	280 (62.2)	53.7 ± 13.2 [a]	49.9 ± 13.5 [b]	52.1 ± 14.4 [a]	45.7 ± 9.3 [a]	43.0 ± 8.9 [b]	44.5 ± 9.9 [a,b]
		$F = 6230.596; p < 0.001; \eta^2 = 0.974$			$F = 16{,}912.648; p < 0.001; \eta^2 = 0.984$		

[a,b] represent the statistically significant differences among the line groups at $p < 0.05$. BMI: body mass index; HEI: Healthy Eating Index; SD: standard deviation; PHDI: Planetary Health Diet Index.

Table 2. Diet quality and sustainable nutrition trends of health workers pre-, during and post-night-shifts according to the HEI-2020 and PHDI.

Indices and Their Components	Pre-Night-Shift ($\bar{x} \pm$ SD)	During Night Shift ($\bar{x} \pm$ SD)	Post-Night-Shift ($\bar{x} \pm$ SD)	F	p	η^2
HEI-2020 score	46.1 ± 9.2 [a]	44.0 ± 8.8 [b]	44.7 ± 9.9 [b]	6.277	0.002	0.014
HEI-2020 components scores [$\bar{x} \pm$ SD]						
Whole grains	0.8 ± 2.5 [a]	0.5 ± 1.9 [b]	0.7 ± 2.3 [b]	3.633	0.027	0.008
Refined grains	7.6 ± 2.9	7.2 ± 2.9	7.3 ± 3.3	2.676	0.069	0.006
Seafood and plant proteins	4.9 ± 0.7 [a]	4.9 ± 0.5 [a]	4.8 ± 0.9 [b]	5.626	0.006	0.012
Sodium	9.4 ± 1.9 [a]	6.7 ± 1.3 [b]	9.4 ± 1.9 [a]	4.428	0.014	0.010
Dairy	3.2 ± 2.1	3.1 ± 2.0	3.4 ± 2.7	1.895	0.153	0.004
Greens and beans	3.5 ± 1.7 [a]	3.5 ± 1.6 [a]	3.2 ± 1.8 [b]	5.796	0.003	0.013
Total vegetable	3.2 ± 1.5	3.2 ± 1.4	3.1 ± 1.6	0.348	0.706	0.001
Whole fruit	3.5 ± 1.9 [a]	2.1 ± 1.7 [b]	2.4 ± 2.0 [a]	6.568	0.001	0.014
Total fruit	1.7 ± 1.6 [a]	1.3 ± 1.2 [b]	1.7 ± 1.7 [a]	10.502	<0.001	0.023
Added sugar	4.9 ± 4.6 [a]	4.1 ± 4.5 [b]	4.6 ± 4.7 [a]	4.662	0.010	0.010
MUFA/PUFA ratio	0.1 ± 0.6 [b]	0.1 ± 0.5 [b]	0.2 ± 1.3 [a]	5.001	0.014	0.011
Saturated fatty acids	0.0 ± 0.0	0.0 ± 0.0	0.1 ± 0.4	1.000	0.318	0.002
PHDI score [$\bar{x} \pm$ SD]	51.9 ± 13.4 [a]	48.3 ± 13.2 [b]	50.6 ± 14.9 [a]	8.208	<0.001	0.018
PHDI components scores [$\bar{x} \pm$ SD]						
Red meat	1.5 ± 3.5 [a]	0.6 ± 2.3 [b]	2.3 ± 4.1 [c]	27.081	<0.001	0.057
Nuts and peanuts	5.3 ± 4.2 [a]	5.6 ± 4.2 [a]	4.7 ± 4.4 [b]	5.163	0.006	0.011
Legumes	3.2 ± 3.8 [b]	3.5 ± 3.8 [a]	2.7 ± 3.8 [b]	4.332	0.013	0.010
Chicken and substitutes	7.7 ± 4.2 [a]	6.6 ± 4.7 [b]	8.0 ± 3.9 [a]	13.943	<0.001	0.030
Fish and seafood	0.0 ± 0.0	0.0 ± 0.0	0.1 ± 0.1	0.640	0.491	0.001
Eggs	0.4 ± 1.5 [a]	0.9 ± 2.4 [b]	2.9 ± 3.7 [a]	106.921	<0.001	0.192
Fruits	6.9 ± 3.7	6.4 ± 3.6	6.4 ± 3.9	2.4560	0.086	0.005
Vegetables	6.7 ± 2.5 [a]	8.7 ± 2.5 [a]	8.3 ± 3.0 [b]	3.469	0.033	0.008
DGV/total ratio	0.5 ± 0.3	0.4 ± 0.3	0.4 ± 0.3	0.056	0.944	0.000
ReV/total ratio	0.8 ± 0.3 [a]	0.9 ± 0.3 [b]	0.8 ± 0.4 [b]	6.928	0.001	0.015
Whole cereals	0.7 ± 1.8 [a]	0.4 ± 0.3 [b]	0.6 ± 0.3 [a,b]	3.633	0.027	0.008
Tubers and potatoes	0.3 ± 0.1	0.4 ± 0.1	0.5 ± 0.8	1.907	0.150	0.004
Dairy	2.7 ± 0.3 [a]	2.9 ± 0.4 [a]	2.3 ± 0.3 [b]	4.613	0.010	0.010
Vegetable oils	3.9 ± 0.6 [a]	3.2 ± 0.7 [b]	3.1 ± 0.4 [b]	6.853	0.001	0.015
Animal fats	5.1 ± 0.9 [a]	4.6 ± 0.4 [b]	5.7 ± 0.9 [c]	7.822	0.001	0.017
Added sugar	4.3 ± 0.6 [a]	3.4 ± 0.4 [b]	4.1 ± 0.6 [a]	5.706	0.003	0.013

[a,b,c] represent the statistically significant differences among the line groups at $p < 0.05$. DGV: dark green vegetables; HEI: Healthy Eating Index; MUFA: monounsaturated fatty acids; PHDI: Planetary Health Diet Index; PUFA: polyunsaturated fatty acids; ReV: red vegetables; SD: standard deviation.

Table 3. Healthy Eating Index 2020 and Planetary Health Diet Index total score differences according to interactions of the night shift working with descriptive variables.

Variables	SS	df	MS	F	p	η_p^2
PHDI total scores						
Night shift working	2933.499	2	1466.750	8.208	<0.001	0.018
Night shift working * Gender	16.190	2	8.095	0.045	0.956	0.000
Night shift working * Age group	513.499	4	128.375	0.717	0.580	0.003
Night shift working * BMI group	581.021	4	145.255	0.812	0.517	0.004
Night shift working * Marital status	5.662	2	2.831	0.016	0.984	0.000
Night shift working * Job title	777.763	6	129.627	0.724	0.630	0.005
Night shift working * Sleeping	20.722	2	10.361	0.058	0.944	0.000
Night shift working * Physical activity	33.696	2	16.848	0.094	0.910	0.000
HEI-2020 total scores						
Night shift working	975.849	2	487.924	6.277	0.002	0.014
Night shift working * Gender	342.720	2	171.360	2.210	0.110	0.005
Night shift working * Age group	425.992	4	106.498	1.372	0.242	0.006
Night shift working * BMI group	142.162	4	35.541	0.456	0.768	0.002
Night shift working * Marital status	14.640	2	7.320	0.094	0.910	0.000
Night shift working * Job title	604.204	6	100.701	1.298	0.255	0.009
Night shift working * Sleeping	6.188	2	3.094	0.040	0.961	0.000
Night shift working * Physical activity	236.282	2	118.141	1.522	0.219	0.003

BMI: body mass index; HEI: Healthy Eating Index; MS: mean square; SS: sum of squares; PHDI: Planetary Health Diet Index. The * symbol shows the combined interactions of the night shift changes with gender, age group, BMI group, marital status, branch of work, sleeping statues, respectively.

3. Results

The descriptive characteristics of the participants and the total PHDI and total HEI-2020 scores pre-, during and post-night-shift, categorized according to these characteristics, are shown in Table 1. It has been shown that total PHDI scores in females were lowest during the night shift (48.2 ± 13.8; $p < 0.001$). Total HEI-2020 scores in females were found to be significantly lower during and post-night-shift than pre-night-shift (43.8 ± 8.8; 44.6 ± 10.2; 46.6 ± 9.4, respectively; $p < 0.001$). There was no significant change in total HEI-2020 scores in men according to shift patterns ($p > 0.05$). However, it was determined that total PHDI scores in males decreased significantly during and post-night-shift (48.8 ± 11.7 and 50.8 ± 14.9, respectively) compared to pre-night-shift (51.9 ± 13.3; $p < 0.001$). It has been shown that the total PHDI and total HEI-2020 scores of healthcare workers according to their age groups decreased significantly during the night shift compared to pre-night-shift. Total PHDI and total HEI-2020 scores of individuals decreased during the night shift in normal-body-weight and overweight groups, and there was still a significant difference post-night-shift compared to pre-night-shift, that is, there was no increase in total PHDI and HEI-2020 scores after the shift. Similarly, it was determined that total HEI-2020 and PHDI scores decreased significantly during the night shift in single and married individuals compared to pre-night-shift ($p < 0.001$). When looked at according to the professions of healthcare workers, it has been shown that both total HEI-2020 and total PHDI scores decrease significantly during the night shift in nurses, doctors, and emergency medical technicians, except for ambulance maintenance technicians ($p < 0.001$). A decrease in total HEI-2020 and PHDI scores was detected in individuals who did not sleep during the night shift and those who slept for 2 h during the night shift, while a similar decrease was observed in those who did sufficient physical activity ($p < 0.001$).

The change in the mean and standard deviation values of the HEI-2020 and PHDI subcomponents of healthcare workers pre-, during and post-night-shift is shown in Table 2. It was revealed that the total HEI-2020 scores of individuals decreased significantly during the night shift (44.0 ± 8.8) compared to pre-night-shift (46.1 ± 9.2; $p = 0.002$) and increased post-night-shift (44.7 ± 9.9), with no statistically significant difference between pre- and post-night-shift. The change observed in subcomponent scores during the night shift compared to the pre-night-shift was similarly demonstrated in the sodium ($p = 0.014$), whole fruit ($p = 0.001$), total fruit ($p < 0.001$), and added sugar ($p = 0.010$) subcomponents. It was revealed that the total PHDI scores of individuals decreased significantly during the night shift (48.3 ± 13.2) compared to pre-night-shift (51.9 ± 13.4; $p < 0.001$) and increased post-night-shift (50.6 ± 14.9), with no statistically significant difference between pre- and post-night-shifts. The change observed in subcomponent scores during the night shift compared to the pre-night-shift was similarly demonstrated in the chicken and substitutes ($p < 0.001$), vegetable oils ($p = 0.001$), animal fats ($p = 0.001$), whole cereals ($p = 0.027$), and added sugar ($p = 0.003$) subcomponents. However, it was found that individuals' legumes ($p = 0.013$), eggs ($p < 0.001$), and dairy ($p = 0.010$) PHDI subcomponent scores increased significantly during the night shift compared to pre-night-shift and decreased again post-night-shift.

The effects of individuals' night shift changes (pre-, during, and post-night-shift) and the interactions of the night shift changes with gender, age group, BMI group, marital status, branch of work, sleeping status during the night shift, and physical activity on the total PHDI and HEI-2020 scores are shown in Table 3. There was a significant main effect of night shift working on total PHDI ($F(896, 2) = 8.208$, $p < 0.001$, $\eta_p^2 = 0.018$) and HEI-2020 scores ($F(894, 2) = 6.277$, $p = 0.002$, $\eta_p^2 = 0.014$). In contrast, there was no significant main effect of night-shift-working interactions with gender, age group, BMI group, marital status, branch of work, sleeping status during the night shift, and physical activity on total PHDI and HEI-2020 scores ($p > 0.05$).

The changes in contributions of individuals' dietary macronutrients to their dietary energy, diet quality, and diet sustainability according to whether they were pre-, during, or post-night-shift are visualized in Figures 1–3. In the figures, the night shift sequence is expressed with moonlight while pre- and post-night-shift are expressed with sunlight. The size of the world map symbolizes diet quality. It is stated that the larger the world map (pre-night-shift), the higher the diet quality. Meanwhile, the smallest world map diameter indicates the lowest diet quality (during night shift) and the medium-sized world map (post-night-shift) indicates a higher diet quality than the lowest diet quality. According to the difference among the shift periods, it is symbolized that as the diameter of the world map decreases, the quality of the diet also decreases. The vibrant shades of green color on tree leaves vary depending on their dietary sustainability. The most vibrant shade of green indicates the highest diet sustainability (pre-night-shift), while paler green indicates lower diet sustainability (post-night-shift), and the palest green indicates the lowest diet sustainability (during night shift). Moreover, the proportional distributions of green colors and the world map diameter are shown for illustrative purposes only, not mathematical purposes. No significant change was observed in the contribution of individuals' dietary protein intake to dietary energy according to whether they were pre-, during, or post-night-shifts. While the contribution of individuals' dietary carbohydrate intake to dietary energy decreased significantly during the night shift (43.7%; $p < 0.001$) compared to pre-night-shift (44.4%), it increased significantly post-night-shift (45.4%; $p = 0.047$) and reached a level where there was no statistical difference compared with pre-night-shift ($p = 0.156$). While the contribution of individuals' dietary fat intake to dietary energy increased significantly during the night shift (41.4%; $p = 0.008$) compared to pre-night-shift (40.7%), it decreased post-night-shift (39.9%; $p < 0.001$) and reached a level where there was no statistical difference compared with before the shift ($p = 0.253$).

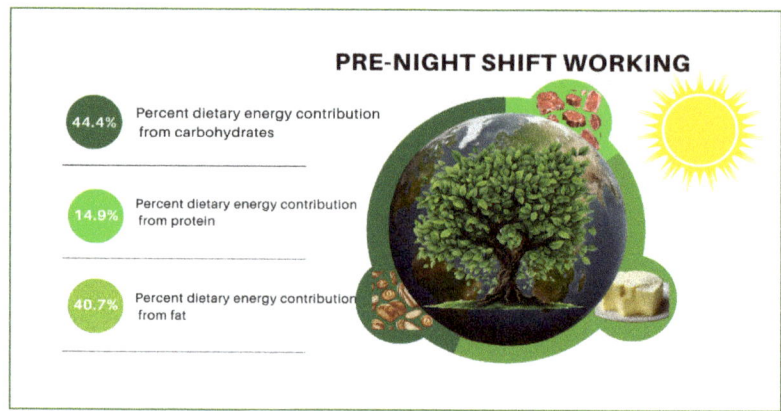

Figure 1. The contributions of individuals' dietary macronutrients to their dietary energy, diet quality, and diet sustainability pre-night-shift.

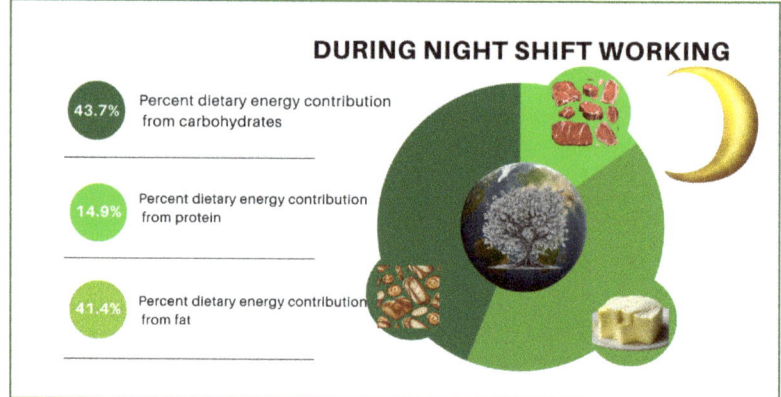

Figure 2. The contributions of individuals' dietary macronutrients to their dietary energy, diet quality, and diet sustainability while working the night shift.

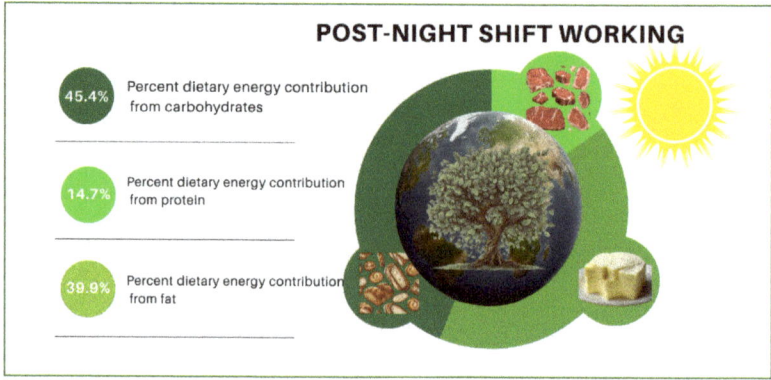

Figure 3. The contributions of individuals' dietary macronutrients to their dietary energy, diet quality, and diet sustainability post-night-shift.

4. Discussion

In this observational follow-up study conducted on healthcare workers working night shifts, it was shown that both the diet sustainability and diet quality of individuals decreased significantly during night shift working compared to before and increased again after the night shift. This change occurred regardless of the healthcare professionals' job title, age, ability to sleep during shifts, and physical activity status.

It has been shown that the circadian rhythm disruption experienced by healthcare professionals as a result of working night shifts causes many negative health consequences, such as impaired glucose tolerance [17], decreased insulin sensitivity [18,19], obesity [20], cardiometabolic diseases [21], and cancer [22]. It was found that the health problems seen in individuals were not only caused by circadian disruptions as a result of changes in the sleep–wake cycle, but night shifts can also cause diseases by changing eating habits in an unhealthy way [20,23–26]. In order to intervene in changing eating habits during a night shift, it is necessary first to reveal the changes. In this study, which examined the diet quality and diet sustainability of the night shift in healthcare workers, a group with basic knowledge about health protection, it was shown that there were negative changes in nutritional status during the night shift. Participants' diet quality measured using HEI-2020 and dietary sustainability measured using PHDI were found to be significantly lower during the night shift compared to pre- and post-night-shift. Similarly, it has been revealed that individuals working night shifts frequently choose unhealthy snacks as a strategy to stay awake during their shifts, and these snacks are often high in fat, sodium, and added sugar [23,27,28]. In this study, it was shown that the index scores of individuals according to their saturated fatty acid intake were low pre-, during, and post-night-shift, without any significant differences among them. Additionally, individuals' diet quality scores from added sugar intake were shown to significantly decrease during night shifts (4.9 ± 4.6, 4.1 ± 4.5, 4.6 ± 4.7, pre-, during, and post-night-shift, respectively; $p = 0.010$), supporting previous studies.

In addition, when it was investigated as to how the effects of a night shift on the decrease in diet quality would change when combined with these sociodemographic data, it was shown that the night shift did not show its effects on diet quality by interacting with these sociodemographic descriptors, and that the night shift was the main influencing factor ($F(894, 2) = 6.277$, $p = 0.002$, $\eta_p^2 = 0.014$, Table 3). Similar to this study, it has been revealed that food intake or eating habits change in an "unhealthy" direction [20,24–31] along the same lines as in this study conducted in healthcare workers. However, studies investigating diet quality in night shift workers are quite limited [8]. The evaluation of the HEI-2020 score and its subcomponents, which allow for comparison of the nutritional status of individuals with more objective criteria, has contributed an essential finding to the literature.

Sustainable nutrition, the importance of which has become more evident with the rapid depletion of natural resources, will be an inevitable strategy of this age, not only because of its low environmental impacts and protection of the ecosystem and biodiversity but also because it is a nutritionally adequate and healthy nutrition model [32]. This should also be recommended for night shift workers. In this way, the health of these individuals in the at-risk group working the night shift will be protected while natural resources will also be protected. Sustainable nutrition models, which will become an inevitable proposal of the age by consensus, are characterized by prominently featuring substantial quantities of plant-based foods, including vegetables, fruits, seeds, nuts, legumes, and whole grains, while incorporating only moderate-to-minimal amounts of animal-based products, such as meat, poultry, seafood, eggs, and dairy [15,32–35]. Considering the foods included in sustainable nutrition recommendations, it appears that they meet the dietary approaches recommended to improve health in individuals working night shifts. Therefore, the implementation of sustainable nutrition approaches in individuals working night shifts reduces the intake of saturated fatty acids and added sugars, which are included in unhealthy eating tendencies in this group [20,23–26], while increasing the intake of fiber, unsaturated fatty acids, fruits, and vegetables. The supporting data in this study demonstrate that sustainable diet quality decreased when healthcare workers switched to night shifts. During the night shift, healthcare workers' sustainable diet quality scores of red meat (0.6 ± 2.3), chicken and substitutes (6.6 ± 4.7), and animal fats (4.6 ± 0.4) decreased significantly ($p < 0.05$) compared to pre-night-shift (1.5 ± 3.5, 7.7 ± 4.2, 5.1 ± 0.9, respectively), meaning their consumption of these foods increased significantly. The significant decrease in the consumption of these foods post-night-shift ($p < 0.05$), that is, the increase in the PHDI subscores (2.3 ± 4.1, 8.0 ± 3.9, 5.7 ± 0.9, respectively), strengthens the hypothesis that the changes occur only during the night shift (Table 2). Similarly, studies have shown that meat consumption increases during the night shift, and that individuals tend to eat meals containing high saturated fat, sodium, red meat, and chicken, and especially "fast" foods [29,36,37].

Studies have shown that females tend to have a higher sustainable diet quality than males and are more prone to plant-based foods [38–40]. For these reasons, in this study, the sustainable diet quality of females increased faster than males' post-night-shift. It is thought that the effect of the increase in sustainable diet quality after the night shift depending on the sleeping state during the night shift is also related to the effect of sleep duration on the feeling of hunger. In individuals with less sleep time, the feeling of hunger increases, and as a result, the tendency to foods with poorer nutritional value including "fast" food increases. Studies supporting this interpretation have shown that the feeling of hunger, which causes unhealthy eating choices, is affected by sleep duration [8,41,42]. It has been shown that decreasing sleep duration affects hunger and satiety levels through the mechanism of changing plasma ghrelin and leptin levels, which are hormones that regulate appetite [8,41,42]. The increase in sustainable diet quality after a night shift in individuals with a normal body weight and adequate physical activity level has been interpreted as being related to the fact that the diet choices of individuals who make healthy lifestyle choices may also be healthy. However, when it was investigated as to how the effects of the night shift on the decrease in sustainable diet quality (total PHDI score) would change when combined with these sociodemographic data, it was shown that the night shift did not show its effects on sustainable diet quality by interacting with these sociodemographic descriptors, and that the night shift was the main influencing factor on sustainable diet quality ($F(894, 2) = 6.277$, $p = 0.002$, $\eta_p^2 = 0.014$, Table 3).

One of the strengths of this study is that it evaluated night shift workers' nutritional status by following a large sample before, during, and after the night shift. In addition, this study, in which the diet quality of the participants was calculated according to HEI-2020, has another strength due to the limited number of studies in the literature that have observed changes in diet quality by following night shift workers. Another of its strengths is that it is the first study to investigate the implementation of sustainable nutrition, which will inevitably become a healthy nutrition strategy for every individual due to today's conditions, including night shift workers. The first limitation of this study is that since the study was conducted only in healthcare workers, the results cannot be generalized to all night shift workers. Secondly, there are limitations in generalizing the findings of the study because the factors affecting individuals' eating habits and food preferences vary across countries and even geographical regions within the same country. Thirdly, considering that the stress experienced by healthcare workers during night shifts may affect their eating behavior, it will be important to include this parameter in future studies. Lastly, healthcare workers may encounter many emergencies during the night shift. Experiencing these emergencies may also affect individuals' food consumption. However, in this study, no evaluation was made regarding the emergency situations encountered by healthcare workers working on night shifts, and it is recommended that future studies include this evaluation and exclude from the study periods when unusual emergencies (long surgeries, etc.) occur.

5. Conclusions

Compared to before the night shift, both the diet quality and diet sustainability of healthcare workers decreased during the night shift, without any differences according to gender, age group, BMI group, marital status, job title, and napping during the night shift. The significant increase in diet quality and diet sustainability scores again after the night shift supports the finding that the night shift is an important factor affecting these two parameters. It is thought that sustainable nutrition, which is a solution-oriented proposal of the age with its health benefits and strengths such as the protection of natural resources and low environmental impact, will be inevitable to be implemented day by day in health professionals working night shifts.

The fact that these negative dietary changes occur during the night shift, even among healthcare workers who have basic knowledge about the factors affecting the protection and promotion of health, reveals that further steps are needed than just providing information on the subject. The first of these should be to increase the chance of accessing healthy alternatives by evaluating the environment in which healthcare workers access food sources. Other suggestions include organizing break times at work by encouraging healthy eating and ensuring that workplace cafeterias and vending machines contain healthy alternatives. Ensuring that not only healthcare professionals but also managers are informed about sustainable nutrition will make it easier to accelerate the steps to be taken. Finally, it is also valuable to evaluate the nutritional knowledge levels of healthcare professionals in future studies and correlate them with diet quality and sustainable nutritional quality, and to develop suggestions for updates to be made in the undergraduate education curriculum of healthcare professionals based on the results of the research.

Author Contributions: Conceptualization, S.N.-V. and H.M.; data curation, S.N.-V.; formal analysis, H.M.; investigation, S.N.-V. and H.M.; methodology, S.N.-V. and H.M.; project administration, S.N.-V.; resources, H.M. and S.N.-V.; software, H.M.; supervision, H.M. and S.N.-V.; validation, H.M.; visualization, H.M.; writing, H.M. and S.N.-V. All authors have read and agreed to the published version of the manuscript.

Funding: This research received no external funding.

Institutional Review Board Statement: The study was conducted in accordance with the Declaration of Helsinki and approved by the Ethics Committee of Gazi University of Ankara/Turkey (Date: 16 April 2024, No: 2023-851-07).

Informed Consent Statement: Informed consent was obtained from all subjects involved in the study.

Data Availability Statement: The data presented in this study are available on request from the corresponding author (handeyilmaz@gazi.edu.tr) due to fact that it is intended to be shared only with researchers working in this field.

Conflicts of Interest: The authors declare no conflicts of interest.

References

1. Labor Force Statistics from the Current Population Survey. Work Schedules (Flexible and Shift Schedules). 2018. Available online: https://www.bls.gov/cps/lfcharacteristics.htm#schedules (accessed on 8 June 2024).
2. Rijk, M.G.; Vries, H.H.M.; Mars, M.; Feskens, E.J.M.; Boesveldt, S. Dietary taste patterns and diet quality of female nurses around the night shift. *Eur. J. Nutr.* **2024**, *63*, 513–524. [CrossRef] [PubMed]
3. Berent, D.; Skoneczny, M.; Macander, M.; Wojnar, M. The association among health behaviors, shift work and chronic morbidity: A cross-sectional study on nurses working in full-time positions. *J. Public Health Res.* **2022**, *11*, 2099. [CrossRef] [PubMed]
4. Mazurek Melnyk, B.; Pavan Hsieh, A.; Tan, A.; Teall, A.M.; Weberg, D.; Jun, J.; Gawlik, K.; Hoying, J. Associations among nurses' mental/physical health, lifestyle behaviors, shift length, and workplace wellness support during COVID-19: Important implications for health care systems. *Nurs. Adm. Q.* **2022**, *46*, 5–18. [CrossRef] [PubMed]
5. Shaw, E.; Dorrian, J.; Coates, A.M.; Leung, G.K.W.; Davis, R.; Rosbotham, E.; Warnock, R.; Huggins, C.E.; Bonham, M.P. Temporal pattern of eating in night shift workers. *Chronobiol. Int.* **2019**, *36*, 1613.e52. [CrossRef]
6. Flanagan, A.; Lowson, E.; Arber, S.; Griffin, B.A.; Skene, D.J. Dietary patterns of nurses on rotational shifts are marked by redistribution of energy into the nightshift. *Nutrients* **2020**, *12*, 1053. [CrossRef] [PubMed]

7. Pepłońska, B.; Nowak, P.; Trafalska, E. The association between night shift work and nutrition patterns among nurses: A literature review. *Medycyna Pracy* **2019**, *70*, 363–376. [CrossRef] [PubMed]
8. Rangel, T.L.; Bindler, T.S.R.; Roney, J.K.; Penders, R.A.; Faulkner, R.; Miller, L.; Sperry, M.; James, L.; Wilson, M.L. Exercise, diet, and sleep habits of nurses working full-time during the COVID-19 pandemic: An observational study. *Appl. Nurs. Res.* **2023**, *69*, 151665. [CrossRef]
9. Farías, R.; Sepúlveda, A.; Chamorro, R. Impact of shift work on the eating pattern, physical activity and daytime sleepiness among chilean healthcare workers. *Saf. Health Work.* **2020**, *11*, 367–371. [CrossRef]
10. Frank, S.M.; Jaacks, L.M.; Adair, L.S.; Avery, C.L.; Meyer, K.; Rose, D.; Taillie, L.S. Adherence to the Planetary Health Diet Index and correlation with nutrients of public health concern: An analysis of NHANES 2003–2018. *Am. J. Clin. Nutr.* **2024**, *119*, 384–392. [CrossRef]
11. World Health Organization (WHO). Fact Sheets. A Healthy Lifestyle-WHO Recommendations. 2010. Available online: https://www.who.int/europe/news-room/fact-sheets/item/a-healthy-lifestyle---who-recommendations (accessed on 8 June 2024).
12. Merdol, T.K. *Standart Yemek Tarifeleri*, 1st ed.; Hatipoğlu Yayınevi: Ankara, Türkiye, 2011; pp. 10–200.
13. Kennedy, E.T.; Ohls, J.; Carlson, S.; Fleming, K. The Healthy Eating Index: Design and applications. *J. Am. Diet. Assoc.* **1995**, *95*, 1103–1108. [CrossRef]
14. Krebs-Smith, S.M.; Pannucci, T.E.; Subar, A.F.; Kirkpatrick, S.I.; Lerman, J.L.; Tooze, J.A.; Wilson, M.M.; Reedy, J. Update of the Healthy Eating Index: HEI-2015. *J. Acad. Nutr. Diet.* **2018**, *118*, 1591–1602. [CrossRef]
15. Cacau, L.T.; Carli, E.; de Carvalho, A.M.; Lotufo, P.A.; Moreno, L.A.; Bensenor, I.M.; Marchioni, D.M. Development and validation of an index based on EAT-Lancet recommendations: The planetary health diet index. *Nutrients* **2021**, *13*, 1698. [CrossRef]
16. Marshall, A.L.; Smith, B.J.; Bauman, A.E.; Kaur, S. Reliability and validity of a brief physical activity assessment for use by family doctors. *Br. J. Sports Med.* **2005**, *39*, 294–297. [CrossRef]
17. Suyoto, P.S.T.; de Rijk, M.G.; de Vries, J.H.; Feskens, E.J.M. The effect of meal glycemic index and meal frequency on glycemic control and variability in female nurses working night shifts: A two-arm randomized cross-over trial. *J. Nutr.* **2024**, *154*, 69–78. [CrossRef]
18. Chellappa, S.L.; Qian, J.; Vujovic, N.; Morris, C.J.; Nedeltcheva, A.; Nguyen, H.; Rahman, N.; Heng, S.W.; Kelly, L.; Kerlin-Monteiro, K.; et al. Daytime eating prevents internal circadian misalignment and glucose intolerance in night work. *Sci. Adv.* **2022**, *7*, eabg9910. [CrossRef]
19. Augustin, L.S.A.; Kendall, C.W.C.; Jenkins, D.J.A.; Willett, W.C.; Astrup, A.; Barclay, A.W.; Björck, I.; Brand-Miller, J.C.; Brighenti, F.; Buyken, A.E.; et al. Glycemic index, glycemic load and glycemic response: An International Scientific Consensus Summit from the International Carbohydrate Quality Consortium (ICQC). *Nutr. Metab. Cardiovasc. Dis.* **2015**, *25*, 795–815. [CrossRef] [PubMed]
20. Heath, G.; Dorrian, J.; Coates, A. Associations between shift type, sleep, mood, and diet in a group of shift working nurses. *Scand. J. Work Environ. Health* **2019**, *45*, 402–412. [CrossRef] [PubMed]
21. Hannemann, J.; Laing, A.; Middleton, B.; Schwedhelm, E.; Marx, N.; Federici, M.; Kastner, M.; Skene, D.J.; Böger, R. Effect of oral melatonin treatment on insulin resistance and diurnal blood pressure variability in night shift workers. A double-blind, randomized, placebo-controlled study. *Pharmacol. Res.* **2024**, *199*, 107011. [CrossRef] [PubMed]
22. Moon, J.; Holzhausen, E.A.; Mun, Y. Risk of prostate cancer with increasing years of night shift work: A two-stage dose-response meta-analysis with duration of night shift work as exposure dose. *Heliyon* **2024**, *10*, e29080. [CrossRef]
23. Habib Rodrigues, G.; de Sousa Duarte, A.; Garrido, A.L.F.; Santana, P.T.; Pellegrino, P.; Nogueira, L.F.R.; Crispim, C.A.; Cipolla-Neto, J.; de Castro Moreno, C.R.; Marqueze, E.C. A putative association between food intake, meal timing and sleep parameters among overweight nursing professionals working night shifts. *Sleep Epidemiol.* **2022**, *2*, 100040. [CrossRef]
24. Chen, Y.; Lauren, S.; Chang, B.P.; Shechter, A. Objective food intake in night and day shift workers: A laboratory study. *Clocks Sleep* **2019**, *1*, 42–49. [CrossRef] [PubMed]
25. Kosmadopoulos, A.; Kervezee, L.; Boudreau, P.; Gonzales-Aste, F.; Vujovic, N.; Scheer, F.A.J.L.; Boivin, D.B. Effects of shift work on the eating behavior of police officers on patrol. *Nutrients* **2020**, *12*, 999. [CrossRef] [PubMed]
26. Jansen, E.C.; Stern, D.; Monge, A.; O'Brien, L.M.; Lajous, M.; Peterson, K.E.; López-Ridaura, R. Healthier dietary patterns are associated with better sleep quality among mid-life Mexican women. *J. Clin. Sleep Med.* **2020**, *16*, 1321–1330. [CrossRef] [PubMed]
27. Crispim, C.A.; Zalcman, I.; Dáttilo, M.; Padilha, H.G.; Tufik, S.; de Mello, M.T. Relação entre sono e obesidade: Uma revisão da literatura. *Arq. Bras. Endocrinol. Metab.* **2007**, *51*, 1041–1049. [CrossRef] [PubMed]
28. Schiavo-Cardozo, D.; Lima, M.M.O.; Parej, J.C.; Geloneze, B. Appetite-regulating hormones from the upper gut: Disrupted control of xenin and ghrelin in night workers. *Clin. Endocrinol.* **2013**, *79*, 807–811. [CrossRef] [PubMed]
29. Balieiro, L.C.; Rossato, L.T.; Waterhouse, J.; Paim, S.L.; Mota, M.C.; Crispim, C.A. Nutritional status and eating habits of bus drivers during the day and night. *Chronobiol. Int.* **2014**, *31*, 1123–1129. [CrossRef] [PubMed]
30. De Freitas, E.S.; Canuto, R.; Henn, R.L.; Olinto, B.A.; Macagnan, J.B.A.; Pattussi, M.P.; Busnello, F.M.; Olinto, M.T.A. Alteração no comportamento alimentar de trabalhadores de turnos de um frigorífico do sul do Brasil. *Ciência Saúde Coletiva* **2015**, *20*, 2401–2410. [CrossRef]
31. Mota, M.C.; De-Souza, D.A.; Crispim, C.A. Dietary patterns, metabolic markers and subjective sleep measures in resident physicians. *Chronobiol. Int.* **2013**, *30*, 1032–1041. [CrossRef]
32. Food and Agriculture Organization. Bioversity International. Sustainable Diets and Biodiversity: Directions and Solutions for Policy, Research and Action. Available online: http://www.fao.org/3/i3004e/i3004e.pdf (accessed on 27 June 2024).

33. Fardet, A.; Rock, E. How to protect both health and food system sustainability? A holistic 'global health'-based approach via the 3V rule proposal. *Public Health Nutr.* **2020**, *23*, 3028–3044. [CrossRef]
34. Steenson, S.; Buttriss, J.L. The challenges of defining a healthy and 'sustainable' diet. *Nutr. Bull.* **2020**, *45*, 206–222. [CrossRef]
35. Meltzer, H.M.; Brantsaeter, A.L.; Trolle, E.; Eneroth, H.; Fogelholm, M.; Ydersbond, T.A.; Birgisdottir, B.E. Environmental sustainability perspectives of the nordic diet. *Nutrients* **2019**, *11*, 2248. [CrossRef]
36. Chaves, D.B.R.; Costa, A.G.S.; Oliveira, A.R.S.; Olivera, T.C.; Araujo, T.L.; Lopes, M.V.O. Risk factors to high blood pressure: Inquiry with bus drivers and collectors. *Rev. Enferm.* **2008**, *16*, 370–376.
37. Cavagioni, L.C. Cardiovascular Risk Profile Observed in Professional Truck Drivers Who Work on Highway BR116 within the Area of the State of São Paulo—Régis Bittencourt. Master's Thesis, Nursing School, University of São Paulo, São Paulo, Brazil, 2008.
38. Seffen, A.E.; Dohle, S. What motivates German consumers to reduce their meat consumption? Identifying relevant beliefs. *Appetite* **2023**, *187*, 106593. [CrossRef] [PubMed]
39. Tobler, C.; Visschers, V.H.M.; Siegrist, M. Eating green Consumers' willingness to adopt ecological food consumption behaviors. *Appetite* **2011**, *57*, 674–682. [CrossRef] [PubMed]
40. Judge, M.; Wilson, M.S. A dual-process motivational model of attitudes towards vegetarians and vegans. *Eur. J. Soc. Psychol.* **2019**, *49*, 169–178. [CrossRef]
41. McHill, A.W.; Hull, J.T.; Klerman, E.B. Chronic circadian disruption and sleep restriction influence subjective hunger, appetite, and food preference. *Nutrients* **2022**, *14*, 1800. [CrossRef]
42. Spiegel, K.; Tasali, E.; Penev, P.; Van Cauter, E. Brief communication: Sleep curtailment in healthy young men is associated with decreased leptin levels, elevated ghrelin levels, and increased hunger and appetite. *Ann. Intern. Med.* **2004**, *141*, 846–850. [CrossRef]

Disclaimer/Publisher's Note: The statements, opinions and data contained in all publications are solely those of the individual author(s) and contributor(s) and not of MDPI and/or the editor(s). MDPI and/or the editor(s) disclaim responsibility for any injury to people or property resulting from any ideas, methods, instructions or products referred to in the content.

MDPI AG
Grosspeteranlage 5
4052 Basel
Switzerland
Tel.: +41 61 683 77 34

Nutrients Editorial Office
E-mail: nutrients@mdpi.com
www.mdpi.com/journal/nutrients

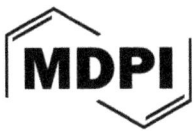

Disclaimer/Publisher's Note: The statements, opinions and data contained in all publications are solely those of the individual author(s) and contributor(s) and not of MDPI and/or the editor(s). MDPI and/or the editor(s) disclaim responsibility for any injury to people or property resulting from any ideas, methods, instructions or products referred to in the content.

www.ingramcontent.com/pod-product-compliance
Lightning Source LLC
LaVergne TN
LVHW070143100526
838202LV00015B/1885